Multimodal Therapy in Oncology Nursing

Multimodal Therapy in Oncology Nursing

Edited by

Marcia C. Liebman, RN, MS, OCN

Oncology Clinical Nurse Specialist
Southwood Community Hospital
Norfolk, Massachusetts

Dawn Camp-Sorrell, RN, MSN, FNP, AOCN

Oncology Nurse Practitioner
University of Alabama at Birmingham Hospital
Birmingham, Alabama

Illustrated

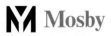 Mosby

St. Louis Baltimore Boston
Carlsbad Chicago Naples New York Philadelphia Portland
London Madrid Mexico City Singapore Sydney Tokyo Toronto Wiesbaden

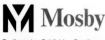

Publisher: *Nancy L. Coon*
Editor: *Jeff Burnham*
Developmental Editor: *Linda Caldwell*
Project Manager: *Carol Sullivan Weis*
Manufacturing: *Dave Graybill*

A NOTE TO THE READER

The authors and publisher have made every attempt to check dosages and nursing content for accuracy. Because the science of pharmacology is continually advancing, our knowledge base continues to expand. Therefore we recommend that the reader always check product information for changes in dosage or administration before administering any medication. This is particularly important with new or rarely used drugs.

Printed in the United States of America
Composition by Penmarin Books
Printing and binding by Courier—
 Westford, Massachusetts

Mosby–Year Book, Inc.
11830 Westline Industrial Drive
St. Louis, Missouri 63146

Library of Congress Cataloging-in-Publication Data

Multimodal therapy in oncology nursing/edited by Marcia C. Liebman,
 Dawn Camp-Sorrell.
   p.   cm.
  Includes bibliographical references and index.
  ISBN 0-8151-5422-4 (pbk.). — ISBN 0-8151-5422-4 (pbk.)
  1. Cancer—Nursing.   2. Cancer—Treatment.   I. Liebman, Marcia C.
II. Camp-Sorrell, Dawn.   III. Liebman, Marcia C.   IV. Camp-Sorrell, Dawn.
  [DNLM: 1. Neoplasms—nursing.   2. Neoplasms—therapy—nurses'
instruction.   3. Combined Modality Therapy—nurses' instruction.
4. Neoplasmas—nursing.   5. Neoplasms—therapy—nurses' instruction.
6. Combined Modality Therapy—nurses' instruction.   WY 156 M961
1996]
RC266.M85   1996
610.73′698—dc20   96-10353

96 97 98 99 00 / 9 8 7 6 5 4 3 2 1

Contributors

Karen H. Baker, RN, MSN, CORLN
Nurse Consultant
Ear, Nose, and Throat Branch
Office of Device Evaluations
Food and Drug Administration
Consultant Clinical Nurse Specialist
Otolaryngology/Head and Neck Surgery
National Naval Medical Center
Bethesda, Maryland

Susan Weiss Behrend, RN, MSN
Clinical Case Manager
Department of Radiation Oncology
Fox Chase Cancer Center
Philadelphia, Pennsylvania

Anne E. Belcher, RN, PhD
Associate Professor and Chairperson
Department of Acute and Long-term Care
American Cancer Society Professor of
    Oncology Nursing
School of Nursing
University of Maryland
Baltimore, Maryland

Kathleen E. Bell, RN, MSN
Department of Radiation Oncology
Butterworth Hospital
Grand Rapids, Michigan

Jeannine M. Brant, RN, MS, AOCN
Oncology Clinical Nurse Specialist/Pain
    Consultant
Saint Vincent Hospital and Health Center
Billings, Montana
Affiliate Assistant Professor
Montana State University
Bozeman, Montana

**Catherine C. Burke, RN, MS, ANP,
    OCN**
Clinical Cancer Detection Specialist
M.D. Anderson Cancer Center
University of Texas
Houston, Texas

Aurelie C. Cormier, RN, CS, MS, OCN
Clinical Nurse Specialist—Women's Health
Stamford Health Systems
Stamford, Connecticut

Ann Marie Dose, RN, MS, OCN
Clinical Nurse Specialist
Women's Cancer Program
Mayo Clinic
Rochester, Minnesota

Mary L. Dougherty, MS
Department of Radiation Oncology
Butterworth Hospital
Grand Rapids, Michigan

Jane E. Feldman, RN, BA, MEd
Oncology Nurse Specialist and Administrative
    Coordinator
Division of Radiation Oncology
Georgetown University Medical Center
Washington, D.C.

Norma J. Fenerty, RN, BSN, OCN
Case Manager
Fox Chase Cancer Center
Philadelphia, Pennsylvania

Rebecca Hawkins, MSN, ANP, AOCN
Oncology Nurse Practitioner
St. Mary Regional Cancer Center
Walla Walla, Washington

Jeanne Held-Warmkessel, MSN,
RN, CS, AORN
Medical Oncology Clinical Nurse Specialist
Albert Einstein Cancer Center
Philadelphia, Pennsylvania

Alice J. Longman, EdD, RN, FAAN
Professor
College of Nursing
The University of Arizona
Tucson, Arizona

Debra J. Luce, RN, BSN, MSN, OCN
Manager, Oncology Home Care Program
Advantage Home Health
Savannah, Georgia

Mary Mrozek-Orlowski, MSN, RN,
AOCN
Clinical Nurse Specialist and Coordinator
Comprehensive Breast Care Program
Section of Hematology and Oncology
Dartmouth-Hitchcock Medical Center
Lebanon, New Hampshire

Robyn Rebl Mundy, RN, MS, CRC,
LPC
Psychooncology Nurse Therapist
Certified Rehabilitation Counselor
Licensed Professional Counselor
Sheridan, Wyoming

Maureen E. O'Rourke, RN, MS, OCN
Doctoral Candidate, School of Nursing
University of North Carolina at Chapel Hill
Chapel Hill, North Carolina

Marcia E. Rostad, RN, MS, NS, OCN
Pediatric Oncology Clinical Nurse Specialist
University of Arizona Medical Center
Tucson, Arizona

Kimberly A. Rumsey, RN, MSN, OCN
Adjunct Faculty
School of Nursing
Houston Baptist University
Houston, Texas

Judith A. Shell, RN, MS, OCN
Oncology Clinical Nurse Specialist
Butterworth Hospital
Grand Rapids, Michigan

Anne T. Slivjak, RN, MSN, OCN
Assistant Clinical Manager
Department of Radiation Oncology
Fox Chase Cancer Center
Philadelphia, Pennsylvania

Patricia A. Spencer-Cisek, MS, RN,
ANP, CS, OCN
Clinical Cancer Detection Specialist
M.D. Anderson Cancer Center
University of Texas
Houston, Texas

Barbara Rassat Tripp, MSN, RN, OCN
Oncology Clinical Nurse Specialist
Cleveland Clinic Foundation
Cleveland, Ohio

Debra Wujcik, RN, MS, AOCN
Clinical Director
Vanderbilt Cancer Center Affiliate Network
Adjunct Faculty
Vanderbilt University School of Nursing
Nashville, Tennessee

Reviewers

Joyce M. Adams, MS, RN, CNS
Department Chairperson
Associate Degree Nursing
San Jacinto College South
Houston, Texas

Sandra A. Mitchell Beddar, RN,
  MScN, OCN
Nurse Practitioner
Bone Marrow Transplant Program
Roswell Park Cancer Center
Buffalo, New York

Patricia J. Bluml, MSN, ARNP, OCN
Bone Marrow Transplant Clinical Nurse
  Specialist
St. Francis Regional Medical Center
Wichita, Kansas

Janet Marie Burns, RN, MSN
Director of Cardiac Education
Delaware Valley Cardiology Group
Philadelphia, Pennsylvania

Patricia Carter, RN, MSN, OCN
Director
Infusion Center
Southwest Internal Medicine Associates
El Paso, Texas

Gwen Killam Corrigan, RN, MSN,
  FNP
Clinical Cancer Detection Specialist
Coordinator, Professional Education for
  Prevention/ Early Detection
M.D. Anderson Cancer Center
Houston, Texas

Margaret Dean, RN, CS, NP, MSN
Nurse Manager
Women's Program
Harrington Cancer Center
Amarillo, Texas

Sharon S. Forrester, RN, BSN, OCN
Oncology Coordinator
St. Anthony's Health Center
Alton, Illinois

Jan Foster, MSN, RN, CCRN
Nurse Manager
Medical Intensive Care Unit
M.D. Anderson Cancer Center
University of Texas
Houston, Texas

Sue L. Frymark, RN, BS
Manager
Clinical and Data Support Services
Good Samaritan Hospital
Portland, Oregon

Sharron R. Havens, RN, BSN
Special Project/Oncology Nurse
Allison Cancer Center
Midland, Texas

Barbara Carlile Holmes, MSN, RN,
  OCN
Oncology Nursing Consultant
San Antonio, Texas
Doctoral Candidate
University of Texas at Austin
Austin, Texas

Lisa M. Howes, RN, MA, MN, OCN
Oncology Clinical Nurse Specialist
Division of Medical Oncology
University of Texas Health Science Center
San Antonio, Texas

Allison B. Jones, RN, MSN
Assistant Professor of Nursing
Troy State University
Montgomery, Alabama

Cynthia R. King, RN, MSN, CNA
Owner and Nurse Consultant
Special Care Consultants
Rochester, New York

Cheryl Lacasse, RN, MS, OCN
Oncology Clinical Nurse Specialist
Dana-Farber Cancer Institute
Boston, Massachusetts

Claudia Loveland, MS, RN, CNA
Assistant Professor
Adult Health Department
School of Nursing
University of Texas
Galveston, Texas

Suzanne M. Mahon, RN, DNSc, OCN
Clinical Coordinator
Cancer Screening Center
Deaconess Health System
St. Louis, Missouri

Shirley E. Otto, MSN, CRNI, AOCN
Clinical Nurse Specialist
Via Christi Regional Medical Center
Wichita, Kansas

Elizabeth M. Outlaw, RN, MA
Per Diem, Oncology
Stamford Hospital
Stamford, Connecticut

Dinah Saunders, RN, EdS
Assistant Professor
Department of Nursing
Norfolk State University
Norfolk, Virginia

Denice Sheehan, RN, MSN, OCN
Hospice Consultant
Cleveland Heights, Ohio

Virginia R. Sicola, RN, OCN, PhD
Oncology Coordinator
Department of Veterans Affairs
Amarillo, Texas
Adjunct Faculty
Division of Nursing
West Texas A&M University
Canyon, Texas

Susan Smith, RN, MSN, OCN
Project Manager, Clinical Trials
Institute for Drug Development
San Antonio, Texas

Susan J. Sturgeon, RN, BS, OCN
Project Director
Indiana Community Cancer Care
Indianapolis, Indiana

Barbara L. Summers, RNCS, MSN, OCN
Clinical Nurse Specialist, Oncology
Fairfax, Virginia

Catherine Ann Ultrino, MSN, OCN, RN
Administrative Coordinator
School of Practical Nursing
Youville Hospital
Cambridge, Massachusetts

Julia Anne Walsh, RN, C, MSN, OCN
Nurse Manager
Hematology/Oncology Outpatient Services
Cancer Management Center
Holy Family Hospital and Medical Center
Methuen, Massachusetts

James R. Wenger, RN, MS
Instructor
Department of Nursing
Truman College
Chicago, Illinois

Vanessa L. Witcher, RN, OCN
Staff Nurse
Oncology Care Center
Maryville, Illinois

Karen Woodward, RN, MSN, OCN
Clinical Nurse Specialist
Harrington Cancer Center
Amarillo, Texas

Emily Yale, RN, MSN
Instructor
Department of Nursing
St. Louis Community College at Meramec
St. Louis, Missouri

Preface

Cancer treatment is changing from a surgically centered approach to a multimodal approach in which any of the four primary treatment modalities (surgery, radiation therapy, chemotherapy, and biotherapy) can play a leading role, supplemented by one or more other modalities. As treatment moves from inpatient to outpatient settings and into the home, and from teaching to community hospital, nurses without an oncology background are asked to coordinate intricate treatment regimens, manage side effects, teach patients, and interpret information from a myriad of sources.

Multimodal therapy is the integration of more than one antineoplastic therapy in order to increase survival, increase the length of disease-free intervals, and improve patients' quality of life. Surgery, radiation therapy, chemotherapy, and biotherapy are used in various combinations and sequences. As the approach to cancer treatment and health care changes, nurses must care for patients with more complex treatment concerns. To assure that nurses have adequate practical information to face this challenge, this reference has been developed to supplement current oncology nursing texts.

This clinical reference is geared toward the practitioner who has basic nursing skills but has not necessarily cared for patients with cancer. It is assumed that the reader understands basic nursing terminology. Terms specific to oncology nursing and cancer treatments are explained in detail. This book is intended to be a reference for nurses who periodically care for patients with cancer (general medical-surgical nurses, outpatient nurses, home care nurses, and long-term care nurses; nurses with family members who have cancer; seniors in nursing school who are thinking of specializing in oncology nursing; and graduate students who are obtaining advanced training in oncology nursing), as well as full-time oncology nurses. In addition, oncology nursing educators will find this book beneficial in preparing oncology classes.

This book discusses the integration of care of the patient receiving multimodal therapy. For example, it does not just address the fact that radiation therapy causes skin changes but discusses the effect on wound healing when surgery is performed at a previously irradiated site. The book is an easy-to-read, comprehensive clinical reference. It has clear explanations of in-depth material. Nursing interventions are described in concrete terms rather than vague generalizations. The chapters can stand alone. Although this leads to some duplication, it accommodates practitioners who, out of the classroom, mostly use books on a need-to-know basis.

The increased use of multimodal treatments has challenged the editors and the authors to provide updated and pertinent material. We believe that this book accomplishes our goals. Unit I presents an overview of cancer and the different treatment modalities. Unit II describes the types of cancers currently being treated with multimodal therapy. Unit III describes the numerous side effects, both acute and long-term, that can result from multimodal therapy. These chapters provide information on nursing assessment and patient management. Unit IV discusses the special considerations faced by the patient undergoing multimodal therapy.

Each chapter has been written by an expert oncology nurse. Boxes and tables are included to emphasize important material and new concepts. Reference lists are provided with each chapter so that the reader can easily find background data. New terms are defined in the text and listed in a glossary in the back of the book.

Several special features present important information in a unique, consistent format. *Patient Education Guidelines* are found in Units II and III. *Nursing Care* tables in Unit II highlight specific nursing care and provide rationales for the care. *Research Highlights* in Unit II emphasize significant multimodal treatment research findings. The *Possible Side Effects from Multimodal Treatment* tables in Unit II detail the enhanced combined side effects of multimodal treatment for site-specific cancers. *Nursing Management* boxes in Unit III summarize nursing care for specific side effects.

The editors gratefully acknowledge the tremendous effort of the chapter authors who shared their knowledge and expertise. We believe that this book will be a valuable resource for nurses caring for cancer patients.

Marcia C. Liebman
Dawn Camp-Sorrell

Contents in Brief

Detailed Contents

OVERVIEW OF CANCER AND TREATMENT

Chapter 1

❖ *Overview of Cancer and Multimodal Therapy*

Dawn Camp-Sorrell
Marcia C. Liebman

Multimodal therapy is the combined use of cancer treatment modalities to improve the outcome for the patient and to keep complications at an acceptable level. Improved outcomes include increased survival, larger disease-free intervals until recurrence, and better quality of life. The components of multimodal therapy include surgery, radiation therapy, chemotherapy (including hormonal therapy), and biotherapy. Individually each of these modalities plays a significant role in cancer treatment. The effectiveness of combining treatment modalities has been demonstrated in clinical trials, and multimodal therapy has become a standard approach to cancer care (Lokich, 1991).

❖ *Overview of Cancer*

Cell Cycle

To understand cancer treatment, it is important first to understand normal cell biology. Both normal cells and cancer cells go through the same cell cycle. The cell cycle consists of phases that control the growth and replication of cells. Most of the replication process occurs in the synthesis phase (S) and the mitosis phase (M), separated by "gap" phases (G_1 and G_2) (Figure 1-1) (Norton and Surbone, 1993). *Generation time* is the term for the length of time required to complete the cell

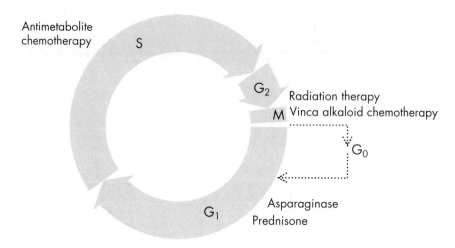

Fig. 1-1.   The cell cycle. Adapted from Goodman MS: Cancer: chemotherapy and care, ed 3, Princeton, 1992, Bristol-Myers Squibb Co.

cycle. Generation time varies among different cell types and depends on the need for new cells by the body tissue (Norton and Surbone, 1993).

G_0 is the resting phase of the cell cycle, when no division takes place (Baserga, 1993; Fingert, Campisi, and Pardee, 1993). Some cells, such as hepatocytes, temporarily step out of the cell cycle but can return when needed; others, such as neurons and most striated muscle cells, are permanently in the G_0 pool (Baserga, 1993; Guyton, 1991; Norton and Surbone, 1993). When in the G_0 phase, cells are resistant to chemotherapy (Baserga, 1993) but still may be sensitive to the biotherapy agent interferon (Perez and Brady, 1992).

In the G_1 phase, synthesis of ribonucleic acid (RNA) and proteins occurs. In addition, many of the enzymes necessary for deoxyribonucleic acid (DNA) synthesis are produced. Cells in the G_1 phase are vulnerable to some chemotherapeutic agents such as asparaginase and prednisone. The time that cells spend in the G_1 phase can vary from several hours to several days (Norton and Surbone, 1993).

During the synthesis phase (S), DNA is synthesized as the cell prepares for cell division. Cells in this phase are most vulnerable to damage from antimetabolite chemotherapy such as 5-fluorouracil (Norton and Surbone, 1993) and are most resistant in some cancers, such as head and neck, to radiation therapy (Quiet, Weichselbaum, and Gardina, 1991). The S phase lasts 12 to 24 hours (Norton and Surbone, 1993).

The G_2 phase is a short phase of about 3 hours during which DNA synthesis is completed and RNA and protein synthesis continues. Cells in the G_2 phase are vulnerable to chemotherapeutic agents such as etoposide and bleomycin. After cells complete the G_2 phase, they enter the mitosis phase (M).

Cellular division actually occurs during the M phase, when two identical daughter cells are created. Many cells are most sensitive to radiation therapy damage (Weichselbaum et al., 1992) and vinca alkaloid chemotherapeutic agents such as vincristine in this phase. This is a relatively short period generally lasting about 60 minutes (Norton and Surbone, 1993).

Only a small proportion of cells, known as *stem cells,* have the continued capability to renew themselves (Fingert, Campisi, and Pardee, 1993). Other cells differentiate and mature (Fingert, Campisi, and Pardee, 1993). *Differentiation* is the term for the process of cells developing into specialized cells, such as breast, lung, or epidermoid cells (Fingert, Campisi, and Pardee, 1993).

Theory of Immune Surveillance

Many researchers believe that cancer begins with an abnormal cell that has lost the ability to control its growth. The theory of immune surveillance is that cancer cells continuously develop in the body but that the immune system normally recognizes cancer cells as foreign and destroys them. However, when the immune system fails, as in states of chronic malnutrition, chronic disease, or advanced age, the cancer cells grow unimpeded and eventually overtake normal cells as they compete for space and nutrition (Perez and Brady, 1992).

Characteristics of Malignant Cells

Cancer cells have certain properties that distinguish them from normal cells. Cancer cells are characterized by a lack of contact inhibition; they do not respond to the presence of other cells and continue to proliferate uncontrollably. Normal cells depend on growth factors to stimulate cell proliferation, but cancer cells have a decreased requirement for growth factors; therefore, cells continue to proliferate with minimal stimulation (Norton and Surbone, 1993). Oncologists theorize that tumors grow in a manner known as *Gompertzian function* (Figure 1-2) (DeVita, 1993; Norton and Surbone, 1993). Normally, cell birth equals cell death (Baserga, 1993). For example, when red blood cells become old and no longer function, they are replaced in equal amounts with new red blood cells. In cancer tumor growth there is rapid proliferation of cells followed by continuous but slowed proliferation. Terms that describe tumor growth include *doubling time* (the time it takes a tumor to double in size) and *growth fraction* (the fraction of cells that are actively cycling at any one time). In early stages, when the tumor volume is low, growth fraction is high and the tumor doubles its volume rapidly. As the tumor grows, space becomes restricted and the tumor outgrows its blood supply so that tumor doubling takes longer. Tumors with a high growth fraction are more sensitive to chemotherapy and radiation therapy because the tumors grow rapidly. Tumors without blood supply are more resistant to chemotherapy and radiation therapy because chemotherapy passes through the tumor via the blood and because radiation therapy needs the oxygen carried by the blood for maximum effectiveness (Hall and Cox, 1994; Perez and Brady, 1992).

Cancer cells lack the ability to differentiate fully. *Differentiation* describes the degree to which the cancer cells resemble the normal cells of the tissue of origin (primary site of disease) in terms of structure, character, and function. The more a cancer cell resembles the normal cell the greater the degree of differentiation.

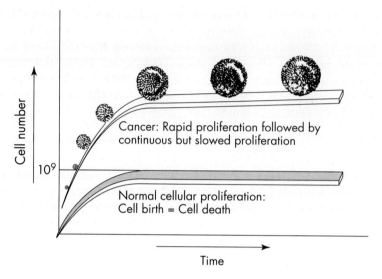

Fig. 1-2. Gompertzian function. From Goodman MS: Cancer: chemotherapy and care, ed 3, Princeton, 1992, Bristol-Myers Squibb Co.

Poorly differentiated or undifferentiated cells have little or no resemblance to normal cells.

Cancer cells are rarely encapsulated; thus they easily invade surrounding tissues. *Direct invasion* is the term used for the local spread of cancer cells into the surrounding tissue.

Cancer cells also lack adhesiveness and are not firmly attached to neighboring cells; this contributes to their ability to metastasize or travel to distant sites. Metastasis occurs simultaneously via the lymphatic and the circulatory systems (Liotta and Statler-Stevenson, 1993). Metastatic tumors tend to grow faster than the original primary tumor (Norton and Surbone, 1993).

Staging of Tumors

Staging is the process of describing the extent of disease at the time of diagnosis to assist in planning the appropriate treatment and to predict a clinical outcome or prognosis. The American College of Surgeons requires that all malignant tumors be staged. The American Joint Committee on Cancer (AJCC) has standardized the definitions for each stage of the various cancers (Beahrs et al., 1992). Each cancer patient is evaluated in terms of tumor size (represented by a *T*), lymphatic spread to lymph nodes (represented by an *N*), and whether or not the disease has metastasized (represented by an *M*). This is known as the *TNM clinical classification*. The T, N, and M categories are then divided into subcategories representing the degree of disease involvement. The range for T is 1 through 4, N is 0 through 3, and M is 0 through 1.

Information from the TNM assessment is used to classify the tumor by stage, which proceeds from I to IV. Stage I is the earliest stage, where the tumor is small and there is no lymph node involvement. Stage II usually means that there is a large tumor with no nodal involvement or a small tumor with some nodal involvement. Stage III is usually a small tumor with a lot of nodal involvement or a large tumor with any amount of nodal involvement, but in both cases there is no metastasis. At stage IV, metastasis has occurred. There are some variations, but most cancers are staged according to this general format.

Standardization of staging allows clinicians to describe the extent of disease not only to the patient but also to other health care professionals. For example, instead of saying that the breast cancer patient had a 0.8-cm tumor at its greatest dimension with no spread to the regional lymph nodes or to surrounding tissues, the patient's disease can be described as $T_{1b}N_0M_0$ or stage I breast cancer (Beahrs et al., 1992).

Staging is discussed in terms of *clinical staging* and *pathologic staging*. Clinical staging is done in the clinic, that is, there is a physical exam followed by diagnostic tests. For example, the clinician may be able to palpate a large tumor in the breast but not feel any enlarged lymph nodes in the axilla or see any evidence of metastasis. This patient might be staged clinically as a stage II. After analyzing a lumpectomy and axillary node dissection, however, the pathologist reports a 5.4-cm tumor with 4 out of 11 positive (diseased) lymph nodes, and the patient is reclassified as a pathological stage III (Beahrs et al., 1992). Once a patient is staged, even if the disease progresses, that patient is always categorized under the stage classified at time of diagnosis. In the case of the patient with breast cancer just described, he or she would be considered a person with stage III cancer that has metastasized.

Tumors are also graded histologically at the time of diagnosis to determine the degree of cell differentiation. G_1 describes a tumor that is well differentiated, meaning that the cancer cell is very similar to the normal cell. G_2 describes a moderately well-differentiated tumor. G_3 describes a poorly differentiated one, and G_4 describes a very poorly differentiated to undifferentiated tumor, where cells bear little resemblance to normal tissue (Beahrs et al., 1992). Usually, the less well differentiated the cells, the poorer the prognosis, because this represents a higher degree of malignancy (Rosai, 1993).

Goals of Therapy

The goals of therapy are cure, control of disease, or palliation of symptoms. *Cure* means that the disease is completely eradicated and the patient dies of something unrelated to the cancer. *Control of disease* means that, although the cancer is not gone, it is not growing. Control generally involves continued treatment that, if stopped, allows the cancer to grow. *Palliation* is the treatment of symptoms to improve the patient's quality of life when the disease is beyond control. Palliative treatment might include surgery to relieve small bowel obstruction caused by a tumor, radiation therapy to relieve spinal cord compression before it causes paralysis, or chemotherapy to shrink a tumor that causes pain by pressing on a nerve. It is important that the health care team discuss the goal of treatment with the patient and family so that there is no confusion or unreal expectation when the patient receives treatment.

Limitations of Single Modality Therapy

The history of the development of surgical therapy, radiation therapy, chemotherapy, and biotherapy parallels their traditional use along the cancer continuum. Surgery, refined in the mid-nineteenth century with the development of anesthesia and infection-control practices, traditionally has been used when cancer is considered "local," that is, it has not spread. The turn of the century marked the beginning of radiation therapy as a cancer treatment. Historically, when cancer spread regionally (but not to distant areas of the body), radiation therapy was used. Chemotherapy first appeared during World War II and had been used only in advanced disease. Biotherapy research began in the 1950s and is now being added to the arsenal of cancer treatments.

Although each treatment modality has advantages, each also has its limitations. Both surgery and radiation therapy are local treatments that can successfully remove or decrease the bulk of a tumor but are ineffective outside the treatment area. In addition, a tumor may be inoperable or incompletely excised if it is too large or if major organs are involved. Surgery can also cause disfigurement or functional loss, greatly affecting the patient's quality of life. Radiation therapy can sometimes reach tumors inaccessible by surgery but cannot totally destroy large tumors that have outgrown their blood supply. Chemotherapy is a systemic treatment that travels throughout the body (although many chemotherapeutic agents do not cross the blood-brain barrier) and fights metastasis and micrometastasis (undetected spread of disease), but it is not as effective as surgery or radiation therapy in treating large bulky tumors (Harris and Mastrangelo, 1993; Perez and Brady, 1992). The role of biotherapy, used to enhance the patient's defense mechanisms against tumors, continues to be explored (Rosenberg, 1993).

In the 1950s, investigators realized that, despite aggressive surgical treatment for local or early disease, cancer still recurred. As more information about cell biology and cancer development became known, it was recognized that many tumors metastasized, or spread to distant areas, during early tumor development (Harris and Mastrangelo, 1991). It has been demonstrated that 60% to 70% of all patients have metastasis or micrometastasis at the time of diagnosis (Liotta, Stetler-Stevenson, and Steeg, 1993). Conflict about giving chemotherapy for nondetectable disease arose. It was based on the fact that the side effects of chemotherapy were harsh and that, because a subgroup of patients could be cured without chemotherapy, some patients would be getting unnecessary treatment. Even today, we are faced with the problem of identifying who will benefit from multimodal treatment in so-called early-stage cancer.

❖ Multimodal Therapy

Benefits of Multimodal Therapy

Multimodal therapy exploits the strengths of each modality to maximize the eradication of cancer cells. Any combination of two, three, or four modalities can be used throughout the cancer continuum (although generally combinations of two or three predominate). Figure 1-3 shows this model as four circles, each representing a different modality, overlapping and combined in multiple ways. The time of diagnosis, regardless of stage of disease, is the time to use the most aggressive treatment possible. The only exception is when the goal of treatment is palliation of symptoms.

Steele and Peckham (1979) are credited as the first oncologists to discuss the theoretical background of multimodal therapy. They described four types of mechanisms that made combined chemotherapy and radiation therapy particularly effective: (1) spatial cooperation, in which one modality is active against tumor cells spatially missed by the other modality; (2) toxicity independence, implying that each modality can be administered at its optimal dose without significantly increasing the toxicity to normal cells; (3) normal tissue protection by the chemotherapy, which allows a higher-than-usual dose of radiation therapy to be given to the tumor cells; and (4) the enhanced effect of the combined use of chemotherapy and radiation therapy.

Combining treatment modalities produces results that may be additive, synergistic, or subadditive. *Additive* results occur when the outcome of the combined therapies is more than the expected outcome from a single modality but is no more than the outcome expected from adding the results of the two therapies. *Synergistic* (or *superadditive*) results occur when the outcome from the combination of modalities is more than expected. Although the exact mechanism of the synergistic response is unclear, various physiologic phenomenon may be influential, including (1) interference with the repair of radiation damage (through enzyme inhibition and/or DNA alterations), (2) alteration in cellular oxygen levels, (3) inducement

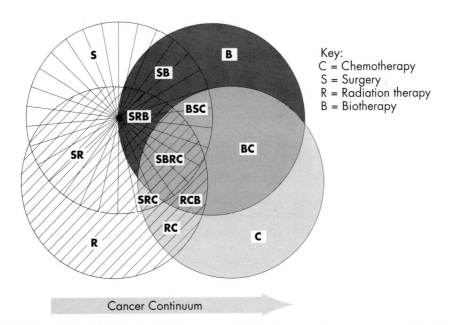

Fig. 1-3. Model of multimodal therapy. The circles represent the individual cancer treatment modalities. The model shows current as well as potential future combined treatments. Adapted with permission from J. Popkin, MD.

of cell cycle progression, (4) changes in receptor sites for radiation therapy, and (5) alteration of vascular supply to the tumor itself (Phillips, 1980; Vokes and Weich-selbaum, 1991). Subadditive results occur when the outcome is more than that expected from a single modality but less than that expected when adding two modalities (Phillips, 1993). Sensitization occurs when one modality, which has no effect on the tumor when used alone, enhances the effect of a second modality when both are given together (Fu, 1985). Some practitioners do not differentiate these terms but refer to the combined effects of multimodal therapy as "enhancement" (Fu, 1985).

Disadvantages of Multimodal Therapy

The disadvantages of multimodal therapy include increased side effects, both acute and long-term; increased cost; compromised staging; and possible inability to deliver all modalities at a single facility.

Acute side effects such as bone marrow depression may occur earlier and be more severe than when single modality therapy is given. So-called new or unex-pected side effects may occur as the use of multiple therapies causes previously sub-clinical side effects (too subtle to be recognized) to become clinically detectable or prominent (Scofield, Liebman, and Popkin, 1991). For example, preoperative radi-ation may cause postoperative complications, such as increased risk of fistula for-mation and delayed wound healing. Long-term side effects also increase because of the simple addition of long-term side effects from each modality and because of increased survival. Some of the acute side effects, such as pulmonary fibrosis, may also become chronic or long-term. If treatment doses are decreased or delayed due to severe side effects, suboptimal dosing may be the result. Suboptimal dosing can lead to a lesser chance of cure (DeVita, 1993). Results may be even less than if only one modality were used (Coleman, 1989).

Staging the disease may be compromised if neoadjuvant chemotherapy or radi-ation therapy is given before surgery. Lymph nodes excised after chemotherapy or radiation therapy may be free of disease, with the only indication of previous dis-ease being evidence of former enlargement. The cause of enlargement is question-able and may be due to factors other than eradicated disease, such as a previous infection or a radiation-induced reaction, leading to reluctance by clinicians to assume that cancer had been present in those lymph nodes. However, current stan-dards dictate that cancer involvement should be presupposed when enlarged lymph nodes are removed after neoadjuvant treatment.

Because not all cancer treatment facilities can provide all therapy modalities, many patients go to multiple facilities for treatment, especially for radiation ther-apy. This can lead to difficulty in patient-care coordination. It also increases the number of caregivers who may give conflicting, or what sounds like conflicting, information as different teaching methods or terminology are used. Even for the patient who receives all treatment within the same institution, different physicians and nurses are involved in the various treatment settings and may face the same chal-lenges in coordinating patient care as caregivers located in different places.

Multimodal therapy costs more than single modality therapy at the outset, because more treatment is provided and because higher intensity of care is needed.

Multimodal therapy is not exempt from other changes occurring in health care, including discharge of sicker patients, increased emphasis on outpatient and home therapy, and insurance denials for coverage of treatment.

Sequencing of Multimodal Therapy

Multimodal therapy can be combined in various ways, based on treatment strategies, convenience, and expected side effects. Table 1-1 gives examples of various sequencing methods. *Adjuvant therapy,* additional therapy given for micrometastasis, usually follows the primary therapy and has the goal of eradicating residual disease. Studies of adjuvant chemotherapy have demonstrated the advantages of adding chemotherapy to surgery: more patients are cured than if either modality is used alone. Animal studies have demonstrated that surgical removal or radiation eradication of the primary tumor can increase the growth rate of the metastasis, proving the importance of giving adjuvant treatment as soon after primary treatment as possible (Harris and Mastrangelo, 1991). Stage III colon cancer, for example, is treated with surgery, followed as soon as surgical healing is completed by chemotherapy and biotherapy.

Neoadjuvant, or induction, *therapy* is given "up front" or before the primary treatment, with the goal of shrinking the tumor to increase the chance of cure from the primary treatment. Studies have demonstrated improved response in neoadjuvant chemotherapy before surgery in head and neck cancers, esophageal cancers, osteosarcomas, and stage III breast cancers (Harris and Mastrangelo, 1991).

Sandwiching refers to giving one modality of therapy between a split course of another modality, for example, two cycles of chemotherapy followed by a complete course of radiation therapy, followed by four cycles of chemotherapy.

Concomitant or *concurrent therapy* refers to two therapies given at the same time with the goal of simultaneously killing cells of both the primary tumor and the spreading disease. *Alternating* or *interdigitating therapy* (a form of concomitant therapy) refers to giving one modality on the non-treatment days of the other modality without causing delay in the schedule of the first modality. It is used in an attempt to maximize the positive aspects of concomitant therapy while minimizing the toxicities. Tables 1-2 and 1-3 list the advantages and disadvantages of different sequencing combinations.

Sequencing depends on how the modalities enhance each other. Some enhancements require direct interaction of modalities, in which case they are given concurrently, whereas others do not (Fu, 1985). For example, when a chemotherapeutic agent enhances the effect of radiation therapy if given together, these two modalities may be given concurrently. If the chemotherapeutic agent is active against the tumor but does not potentiate the effects of radiation, the treatments may be given sequentially. Cyclophosphamide, for instance, enhances the effect when radiation is given to the lung and the bladder, but not when given to the small intestine or the esophagus (Fu, 1985).

When modalities follow each other, timing is of the utmost importance. Prolonged delays between modalities can compromise the outcome by giving cancer cells time to repair and grow (Fowler and Lindstrom, 1992; Pajak et al., 1991). Generally 3 to 4 weeks allows time for normal tissue to heal but does not allow for

Table 1-1 Examples of Multimodal Therapy

Sequence	Cancer	Protocol	Reference
Adjuvant	Breast	Surgery followed by cyclophosphamide, methotrexate, 5-fluorouracil, prednisone (followed by radiation therapy if partial mastectomy done)	Fisher, Wickerham, and Redmond, 1992; Haffty et al., 1994
	Colon	Surgery followed by radiation therapy	Willett et al., 1993
	Colon	Surgery followed by 5-fluorouracil	Fuchs and Mayer, 1993
	Esophagus	Cisplatin, bleomycin followed by radiation therapy	Izquierdo et al., 1993
Neoadjuvant	Head and neck	Cisplatin, bleomycin followed by surgery	Baker, Makuch, and Wolf, 1981; Hong et al., 1979
	Larynx	Cisplatin, 5-fluorouracil followed by radiation therapy	Dept. of Veterans Affairs, 1991
	Pineoblastoma	Cisplatin, etoposide, vincristine followed by radiation therapy	Ghim et al., 1993
Concomitant	Esophagus	Cisplatin, 5-fluorouracil, radiation therapy	Forastiere, 1992; Naunheim et al., 1992
	Esophagus	Cisplatin, radiation therapy	Mandard et al., 1994
	Head and neck	Cisplatin, 5-fluorouracil, radiation therapy	Adelstein et al., 1992; Taylor et al., 1994
	Head and neck	Carboplatin, radiation therapy	Eisenberger and Jacobs, 1992
	Head and neck	5-Fluorouracil, mitomycin-C, radiation therapy	Coia et al., 1991
	Anus	5-Fluorouracil, mitomycin-C, radiation therapy	Cummings, 1992
	Colon	5-Fluorouracil, leucovorin, interferon alfa-2a	Grem et al., 1993
	Pancreas	Intraoperative radiation therapy	Zerbi et al., 1994
	Lung (small cell)	Cisplatin, etoposide, radiation therapy	Turrisi, Glover, and Mason, 1990
	Lung (non–small cell)	Cisplatin, radiation therapy	Schaake-Koning et al., 1990
	Lymphoma	Cyclophosphamide, doxorubicin, teniposide, prednisone, interferon alfa-2b alfa-2b	Soloa-Celigny, 1993
	Melanoma	Dacarbazine, interferon alfa-2b	Falkson, Falkson, and Falkson, 1991
	Melanoma	Cisplatin, interleukin-2	Demchak et al., 1991
	Melanoma	Dacarbazine, cisplatin, interleukin-2, interferon alfa	Richards et al., 1992

Neoadjuvant	Pancreas	5-Fluorouracil, mitomycin-C, radiation therapy followed by surgery	Yeung et al., 1993
Concomitant	Rectum	5-Fluorouracil, mitomycin-C, radiation therapy followed by surgery	Chan et al., 1993
	Rectum	5-Fluorouracil, leucovorin followed by surgery	Minsky et al., 1992
Sandwich	Rectum	5-Fluorouracil, leucovorin followed by surgery followed by 5-fluorouracil, leucovorin	Minsky et al., 1993
Concomitant followed by adjuvant therapy	Pancreas	Intraoperative radiation therapy followed by radiation therapy	Dobelbower et al., 1991
	Colon	5-Fluorouracil, leucovorin, radiation therapy followed by 5-fluorouracil, leucovorin	Moertel et al., 1994
	Sarcoma (retroperitoneal)	Intraoperative radiation therapy followed by radiation therapy	Johnstone, Sindelar, and Kinsella, 1994

Table 1-2   **Advantages and Disadvantages of Neoadjuvant Chemotherapy in Previously Untreated Patients**

Advantages	*Disadvantages*
Better performance status and good nutritional status will increase tolerance of chemotherapy in the preoperative patient	Delay of surgery from complications of chemotherapy
Intact blood supply of previously untreated tumors has the potential to deliver high concentrations of the drug to the tumor site	Inaccurate knowledge of tumor margins
Increased tumor cell kill in rapidly growing tumor cells	Increased immunosuppression
Potential eradication of subclinical microscopic metastatic disease that is not exposed to local treatment	
Enhanced efficacy of planned definitive local treatment by cytoreduction of the primary tumor and nodal metastases	
Continued use of a chemotherapeutic regimen as a maintenance regimen in patients who initially achieved significant response	

From Scofield RP, Liebman MC, and Popkin JD: Multimodal therapy. In Baird SB, McCorkle R, and Grant M, editors: Cancer nursing: a comprehensive textbook, Philadelphia, 1991, WB Saunders Co.

tumor cell regeneration (Sause, 1994). Optimal scheduling of multimodal therapy has not been determined in most cases (Buchholz, 1993; Townsend, Abston, and Fish, 1985; Tupchong et al., 1991).

Mechanisms of Multimodal Therapy

Surgery and radiation therapy can enhance each other in several ways. Surgery can remove gross disease, whereas radiation therapy destroys microscopic disease in the surgical bed and disease inaccessible to the surgeon (Sause, 1994). Preoperative radiation therapy can shrink inoperable tumors and make them operable. Postoperative radiation therapy can destroy any tumor cells left after surgery. Although preoperative radiation therapy may be more effective than postoperative radiation therapy, larger radiation doses can be given postoperatively, leading to increased cell kill (Perez and Brady, 1992). Surgery and radiation therapy can also be combined so that less radical surgery is necessary, resulting in disease control and organ preservation or function, such as a lumpectomy followed by radiation therapy for breast cancer.

Intraoperative radiation therapy (IORT) is radiation therapy given directly to the tumor during surgery. It delivers the maximum dose of radiation to the tumor while minimizing side effects to healthy tissues (Cox, 1994; Johnstone, Sindelar, and Kinsella, 1994; Tepper and Calvo, 1992).

Table 1-3   Advantages and Disadvantages of Preoperative and Postoperative
Radiation Therapy

Advantages	Disadvantages
Preoperative Radiation Therapy	
Decreased tumor size and increased resectability	Greater chance of postoperative complications
	♦ Delayed wound healing
Intact blood supply; tumor more responsive to radiation therapy	♦ Increased risk of fistula formation
	♦ Increased risk of wound infection
Usually requires smaller treatment area	Compromise of accurate staging— "pathologic downstaging"
Fewer small bowel adhesions and less incidence of future small bowel obstruction	Radiation therapy doses are minimized to lessen risk of surgical complications
Postoperative Radiation Therapy	
Surgical margins and extent of the tumor defined	Tumor may be poorly oxygenated due to disrupted blood supply
Organs may be removed from radiation field during surgery to prevent unnecessary toxicity	Usually requires larger radiation therapy field due to possible seeding of the tumor during surgery
Higher doses of radiation can be given if surgical margins are not clean	Radiation therapy may be delayed if patient doesn't heal as expected from surgery
Staging is not compromised	In radiation therapy to the bowel, there is an increased incidence of small bowel obstruction

Data taken from Koops and Hoekstra, 1994; Sause, 1994; Scofield, Liebman, and Popkin, 1991; Stevens, 1994; and Tupchong et al., 1991.

Chemotherapy can be given before surgery to shrink the tumor and enhance operability (Perez and Brady, 1992). Benefits have been demonstrated in head and neck, esophageal, and breast cancers and in osteosarcoma (Harris and Mastrangelo, 1991).

Chemotherapy used in conjunction with surgery or radiation therapy can simultaneously treat distant disease and local disease. Combining chemotherapy and radiation therapy increases cell kill by attacking the cell in different phases of the cell cycle. Chemotherapy has also been shown to inhibit sublethal repair of damage to cancer cells caused by radiation therapy (Fu, 1985; Phillips, 1993; Rotman, 1992). Chemotherapy and radiation therapy also enhance each other by decreasing tumor mass and therefore increasing the blood supply to the tumor. An increased blood supply means increased oxygenation of tumor cells, making them more responsive to the other modality (Phillips, 1993). Chemotherapeutic agents such as cisplatin, 5-fluorouracil, mitomycin-C, hydroxyurea, paclitaxel, doxorubicin, cyclophosphamide, and bleomycin have been shown to increase tumor cell radiosensitivity by disrupting normal cell kinetics (Fu, 1985; Hall and Cox, 1994; Perez and Brady, 1992; Rotman, 1992; and Schilsky, 1992).

Chemotherapy is combined with biotherapy to reduce the size of the tumor (via chemotherapy) and to enhance the body's immune system (via biotherapy) in an attempt to eradicate the remaining cancer cells (Wadler, 1992). Carmustine, cisplatin, cyclophosphamide, dacarbazine, and doxorubicin have each demonstrated either additive or synergistic effects when given with interleukin-2 (Sznol and Longo, 1993). Interferon-alfa,* given after 5-fluorouracil, decreases related bone-marrow depression and allows for increased doses of 5-fluorouracil to be given (Sznol and Longo, 1993; Wadler, 1992). Biotherapy has also been combined with radiation therapy (Hendry, 1994; Weichselbaum et al., 1992). Interleukin-1 has been shown to provide protection from radiation damage to normal cells in mice (Coleman, 1989). The role of biotherapy in combination with other modalities is still in its infancy (Gilewski and Golomb, 1990; Rosenberg, 1993).

Assessment Tools

The standardization of assessment and the documentation of side effects are crucial in evaluating treatment. Functional status should be evaluated before treatment is initiated to determine if the patient is "a viable candidate" for treatment. Factors to consider include: (1) the patient's ability to tolerate treatment and (2) the possible improvement of functional status if the patient is treated. The Karnofsky Performance Scale (Box 1-1), first developed in 1948, is frequently used today to assess functional ability of cancer patients. The scale ranges from 0 to 100, with 0 representing no life and 100 representing "normal" functional status. Generally, patients with a rating of less than 60 are not considered candidates for treatment other than palliation of symptoms.

Box 1-1   Karnofsky Performance Scale

Functional Status	*Rating*
No complaints; no evidence of disease	100
Able to carry on normal activity; minor signs or symptoms of disease	90
Some signs or symptoms of disease with effort	80
Cares for self but is unable to carry on normal activity or to do active work	70
Requires occasional assistance but is able to care for most personal needs	60
Requires considerable assistance and frequent medical care	50
Disabled; requires special care and assistance	40
Severely disabled; hospitalization indicated, although death not imminent	30
Very sick; hospitalization necessary; requires active supportive treatment	20
Moribund; fatal processes progressing rapidly	10
Dead	0

---

*Interferon-alfa is the form of interferon-α created by recombinant DNA technology (Dorr RT and Von Hoff DD: Cancer chemotherapy handbook, ed 2, Norwalk, Connecticut, 1994, Appleton & Lange).

Several tools have been developed to define the degree of toxicity experienced by the cancer patient and to provide consistency in documenting acute and chronic side effects (Tables 1-4 to 1-6). The scales commonly used for grading toxicity, although developed by committees that recognized the multimodality of cancer treatment, were for separate use by the modalities. Currently representatives from the Radiation Therapy Oncology Group, the European Organization for Research on Treatment of Cancer, and the National Cancer Institute are developing a new set of toxicity criteria to reflect the side effects of combination chemotherapy and radiation therapy (John, 1993). Adequate assessment and documentation of side effects and the subsequent quality of life for the patient are essential for evaluating the impact of treatment.

Patient Response to Treatment

After treatment, patient response is evaluated subjectively and objectively. A subjective response might be indicated by a patient's report of pain relief. An objective, or measurable, response compares results of diagnostic tests (scans, laboratory tests, tumor markers) to results of pretreatment tests.

Complete response is the term used to describe the patient who shows no detectable disease for a period of at least a month after treatment. *Partial response* refers to a decrease of tumor size by at least 50% and the absence of new areas of tumor. *Minimal response* is a 25% to 50% reduction of tumor size, and *stable disease* describes a tumor that has remained the same, decreased by less than 25%, or increased by less than 25% after treatment. *Progressive disease* is an increase of tumor mass by at least 25% and/or the appearance of new areas of cancer.

Nursing Management

Nursing management of patients receiving multimodal therapy focuses on prevention and the early detection of treatment side effects, and on symptom management, patient/family education, coordination of care, and emotional support. Nursing management will not be discussed here because it is addressed in depth in Units III and IV.

Future of Cancer Treatment and Multimodal Therapy

What does the future hold? As specialty care reverts to primary-care physicians and the role of the oncologist becomes more consultative, nurses may play a bigger role in monitoring side effects, patient teaching, and even ensuring that treatment referrals are made appropriately. Cancer treatment has become more complex at a time when payment for the care demands less patient contact with the health care system. Health care providers must broaden their scope of knowledge because patients who were formerly cared for in teaching hospitals are now treated in community hospitals and physicians' offices with follow-up care by home-care nurses, office nurses, or clinic nurses. Family members or significant others are given the responsibility to provide direct care or to give information or guidance in decision making. Nursing

Table 1-4 Common Toxicity Criteria of the Eastern Cooperative Oncology Group (National Cancer Institute)

Toxicity	Grade				
	0	*1*	*2*	*3*	*4*
Blood, Bone Marrow					
WBC	≥4.0	3.0–3.9	2.0–2.9	1.0–1.9	<1.0
Platelets	WNL	75.0–normal	50.0–74.9	25.0–49.9	<25.0
Hemoglobin	WNL	10.0–normal	8.0–10.0	6.5–7.9	<6.5
Granulocytes/Bands	≥2.0	1.5–1.9	1.0–1.4	0.5–0.9	<0.5
Lymphocytes	≥2.0	1.5–1.9	1.0–1.4	0.5–0.9	<0.5
Hemorrhage (clinical)	None	Mild, no transfusion	Gross, 1–2 units transfusion per episode	Gross, 3–4 units transfusion per episode	Massive, >4 units transfusion per episode
Infection	None	Mild	Moderate	Severe	Life-threatening
Gastrointestinal					
Nausea	None	Able to eat reasonable intake	Intake significantly decreased but can eat	No significant intake	
Vomiting	None	1 episode in 24 hrs	2–5 episodes in 24 hrs	5–10 episodes in 24 hrs	>10 episodes in 24 hrs or requiring parenteral support
Diarrhea	None	Increase of 2–3 stools/day over pre-Rx	Increase of 4–5 stools/day, or nocturnal stools, or moderate cramping	Increase of 7–9 stools/day, or incontinence, or severe cramping	Increase of ≥10 stools/day or grossly bloody diarrhea, or need for parenteral support
Stomatitis	None	Painless ulcers, erythema, or mild soreness	Painful erythema, edema, or ulcers, but can eat	Painful erythema, edema, or ulcers, and cannot eat	Requires parenteral or enteral support
Liver					
Bilirubin	WNL	—	$<1.5 \times N$	$1.5–3.0 \times N$	$>3.0 \times N$

Transaminase (SGOT, SGPT)	WNL	≤2.5 × N	2.6–5.0 × N	5.1–20.0 × N	>20.0 × N
Alkaline phosphatase or 5' nucleotidase	WNL	≤2.5 × N	2.6–5.0 × N	5.1–20.0 × N	>20.0 × N
Neurologic					
Sensory	None or no change	Mild paresthesia, loss of deep tendon reflexes	Mild or moderate objective sensory loss; moderate paresthesia	Severe objective sensory loss or paresthesia that interferes with function	—
Motor	None or no change	Subjective weakness; no objective findings	Mild objective weakness without significant impairment of function	Objective weakness with impairment of function	Paralysis
Cortical	None	Mild somnolence or agitation	Moderate somnolence or agitation	Severe somnolence, agitation, confusion, disorientation, or hallucinations; aphasia—transient	Coma, seizures, toxic psychosis; aphasia—permanent (>1 week)
Cerebellar	None	Slight uncoordination, dysdiadokinesis	Intention tremor, dysmetria, slurred speech, nystagmus	Locomotor ataxia	Cerebellar necrosis
Mood	No change	Mild anxiety or depression	Moderate anxiety or depression	Severe anxiety or depression	Suicidal ideation
Headache	None	Mild	Moderate or severe but transient	Unrelenting and severe	—
Constipation	None or no change	Mild	Moderate	Severe	Ileus >96 hrs
Hearing	None or no change	Asymptomatic, hearing loss on audiometry only	Tinnitus	Hearing loss interfering with function but correctable with hearing aid	Deafness not correctable

Continued

Table 1-4 Common Toxicity Criteria of the Eastern Cooperative Oncology Group (National Cancer Institute)—cont'd

Toxicity	0	1	Grade 2	3	4
Vision	None or no change	—	—	Symptomatic nontotal loss of vision	Blindness
Skin	None or no change	Scattered macular or papular eruption or erythema that is asymptomatic	Scattered macular or papular eruption or erythema with pruritus or other associated symptoms	Generalized symptomatic macular, papular, or vascular eruption	Exfoliative dermatitis or ulcerating dermatitis
Allergy	None	Transient rash, drug fever <38°C, 100.4°F	Urticaria, drug fever = 38°C, 100.4°F, mild bronchospasm	Serum sickness, bronchospasm, requiring parenteral medication	Anaphylaxis
Fever in absence of infection	None	37.1°–38.0°C 98.7°–100.4°F	38.1°–40.0°C 100.5°–104.0°F	>40.0°C >104.0°F for less than 24 hrs	>40.0°C (104.0°F) for more than 24 hrs or fever accompanied by hypotension
Kidney/Bladder					
Creatinine	WNL	<1.5N	$1.5 - 3.0 \times N$	$3.1 - 6.0 \times N$	$<6.0 \times N$
Proteinuria	No change	1+ or <0.3 g% or <3 g%/1	2–3+ or 0.3–1.0 g% or 3–10 g/1	4+ or >1.0 g% or >10 g/1	Nephrotic syndrome
Hematuria	Negative	Micro only	Gross, no clots	Gross + clots	Requires transfusion
Alopecia	No loss	Mild hair loss	Pronounced or total hair loss	—	—
Pulmonary	None or no change	Asymptomatic, with abnormality in PFTs	Dyspnea on significant exertion	Dyspnea at normal level of activity	Dyspnea at rest

Heart				
Dysrhythmias	None	Asymptomatic, transient, requiring no therapy	Recurrent or persistent, but no therapy required	Requires treatment	Requires monitoring; or hypotension, or ventricular tachycardia, or fibrillation
Function	None	Asymptomatic, decline of resting ejection fraction by less than 20% of baseline value	Asymptomatic, decline of resting ejection fraction by more than 20% of baseline value	Mild CHF, responsive to therapy	Severe or refractory CHF
Ischemia	None	Nonspecific T-wave flattening	Asymptomatic, ST and T-wave changes suggesting ischemia	Angina without evidence of infarction	Acute myocardial infarction
Pericardial	None	Asymptomatic effusion; no intervention required	Pericarditis (rub. chest pain, ECG changes)	Symptomatic effusion; drainage required	Tamponade; drainage urgently required
Blood Pressure				
Hypertension	None or no change	Asymptomatic, transient increase by greater than 20 mm Hg(D) or to >150/100 if previously WNL; no treatment required	Recurrent or persistent increase by greater than 20 mm Hg(D) or to >150/100 if previously WNL; no treatment required	Requires therapy	Hypertensive crisis
Hypotension	None or no change	Changes requiring no therapy (including transient orthostatic hypotension)	Requires fluid replacement or other therapy but not hospitalization	Requires therapy and hospitalization; resolves within 48 hrs of stopping the agent	Requires therapy and hospitalization for >48 hrs after stopping the agent
Local	None	Pain	Pain and swelling, with inflammation or phlebitis	Ulceration	Plastic surgery indicated
Weight gain/loss	<5.0%	5.0–9.9%	10.0–19.9%	≥20.0%	—
Hyperglycemia	<116	116–160	161–250	251–500	>500 or ketoacidosis

Continued

Table 1-4 Common Toxicity Criteria of the Eastern Cooperative Oncology Group (National Cancer Institute)—cont'd

Toxicity	0	1	Grade 2	3	4
Hypoglycemia	>64	55-64	40-54	30-39	<30
Amylase	WNL	<1.5 × N	1.5-2.0 × N	2.1-5.0 × N	>5.1 × N
Hypercalcemia	<10.6	10.6-11.5	11.6-12.5	12.6-13.5	≤13.5
Hypocalcemia	>8.4	8.4-7.8	7.7-7.0	6.9-6.1	≤6.0
Hypomagnesemia	>1.4	1.4-1.2	1.1-0.9	0.8-0.6	≤0.5
Fibrinogen	WNL	0.99-0.75 × N	0.74-0.50 × N	0.49-0.25 × N	≤0.24 × N
Prothrombin time	WNL	1.01-1.25 × N	1.26-1.50 × N	1.51-2.00 × N	>2.00 × N
Partial thromboplastin time	WNL	1.01-1.66 × N	1.67-2.33 × N	2.34-3.00 × N	>3.00 × N
Vascular serum albumin (gm%)	>2.8	2.4-2.7	2.0-2.3	<2.0 with supplements	<2.0 with pulmonary edema and/or 4+ leg edema
Muscle	None	Myalgia	Myalgia requiring therapy	CPK or aldolase elevations >2 × N and <5 × N	CPK or aldolase elevations >5 × N

Table 1-5   Acute Radiation Morbidity Scoring Criteria of the Radiation Therapy Oncology Group

Toxicity Site	0	1	Grade 2	3	4
Skin	No change over baseline	Follicular, faint or dull erythema; epilation; dry desquamation; decreased sweating	Tender or bright erythema, patchy moist desquamation; moderate edema	Confluent, moist desquamation other than skin folds, pitting edema	Ulceration, hemorrhage, or necrosis
Mucous membrane	No change over baseline	Injection; may experience mild pain not requiring analgesic	Patchy mucositis that may produce an inflammatory serosanguinous discharge; may experience moderate pain requiring analgesic	Confluent fibrinous mucositis; may include severe pain requiring narcotic	Ulceration, hemorrhage, or necrosis
Eye	No change	Mild conjunctivitis with or without scleral injection; increased tearing	Moderate conjunctivitis with or without keratitis requiring steroids and/or antibiotics; dry eye requiring artificial tears; iritis with photophobia	Severe keratitis with corneal ulceration; objective decrease in visual acuity or in visual fields; acute glaucoma; panophthalmitis	Loss of vision (unilateral or bilateral)
Ear	No change over baseline	Mild external otitis with erythema, pruritus, secondary to dry desquamation not requiring medication; audiogram unchanged from baseline	Moderate external otitis requiring topical medication; serous otitis medium; hypoacusis on testing only	Severe external otitis with discharge or moist desquamation; symptomatic hypoacusis; tinnitus, not drug related	Deafness
Salivary gland	No change over baseline	Mild mouth dryness; slightly thickened saliva; may have slightly altered taste such as metallic taste; these changes not reflected in alteration in baseline feeding behavior, such as increased use of liquids with meals	Moderate to complete dryness; thick, sticky saliva; markedly altered taste	—	Acute salivary gland necrosis

Continued

Table 1-5 Acute Radiation Morbidity Scoring Criteria of the Radiation Therapy Oncology Group—cont'd

Toxicity Site	Grade 0	1	2	3	4
Pharynx and esophagus	No change over baseline	Mild dysphagia or odynophagia; may require topical anesthetic or nonnarcotic analgesics; may require soft diet	Moderate dysphagia or odynophagia; may require narcotic analgesics; may require puree or liquid diet	Severe dysphagia or odynophagia with dehydration or weight loss (>15% from pretreatment baseline requiring N-G feeding tube, IV fluids, or hyperalimentation	Complete obstruction, ulceration, perforation, fistula
Larynx	No change over baseline	Mild or intermittent hoarseness; cough not requiring antitussive; erythema of mucosa	Persistent hoarseness but able to vocalize; referred ear pain, sore throat, patchy fibrinous exudate or mild arytenoid edema not requiring narcotic; cough requiring antitussive	Whispered speech, throat pain or referred ear pain requiring narcotic; confluent fibrinous exudate, marked arytenoid edema	Marked dyspnea, stridor or hemoptysis with tracheostomy or intubation necessary
Upper GI tract	No change	Anorexia with ≤5% weight loss from pretreatment baseline; nausea not requiring antiemetics; abdominal discomfort not requiring parasympathetic drugs or analgesics	Anorexia with ≤15% weight loss from pretreatment baseline; nausea and/or vomiting requiring antiemetics; abdominal pain requiring analgesics	Anorexia with >15% weight loss from pretreatment baseline or requiring N-G tube or parenteral support; nausea and or vomiting requiring N-G tube or parenteral support; abdominal pain, severe despite medication; hematemesis or melena; abdominal distention (flat-plate radiograph demonstrated distended bowel loops)	Ileus, subacute or acute obstruction, perforation, GI bleeding requiring transfusion; abdominal pain requiring tube decompression or bowel diversion

Lower GI tract, including pelvis	No change	Increased frequency or change in quality of bowel habits not requiring medication; rectal discomfort not requiring analgesics	Diarrhea requiring parasympatholytic drugs (e.g., Lomotil); mucous discharge not necessitating sanitary pads; rectal or abdominal pain requiring analgesics	Diarrhea requiring parenteral support; severe mucous or blood discharge necessitating sanitary pads; abdominal distention (flat-plate radiograph demonstrates distended bowel loops)	Acute or subacute obstruction, fistula or perforation GI bleeding, requiring transfusion; abdominal pain or tenesmus requiring tube decompression or bowel diversion
Lung	No change	Mild symptoms of dry cough or dyspnea on exertion	Persistent cough requiring narcotic, antitussive agents; dyspnea with minimal effort but not at rest	Severe cough unresponsive to narcotic antitussive agent or dyspnea at rest; clinical or radiologic evidence of acute pneumonitis; intermittent O_2 or steroids may be required	Severe respiratory insufficiency; continuous oxygen or assisted ventilation
Genitourinary	No change	Frequency of urination or nocturia twice pretreatment habit; dysuria, urgency not requiring medication	Frequency of urination or nocturia that is less frequent than every hour; dysuria, urgency, bladder spasm requiring local anesthetic (e.g., Pyridium)	Frequency with urgency and nocturia hourly or more frequently; dysuria, pelvis pain, or bladder spasm requiring regular, frequent narcotic; gross hematuria with or without clot passage	Hematuria requiring transfusion; acute bladder obstruction not secondary to clot passage, ulceration or necrosis
Heart	No change over baseline	Asymptomatic but objective evidence of ECG changes or pericardial abnormalities without evidence of other heart disease	Symptomatic with ECG changes and radiologic findings of congestive heart failure or pericardial disease; no specific treatment required	Congestive heart failure, angina pectoris, pericardial disease responding to therapy	Congestive heart failure, angina pectoris, pericardial disease, arrhythmias not responsive to nonsurgical measures

Continued

Table 1-5 Acute Radiation Morbidity Scoring Criteria of the Radiation Therapy Oncology Group—cont'd

Toxicity Site	Grade				
	0	1	2	3	4
CNS	No change	Fully functional status (i.e., able to work) with minor neurologic findings; no medication needed	Neurologic findings present sufficient to require home care; nursing assistance may be required; medications including steroids or anti-seizure agents may be required	Neurologic findings requiring hospitalization for initial management	Serious neurologic impairment, which includes paralysis, coma, or seizures >3 per week despite medication; hospitalization required
Hematologic WBC (×1000)	≥4.0	3.0–<4.0	2.0–<3.0	1.0–<2.0	<1.0
Platelets (×1000)	>100	75–<100	50–<75	25–<50	<25 or spontaneous bleeding
Neutrophils (×1000)	≥1.9	1.5–<1.9	1.0–<1.5	0.5–<1.0	<0.5 or sepsis
Hemoglobin (gm %)	>11	11–9.5	<9.5–7.5	<7.5–5.0	—
Hematocrit (%)	≥32	28–<32	28	Packed cell transfusion required	—

Guidelines: The acute morbidity criteria are used to score or grade toxicity from radiation therapy. The criteria are relevant from day 1, the commencement of therapy, through day 90. Thereafter, the EORTC/RTOG Criteria for Late Effects are to be utilized.
The evaluator must attempt to discriminate between disease and treatment-related signs and symptoms.
An accurate baseline evaluation before commencement of therapy is necessary.
All toxicities Grade 3, 4, or 5 must be verified by the principal investigator. Any toxicity that caused death is graded 5.
From the Radiation Therapy Oncology Group (RTOG) and the European Organization for Research on Treatment of Cancer (EORTC).

Table 1-6 Late Radiation Morbidity Scoring Criteria of the Radiation Therapy Oncology Group/European Organization for Research on Treatment of Cancer

Organ/Tissue	0	1	2	Grade 3	4	5
Skin	None	Slight atrophy; pigmentation change; some hair loss	Patchy atrophy; moderate telangiectasia; total hair loss	Marked atrophy; gross telangiectasia	Ulceration	Death directly related to late radiation effect in all Grade 5 cases
Subcutaneous tissue	None	Slight induration (fibrosis) and loss of subcutaneous fat	Moderate fibrosis but asymptomatic; slight field contracture; <10% linear reduction	Severe induration and loss of subcutaneous tissue; field contracture >10% linear measurement	Necrosis	
Mucous membrane	None	Slight atrophy and dryness	Moderate atrophy and telangiectasia; little mucus	Marked atrophy with complete dryness; severe telangiectasia	Ulceration	
Salivary glands	None	Slight dryness of mouth; good response on stimulation	Moderate dryness of mouth; poor response on stimulation	Complete dryness of mouth; no response on stimulation	Fibrosis	
Spinal cord	None	Mild L'hermitte's syndrome	Severe L'hermitte's syndrome	Objective neurological findings at or below cord level treated	Mono-, para-, or quadriplegia	
Brain	None	Mild headache; slight lethargy	Moderate headache; great lethargy	Severe headache; severe CNS dysfunction (partial loss of power or dyskinesia)	Seizures or paralysis; coma	
Eye	None	Asymptomatic cataract; minor corneal ulceration or keratitis	Symptomatic cataract; moderate corneal ulceration; minor retinopathy or glaucoma	Severe keratitis; severe retinopathy or detachment; severe glaucoma	Panophthalmitis; blindness	
Larynx	None	Hoarseness; slight arytenoid edema	Moderate arytenoid edema; chondritis	Severe edema; severe chondritis	Necrosis	

Continued

Table 1-6 Late Radiation Morbidity Scoring Criteria of the Radiation Therapy Oncology Group/European Organization for Research on Treatment of Cancer—cont'd

Organ/Tissue	Grade					
	0	1	2	3	4	5
Lung	None	Asymptomatic or mild symptoms (dry cough); slight radiographic appearances	Moderate symptomatic fibrosis or pneumonitis (severe cough); low-grade fever; patchy radiographic appearances	Severe symptomatic fibrosis or pneumonitis; dense radiographic changes	Severe respiratory insufficiency; continuous O_2; assisted ventilation	Death directly related to late radiation effect in all Grade 5 cases
Heart	None	Asymptomatic or mild symptoms; transient T-wave inversion and ST changes; sinus tachycardia >110 (at rest)	Moderate angina on effort; mild pericarditis; normal heart size; persistent abnormality T-wave and ST changes; low QRS	Severe angina; pericardial effusion; constrictive pericarditis; moderate heart failure; cardiac enlargement; ECG abnormalities	Tamponade; severe heart failure; severe constrictive pericarditis	
Esophagus	None	Mild fibrosis; slight difficulty in swallowing solids; no pain on swallowing	Unable to take solid food normally; swallowing semisolid food; dilatation may be indicated	Severe fibrosis; able to swallow only liquids; may have pain on swallowing; dilatation required	Necrosis; perforation; fistula	
Small/large intestine	None	Mild diarrhea; mild cramping; bowel movement 5 times daily; slight rectal discharge or bleeding	Moderate diarrhea and colic; bowel movement >5 times daily; excessive rectal mucus or intermittent bleeding	Obstruction or bleeding requiring surgery	Necrosis; perforation; fistula	
Liver	None	Mild lassitude; nausea and dyspepsia; slightly abnormal liver function	Moderate symptoms; some abnormal liver function tests; serum albumin normal	Disabling hepatitic insufficiency; liver function tests grossly abnormal; low albumin; edema or ascites	Necrosis; hepatic coma or encephalopathy	
Kidney	None	Transient albuminuria; no hypertension; mild impairment of renal function; urea 25–35 mg%; creatinine 1.5–2.0 mg%; creatinine clearance >75%	Persistent moderate albuminuria (2+); mild hypertension; no related anemia; moderate impairment of renal function; urea >36–60 mg%; creatinine clearance 50–74%	Severe albuminuria; severe hypertension; persistent anemia (<10 g%); severe renal failure; urea >60 mg%; creatinine >4.0 mg%; creatinine clearance <50%	Malignant hypertension; uremic coma; urea >100%	

	None				Death directly related to late radiation effect in all Grade 5 cases
Bladder	None	Slight epithelial atrophy; minor telangiectasia (microscopic hematuria)	Moderate frequency; generalized telangiectasia; intermittent macroscopic hematuria	Severe frequency and dysuria; severe generalized telangiectasia (often with petechiae); frequent hematuria; reduction in bladder capacity (<150 cc)	Necrosis; contracted bladder capacity (<100 cc); severe hemorrhagic cystitis
Bone	None	Asymptomatic; no growth retardation; reduced bone density	Moderate pain or tenderness; growth retardation; irregular bone sclerosis	Severe pain or tenderness; complete arrest of bone growth; dense bone sclerosis	Necrosis; spontaneous fracture
Joint	None	Mild joint stiffness; slight limitation of movement	Moderate stiffness; intermittent or moderate joint pain; moderate limitation of movement	Severe joint stiffness; pain with severe limitation of movement	Necrosis; complete fixation

From the Radiation Therapy Oncology Group (RTOG) and the European Organization for Research on Treatment of Cancer (EORTC).

research must address the testing of newer models of cancer care that promote integration rather than fragmentation, and the development of ways to educate patients and families about complex multimodal treatment. The role of the nurse in multimodal therapy within the framework of today's changes in health care is still to be defined. It will require up-to-date factual information about the totality of cancer-patient care and not just one aspect of treatment, as has been the tradition. It will require strong patient advocacy and much networking among the multiple nurses involved in the care of each patient.

❖ References

Adelstein DJ, Sharan VM, Damm C, Earle AS, Shah AC, Haria CD, Trey JE, Carter SG, and Hines JD: Concurrent radiation therapy, 5-fluorouracil and cisplatin for stage II, III, and IV, node-negative, squamous cell head and neck cancer, Cancer 70:2685–2690, 1992.

Baker SR, Makuch RW, and Wolf GT: Preoperative cisplatin and bleomycin therapy in head and neck squamous carcinoma, Arch Otolaryngol 107:683–689, 1981.

Baserga R: Principles of molecular cell biology of cancer: the cell cycle. In DeVita VT Jr, Hellman S, and Rosenberg SA, editors: Cancer: principles and practice of oncology, ed 4, Philadelphia, 1993, JB Lippincott Co, pp. 60–66.

Beahrs OH, Henson DE, Hutter RVP, and Kennedy BJ, editors: Manual for staging cancer, ed 4, Philadelphia, 1992, JB Lippincott Co.

Buchholz TA: Letter in response to Drs. Harris and Recht: Optimal sequencing of chemotherapy and radiation, Int J Radiation Oncol Biol Phys 26:189, 1993.

Chan A, Wong A, Langevin J, and Khoo R: Preoperative concurrent 5-fluorouracil infusion, mitomycin-C and pelvic radiation therapy in tethered and fixed rectal carcinoma, Int J Radiation Oncol Biol Phys 25:791–799, 1993.

Coia LR, Engstrom PF, Pau AR, Stafford PM, Hanks G: Long-term results of infusional 5-FU, mitomycin-C, and radiation as primary management of esophageal carcinoma, Int J Radiation Oncol Biol 20:29–36, 1991.

Coleman CN: Modification of radiotherapy by radiosensitizers and cancer chemotherapy agents. I. Radiosensitizers, Sem Oncol 16:169–175, 1989.

Cox JD: Clinical applications of new modalities. In Cox JD, editor: Moss' radiation oncology: rationale, technique, results, ed 7, St. Louis, 1994, Mosby, pp. 971–986.

Cummings BJ: Concomitant radiotherapy and chemotherapy for anal cancer, Sem Oncol 19(Suppl 11):102–108, 1992.

Demchak PA, Mier JW, Robert NJ, O'Brien K, Gould JA, and Atkins MB: Interleukin-2 and high-dose cisplatin in patients with metastatic melanoma: a pilot study, J Clin Oncol 9:1821–1830, 1991.

Department of Veterans Affairs Laryngeal Cancer Study Group: Induction chemotherapy plus radiation compared with surgery plus radiation in patients with advanced laryngeal cancer, N Eng J Med 324:1685–1690, 1991.

DeVita VT Jr: Principles of chemotherapy. In DeVita VT Jr, Hellman S, and Rosenberg SA: Cancer: principles and practice of oncology, ed 4, Philadelphia, 1993, JB Lippincott Co, pp. 276–292.

Dobelbower RR, Konski AA, Merrick HW III, Bronn DG, Schifeling D, and Kamen C: Intraoperative electron beam radiation therapy (IOEBRT) for carcinoma of the exocrine pancreas, Int J Radiation Oncol Biol Phys 20:113–119, 1991.

Eisenberger M and Jacobs M: Simultaneous treatment with single-agent chemotherapy and radiation for local advanced cancer of the head and neck, Sem Oncol 19(suppl 11):41–46, 1992.

Falkson CI, Falkson F, and Falkson HC: Improved results with the addition of interferon alfa-2b to dacarbazine in the treatment of patients with metastatic malignant melanoma, J Clin Oncol 9:1403–1408, 1991.

Fingert HJ, Campisi J, and Pardee AB: Cell proliferation and differention. In Holland JF, Frei E III, Bast RC Jr, Kufe DW, Morton DL, and Weichselbaum RR, editors: Cancer medicine, ed 3, Philadelphia, 1993, Lea & Febiger, pp. 1–14.

Fisher B, Wickerham DL, and Redmond C: Recent developments in the use of systemic adjuvant therapy for the treatment of breast cancer, Sem Oncol 19:263–277, 1992.

Forastiere AA: Treatment of locoregional esophageal cancer, Sem Oncol 19(suppl 11):57–63, 1992.

Fowler JF and Lindstrom MJ: Loss of local control with prolongation in radiotherapy, Int J Radiation Oncol Biol Phys 23:457–467, 1992.

Fu KK: Biological basis for the interaction of chemotherapeutic agents and radiation therapy, Cancer 55:2123–2130, 1985.

Fuchs CS and Mayer RJ: Adjuvant chemotherapy for colon and rectal cancer, Sem Radiation Oncol 13:29–41, 1993.

Ghim TT, Davis P, Seo J, Crock I, O'Brien M, and Krawiecki N: Response to neoadjuvant chemotherapy in children with pineoblastoma, Cancer 73:1795–1800, 1993.

Gilewski TA and Golomb HM: Design of combination biotherapy studies: future goals and challenges, Sem Oncol 17(suppl 1):3–10, 1990.

Goodman MS: Cancer: chemotherapy and care, ed 3, Princeton, NJ, 1992, Bristol-Myers Squibb Co.

Grem JL, Jordan E., Robson ME, Binder RA, Hamilton JM, Steinberg SM, Arbuck SG, Beveridge RA, Kales AN, Miller JA, Weiss RB, McAtee N, Chen A, Goldspiel B, Sover E, and Allegra DJ: Phase II study of fluorouracil, leucovorin, and interferon alfa-2a in metastatic colorectal carcinoma, J Clin Oncol 11:1737–1745, 1993.

Guyton AD: Textbook of medical physiology, ed 8, Philadelphia, 1991, WB Saunders Co.

Haffty BG, Wilmarth K, Wilson L, Fischer D, Beinfield M, and McKhann C: Adjuvant systemic chemotherapy and hormonal therapy, Cancer 73:2543–2548, 1994.

Hall EJ and Cox JD: Physical and biologic basis of radiation therapy. In Cox JD, editor: Moss' radiation oncology: rationale, techniques, results, ed 7, St. Louis, 1994, Mosby, pp. 3–66.

Harris DT and Mastrangelo MJ: Theory and application of early systemic therapy, Sem Oncol 18:493–503, 1991.

Hendry JH: Biological response modifiers and normal tissue injury after irradiation, Sem Rad Oncol 4:123–132, 1994.

Hong WK, Shapshay SM, Bhutani R, Craft ML, Ucmakli A, Yamaguchi KT, Vaughan CW, and Strong MS: Induction chemotherapy in advanced squamous head and neck carcinoma with high-dose cisplatinum and bleomycin infusion, Cancer 44:19–25, 1979.

Izquierdo MA, Marcuello E, deSegura GG, Blanco R, Canals E, Gomez A, and Sampedro F: Unresectable monmetastatic squamous cell carcinoma of the esophagus managed by sequential chemotherapy (cisplatin and bleomycin) and radiation therapy, Cancer 71:287–292, 1993.

John MJ: Grading of chemoradiation toxicity. In John MJ, Flam MS, Legha SS, and Phillips TL, editors: Chemoradiation: an integrated approach to cancer treatment, Philadelphia, 1993, Lea & Febiger, pp. 601–606.

Johnstone PAS, Sindelar WF, and Kinsella TJ: Experimental and clinical studies of intraoperative radiation therapy, Current problems in cancer 18:249–292, 1994.

Koops HS and Hoekstra HJ: Surgical prevention and treatment of late normal tissue injury, Sem Radiation Oncol 4:119–122, 1994.

Liotta LA and Stetler-Stevenson WG: Principles of molecular cell biology of cancer: cancer metastasis. In DeVita VT Jr, Hellman S, and Rosenberg SA, editors: Cancer: principles and practice of oncology, ed 4, Philadelphia, 1993, JB Lippincott Co, pp. 134–149.

Liotta LA, Stetler-Stevenson WG, and Steeg PS: Invasion and metastasis. In Holland JF, Frei E III, Bast RC Jr, Kufe DW, Morton DL, and Weichselbaum RR, editors: Cancer medicine, ed 3, Philadelphia, 1993, Lea & Febiger, pp. 138–153.

Lokich JJ: Combined modality chemoradiation therapy: state of the art. In Lokich JJ and Byfield JE, editors: Combined modality cancer therapy: radiation and infusional chemotherapy, 241–244, Chicago, 1991, Precept Press.

Mandard A, Dalibard F, Mandard J, Marnay J, Henry-Amar M, Petiot J, Roussel A, Jacob J, Segol P, Samama G, Ollivier J, Bonvalot S, and Gignoux M: Pathologic assessment of tumor regression after preoperative chemoradiotherapy of esophageal carcinoma, Cancer 73:2680–2686, 1994.

Minsky BD, Cohen AM, Kemeny N, Enker WE, Kelsen DP, Reichman B, Saltz L, Sigurdson ER, and Frankel J: Enhancement of radiation-induced downstaging of rectal cancer by fluorouracil and high-dose leukovoran chemotherapy, J Clin Oncol 10:79–84, 1992.

Minsky BD, Cohen AM, Kemeny N, Enker WE, Kelsen DP, Schwartz G, Saltz L, Dougherty J, Frankel J, and Wiseberg J: Pre-operative combined 5-FU, low dose leucovorin, and sequential radiation therapy for unresectable rectal cancer, Int J Radiation Oncol Biol Phys 25:821–827, 1993.

Moertel CG, Bunderson LL, Mailliard JA, McKenna PJ, Martenson JA Jr, Burch PA, and Cha SS: Early evaluation of combined fluorouracil and leucovorin as a radiation enhancer for locally unresectable, residual, or recurrent gastrointestinal carcinoma, J Clin Oncol 12:21–27, 1994.

Naunheim KS, Petruska PJ, Roy TS, Andrus CH, Johnson FE, Schlueter JM, and Baue AE: Preoperative chemotherapy and radiotherapy for esophageal carcinoma, J Thorac Cardiovasc Surg 103:887–895, 1992.

Norton L and Surbone A: Principles of chemotherapy: cytokinetics. In Holland JF, Frei E III, Bast RC Jr, Kufe DW, Morton DL, and Weichselbaum RR, editors: Cancer medicine, ed 3, Philadelphia, 1993, Lea & Febiger, pp. 598–617.

Pajak TF, Laramore GE, Marcial VA, Fazekas JT, Cooper J, Rubin P, Curran WJ Jr, and Davis LW: Elapsed treatment days—a critical item for radiotherapy quality control review in head and neck trials: RTOG report, Int J Radiation Oncol Biol Phys 20:13–20, 1991.

Perez CA and Brady LW: Overview. In Perez CA and Brady LW, editors: Principles and practice of radiation oncology, ed 2, Philadelphia, 1992, JB Lippincott Co, pp. 1–63.

Phillips TL: Tissue toxicity of radiation-drug interactions. In Sokol GH and Maickel RP, editors: Radiation drug interactions in the treatment of cancer, New York, 1980, John Wiley & Sons, Inc, pp. 175–200.

Phillips TL: Terminology for chemoradiation effects. In John MJ, Flam MS, Legha SS, and Phillips TL, editors: Chemoradiation: an integrated approach to cancer treatment, Philadelphia, 1993, Lea & Febiger, pp. 11–17.

Quiet C, Weichselbaum RR, and Gardina D: Variation in radiation sensitivity during the cell cycle of two human squamous cell carcinomas, Int J Radiation Oncol Biol Phys 20:733–738, 1991.

Richards JM, Mehta M, Ramming K, and Skosey P: Sequential chemoimmunotherapy in the treatment of metastatic melanoma, J Clin Oncol 10:1338–1343, 1992.

Rosai J: Principles of oncologic pathology. In DeVita VT Jr, Hellman S, and Rosenberg SA, editors: Cancer: principles and practice of oncology, ed 4, Philadelphia, 1993, JB Lippincott Co, pp. 228–237.

Rosenberg SA: Principles and applications of biology therapy. In DeVita VT Jr, Hellman S, and Rosenberg SA, editors: Cancer: principles and practice of oncology, ed 4, Philadelphia, 1993, JB Lippincott Co, pp. 293–324.

Rotman MZ: Chemoirradiation: a new initiative in cancer treatment, Radiology 184:319–327, 1992.

Sause WT: Principles of combining radiation therapy and surgery. In Cox JD, editor: Moss' radiation oncology: rationale, techniques, results, ed 7, St. Louis, 1994, Mosby, pp. 67–78.

Schaake-Konig C, Maat B, van Houtte P, van den Bogaert W, Dalesio O, Kirkpatrick A, and Bartelink H: Radiotherapy combined with low-dose cis-diammine dichloroplatinum (II) (CDDP) in inoperable nonmetastatic non-small cell lung cancer (NSCLC): a randomized three arm phase II study of the EORTC lung cancer and radiotherapy cooperative groups, Int J Radiation Oncol Biol Phys 19:967–972, 1990.

Schilsky RL: Biochemical pharmacology of chemotherapeutic drugs used as radiation enhancers, Sem Oncol 19(suppl 11):2–7, 1992.

Scofield RP, Liebman MC, and Popkin JD: Multimodal therapy. In Baird SB, McCorkle R, and Grant M, editors: Cancer nursing: a comprehensive textbook, Philadelphia, 1991, WB Saunders Co, pp. 344–354.

Solol-Celigny P, Lepage E, Brousse N, Reyes F, Haioun C, Leporrier M, Peuchmaur M, Bosly A, Parlier Y, Brice P, Coiffier B, Gisselbrecht, C: Recombinant interferon alfa-2b combined with a regimen containing doxorubicin in patients with advanced follicular lymphoma, N Eng J Med 329:1608–1614, 1993.

Steele GG and Peckham MJ: Exploitable mechanisms in combined radiotherapy-chemotherapy: the concept of additivity, Int J Radiation Oncol Biol Phys 5:85–91, 1979.

Stevens KR Jr: The colon and rectum. In Cox JD, editor: Moss' radiation oncology: rationale, techniques, results, ed 7, St. Louis, 1994, Mosby, pp. 462–486.

Sznol M and Longo DL: Chemotherapy drug interactions with biological agents, Sem Oncol 20:80–93, 1993.

Taylor SG IV, Murthy AK, Vannetzel JM, Colin P, Dray M, Caldarelli DD, Shott S, Vokes E, Showel JL, Hutchinson JC, Witt TR, Griem KL, Hartsell WF, Kies MS, Mittal B, Rebischung JL, Coupez DJ, Desphiwux JL, Bobin S, and LePajolec C: Randomized comparison of neoadjuvant cisplatin and fluorouracil infusion followed by radiation versus concomitant treatment in advanced head and neck cancer, J Clin Oncol 12:385–395, 1994.

Tepper JE and Calvo FA: Intraoperative radiation therapy. In Perez CA and Brady LW, editors: Principles and Practice of Radiation Oncology, ed 2, Philadelphia, 1992, JB Lippincott Co, pp. 388–395.

Townsend CM Jr, Abston S, and Fish JD: Surgical adjuvant treatment of locally advanced breast cancer, Ann Surg 201:604–610, 1985.

Tupchong L, Scott CB, Blitzer PH, Marcial VA, Lowry LD, Jacobs JR, Stetz J, Davis LW, Snow JB, Chandler R, Kramer S, and Pajak TF: Randomized study of preoperative versus postoperative radiation therapy in advanced head and neck carcinoma: long-term follow-up of RTOG 73–03, Int J Radiation Oncol Biol Phys 20:21–28, 1991.

Turrisi AT III, Glover DJ, and Mason BA: A preliminary report: concurrent twice-daily radiotherapy plus platinum-etoposide chemotherapy for limited small cell lung cancer, Int J Radiation Oncology Biol Phys 15:183–187, 1988.

Vokes EE and Weichselbaum RR: Experimental basis for radiation and chemotherapy. In Lokich JJ and Byfield JE, editors: Combined modality cancer therapy: radiation and infusional chemotherapy, Chicago, 1991, Precept Press, pp. 1–14.

Wadler S: Antineoplastic activity of the combination of 5-fluorouracil and interferon: preclinical and clinical results, Sem Oncol 19(suppl 4):38–40, 1992.

Weichselbaum RR, Beckett MA, Hallahan DE, Kufe DW, and Vokes EE: Molecular targets to overcome radioresistance, Sem Oncol 19(suppl 11):14–20, 1992.

Willett CG, Tepper JE, Kaufman DS, and Shellito PC: Adjuvant postoperative radiation therapy for colonic carcinoma, Sem Radiation Oncol 3:64–67, 1993.

Yeung RS, Weese JL, Hoffman JP, Solin LJ, Paul AR, Engstrom PF, Litwin S, Kowalyshyn MJ, and Eisenberg BL: Neoadjuvant chemoradiation in pancreatic and duodenal carcinoma, Cancer 72:2124–2133, 1993.

Zerbi A, Fossati V, Parolini D, Carlucci M, Balzano G, Bordogna G, Staudacher C, and DiCarlo V: Intraoperative radiation therapy adjuvant to resection in the treatment of pancreatic cancer, Cancer 73:2930–2935, 1994.

Chapter 2

❖ *Surgery*

Catherine C. Burke

❖ *Role of Surgical Procedures in Cancer*

In cancer treatment, diagnosis, staging, treatment, and symptom relief involve the use of surgical procedures. New technologies, such as laser therapy, cryotherapy, ultrasonic aspiration, and multimodal treatment, have allowed for less radical surgery. Approximately 70% of patients will have micrometastases beyond the primary site at diagnosis. This requires interdisciplinary collaboration and treatment planning tailored to the individual patient. Multimodal treatment improves cure rates for patients who would otherwise fail if treated by surgery alone.

Diagnosis

Diagnosis requires the pathologic examination of a tissue sample. Originally, biopsy for diagnosis involved removing a portion of tumor that was then processed to obtain a histologic diagnosis. However, with the advent of reliable and accurate cytological techniques, many tumors can now be identified by examining cellular materials obtained from needle aspirations, effusions, or washes from body cavities (Hindle, Payne, and Pan, 1993; Staerkel, 1993; Westcott, 1980).

The surgeon selects the biopsy technique most appropriate in each clinical setting by considering the site to be biopsied, the size of the tumor, the suspected diagnosis, and the patient's physical status. In general, for an initial diagnosis, the simplest procedure that provides a tissue sample adequate for analysis is selected. Tumors arising on or near the body surface that are easily visualized or palpated can be biopsied directly by incisional, excisional, or needle biopsy. An *incisional biopsy* involves removing a piece of tumor from a larger mass. An *excisional biopsy* involves complete tumor removal, and in some situations it may be all the surgery needed for treatment. However, wide excision margins are not normally used for the biopsy, and a repeat resection may be necessary after the diagnosis is made.

Two needle biopsy techniques are available for sampling palpable tumors near the skin surface. *Fine-needle aspiration* (FNA) involves placing a small-gauge needle into the tumor mass and removing cellular material by suctioning it into a syringe. Repeating the process multiple times ensures that the sample is representative of all cells. Although an aspiration biopsy with positive results is diagnostic, a negative result does not necessarily rule out cancer, because FNA may sometimes miss malignant cells. If a clinician strongly suspects malignancy, alternate diagnostic approaches must be considered.

Many tumors are identified by imaging studies (e.g., computerized axial tomography [CT] scanning, magnetic resonance imaging [MRI], and ultrasound) and are located in deep organ sites that can be diagnosed only by deep biopsy techniques. A recent refinement of directed FNA is the stereotactic biopsy, which three-dimensional imaging directs precise placement of the biopsy needle (Ranjan et al., 1993; Schmidt, 1994).

Core needle biopsy involves inserting a specialized large-gauge needle into the tumor mass. This provides a tissue specimen whose cellular architecture is not disrupted; consequently, a histologic sample is possible.

Fiberoptic biopsy is used for sampling intraluminal tumors of the respiratory, genitourinary, and gastrointestinal tracts. A flexible fiberoptic scope enables the clinician to view the tumor; specialized instruments are then passed through a channel to obtain a tissue biopsy while the patient is under intravenous sedation. Fiberoptic biopsy (e.g., endoscopy and bronchoscopy) is the diagnostic method of choice for cancers of the bladder, stomach, colon, and lungs (Sugarbaker and Roth, 1989).

When tissue samples from a tumor in a body cavity are required, *open biopsy,* a major surgical procedure usually performed under general anesthesia, is performed. Previously, diagnostic thoracotomy and laparotomy were commonly used; however, open biopsies are necessary now only in rare situations. Minimally invasive procedures, such as laparoscopy and thoracoscopy, can provide information equivalent to that of open biopsy in most cases. A rigid fiberoptic scope is introduced into the body cavity through a small incision. Additional instruments are inserted through separate punctures to permit examination of organs and to obtain biopsy materials.

Staging

If a cancer diagnosis is confirmed, the disease must be staged. While some cancers are clinically staged by noninvasive diagnostic modalities, many must be staged by *pathologic staging,* an operative procedure that provides more accurate information. Components of pathologic staging are specified by the type of cancer and the tumor site. During the surgical procedure the areas of disease spread are evaluated.

Many surgical staging procedures assess the abdominal (peritoneal) cavity because tumors and their metastases are inaccessible and difficult to evaluate by other means. Such tumors are usually accessed by a general staging laparotomy. This procedure begins with a large vertical incision that provides access to the entire peritoneal cavity. One or more saline washes for cytologic analysis are taken before exploration. These washes provide cellular samples from a large surface area and are useful in detecting microscopic, serosal, and peritoneal metastases. Next, the abdominal organs and peritoneal surfaces are systematically examined for visual and palpable abnormalities. A biopsy is performed on all suspicious areas. Finally, retroperitoneal lymph nodes in the drainage routes of the primary tumor are exposed and a biopsy performed. Examples of surgically staged cancers include cancers of the lymph nodes, testicles, endometrium, and ovaries.

An alternative to laparotomy is a minimally invasive surgical procedure such as laparoscopy. Laparoscopy allows assessment of the peritoneal cavity but makes accurate lymph node evaluation technically difficult. However, for pancreatic and gastric cancers, laparoscopy has been successfully used to evaluate resectability. Staging by laparoscopy also avoids the morbidity of laparotomy in patients with unresectable disease (Greene and Dorsey, 1993). Second-look operations are sometimes undertaken after primary therapy to measure tumor response, such as in ovarian cancer. The second-look surgical technique is identical to that for laparotomy (Barnhill et al., 1984; Podratz et al., 1989).

For some malignancies such as melanoma, breast cancer, and vulvar cancer, a biopsy of regional lymph nodes may be combined with a primary tumor resection. Excision of the regional lymph nodes is technically a staging procedure, because nodal status affects subsequent therapeutic decisions.

Primary Treatment

The goal of primary curative resection is the complete removal of the tumor with an adequate margin of normal tissue. The extent of primary resection varies greatly. A small superficial melanoma can be curatively excised by removing the lesion and a 2-cm margin of skin in an outpatient setting. In contrast, a radical hysterectomy involves removing the uterus and its supporting ligaments with the pelvic lymph nodes and upper vagina and requires a hospital stay.

Much of the current focus in surgery is on expanding the impact of primary resection while maintaining cosmetic appearance and functional integrity. Most of these efforts involve combining surgery with radiation therapy and/or chemotherapy. Concepts under investigation include: (1) preoperative therapy aimed at shrinking large tumors and making surgical excision possible or simpler; (2) intraoperative therapy aimed at reducing the incidence of local recurrence; and (3) postoperative treatment aimed at reducing the need for radical resections.

Cytoreductive Surgery

Cytoreductive surgery, or debulking, refers to the removal of as much tumor as possible when complete excision is clearly impossible. Major cytoreductive procedures are limited to patients who can physically tolerate an extensive procedure and whose survival would benefit from tumor removal. In most current clinical settings, cytoreductive operations are attempted in patients with bulky primary tumors and substantial regional spread.

Cytoreduction has been widely applied in women with advanced ovarian cancer. Numerous studies document enhanced survival for women with small-volume tumors after primary cytoreduction, with approximately 75% of tumors responding to postoperative platinum-based chemotherapy (Griffiths, Parker, and

Fuller, 1979). Cytoreductive surgery also provides a survival benefit in patients with lymphoma, testicular germ-cell tumor, neuroblastoma, and rhabdomyosarcoma (Silberman, 1982; Wong and Decosse, 1990).

Ablative Techniques

Several advanced technologies designed to ablate, or destroy, tumor masses can be used alone or in conjunction with exploratory surgery. Ablative techniques currently in use include laser therapy, cryotherapy, and ultrasonic surgical aspiration. In most cases these techniques are used in situations where classical resection is not feasible. Many of these applications are currently experimental or palliative.

Lasers generate a high-energy light beam that can be focused on specific tissues and that causes destruction from the tissue's absorption of the light energy. Three types of lasers are in clinical use: the carbon dioxide (CO_2) laser, the argon laser, and the neodymium YAG laser (Dixon, 1988; Lehr, 1989). The CO_2 laser is best suited for vaporization of tissue and is particularly useful in vaporizing surface lesions of the head, neck, and genital tracts. Laser vaporization permits precise removal of tissue with minimal blood loss and rapid healing. The argon laser is best suited for vascular lesions in which minimal penetration is desirable. Most applications are for palliative control of bleeding. On the other hand, the neodymium YAG laser can penetrate more deeply. It is used primarily for palliative control of bleeding and relief of obstruction in gastrointestinal lesions.

Cryotherapy involves operative placement of a probe within a tumor mass followed by the circulation of a refrigerant to cause freezing and necrosis of adjacent tissue. The extent of necrosis depends on how long the freezing lasts, with the best results achieved using a freeze-thaw-refreeze technique. For example, cryoprobes may be used to cause necroses in unresectable hepatic tumors (Ravikumar et al., 1991).

Ultrasonic aspiration is sometimes used as an adjunct to cytoreductive surgery. A specialized probe emits high-frequency ultrasonic vibrations that fragment the tumor while leaving vascular structures intact. It is most commonly used to remove tumor tissue from intraabdominal organs and surfaces (Deppe et al., 1989).

Reconstruction

Only recently have plastic surgery and reconstructive procedures been offered to cancer patients in conjunction with radical resections. The previous focus of surgical therapy was on curing the cancer, with less concern for cosmetic and functional outcome. Even in settings where reconstruction was possible, patients were encouraged to wait until they were free of disease for a specified period before undergoing a reconstructive procedure.

Today reconstruction is an integral part of primary treatment planning, due to increased long-term survival, development and refinement of plastic surgery techniques, greater focus on quality-of-life issues, and patient interest. The reconstructive surgeon participates in a multidisciplinary preoperative evaluation to select the most appropriate reconstructive procedure and to ensure that primary resection will facilitate reconstruction. For example, selection criteria for immediate breast reconstruction include psychologic suitability and motivation; oncologic considerations such as tumor size, location, and status of the regional lymph nodes and the opposite breast; the need for adjuvant therapy; and the probability of an acceptable cosmetic result (Bostwick, 1990). Equally important is the fact that many primary resections cannot be attempted without simultaneous reconstruction to maintain anatomic integrity and function. The end result is that a patient with a mastectomy can have a cosmetically acceptable breast (Figure 2-1), the patient with oral cancer can eat, and a patient with pelvic cancer can function sexually. These outcomes may be as important to patients as the curative resection of their tumors.

Palliation

Surgical procedures designed to relieve suffering, to minimize symptoms, or to improve the patient's quality of life are termed *palliative*. It is important that the patient and family have a clear understanding of what the procedure is designed to accomplish and that they have realistic expectations of the anticipated outcome. Palliative operations should be considered only if the patient's symptoms cannot be relieved by more conservative means. For example, surgical relief of bowel obstruction may prevent a morbid terminal phase of disease and allow the patient to return

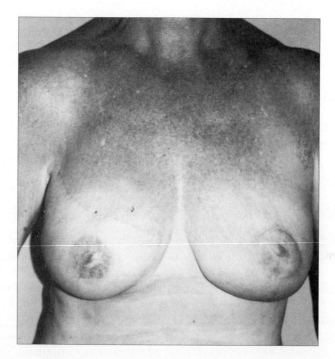

Fig. 2-1.   Photograph of breast reconstruction performed in conjunction with mastectomy. Reconstruction is considered an integral part of primary cancer treatment.

to home care. Overall life expectancy is also an important consideration. For example, subjecting a patient with limited life expectancy to a relatively minor procedure to relieve intractable pain is quite reasonable. However, subjecting the same patient to a major operation and recovery merely prolongs life without providing a tangible benefit.

A wide range of surgical procedures such as operations to relieve pain, restore function, and prevent impairment of organ function from denervation can be considered palliative (Dyck, 1991; Held and Peahota, 1993). For instance, excision of an isolated tumor mass causing nerve compression can dramatically reduce pain and maintain the function of the entrapped nerve. Bowel obstructions may be decompressed by resection, diversion to an ostomy, or placement of a drainage tube (gastrostomy). Fistulas require operative resection or bypass proximal to the fistula tract. In selected patients, a surgically placed feeding tube or a central venous catheter may be used to provide nutritional support or pain medications.

❖ Factors Influencing Treatment

A key principle of cancer therapy is that the first treatment has the best chance of success. Thus multidisciplinary planning is necessary to ensure that the chance for cure is not compromised. Surgery as a treatment option is influenced by three factors: (1) tumor characteristics, (2) tumor location, and (3) host characteristics.

The use of surgery as a therapeutic option depends on the tumor's growth rate, invasiveness, and metastatic potential. In general, slow-growing tumors with prolonged cell cycles are more amenable to surgical resection because they tend to be locally or regionally confined. Examples of slow-growing tumors include sarcomas, basal and squamous cell skin cancers, and tumors of the colon and rectum.

The invasive pattern of the tumor must also be considered. To achieve a curative surgical resection, the entire tumor, along with a margin of normal tissue, must be removed. Many cancers have a predictable pattern of local spread, which must be assessed before attempting a resection. Surgical resection of tumors with extensive local spread is technically difficult and not always possible. The use of other therapies, such as chemotherapy and radiation therapy, may justify less radical or incomplete resections. Using these additional therapies before or after surgery, may reduce tumor bulk and control micrometastases, thus allowing cure by a less radical surgical procedure.

The metastatic potential of the tumor must also be evaluated with consideration of the timing and location of metastases. Tumors that metastasize early or that have a propensity to spread to distant sites are generally not amenable to a curative surgical resection. Some tumors, however, do not readily metastasize or metastasize late in the course of the disease, leaving curative surgery as a viable option. A thorough search for metastases should be performed before any mode of treatment is recommended. For some cancers, such as lung or stomach cancers, the presence of metastatic disease may eliminate surgery as a treatment option. For other tumors, such as breast or colon cancers, surgery may provide local disease control despite the presence of metastatic disease. For example, removal of a primary breast tumor prevents skin ulcerations and breakdown; systemic therapy can be given to treat distant disease. Similarly, excision of a primary colon cancer, while not curative, decreases the probability of bleeding and colonic obstruction.

Another major factor in determining operative status is the tumor site. To be resectable, the tumor must be anatomically accessible. Resection of tumors that encase major blood vessels or that involve vital structures is not technically feasible. Tumor location becomes an issue when the organ of origin is difficult to approach or when extensive local growth has occurred. An example is pancreatic cancer. Anatomically, the pancreas is surrounded by the duodenum, stomach, biliary ducts, gallbladder, spleen, lymph nodes, and major vascular structures (the hepatic and superior mesenteric arteries and the portal and superior mesenteric veins). Because of these close anatomic relationships, local tumor infiltration rapidly involves one or more unresectable structures, which limits the feasibility of surgery. Current efforts to enhance resectability using preoperative concomitant chemotherapy and radiation therapy may ultimately expand the role of surgery in this disease (Warshaw and Castillo, 1992).

The patient's ability to withstand the proposed operation must be evaluated. Determinants of operative risk include age (older than 65), current health status (a history of smoking, obesity, immunosuppression, malnutrition, a large tumor burden, or previous chemotherapy), the presence and severity of concomitant illnesses, and the extent of the proposed surgery. Many patients diagnosed with cancer are over age 65 (Dellefield, 1986). Although advanced age is not a contraindication to surgery, older people are more likely to have other medical conditions and less physiologic reserve than younger people (Derby, 1991; Patterson, 1989).

All patients require a thorough preoperative evaluation focusing on the status of the patient's major organ systems (Polomano, Weintraub, and Wurster, 1994). The extent of preoperative laboratory and diagnostic testing required for risk evaluation is dictated by the findings of the medical history and physical examination (Ewer and Ali, 1990). Healthy patients with a medical history clear of chronic disease and a normal physical examination require minimal preoperative testing. In contrast, a patient with an existing chronic illness requires more detailed testing (e.g., arterial blood gases, spirometry, echocardiogram) to evaluate organ function and to estimate surgical risk.

Operative risk may be reduced by controlling or correcting physiologic abnormalities by appropriate medical management before surgery. Examples include correction of fluid and electrolyte imbalances, control of hyperglycemia and hypertension, and reversal of malnutrition. Ultimately the decision to perform surgery must weigh the estimated risks to the patient against the proposed advantages. When the risk/benefit ratio is too high, alternate treatment options should be considered.

❖ Nursing Considerations

Many aspects of nursing care for the patient undergoing oncology surgery are identical to those associated with routine preoperative care for any patient undergoing surgery. Surgical procedures in the patient with cancer tend to be complex and may produce major physiologic alterations that require the patient or caregiver to perform new tasks and to develop problem-solving skills. Examples include administering nutritional supplements, giving injections, and caring for wounds or drains. There is also a trend to reduce each patient's length of hospital stay. Not only are major postoperative stays shorter but many procedures that previously required hospitalization (e.g., mastectomy, lymph node biopsy, simple hysterectomy) are now performed in an outpatient setting (Burke, Zabka, and McCarver, 1995). To accomplish their patient-education and patient-care goals, the multidisciplinary team must plan carefully for successful implementation.

Preoperative Preparation

After the decision to proceed with surgery is made, the patient's physical and psychosocial needs are assessed in detail. This nursing assessment begins with an evaluation of general health status and should include information about concomitant disease and existing organ impairment. Special attention should be directed toward factors most likely to influence the course of surgery and recovery in an adverse way. Wound healing is impaired by factors such as diabetes, obesity, malnutrition, previous radiation therapy to the surgical field, cardiovascular disease, and recent treatment with cytotoxic drugs or steroids (Barber and Brown, 1993; Erlichman et al., 1991; Falcone and Nappi, 1984). The pulmonary complications of general anesthesia increase in patients with chronic lung disease and previous chest radiation or bleomycin therapy. Cardiac reserve may be diminished in patients with coronary artery disease, congestive heart failure, valvular problems, or prior anthracycline-based chemotherapy. The risks of perioperative infections are higher in patients who have immunosuppression as a result of previous treatment, malnutrition, advanced age, or the tumor itself.

The preoperative assessment must also consider the severity of the cancer and the extent of the planned operation. These features tend to be complementary in that patients with large tumors require more extensive operations.

Basic Postoperative Care

The goal of postoperative nursing care is to provide the physical and psychosocial support necessary to restore the patient to optimal functioning. Care focuses on monitoring vital functions, maintaining tubes and drains, providing pain control, reestablishing nutritional balance, and preventing surgical complications. Meticulous postoperative care is particularly important for the cancer patient who may be at greater risk for surgical problems as a result of immunosuppression, prior treatment, organ dysfunction, or an extensive surgical procedure. Table 2-1 lists potential postoperative complications.

Discharge Planning

Most patients will not have recovered from surgery completely at the time of hospital discharge. With today's emphasis on shortening the length of the hospital stay,

Table 2-1   **Potential Postoperative Complications**

Cardiovascular	*Pulmonary*	*Surgical*
Pulmonary edema; congestive failure	Pneumonia	Infection; abscess
Myocardial infarction	Atelectasis	Ileus; obstruction
Thromboembolism	Pulmonary embolism	Bleeding; hematoma
Arrhythmia	Pleural effusion	Wound separation; dehiscence
Coagulopathy	Pneumothorax	Pressure injuries
	Adult Respiratory Distress Syndrome (ARDS)	Malnutrition

more care must be provided outside of the acute-care setting. The goal of discharge planning is to assess and coordinate resources so that patient care is not compromised during this transition. Ideally, discharge planning begins before the operation. Assessment should address the following questions: (1) Who is the primary caregiver? (2) What are the patient-care needs? (3) Is the caregiver capable of providing the patient-care needs? (4) Does the caregiver need special training or home-care resources (e.g., a Visiting Nurse Association)? (5) How will discharge resources be provided?

After development of the discharge plan, nursing care is coordinated to ensure its implementation. Most patients require limited teaching and have adequate resources for home care. In these situations, the primary nurse can successfully accomplish the discharge planning. However, for patients with complicated discharge needs, a nurse specialized in discharge planning may be consulted. When a workable plan is not feasible because of excessive care requirements or inadequate resources, an extended-care facility should be considered. Finally, the surgical nurse should coordinate the follow-up and subsequent referral for further treatment when multimodal therapy is planned. When no further therapy is needed, the patient is referred to the primary physician for long-term follow-up.

❖ Summary

Surgery at one time was the primary modality for cancer treatment. Today an understanding of tumor biology and metastasis patterns, coupled with effective surgery, radiotherapy, chemotherapy, and biotherapy, form the basis of current oncologic practice. Multimodal therapy has improved cure rates with the use of less radical surgeries, which ultimately improve patients' quality of life. Successful implementation of the multidisciplinary team plan of care requires the combined efforts of the inpatient nurse, the clinic nurse, and the home health care nurse to promote continuity of care to the patient recovering from oncology surgery. Because surgery is no longer the only treatment for the majority of patients with cancer, the nurse must understand the complete treatment plan. This knowledge can be used to minimize postoperative complications and to avoid treatment delays.

❖ *References*

Barber GR and Brown AE: Surveillance of surgical wound infections in cancer patients, Canc Prac 1:72–76, 1993.

Barnhill DR, Hoskins WJ, Heller PB, and Park RC: The second-look surgical reassessment for epithelial ovarian carcinoma, Gynecol Oncol 19:148–154, 1984.

Bostwick J III: Plastic reconstructive breast surgery, St. Louis, 1990, Quality Medical Publishing, Inc, pp. 967–969.

Burke CC, Zabka CL, and McCarver K: Patients respond positively to nurse-initiated short-stay program following breast cancer surgery, Oncol Nurs Forum 22:148–149, 1995.

Dellefield ME: Caring for the elderly patient with cancer, Oncol Nurs Forum 13(3):19–27, 1986.

Deppe G, Malviya VK, Boike G, and Malone JM Jr: Use of cavitron surgical aspirator for debulking of diaphragmatic metastasis in patients with advanced carcinoma of the ovaries, Surg Gynecol Obstet 168:455–456, 1989.

Derby SE: Ageism in cancer care of the elderly, Oncol Nurs Forum 18:921–926, 1991.

Dixon JA: Current laser applications in general surgery, Ann Surg 207:355–370, 1988.

Dyck S: Surgical instrumentation as a palliative treatment for spinal cord compression, Oncol Nurs Forum 18:515–521, 1991.

Ehrlichman RJ, Seckel BR, Bryan DJ, and Moschella CJ: Common complications of wound healing, Surg Clin North Am 71:1323–1348, 1991.

Ewer MS and Ali MS: Surgical treatment of the cancer patient: preoperative assessment and perioperative medical management, J Surg Oncol 44:185–190, 1990.

Falcone RE and Nappi JF: Chemotherapy and wound healing, Surg Clin North Am 64:779–790, 1984.

Greene FL and Dorsey D: Laparoscopic evaluation of abdominal malignancy, Canc Prac 1:29–34, 1993.

Griffiths CT, Parker LM, and Fuller AF Jr: Role of cytoreductive surgical treatment in the management of advanced ovarian cancer, Cancer Treatment Rep 63:235–240, 1979.

Held JL and Peahota A: Nursing care of the patient with spinal cord compression, Oncol Nurs Forum 20:1507–1514, 1993.

Hindle WH, Payne PA, and Pan EY: The use of fine-needle aspiration in the evaluation of persistent palpable dominant breast masses, Amer J Obstet Gynecol 168:1814–1819, 1993.

Lehr PS: Surgical lasers: how they work, current applications, AORN J 50:972–977, 1989.

Patterson WB: Surgical issues in geriatric oncology, Semin Oncol 16:57–65, 1989.

Podratz KC, Malkasian GD, Hilton JF, Harris EA, and Gaffey TA: Second-look laparotomy in ovarian cancer: evaluation of pathologic variables, Amer J Obstet Gynecol 152:230–238, 1989.

Polomano R, Weintraub FN, and Wurster A: Critical surgical care for cancer patients, Semin Oncol Nurs 10:165–176, 1994.

Ranjan A, Rajshekhar V, Joseph T, Chandy MJ, and Chandi SM: Nondiagnostic CT-guided stereotactic biopsies in a series of 407 cases: influence of CT morphology and operator experience, J Neurosurg 79:839–844, 1993.

Ravikumar TS, Kane R, Cady B, Jenkins R, Clouse M, and Steele G Jr: A 5-year study of cryosurgery in the treatment of liver tumors, Arch Surg 126:1520–1524, 1991.

Schmidt RA: Stereotactic breast biopsy, CA 44:172–191, 1994.

Silberman AW: Surgical debulking of tumors, Surg Gynecol Obstet 155:577–584, 1982.

Staerkel GA: Fine-needle aspiration: technique and application in the evaluation of malignancies, Cancer Bull 46(1):8–12, 1993.

Sugarbaker PH and Roth JA: Specialized techniques of cancer management: endoscopy. In DeVita VT, Hellman S, and Rosenberg SA, editors: Cancer: principles and practice of oncology, ed 3, Philadelphia, 1989, JB Lippincott Co, pp. 423–438.

Warshaw AL and Castillo CF: Pancreatic carcinoma, N Eng J Med 326:455–465, 1992.

Westcott JL: Direct percutaneous needle aspiration of localized pulmonary lesions: results in 422 patients, Radiology 137:31–35, 1980.

Wong RJ and DeCosse JJ: Cytoreductive surgery, Surg Gynecol Obstet 170:276–281, 1990.

Chapter *3*

❖ *Radiation Therapy*

Susan Weiss Behrend
Anne T. Slivjak

Radiation therapy is the treatment of cancer with ionizing radiation. It is a local-regional therapeutic method that utilizes high-energy rays to target tumors located in a variety of anatomic areas, which can achieve the goals of cure, control, or palliation of many types of cancer. Radiation is administered as a primary treatment for cancer and in combination with other treatments. The sequencing of radiation treatments depends on the tumor type, the anatomic location, and the availability of other treatment options. The mechanism of action of radiation therapy is based on the disciplines of physics and biology. The intermeshing of these sciences provides the basis for both theoretical and clinical practice.

❖ *Physics of Radiation Oncology*

Electromagnetic Radiation

The two major sources of radiation are electromagnetic and particulate. Electromagnetic energy is characterized by vibrations of electric and magnetic energy in space called electromagnetic waves (Hilderley, 1992a). There is an inverse relationship between wavelength and energy; that is, the shorter the wavelength, the greater the energy. This concept is explained by the fact that as an electromagnetic beam travels farther from its source, a broader area of spread occurs (Hilderley, 1992a). Infrared (heat) waves are long in length, ultraviolet rays (sun) are short, and visible light rays lie in between (Yasko, 1982). X rays and gamma rays are short, high-energy rays that can produce cellular ionization. The electromagnetic energy spectrum ranges from low-energy radio waves of long wavelength and low frequency to high-energy ionizing radiation of short wavelength and high frequency (Coia and Moylan, 1994).

Ionizing radiation is electromagnetic energy of short wavelength and high energy. X rays and gamma rays are the most widely used types of ionizing radiation. They differ only in the way they are produced (Coia and Moylan, 1994; Hall, 1994). X rays are produced from electrical sources in machines and, when generated by megavoltage machines, are often referred to as photons. *Photons* have been defined as packets of energy. The absorption of X rays in living material causes energy to be deposited unevenly in packets that can break chemical bonds and initiate biological change. X-ray potency is a function of the size of the energy packets and not of the total energy absorbed (Hall, 1994). Gamma rays are spontaneously emitted by radioactive isotopes (atoms of an element that have different numbers of neutrons and hence different masses) when an unstable nucleus gives off excess energy as the atom decays over time to a more stable form (Coia and Moylan, 1994; Hall, 1994).

Particulate Radiation

All matter is comprised of atoms, which combine to form molecules. Atoms are comprised of various particles that are sometimes emitted as radiation. The nucleus of the atom has protons, which are positively charged, and neutrons, which lack any charge. Negatively charged electrons orbit the nucleus, and there is always an equal number of electrons and protons, yielding a net atomic charge of 0.

If an atom has a charge other than 0, it is an *ion*. To free an electron from its orbital location around the nucleus, energy is supplied to overcome the attraction that binds the electron to its orbit. As the electron leaves the orbit, the atomic charge changes, and ionization occurs. When an electron is stripped from an atom, the free electron has a charge of -1 and the remaining ion has a charge of $+1$; this is identified as a ion pair (Yasko, 1982).

Throughout the process of nuclear emission, natural and artificial radioisotopes emit two types of particulate radiation: alpha radiation, which is the helium nucleus, and beta radiation, which is an electron equivalent. In addition, gamma radiation, which is electromagnetic, is emitted. The ability of each type of radiation to penetrate depends on the propulsion force as well as the depth of the target substance. Alpha radiation has poor penetration properties and a rapid energy loss. Beta radiation has deeper penetrating abilities and is used in *brachytherapy*, a type of radiation where the source is placed within the body or body cavity. Gamma radiation has great range and penetration and is used in external-beam-radiation treatment.

❖ Biological Effects of Radiation

The biological effects of radiation are responsible for the therapeutic outcome: tumor cells killed, cessation of further malignant growth, and sparing normal tissue in the host. *Radiobiology* is the study of the action of ionizing radiation on living tissue, in terms of its physical, chemical, and biological effects (Hall, 1994).

Cellular Response to Radiation

The mitosis phase of the cell cycle is the phase most sensitive to the biological damage of radiation (see Chapter 1, Overview of Cancer and Multimodal Therapy).

DNA (deoxyribonucleic acid) is the principal structure damaged by radiation treatment. This may occur through direct or indirect cellular action. Direct action occurs when radiation particles are absorbed into the cells, causing damage to the DNA helix by creating breaks in the crosslinked base pairs, damage to the nitrogenous bases, and breaks in the hydrogen ion bonds (Hall, 1994; Hilderley, 1992a).

Indirect action occurs when radiation particles interact with components surrounding the cell (commonly water) to produce free radicals that diffuse and damage critical cellular components (Hall, 1994). A free radical is a free atom carrying an unpaired electron. In their orbitals, electrons typically are paired; this provides a stable environment. However, an unpaired electron is associated with chemical reactivity (Hall, 1994). This chemical process is complex, because the ionization of water by radiation occurs in the extracellular compartment. Ionization of water can trigger many reactions capable of causing significant cellular destruction and death (Hilderley, 1992a).

Tissue and Organ Response to Radiation

Tissues are made up of the following two distinct systems: nonrenewable and renewable. Nonrenewable tissue systems are comprised of cells that are nondividing and have a slow generation time. These cells are found in muscles, tendons, and nerves. The response to radiation by these tissues is weak and is characterized by capillary destruction, edema, and inflammation. The nonrenewable tissue is identified as radioresistant (Coia and Moylan, 1994).

Renewable tissue systems are characterized by fast cell turnover and high proliferation rates. These tissues are sensitive to radiation and include bone marrow and epithelial cells lining the gastrointestinal and genitourinary tracts, the gonads, and hair follicles. Exposing these tissues to radiation causes the release of toxic waste products with concomitant edema, cell sloughing, and ulceration. This process is responsible for many generalized radiation-induced side effects. The ability of these tissues to heal is due to the rapid rate of new cell production and tissue formation (Coia and Moylan, 1994).

Tissue response to radiation has been divided into phases. The early/acute phase occurs within the first 6 months of treatment; the subacute phase occurs 6 months to 1 year after treatment; and the late phase occurs several months or more after completion of radiation treatment. Not all early reactions result in a late effect, and not all late effects are preceded by early reactions. In addition, the severity of late reactions depends on the dose per treatment, not the degree of acute reactions (Coia and Moylan, 1994). Since radiation is a local treatment, tissue response occurs only in the treatment field.

Tumor Response to Radiation

The four *R*'s of radiobiology are repair, repopulation, reoxygenation, and reassortment (or redistribution). *Repair* indicates cellular recovery after radiation. *Repopulation* refers to the ability of cells exposed to radiation to regenerate and to reproduce between doses of radiation. *Reoxygenation* occurs when hypoxic tumor cells become oxygenated and subsequently radiosensitive. *Reassortment* occurs as an increased number of cells moves into the radiosensitive mitotic phase of the cell cycle.

Reoxygenation is the only one of the four *R*'s that occurs in tumors and not in normal tissue (Coia and Moylan, 1994). Normal tissue does not contain hypoxic cells; tumors may contain up to 20% hypoxic cells because of inadequate vascular supply. The ability of a tumor to reoxygenate during a course of radiation determines the degree of tumor eradication (Coia and Moylan, 1994).

❖ *A Walk Through Treatment*

At the initial meeting of the patient and family with the radiation oncologist and the radiation nurse, the patient's presenting diagnosis, past medical history, operative and pathology reports, and radiologic reports and films are reviewed. A complete physical examination is performed. After reviewing the data, the radiation oncologist outlines and discusses the plan of care, which normally includes the goals of treatment, the number of days or weeks of therapy, and the anticipated short- and long-term side effects.

The nurse is responsible for completing a nursing assessment, which includes vital signs, medical allergies, current medications, baseline weight, a review of systems, and pertinent family and psychosocial history. The patient is educated about all aspects of the proposed treatment, including the simulation process, the daily treatment schedule, general and site-specific treatment side effects, and self-care measures (Sporkin, 1992).

The radiation oncology team includes a variety of professional members. The radiation oncologist is a physician responsible for prescribing the appropriate treatment, monitoring the patient's medical status during treatment, managing treatment side effects, and evaluating patient outcomes. Registered radiation therapists (RRTs) assist in the technical planning of treatment during simulation and are responsible for delivering the daily prescribed dose of radiation. Medical physicists and dosimetrists collaborate with the physician to establish the most suitable direction and size of the radiation beams. They also calculate the time necessary for each radiation treatment and ensure that the radiation is being properly delivered.

Simulation is the initial part of the treatment-planning process. Depending on the complexity of the treatment plan, it may last from 15 minutes to $1\frac{1}{2}$ hours. Simulation precisely defines the field to be treated and areas to be shielded. This is accomplished using X rays, scans, and anatomic landmarks to define the field. The simulator machine does not administer radiation but mimics the physical characteristics of the treatment machine and provides a mock-up. The patient is gowned and draped to expose the treatment area and lies on a hard, narrow couch similar to an X-ray table. The simulation machine provides a series of radiographs (simulation X rays) (Hilderley, 1992a).

The treatment area includes the tumor itself plus adjacent areas of potential disease such as local and regional lymph nodes. The area to be treated is outlined with semipermanent markers that gradually wash off. Tattoos, which are tiny permanent black or blue dots, are placed with a fine needle at the edges of the treatment area to ensure accurate daily replication of the treatment field (Dunne-Daly, 1994a).

Immobilization and positioning devices help to ensure that the patient's position during treatment does not vary and that the target area is treated precisely as planned. Examples of immobilization devices include casts or alpha cradles, which help to maintain a prone or supine position, plastic masks and bite blocks to maintain the head's position, arm boards, belly boards, and tape for securing positions (Dunne-Daly, 1994a). Cerrobend blocks are designed to modify the treatment field and to shield critical structures. These blocks, commonly called "lead" blocks are built specifically for the individual and are mounted daily on the treatment machine. Wedge filters and tissue compensators are sometimes used to alter the radiation beam to provide a more uniform distribution of the dose over the treatment field (Coia and Moylan, 1994).

Before the start of daily treatments, the patient goes through a half-hour mock treatment. During this dry run the treatment plan is technically checked and the radiation oncologist makes final adjustments. Routine treatment checks are essential to providing consistent, high-quality care to patients and are monitored by departmental quality-assurance audits. On a scheduled basis, portal films are taken to verify treatment accuracy and to check beam and block placement (Coia and Moylan, 1994).

The total dose is divided into fractions given daily (the *fractionation schedule*) and is prescribed by the radiation oncologist. In general, treatments are administered daily, 5 days a week. The course of treatment may be as short as one fraction for treatment in certain palliative cases or up to 7 weeks for a curative treatment. The total dose and the treatment schedule depend on the goal of treatment (cure, control, or palliation) and the type and location of the tumor, because different organs tolerate different amounts of radiation.

❖ Treatment Techniques

Teletherapy

Teletherapy is the term used for external-beam radiation therapy. The radiation dose is frequently delivered from machines called linear accelerators (LINACs), which usually emit either photons or beta radiation. Although linear accelerators predominate today, many institutions still use cobalt-60 machines, which generate radiation from that indwelling radioactive source.

Brachytherapy

Brachytherapy, often referred to as internal or implant therapy, is the placement of radioactive sources within cavities, lumens, or tissue or on the surface of the body. Its major advantage is that a high dose of radiation can be delivered directly to the target tissue with a rapid falloff in dose outside the implanted area, thus sparing adjacent normal tissue (Jordan and Mantravadi, 1991). Frequently brachytherapy is used before or after teletherapy to improve local control of disease. Currently brachytherapy techniques are used to treat a broad range of cancers, including malignancies of the breast, lung, head and neck, esophagus, brain, prostate, and female reproductive system.

Most often brachytherapy implants utilize sealed radioactive sources such as radium-227, iridium-192, or cesium-137. These sources deliver a low-dose rate (LDR) of 0.5 to 0.7 Gy (Gray) per hour at 1 cm from the source. Treatment time for these indwelling sources ranges from 30 to 50 hours (Jordan and Mantravadi, 1991).

Intracavitary
Brachytherapy has been most widely used to treat gynecologic malignancies. Gynecologic cancers are often treated with a multiweek course of external-beam radiation followed by an intracavitary implant. Intracavitary applications use an applicator device to hold the radioactive source in place within the body cavity. Hollow applicators, or tandems, are inserted into the uterine canal, and colpostats into the vaginal fornices during the implant procedure in the operating suite. A pelvic exam under anesthesia is performed by the gynecologic and radiation oncologists. The patient is then transferred to the simulation area in the radiation oncology department and simulation radiographs are taken to verify proper placement of "dummy" sources loaded into the applicators (Coia and Moylan, 1994). These Xrays are used to plan an optimum dose distribution from the radioactive sources. The applicators are loaded with the radioactive source upon the patient's return to her room. During this hospitalization, restrictions are placed on mobility, activity, and visitors.

Preimplant education offers the patient clear, concise information about the operative and hospitalization period and is intended to dispell fears and myths about radiation. Teaching includes information about preoperative care such as preadmission testing and bowel prep and about the limited visitation policy. Visitors must not be pregnant, must be at least 18 years of age, and can generally visit no longer than 30 minutes per day. Patients are encouraged to bring reading materials or other quiet activities to occupy themselves during the period of imposed bedrest. Phone contact with family and friends is unlimited. The patient must be reassured that care and safety needs will be addressed.

In the event of a medical emergency, appropriate emergency procedures come first and then prompt notification of the radiation safety officer for immediate removal of the radiation sources. A lead container, or "pig," and long-handled forceps are kept in the patient's room in the event that unloading is necessary. The sources must never be touched directly.

After the prescribed implant time, usually 48 to 72 hours, the sources are unloaded by the radiation oncologist. The patient and her room are surveyed to ensure that there is no residual radiation remaining, then the radioactive precautions are discontinued (Shell and Carter, 1987).

Nurses caring for patients with radioactive implants must be familiar with radiation safety principles. The goal is to minimize staff to radiation exposure during radiation applications and time, distance, and shielding are used to reduce the exposure. As distance increases, the amount of radiation exposure decreases; nurses can limit exposure by standing several feet from patients when possible, especially when performing indirect care. Shielding refers to the use of protective materials between the radioactive source and personnel. Hospital room walls may be lead-lined to protect people outside the room; more commonly, movable lead shields are positioned around the patient's bed.

General guidelines suggest that nurses limit direct care to $\frac{1}{2}$ hour a day (Dunne-Daly, 1994b). Staff are monitored for radiation exposure by wearing film badges or dosimeters (these devices do not offer protection from radiation; they simply record occupational exposure). Radiation-exposure records are maintained by the radiation-safety officer and are part of the institution's permanent records. Pregnant nurses or those trying to conceive should not care for brachytherapy patients. Strategies to decrease fears include holding staff in-service days to review basic radiation biology, safety, brachytherapy, and emergency measures and peer discussions to explore fears and misconceptions (Sticklin, 1994).

High-Dose-Rate Brachytherapy
High-dose-rate (HDR) brachytherapy allows rapid treatment time (measured in minutes), decreased staff exposure to radiation, and the convenience of outpatient treatment in the radiation oncology facility. HDR brachytherapy delivers a dose rate of 0.2 to 0.5 Gy per minute. In remote, after-loading devices such as these, the radioactive material (cobalt-60 or iridium-192) is stored in pellet form inside a shielded container. These containers are connected to applicators and are loaded by pneumatic tubes after the staff has placed the applicator in the body cavity and left the room. These techniques are used for a variety of sites, including esophageal and bronchial tumors and gynecologic cancers.

Interstitial
Interstitial implant sources may be radioactive seeds, catheters, wires, or needles that are loaded with a radioactive isotope and placed directly into tissue. This application is commonly seen in head and neck cancers, prostate cancer, sarcomas, and breast cancer.

Most brachytherapy applications are temporary and thus are removed after the prescribed dose has been delivered. However, for prostate cancer, sources such as iodine-125 seeds are permanently implanted. The sources decay rapidly, and though they remain implanted at the time of hospital discharge, there is little risk of significant exposure with patient contact (Dow, 1992).

Unsealed Sources
Unsealed sources are radioactive substances in a colloidal suspension placed directly in contact with tissue by oral, intravenous, intrapleural, or intraperitoneal routes. For example, iodine-131 is used to treat thyroid cancer. It is administered orally and is excreted in body fluids, feces, urine, emesis, saliva, and perspiration.

Unsealed sources present a potential contamination hazard, and special handling is required. Gloves are worn when providing direct patient care, and double flushing after toileting should be enforced. One half of the radioactive iodine is excreted within 2 days after ingestion (Dunne-Daly, 1994c). Linens and patient gowns are placed in separate isolation bags, because they may be contaminated. Disposable utensils, plates, and cups are used for dietary trays. Items such as the telephone, call bell, and floor may be covered with plastic to reduce the risk of contamination (Dow, 1992). Blood should be drawn before the radiation is administered. If necessary, it may be sampled during treatment; however, the lab must be notified of its radioactivity. The Nuclear Regulatory Commission has established safe parameters for patient discharge (Coia and Moylan, 1994).

Strontium-89, used to palliate intractable pain caused by bone metastases, is a radioactive calcium analog, meaning that it acts as a calcium imitator and is taken up and retained at sites of increased bone metabolism or metastases. Patients who have previously received chemotherapy may experience a significant decrease in their white blood cell counts (Robinson, 1993). Strontium therapy can be repeated at 3-month intervals. Staff should exercise appropriate precautions such as gloving and double flushing for the first several days after an injection because strontium is excreted through urine and feces (Porter et al., 1993).

Hyperthermia

Hyperthermia is the use of heat to kill tissue, and in combination with radiation therapy it increases the number of tumor cells killed. Generally, patients receiving this type of treatment are enrolled in investigational protocols that study the synergistic interaction between the two therapies. Superficial malignancies, including melanomas, locally recurrent breast cancers, and head and neck cancers, have been successfully treated with hyperthermia and radiation (Girizos, Order, and Moylan, 1994). Nursing care is directed to meticulous wound and skin care in addition to symptom management and patient education.

Intraoperative Radiation Therapy

Intraoperative radiation therapy (IORT) is used to deliver a single dose of radiation directly to the exposed tumor or tumor bed. The advantage of IORT is the ability to remove or protect normal tissue from the radiated field. This investigational treatment involves surgical exposure of the tumor bed in the operating suite. IORT may take place in an operating suite equipped with a radiation machine, or the surgical site may be temporarily closed and the patient may be transported to the radiation oncology department. In either case, the machine is fitted with a special plastic cone-shaped device that delivers a dose of radiation to a circumscribed anatomic area. The patient is then transported back to the operating suite for completion of the surgical procedure. IORT has been used to treat locally advanced primary and recurrent colorectal cancers, unresectable pancreatic cancers, and gastric cancers.

Radiosensitizers

Radiosensitizers are chemical or pharmacologic agents that increase the lethal effects of radiation on tumor cells when administered concurrently with radiation (Hall, 1994). Oxygen, the most important radiosensitizer, enhances cell damage by producing radiation-induced free radicals that interact with DNA (Girizos, Order, and Moylan, 1994). Hypoxic cells are relatively resistant to radiation. Therefore, attempts to increase oxygenation of the cells have focused on the use of hyperbaric oxygen and on the development of agents that mimic oxygen's effect in the cells. It has been demonstrated that small, daily doses of radiation, which allow for reoxygenation of the tumor, lead to better tumor control than fewer, larger fractions do (Noll, 1992).

Radioprotectors

Radioprotectors are compounds that reduce the effect of radiation on cells and tissue. Most promising is the group known as sulfhydryl compounds (Hall, 1994). Many compounds have been synthesized, but the most effective appears to be WR-1065. This drug is able to rapidly flood normal tissue while penetrating the tumor more slowly. In addition, it protects the blood-forming organs, the gut, and the salivary glands if administered within minutes of the radiation dose (Hall, 1994).

❖ Nursing Considerations

The nurse caring for an individual receiving radiation treatment should know the possible general and site-specific reactions, and patients should be taught appropriate self-care measures. Site-specific side effects occur in the treatment field (Table 3-1). In contrast, general side effects occur independent of the treatment site.

General side effects include skin reactions, fatigue, bone marrow depression, and nutritional deficits. The degree of reaction is individual, with some patients experiencing tremendous debilitation and others only minor effects. Usually these side effects depend on the patient's pretreatment performance status, the duration of treatment, the location and size of the tumor, the timing of multimodal treatment, the type of treatment machine used, and the dose of radiation given.

Skin Reaction

Most individuals receiving radiation treatment will experience side effects in the skin. The skin serves as a protective barrier for the body's internal organs. It has two layers; the dermis and the epidermis (McDonald, 1992). The epidermis is the outermost layer and is more frequently affected by radiation than the dermis because of the rapid mitotic rate of cells in this skin layer. The common types of skin reactions are erythema and dry or moist desquamation.

Erythema, a generalized reddening of the skin in the treatment field, may occur after five to ten treatments and is characterized by itchy, red, raised vesicles. Erythema occurs in response to increased capillary blood flow that progresses from vasodilation to vascular congestion (McDonald, 1992).

Dry desquamation appears as scaly, flaky skin, which causes itching, peeling, and shedding. This reaction occurs in response to radiation damage to the basal cells of the epidermis and decreased functioning of the sweat glands (Dunne-Daly, 1994b).

Moist desquamation is characterized by reddened, weeping skin that often is warm and taut to the touch and has a shiny appearance. The exudate frequently is serous, with random areas of crust or scab formation. This reaction occurs in response to almost complete destruction of the protective epidermis skin layer. Often it is preceded by erythema, looks like a second-degree burn, is painful, and

Table 3-1   Site-specific Side Effects of Radiation

Radiation Site	*Side Effect*
Head and neck	Xerostomia Dysphagia Weight loss Depression Mucositis Altered taste Skin breakdown Dental caries Osteoradionecrosis Trismus
Brain	Severe headache Alopecia Neurologic impairment
Lung	Dermatitis Fatigue Anorexia Dysphagia Esophagitis Cough Pneumonitis Pulmonary fibrosis
Breast	Fatigue Skin reaction Breast and arm edema Breast tenderness Lymphedema Breast hyperpigmentation Breast fibrosis
Pelvis	Fatigue Diarrhea Cystitis Altered sexual function Nausea (if includes paraaortic lymph nodes) Anorexia
Prostate	Dysuria Diarrhea Proctitis Altered sexual function
Upper gastrointestinal tract	Pharyngitis Esophagitis Nausea Vomiting Anorexia

has the potential to become infected (McDonald, 1992). To promote skin regeneration, patients are occasionally offered short treatment breaks or an adjustment of the treatment field to block the sensitive area (Dunne-Daly, 1994c).

Nursing assessment of the skin must be done throughout the course of treatment. It is advisable to assess the following points prior to teaching self-management skills:

◆ Anatomic location of the skin in the treatment field
◆ Pretreatment skin conditions; history of collagen vascular disease
◆ Physical parameters such as age, nutritional status, and prior sun exposure
◆ Documentation of recent chemotherapy or surgery (Dunne-Daly, 1994b)

Skin integrity may be characterized as follows:

0 No changes
1 Faint or dull erythema; follicular reaction; dry desquamation
2 Bright erythema; tender to the touch; patchy moist desquamation
3 Confluent moist desquamation; edema
4 Ulceration, hemorrhage, necrosis (Bruner et al., 1992)

After the patient's skin is assessed, general skin care guidelines are taught. These include (1) avoiding temperature changes, (2) using only approved skin products, (3) avoiding sun exposure, and (4) reporting symptoms of erythema and dry or moist desquamation (Bruner et al., 1992). Management of skin reactions is covered in Chapter 21, Cutaneous Reactions.

Fatigue

Fatigue is common among individuals with cancer. It is difficult to manage and may be variously attributed to the effect of multimodal treatment, the physiologic process of cancer, or individual lifestyle. The general feelings that patients describe include malaise, decreased energy, inability to perform activities of daily living, and exhaustion. Fatigue as a symptom of cancer treatment has become a clinical management priority due to its prevalence, the lack of available interventions, and a limited research base (Winninghan et al., 1994).

The exact mechanism of radiation-induced fatigue is unknown. It has been theorized that an increase in basal metabolic rate occurs during radiation treatment in order to eliminate toxic tumor by-products. Energy is therefore required to repair damaged tissues and cells (Bruner et al., 1992). The patient's energy reserves are often weakened from utilization for other physiologic and psychologic needs. It has also been theorized that a relationship exists between radiation dose, field size, and degree of fatigue. For example, a patient who receives treatment to a deeply seated tumor with a large field at a high dose is more susceptible to fatigue than a patient who receives smaller doses to a surface tumor with a smaller field (Hilderley, 1992b). Additional factors include chemotherapy, surgery, medications such as antiemetics and narcotics, pain, anemia, respiratory compromise, distance from home, the duration of the treatments, and pressure to maintain a normal life-style (Hilderley, 1992b).

Nursing assessment of fatigue includes the duration and intensity of fatigue, factors that increase or decrease fatigue, the patient's nutritional status and emotional status, laboratory studies, the effect of fatigue on daily activities, and assessment of the patient's usual rest and sleep patterns (Bruner et al., 1992). Nursing management of fatigue is discussed in Chapter 25, Other Side Effects.

Bone Marrow Depression

Bone marrow depression during radiation treatment is related to the amount of proliferating bone marrow within the treatment field. Additional risk factors include recent chemotherapy, surgery, the patient's age and performance status, and any prior history of chronic blood dyscrasia. The bone marrow contains highly radiosensitive cells. When areas of bone marrow are within the treatment field, each daily treatment dose has been associated with bone marrow injury (McDonald, 1992). White cells and platelets are most commonly affected by radiation. If the number of white cells decreases (leukopenia), the risk of infection is high. If the number of platelets decreases (thrombocytopenia), there is a risk of bleeding. Red blood cells are affected less, although anemia may arise if chemotherapy is given concomitantly.

Treatment that affects areas with bone marrow, such as the skull, pelvis, spine, sternum, ribs, and long bones, puts the patient at risk for marrow suppression. It is advisable to obtain weekly blood counts (Hilderley, 1993). For individuals with treatment fields containing less proliferating marrow, blood counts may be obtained every other week or as needed. If the patient is receiving total body irradiation or splenic irradiation, daily blood counts are recommended (Hilderley, 1993). Nursing management is discussed in Chapter 22, Hematologic Toxicities.

Nutritional Deficits

Radiation therapy can destroy nutritional well-being. Radiation to the gastrointestinal organs commonly causes nausea, vomiting, diarrhea, and intestinal malabsorption in response to mucosal toxicity (Skipper, Szeluga, and Groenwald, 1993). Altered bowel function frequently resolves shortly after completion of radiation treatment. Radiation given to the lungs, chest wall, and mediastinum can cause dysphagia, which is attributed to esophageal irritation. This can be an uncomfortable side effect requiring the use of systemic antacids, a soft diet, and pain medication. Radiation to the head and neck may cause a dry mouth, dental caries, fungal infections, and diminished ability to chew, swallow, or taste. Early identification by the nurse caring for the individual at risk for radiation-induced nutritional depletion will lessen the morbidity and mortality of treatment regimens. The characteristic complications that occur must be thoroughly assessed utilizing a team approach. Nursing management of nutritional deficits is discussed in detail in Unit III, Side Effects.

❖ Age-specific Considerations

Because cancer may strike a person anywhere along life's continuum, it is important to review briefly the special needs of pediatric, adult, and geriatric populations. Age-specific considerations regarding radiation therapy have been well documented.

Issues that must be addressed when treating children include departmental procedures for pediatric emergencies, the ability to administer and monitor appropriate pediatric sedatives, and staff preparation and experience in meeting the developmental and emotional needs of the child. Attention must be focused on the unique developmental tasks of childhood in order to adequately prepare and support the child during treatment. Parents are an integral part of the process of patient education; they must be encouraged to express their fears and concerns and help the child feel more confident during treatment (Lew, 1992). Preparation strategies range from use of age-appropriate comic books and directed play with dolls, puppets, and medical equipment to individualized teaching plans, and behavioral training so the child lies still during treatments (Bucholz, 1994).

The informed-consent process includes giving information about acute and late effects of radiation therapy. The issue of late effects of treatment immediately affects children immensely, because they have not completed their physical, emotional, and cognitive growth and development. Because learning this information may be stressful, care must be taken to balance immediate treatment needs and the need to know about possible future side effects.

Adults receiving radiation therapy may be divided into younger and older (greater than 65 years old) populations. The physiologic and psychologic responses of older adults to radiation therapy have been documented (Dellefield, 1992). Documentation that the elderly may be at higher risk for cancer-related weight loss has demonstrated several age-related factors such as physiologic change, depletion of iron, and a natural tendency to ingest less food (Brown, 1993).

Coordinating the care of older adults receiving radiation involves management of age-specific side effects along with social-service planning for daily transportation and adequate home support. Many older adults reside in isolation without adequate financial support to provide the basic comforts that could assist them to survive a course of radiation. The nurse should be aware of these complex needs as the care plan is created and actualized for patients in this special population.

❖ Patient Education

A study of patients' perceived knowledge and learning needs concerning radiation therapy demonstrated that effective teaching can enhance patient knowledge regarding radiation treatment (Campbell-Forsyth, 1990). Dispelling myths, misconceptions, and fears is vital for relief of anxiety. The following misconceptions have been identified and must be clarified for the patient: (1) Radiation is a last resort for incurable disease; (2) radiation causes side effects similar to those of chemotherapy, (3) radiation causes skin burns, (4) the patient will become radioactive, and (5) because it is impossible to touch, feel, smell, or see the beams of radiation, the wrong treatment may inadvertently be given. Patients and families must be encouraged to express their concerns and to ask questions. After underlying anxieties are allayed, the educational process can go forward.

Most individuals invite information; however, some individuals prefer less detail than others because it has the potential for stimulating anxiety in them. It is for this reason that the educational plan must be tailored to the needs of each patient and family. The patient should be told that the clinical evaluation includes weekly scheduled visits with the radiation oncologist and the nurse for the assessment of treatment-related side effects and for the development of management interventions. Patients should be encouraged to contact the team on a more frequent basis should any questions or needs arise. An emergency number must be provided for evening and weekend occasions.

Time must be allowed for the exchange of educational material, and the environment must be conducive to teaching the complex aspects of care. The patient waiting room has been identified as an inappropriate setting to meet families, friends, relatives, and patients who may be weary from travel, anxiety-ridden, angry due to unexplained delays, and brimming with questions. Privacy should be provided during the educational process (Copp, 1993).

Because health care can be perceived as fragmented, patients and families may be confused regarding plans for evaluation after the treatment course is completed. Therefore the patient must be reassured that follow-up appointments will be scheduled and appropriate diagnostic studies ordered. Self-evaluation forms are helpful documentation tools that are given to patients at follow-up meetings and that provide the team with valuable insight into the patient's functional status and the side effects of radiation therapy.

❖ Summary

Radiation oncology is an exciting, intricate, precise science that evolved from unrefined historical experimentation to an effective method of cancer treatment. To the individuals receiving radiation therapy and to the persons who support them through the process, treatment may seem arduous, frightening, mysterious, and replete with painful side effects. A cohesive team of nursing and medical professionals is integral to the planning and management of patient-related issues. The management of side effects has become the domain of the professional radiation oncology nurse. As the future evolves, so too should the role of professional nurses at institutions offering radiation therapy.

❖ References

Brown JK: Gender, age, usual weight, and tobacco use as predictors of weight loss in patients with lung cancer, Oncol Nurs Forum 20:466–472, 1993.

Bruner DW, Iwamoto R, Keane K, and Strohl R, editors: Manual for radiation oncology nursing practice and education, Pittsburgh, 1992, Oncology Nursing Society.

Bucholz JD: Comforting children during radiotherapy, Oncol Nurs Forum 21:987–944, 1994.

Campbell-Forsyth L: Patient's perceived knowledge and learning needs concerning radiation therapy, Ca Nurs 13:81–89, 1990.

Coia LR and Moylan DJ: Introduction to clinical radiation oncology, ed 2, Madison, 1994, Medical Physics.

Copp LA: Teaching site: the waiting room, J Prof Nurs 9(1): 1–2, 1993.

Dellefield ME: Special needs of elderly patients. In Dow KH and Hilderley LJ, editors: Nursing care in radiation oncology. Philadelphia, 1992, WB Saunders Co, pp. 203–211.

Dow KH: Principles of brachytherapy. In Dow KH and Hilderly LJ, editors: Nursing care in radiation oncology, Philadelphia, 1992, WB Saunders Co, pp. 16–29.

Dunne-Daly, CF: Brachytherapy, Ca Nurs 17:355–634, 1994c.

Dunne-Daly CF: External radiation therapy self-learning module, Ca Nurs 17:156–169, 1994a.

Dunne-Daly, CF: Nursing care and adverse reactions of external radiation therapy: a self-learning module, Ca Nurs 17:236–255, 1994b.

Girizos WT, Order SE, and Moylan DJ: New developments in radiation oncology. In Coia LR and Moylan DJ, editors: Introduction to clinical radiation oncology, Madison, 1994, Medical Physics, pp. 513–526.

Hall EJ: Radiobiology for the radiologist, Philadelphia, 1994, JB Lippincott Co.

Hilderley LJ: Radiation oncology: historical background and principles of teletherapy. In Dow KH and Hilderley LJ, editors: Nursing care in radiation oncology, Philadelphia, 1992a, WB Saunders Co, pp. 3–15.

Hilderley LJ: Pain and fatigue. In Dow KH and Hilderley LJ, editors: Nursing care in radiation oncology, Philadelphia, 1992b, WB Saunders Co, pp. 57–68.

Hilderley LJ: Radiotherapy. In Groenwald SL, Frogge MH, Goodman M, and Yarbro CH, editors: Cancer nursing: principles and practice, Boston, 1993, Jones & Bartlett, pp. 235–269.

Jordan LN and Mantravadi RVP: Nursing care of the patient receiving high dose rate brachytherapy, Oncol Nurs Forum 18:1167–1171, 1991.

Lew CC: Special needs of children. In Dow KH and Hilderley LJ, editors: Nursing care in radiation oncology, Philadelphia, 1992, WB Saunders Co, pp. 177–202.

McDonald A: Altered protective mechanisms. In Dow KH and Hilderley LJ, editors: Nursing care in radiation oncology, Philadelphia, 1992, WB Saunders Co, pp. 96–125.

Noll L: Chemical modifiers of radiation therapy. In Dow KH and Hilderley LJ, editors: Nursing care in radiation oncology, Philadelphia, 1992, WB Saunders Co, pp. 264–274.

Porter AT, McEwan AJB, Powe JE, Reid R, McGowan DG, Lukka H, Sathyanarayana JR, Yakemchuk KY, Hong KE, and Yardley J: Results of randomized phase-III trails to evaluate the efficacy of strontium-89 adjuvant to local-field external-beam irradiation in the management of endocrine resistant metastatic prostate cancer, Int J Radiat Oncol Biol Phys 25:805–813, 1993.

Robinson RG: Strontium-89-precursor targeted therapy for pain relief of blastic metastatic disease, Cancer 72:3433–3435, 1993.

Shell JA and Carter JC: The gynecological implant patient, Semin Oncol Nurs, 3:54–66, 1987.

Skipper A, Szeluga DJ, and Groenwald SL: Nutritional disturbances. In Groenwald SL, Frogge MH, Goodman M, and Yarbro CH, editors: Cancer nursing: principles and practice, Boston, 1993, Jones & Bartlett, pp. 620–643.

Sporkin E: Patient and family education. In Dow KH and Hilderley LJ, editors: Nursing care in radiation oncology, Philadelphia, 1992, WB Saunders Co, pp. 33–44.

Sticklin LA: Strategies for overcoming nurses' fear of radiation exposure, Cancer Prac 2:275–277, 1994.

Winningham ML, Nail LM, Burke MB, Brophy L, Comprich B, Jones LS, Pickard-Holley S, Rhodes V, St. Pierre B, Beck S, Glass EC, Mock VL, Mooney KH, and Piper B: Fatigue and the cancer experience: the state of the knowledge, Oncol Nurs Forum, 21:23–36, 1994.

Yasko J: Care of the client receiving external radiation therapy, Reston, VA, 1982, Prentice-Hall.

Chapter 4

❖ Chemotherapy

Barbara Rassat Tripp

Chemotherapy by definition is the treatment of disease with chemical substances. In common usage the term has come to mean drugs used to treat cancer. Chemotherapeutic agents are also used in the treatment of nonmalignant diseases such as rheumatoid arthritis and psoriasis and other conditions such as ectopic pregnancy. For the purposes of this text the term chemotherapy refers exclusively to drugs used in the treatment of cancer.

❖ Role of Chemotherapy in Cancer Treatment

Chemotherapy plays an important role in the treatment of cancer. Whether utilized alone or in combination with surgery, radiation therapy, or biotherapy, it can achieve significant improvement in both the cure rate and the length of survival of persons with cancer (Krakoff, 1991).

Chemotherapy interferes with the cell's ability to divide. Chemotherapeutic agents either cause the cell to die (cytocidal agents) or render the cell incapable of dividing (cytostatic agents). Chemotherapeutic agents are classified as either *cell-cycle-phase-specific* (meaning they are effective only when a cell is in a particular phase of the cell cycle) or *cell-cycle-phase-nonspecific* (effectiveness is not affected by cell-cycle phase). (For a discussion of the cell cycle, see Chapter 1, Overview of Cancer and Multimodal Therapy.) Cell-cycle-phase-specific drugs work best on rapidly dividing tumors (Bender, 1992) and are usually given in divided doses or by continuous infusion in order to "catch" cells as they move through the cell cycle (Ratain, 1992). For example, 5-fluorouracil affects cells during the synthesis (S) phase. Because 20% of reproducing cells are in the S phase at any given time (DeVita, 1993), 5-fluorouracil must be given at repeated intervals or continuously to be effective.

Cell-cycle-phase-nonspecific drugs are most effective if given in large single doses because the more drug that is given, the greater the number of tumor cells killed (Ratain, 1992). The cytotoxic effect occurs during the cell cycle and is expressed when cell division is attempted.

Chemotherapeutic agents are also classified by their pharmacologic mechanism of action. Alkylating agents alter DNA structure and interfere with its template functions; antimetabolites mimic natural nutrients needed by the cell to divide; vinca alkaloids bind to the cellular structure required for mitosis; and hormonal agents modulate the endogenous hormonal environment.

Because chemotherapeutic agents have such varying mechanisms of action, they are frequently used in combination. Combination chemotherapy offers the potential for the greatest destruction of cancer cells by affecting them at different points of the cell cycle. Each drug used in combination chemotherapy is generally chosen because of a demonstrated individual effect against the tumor, different side effects (or severity of side effects), and a mechanism of action that varies from the other drugs in that combination (DeVita, 1993). Examples of common combination chemotherapy protocols are listed in Table 4-1.

The ultimate effectiveness of chemotherapy is related to the *total tumor mass* (also called the *tumor burden*). When a tumor is first detected it most likely consists of more than a billion cells. These cells fall into three categories: those that are actively dividing; those that have the ability to divide but are resting; and those cells that have lost the ability to divide. Tumors that have a large proportion of cells that are dividing have a greater susceptibility to chemotherapeutic agents.

The need for repeated and prolonged therapy is based on the *tumor-cell-kill hypothesis*. According to this hypothesis, with each cycle of chemotherapy a certain percentage of cells is destroyed. If a chemotherapeutic regimen has a 90% rate of success in killing cancer cells, and if there are a billion cells present, 10% of the cells, or one hundred million, would remain. The next cycle would kill 90% of those cells, and subsequent cycles would continue killing 90% of the surviving cells until only a few malignant cells remained. At this point the immune system would destroy the final cells that remained.

Unfortunately this theory does not hold true in all cases, because not all persons with the same type and stage of tumor have the same response to chemotherapy. There are many reasons for this: (1) tumor cells may be able to continue dividing between chemotherapy cycles, and this growth may outpace the killing; (2) not all tumor cells are equally chemosensitive; and (3) tumor cells may change or mutate, and their chemosensitivity may diminish or even cease, that is, the tumor cells may develop single-drug or multidrug resistance. This drug resistance may operate by one or more recognized mechanisms: (1) decreased drug entry into cancer cells, (2) increased drug efflux from the cancer cell, (3) increased intracellular degradation of the drug, (4) enhanced repair of drug injury to the cancer cell, (5) inadequate conversion of the drug to its active derivative, and (6) utilization of alternate biochemical pathways not inhibited by the drug (Weiss, 1993).

The limitations of chemotherapy continue to be a frustration for clinicians and a powerful motivator for researchers. The major limitations include (1) the inability to know which cancers have metastasized, to which site(s), and at what point during the tumor's development or treatment; (2) the inability to detect minimal residual disease after apparently successful treatment; (3) the inability to increase doses of effective chemotherapy or administer enough cycles of the regimen to reach the hypothesized death of the cancer cells; (4) the inability to treat chemoresistant

Table 4-1   Common Chemotherapeutic Protocols

Disease Site	Chemotherapeutic Drug Regimen	Frequency of Administration
Breast	Cyclophosphamide 100 mg/m² po, days 1–14 Doxorubicin 30 mg/m² IV, days 1 and 8 Fluorouracil 400–500 mg/m² IV, days 1 and 8 (CAF)	Repeat cycle every 28 days
	or	
	Cyclophosphamide 500 mg/m² IV, day 1 Doxorubicin 50 mg/m² IV, day 1 Fluorouracil 500 mg/m² IV, day 1	Repeat cycle every 21 days
	Cyclophosphamide 100 mg/m² po, days 1–14 Methotrexate 40–60 mg/m² IV, days 1 and 8 Fluorouracil 400–600 mg/m² IV, days 1 and 8 (CMF)	Repeat cycle every 28 days
Colon	Fluorouracil 370–400 mg/m²/d IV, days 1–5 Calcium leucovorin 200 mg/m²/d IV, days 1–5 (F-CL*)	Repeat cycle every 28 days
Gastric	Fluorouracil 600 mg/m² IV, days 1, 8, 29, and 36 Doxorubicin 30 mg/m² IV, days 1 and 29 Mitomycin-C 10 mg/m² IV, day 1 (FAM)	Repeat cycle every 8 weeks
Hodgkin's Disease	Mechlorethamine 6 mg/m² IV, days 1 and 8 Vincristine 1.4 mg/m² (maximum 2.5 mg) IV, days 1 and 8 Procarbazine 100 mg/m² po, days 1–14 Prednisone 40 mg/m² po, days 1–14 (MOPP)	Repeat cycle every 28 days
	Doxorubicin 25 mg/m² IV, days 1 and 15 Bleomycin 10 units/m² IV, days 1 and 15 (ABVD)	Repeat cycle every 28 days
	Vinblastine 6 mg/m² IV, days 1 and 15 Dacarbazine 150 mg/m² IV, days 1–5	Repeat cycle every 28 days
	or	
	Dacarbazine 350 mg/m² IV, days 1 and 15	
Lung cancer (non-small-cell)	Cyclophosphamide 400 mg/m² IV, day 1 Doxorubicin 40 mg/m² IV, day 1 Cisplatin 60 mg/m² IV, day 1 (CAP)	Repeat cycle every 28 days

Continued

*Also abbreviated LVR; infuse prior to 5-fluorouracil.

Table 4-1   Common Chemotherapeutic Protocols—cont'd

Disease Site	Chemotherapeutic Drug Regimen		Frequency of Administration
Lung cancer (small-cell)	CV	Cisplatin 50 mg/m^2 IV, day 1 Etoposide 60 mg/m^2 IV, days 1–5 or Cisplatin 75 mg/m^2 IV, day 2 Etoposide 125 mg/m^2 IV, days 1–3	Repeat cycle every 21–28 days Repeat cycle every 28 days
Lymphoma	CHOP	Cyclophosphamide 750 mg/m^2 IV, day 1 Doxorubicin 50 mg/m^2 IV, day 1 Vincristine 1.4 mg/m^2 (maximum 2 mg) IV, day 1 Prednisone 100 mg po, days 1–5 (dose may be 100 mg/m^2)	Repeat cycle every 21 days
	CHOP-Bleo	Cyclophosphamide 750 mg/m^2 IV, day 1 Doxorubicin 50 mg/m^2 IV, day 1 Vincristine 2 mg IV, days 1 and 5 Prednisone 100 mg po, days 1–5 Bleomycin 15 units IV, days 1 and 5	Repeat cycle every 21–28 days
Ovary	CP	Cyclophosphamide 1000 mg/m^2 IV, day 1 Cisplatin 50–60 mg/m^2 IV, day 1	Repeat cycle every 21 to 28 days
	AP	Doxorubicin 50–60 mg/m^2 IV, day 1 Cisplatin 50–60 mg/m^2 IV, day 1	Repeat cycle every 21 days
Sarcoma (soft tissue)	MAID	± GM-CSF Mesna 2500 mg/m^2/d IV, days 1–4 Doxorubicin 20 mg/m^2/d IV, days 1–3 Ifosfamide 2500 mg/m^2/d IV, days 1–3 Dacarbazine 300 mg/m^2/d IV, days 1–3	Repeat cycle every 4–6 weeks

tumors; and (5) the inability to measure the moment-to-moment impact of treatment on tumor cells (DeVita, 1993).

Researchers have sought to overcome these limitations through various means. Monoclonal antibodies are administered before body scans in an attempt to visualize areas of metastasis at the time of diagnosis (Holleb, Fink, and Murphy, 1991). They can identify minute areas of metastasis, making possible, for example, a small-wedge liver resection at the same time as the initial colon resection, further reducing the tumor burden before adjuvant chemotherapy and potentially increasing long-term survival. Second-look laparotomies are performed to determine the effectiveness of chemotherapy in ovarian cancer that may avoid unnecessary prolongation of repeated chemotherapy cycles (Weiss, 1993).

❖ Side Effects of Chemotherapy

Chemotherapy affects not only cancer cells but other rapidly growing cells, especially those of the gastrointestinal system (oral, gut, and rectal mucosa), the integumentary system (particularly hair follicles of the scalp), and the hematopoietic system (especially neutrophils and platelets). Some chemotherapeutic agents also affect specific organs; for example, bleomycin can cause pulmonary fibrosis.

Side effects range from mild to severe and can include bone marrow depression (with increased risk of infection and bleeding), fatigue, nausea, vomiting, anorexia, mucositis, stomatitis, esophagitis, diarrhea, constipation, rectal sores, alopecia, hemorrhagic cystitis, renal failure, pulmonary fibrosis, pneumonitis, cardiac arrhythmia, congestive heart failure, paralytic ileus, peripheral neuropathy, hearing loss, sterility, loss of libido, and menopause.

Administering a *chemoprotectant,* a medication given before and after or concurrently with a chemotherapeutic agent, eliminates or minimizes the organ toxicity associated with chemotherapy drugs. For example, mesna, a uroprotectant, blocks damage to the bladder wall that can lead to hemorrhagic cystitis following treatment with either ifosfamide or cyclophosphamide.

Whereas chemoprotectants have proven effective with some agents, other chemoprotectants have been or are currently under investigation (Dorr and Von Hoff, 1994). Diethyldithiocarbamate (DDTC) reduces the nephrotoxicity and gastrointestinal toxicity of the platinum-containing drugs cisplatin and carboplatin and the hematopoietic toxicity of alkylating agents like cyclophosphamide without compromising the antitumor effects of these agents. Ethiofos (WR-2721) modulates the hematologic effects of ionizing radiation and DNA alkylating agents and the nephrotoxicity and neurotoxicity of cisplatin and carboplatin. Table 4-2 lists side effects for each chemotherapeutic agent. Nursing assessment and management of side effects are discussed in Units II and III.

❖ Nursing Considerations for Administration of Chemotherapeutic Agents

Every institution, agency, or private practice should have written policies and procedures that deal specifically with the administration of chemotherapeutic agents.

Table 4-2 Chemotherapeutic Agents and Their Side Effects

Agent	Dose	Side Effect	Comments
Alkylating Agents			
Busulfan	4–6 mg/d po HD = 8–16 mg/kg	Myelosuppression, pulmonary toxicity, amenorrhea, anorexia, nausea, vomiting, cateracts	WBC may continue to decrease 2 weeks after discontinuing
Carboplatin	400–500 mg/m² IV, q 4 wks HD = 175 mg/m² q wk	Myelosuppression, nausea, vomiting, nephrotoxicity, taste alterations, anorexia, alopecia, peripheral neuropathy, hepatotoxicity	Facial flushing may occur with alcohol diluent
Chlorambucil	0.4–0.5 mg/kg po q 2–3 wks 0.1–0.2 mg/kg/d po for 3–6 wks	Myelosuppression, mucositis, pulmonary fibrosis, amenorrhea, dermatitis, seizures	Increased toxicity with simultaneous use of barbituates
Cisplatin	50–120 mg/m² IV q 3–4 wks HD = 200 mg/m²	Myelosuppression, nephrotoxicity, peripheral neurotoxicity, nausea, vomiting, ototoxicity, mucositis, hypomagnesemia, hypocalcemia, hypokalemia, encephalopathy	Hypertonic saline-and-mannitol diuresis to prevent renal toxicity
Cyclophosphamide	600–1500 mg/m² q 3–4 wks 100 mg/m²/d po for 14 d HD = 5–8 gm/m²	Myelosuppression, hemorrhagic cystitis, cardiotoxicity, pneumonitis, alopecia, nausea, vomiting, mucositis, amenorrhea, azoospermia, metallic taste, hyperpigmentation, nasal congestion	In high doses, administer with uroprotectant
Dacarbazine	250 mg/m²/d for 5 d q 3 wks HD = 400 mg/m²	Myelosuppression, nausea, vomiting, flulike syndrome, phlebitis, pain upon administration, metallic taste	Irritant
Ifosfamide	1500–1800 mg/m²/d IV for 5 d HD = 8–18 gm/m²	Myelosuppression, hemorrhagic cystitis, nephrotoxicity, hepatotoxicity, sleepiness, confusion, lethargy, ataxia, nausea, vomiting, alopecia	Use with Mesna, a uroprotectant
Mechlorethamine	16 mg/m²/d	Myelosuppression, nausea, vomiting, extravasation, rashes, alopecia, menstrual irregularities, hyperpigmentation, metallic taste	Vesicant
Melphalan	2–10 mg po HD = 0.5–50 mg/m² IV	Myelosuppression, nausea, vomiting, mucositis, anorexia, alopecia	
Thiotepa	5–20 mg/m² IV HD = 900 mg/m² IV	Myelosuppression, headaches, fever, amenorrhea, chemical cystitis, nausea, vomiting, alopecia	Intravesical 60 mg

Antimetabolites	Dose	Toxicities	Comments
Cytarabine	3 g/m² IV q 12 hrs HD = 100–200 mg/m²/d for 7 d	Peripheral neuropathy, encephalopathy, myelosuppression, mucositis, nausea, vomiting, hepatotoxicity, headache, alopecia, photophobia, diarrhea, ocular toxicity, maculopapular rash, erythema on palms and soles	With high dose, give steroid eye drops
Floxuridine	16–24 mg/m² daily	Nausea, vomiting, diarrhea, dermatitis, chemical hepatitis, myelosuppression	Arterial administration
5-Fluorouracil	12 mg/kg/d for 5 d q 4 wks IV 15 mg/kg/wk IV 500–1000 mg	Myelosuppression, mucositis, nausea, vomiting, diarrhea, alopecia, diplopia, hyperpigmentation, photosensitivity, cerebellar dysfunction, ataxia	Leucovorin or levamisole enhances effect, but with increased toxicity
Hydroxyurea	8–12 mg/d po	Myelosuppression, nausea, vomiting, diarrhea, radiation recall, mucositis, pruritus	
Mercaptopurine	100 mg/m²/d po	Myelosuppression, hepatoxicity, nausea, vomiting, mucositis, diarrhea, anorexia, hyperuricemia	Reduce dose when allopurinol is given concurrently
Thioguanine	80 mg/m²/d po	Nausea, vomiting, myelosuppression, anorexia, diarrhea, mucositis, hepatotoxicity	
5-Azacytacine (azacytidine)	150–300 mg/m² IV	Myelosuppression, nephrotoxicity, nausea, vomiting, increase in liver enzymes, lethargy, confusion	
Fludarabine	25 mg/m² IV	Pulmonary toxicity, headache, visual loss, seizures, neuropathy, myelosuppression, diarrhea, nausea, vomiting	Decreases CD-4 lymphocytes
Pentostatin	4 mg/m² IV	Nephrotoxicity, increase in liver enzymes, fever, confusion, nausea, vomiting, rash, myelosuppression, diarrhea	
Cladribine	4 mg/m² IV	Myelosuppression, nausea, vomiting, headache, paresthesia, fever, chills, pancreatitis	
Methotrexate	50 mg/m² q 7 d po 20–200 mg/m² IV q 7 d HD = 12 g/m² IV	Myelosuppression, mucositis, rash, nephrotoxicity, encephalopathy, seizures, nausea, vomiting, diarrhea, urticaria, pneumonitis, hepatictoxicity, photosensitivity, radiation recall	1 gm/m² or greater requires hydration, folinic acid rescue, and urine alkaline. HD requires simultaneous bicarb administration

HD = High dose

Continued

Table 4-2 **Chemotherapeutic Agents and Their Side Effects—cont'd**

Agent	Dose	Side Effect	Comments
Antitumor Antibiotic			
Bleomycin	5–15 units/m^2 IV, IM, SC	Pneumonitis, pulmonary toxicity, flulike syndrome, hyperkeratosis, mucositis, diarrhea, nausea, vomiting, alopecia, hyperpigmentation	Test dose may be given in lymphoma patients. Lifetime cumulative dose: 440 u/m^2
Dactinomycin	500 mg/d IV for 5 d 1–2 mg/m^2 IV q 3 wks	Myelosuppression, mucositis, alopecia, flulike syndrome, radiation recall, nausea, vomiting, extravasation, acne, hypocalcemia	Vesicant
Daunorubicin	30–75 mg/d IV for 3 d	Myelosuppression, cardiotoxicity, red urine, nausea, vomiting, extravasation, mucositis, alopecia, radiation recall, diarrhea, hepatotoxicity	Vesicant. Cumulative lifetime dose: 600 mg/m^2
Doxorubicin	60–75 mg/m^2 IV q 3 wks 20 mg/m^2/wk	Myelosuppression, cardiotoxicity, red urine, mucositis, nausea, vomiting, alopecia, extravasation, radiation recall, hyperpigmentation, hepatotoxicity	Vesicant. Cumulative lifetime dose: 550 mg/m^2
Mitomycin-C	10–20 mg/m^2 IV q 6–8 wks	Myelosuppression, nausea, vomiting, purple urine, extravasation, malaise, nephrotoxicity, mucositis, alopecia, fever, pulmonary fibrosis	Vesicant
Plicamycin	25 mg/kg IV q 3–4 d	Myelosuppression, hypocalcemia, nausea, vomiting, extravasation, metallic taste, mucositis, headaches, confusion, nephrotoxicity, fever, hepatotoxicity	Vesicant. Contraindicated in patients with coagulation disorders
Mitoxantrone	12–14 mg/m^2 IV q 3 wks	Myelosuppression, mucositis, alopecia, cardiotoxicity, blue-green urine, nausea, vomiting, hyperpigmentation	
Idarubicin	18–25 mg/m^2 IV 45–60 mg/m^2	Myelosuppression, alopecia, anorexia, nausea, vomiting, cardiotoxicity, mucositis, radiation recall, extravasation	Vesicant
Hormones			
Flutamide (antiandrogen)	250 mg po tid	Abdominal cramps, gynecomastia, diarrhea	
Leuprolide (luteinizing hormone–releasing hormone)	1 mg/d SC or IV	Hot flashes, bone pain, peripheral edema, nausea, vomiting	

Drug	Dose	Toxicity	Comments
Fluoxymestrone (androgen)	10–30 mg po q d	Nausea, vomiting, edema, hair growth on face and body	
Diethylstilbestrol (estrogen)	1–3 mg po q d (prostate) 1–5 mg po tid (breast)	Nausea, vomiting, edema, hot flashes, enlarged tender breasts, uterine bleeding, hypercalcemia	
Premarin (estrogen)	1.25–2.5 mg tid po (prostate) 10 mg tid po (breast)	Nausea, vomiting, edema, hot flashes, enlarged tender breasts, uterine bleeding, hypercalcemia	
Prednisone (corticosteroid)	20–100 mg/m² /d po for 5 d	Myelosuppression, gastric irritation, edema, anxiety, mood alteration, hyperglycemia, acne, insomnia	Long-term use must taper before discontinuing
Tamoxifen (antiestrogen)	10 mg po bid	Menopausal symptoms, nausea, uterine bleeding, bone pain, headaches, hot flashes, hypercalcemia	Monitor for vaginal bleeding. Recommend annual gynecologic exam for uterine cancer
Megestrol (progestin)	80 mg po bid 160 mg po q d	Edema, carpal tunnel syndrome, deep vein thrombosis, increased appetite	Crosses blood-brain barrier
Nitrosoureas Lomustine	130 mg/m² po q 6 wks	Myelosuppression, nausea, vomiting, mucositis, alopecia, nephrotoxicity, hepatotoxicity	Administer on empty stomach
Streptozocin	500 mg/m²/d IV for 5 d q 6 wks	Myelosuppression, nausea, vomiting, painful administration, diarrhea, nephrotoxicity, altered glucose metabolism	Irritant. Monitor blood-glucose level
Carmustine	200 mg/m² IV q 6–8 wks	Myelosuppression, pneumonitis, nausea, vomiting, pulmonary toxicity, nephrotoxicity, painful infusion, hyperpigmentation, photosensitivity, encephalopathy, confusion	Irritant. Diluent with alcohol
Hexamethylmelamine	150 mg/m² po 4–12 mg/kg IV	Confusion, ataxia, depression, peripheral neuropathy, diarrhea, myelosuppression, nausea, vomiting	Vitamin B may decrease neurotoxicity
Semustine	150–200 mg/m² po	Myelosuppression, nausea, vomiting, nephrotoxicity, pulmonary fibrosis	Administer on empty stomach

Continued

Table 4-2   Chemotherapeutic Agents and Their Side Effects—cont'd

Agent	Dose	Side Effect	Comments
Vinca Alkaloids			
Etoposide	50–100 mg/m² IV for 3–5 d q 4 wks HD = 800–2400 mg/m² IV	Myelosuppression, alopecia, fever, broncospasm, hypotension, chills, nausea, vomiting, anorexia, mucositis, encephalopathy, periperal neuropathy	Irritant. Rapid infusion >60 min. causes bronchospasm and hypotension
Vinblastine	4–6 mg/m² IV q wk .3 mg/kg IV q 3 wks	Myelosuppression, neurotoxicity, constipation, extravasation, nausea, vomiting, alopecia, mental depression	Vesicant. Decreases the effect of phenytoin
Vincristine	1.4 mg/m²/wk IV	Neurotoxicity, myelosuppression, extravasation, jaw pain, mental depression, anorexia, diplopia, alopecia, constipation	Vesicant
Paclitaxel	200–250 mg/m² IV	Neurotoxicity, hypotension, mucositis, nausea, vomiting, dyspnea, myalgia, myelosuppresion, cardiac arrhythmia, alopecia	Vesicant with HD. Administer with polyethylene tubing
Teniposide	50–130 mg/m² IV	Myelosuppression, nausea, vomiting, diarrhea, peripheral neuropathy, anaphylaxis, alopecia	Hypotension with rapid infusion
Vindesine	3–4 mg/m² IV	Neurotoxicity, nausea, vomiting, alopecia, myelosuppression, mucositis, diarrhea, erythematous maculopapular rash	Vesicant
Vinorelbine	30 mg/m² IV 80 mg/m² po	Myelosuppression, nausea, vomiting, alopecia, elevation in liver enzymes, neurotoxicity, dyspnea	Vesicant
Miscellaneous Agents			
Aminoglutethimide	250 mg/q 6 h po	Drowsiness, cytopenia, skin rash, anorexia, adrenal insufficiency, thyroid suppression	May need steroid replacement
Asparaginase	6000 IU/m² q o d for 3–4 wks	Somnolence, confusion, neurotoxicity, nausea, vomiting, fever, malaise, hypoalbuminemia, anaphylaxis	Incidence of anaphylaxis increases with subsequent doses
Procarbazine	100 mg/m² po, d1 and 14 of 28	Myelosuppression, nausea, vomiting, stomatitis, diarrhea, myalgia, arthralgia, encephalopathy	Interacts with MAO inhibitors or food with tyramine
Mitotane	2–6 gm/d po 9–10 gm/d po	Adrenal insufficiency, anorexia, nausea, vomiting, diarrhea, lethargy, depression, sedation, vertigo, ataxia, visual disturbances0	May need steroid replacement

Investigational Agents

Diaziquone (alkylating)	To be determined	Nephrotoxicity, myelosuppression, stomatitis, nausea, vomiting, increase in liver enzymes
Acivicin (antimetabolite)	To be determined, IV	Headache, confusion, ataxia, aphasia, neurotoxicity
Trimetrexate (antimetabolite)	8–12 mg/m² IV	Myelosuppression, stomatitis, nausea, vomiting, diarrhea, hypoalbuminemia
Epirubicin (antitumor antibiotic)	85–90 mg/m² q 3 wks IV	Nausea, vomiting, myelosuppression, mucositis, fever, alopecia
Amsacrine	90–150 mg/m² IV	Mucositis, nausea, vomiting, diarrhea, burning sensation upon administration, orange-red urine, cardiotoxicity, vertigo, headaches — Vesicant
Topotecan	1.3–1.6 mg/m² IV	Myelosuppression, nausea, vomiting, diarrhea, mucositis, alopecia, elevated liver enzymes, headaches, peripheral neuropathy

The responsibility for administering chemotherapy most frequently is that of the registered nurse. Special considerations include safe handling, vesicant administration, and anaphylaxis.

Safe Handling

Chemotherapeutic agents may be (1) *mutagenic,* able to change genetic material and pass on mutations through the process of cell replication; (2) *carcinogenic,* able to cause the development of cancer; and (3) *teratogenic,* able to cause fetal abnormality. Health care providers can be directly exposed to these agents while preparing or administering the drugs or while caring for the patient who has received the drugs through contact with the patient's body fluids. Uptake may occur by absorption through the skin, inhalation of drug aerosols, ingestion of drug droplets, or inoculation by exposed needles. The degree of uptake is measured by nonspecific biologic markers such as urine mutagenicity and sister-chromatid-exchange studies. Although the results of studies utilizing these measures are conflicting (Cloak et al., 1985; Falck et al., 1979; Hoffman, 1983; Waksvik, Klepp, and Brogge, 1981) and the link between actual health hazards and exposure to these agents is not well established, it is prudent to follow protective measures whenever there is the potential for exposure. Guidelines for protective behavior are issued by the Occupational Safety and Health Administration (Office of Occupational Medicine, 1986), the Oncology Nursing Society (ONS, 1989), and the American Society of Hospital Pharmacists (ASHP, 1993). Personnel dealing with these agents should be taught safe handling procedures and later receive periodic updates on current trends and research.

Vesicant Administration

Parenteral chemotherapy drugs can be divided into three categories: vesicants, irritants, and nonvesicants. A *vesicant* is a drug that can cause tissue necrosis when it leaks out of the vein or infiltrates the subcutaneous tissue. An *irritant* may cause achiness, burning, or phlebitis at the injection site or along the vein tract with or without a self-limiting inflammation (Table 4-3).

The detrimental consequences of tissue damage are possible physical or functional deformity. There are pharmacologic and nonpharmacologic ways to manage vesicants. Perhaps the most beneficial aspect of vesicant management is awareness and prevention. Procedures and policies that decrease the likelihood of extravasation include the following:

♦ Administration of vesicants by trained oncology registered nurses.
♦ Constant monitoring of the infusion site to assure minimum extravasation risk and immediate recognition of site changes.
♦ Cooperation and education of the patient to maintain stabilization of the site of injection and to report promptly any changes in feeling or sensation at the injection site.
♦ The appropriate use of venous access devices. The use of venous access devices provides more durable and reliable venous access but is not without risk of extravasation.

Table 4-3 Nursing Assessment of Extravasation Versus Other Reactions

Assessment Parameter	Extravasation		Irritation of the Vein	Flare Reaction
	Immediate Manifestations of Extravasation	Delayed Manifestations of Extravasation		
Pain	Severe pain or burning that lasts minutes or hours and eventually subsides; usually occurs while the drug is being given and around the injection site	Up to 48 hours	Aching and tightness along the vein	No pain
Redness	Blotchy redness around the injection site; it is not always present at time of extravasation	Later occurrence	The full length of the vein may be reddened or darkened	Immediate blotches or streaks along the vein, which usually subside within 30 minutes with or without treatment
Ulceration	Develops insidiously; usually occurs 48–96 hours later	Later occurrence	Not usually	Not usually
Swelling	Severe swelling; usually occurs immediately	Up to 48 hours	Not likely	Not likely; wheals may appear along vein line
Blood return	Inability to obtain blood return	Good blood return during drug administration	Usually	Usually
Other	Change in the quality of infusion	Local tingling and sensory deficits	—	Urticaria

From Oncology Nursing Society: Cancer chemotherapy guidelines. Recommendations for the management of vesicant extravasation, hypersensitivity, and ana-phylaxis, Pittsburgh, 1992, Oncology Nursing Society, p. 11.

Antidotes may help control some vesicant extravasations. For example, sodium thiosulfate is recommended for mechlorethamine extravasation and hyaluronidase is recommended for vincristine or vinblastine extravasation (Oncology Nursing Society, 1992).

Several of the chemotherapeutic agents are irritants; that is, they may cause pain or a burning sensation at the injection site and along the vein during administration. An irritant reaction is similar to the complaints many patients have during peripheral potassium infusions or high pH antibiotic infusion such as nafcillin and erythromycin. Irritant chemotherapeutic agents such as carmustine and dacarbazine can be diluted in 250 to 500 ccs, the infusion rate can be slowed when the patient complains of discomfort, a second intravenous line can further dilute the drug, and a steroid, usually hydrocortisone, can be added to the chemotherapy regimen to decrease or eliminate irritation.

A distressing but not serious reaction that may be associated with the administration of chemotherapy (usually doxorubicin) is a "flare" reaction. A *flare reaction* is characterized by complaint of itching above the injection site with or without the appearance of blotchy, hivelike lesions along the track of the vein. There is typically no swelling at the injection site and no pain, and there is a blood return present. The distress comes from the concern that the drug has extravasated. Comparing and contrasting the symptoms should alleviate the nurse's concern about extravasation. Use of the drug should be stopped and intravenous fluid infused until the reaction subsides. If the symptoms are severe, administration of an antihistamine may resolve any hivelike areas and alleviate the itching.

Anaphylaxis

Some individuals may experience anaphylactoid reactions, most notably with asparaginase, bleomycin, and paclitaxel. Signs and symptoms range from dyspnea, bronchospasm, and hypotension to less severe reactions like agitation, pruritus, urticaria, rash, and diaphoresis. Test doses are sometimes given before a full dose of asparaginase or bleomycin. These test doses may be administered as an intradermal injection, which is then monitored for redness and swelling at the test site, or as an injection of 1 to 2 units subcutaneously, intramuscularly, or intravenously. The patient is then monitored from 1 to 24 hours for any sign of reaction prior to administering the full dose. Premedication with dexamethasone, diphenhydramine, and cimetidine have successfully controlled or prevented the hypersensitivity reaction for most individuals receiving paclitaxel. Lengthening the infusion time may decrease the need for premedication for some individuals (Dorr and Von Hoff, 1994).

❖ Summary

Effective patient care begins with knowledge about chemotherapy. Prevention or assessment and management of side effects, the safe handling of drugs, recognition of extravasation, and quick action during anaphylaxis are essential roles of the chemotherapy nurse.

❖ References

American Society of Hospital Pharmacists: ASHP technical assistance bulletin on handling cytotoxic and hazardous drugs. In Practice Standards of ASHP, 1993–1994, Bethesda, MD, 1993, American Society of Hospital Pharmacists.

Bender B: Implications of antineoplastic therapy for nursing. In Clark JC and McGee RF, editors: Oncology Nursing Society: core curriculum for oncology nursing, ed 2, Philadelphia, 1992, WB Saunders Co, pp. 329–340.

Cloak MM, Connor TH, Stevens JC, Alt JM, Matney TS, and Anderson RW: Occupational exposure of nursing personnel to antineoplastic agents, Oncol Nurs Forum 12:33–39, 1985.

DeVita VT Jr.: Principles of chemotherapy. In DeVita VT Jr., Hellman S, and Rosenberg SA, editors: Cancer: principles and practice of oncology, ed 4, Philadelphia, 1993, JB Lippincott Co, pp. 276–292.

Dorr RT and Von Hoff DD: Cancer chemotherapy handbook, ed 2, Norwalk, Connecticut, 1994, Appleton & Lange.

Falck K, Grohn P, Sorsa M, Vainio H, Heinonen E, and Holsti LR: Mutagenicity in urine of nurses handling cytostatic drugs, Lancet 1:1250–1251, 1979.

Hoffman D: Lack of urine mutagenicity of nurses administering pharmacy-prepared doses of antineoplastic agents, Am J Intravenous Therapy Clin Nutrition 10(8): 29–31, 1983.

Holleb AI, Fink DJ, and Murphy GP: Textbook of clinical oncology, Atlanta, 1991, American Cancer Society.

Krakoff IH: Cancer chemotherapeutic and biologic agents. CA- Cancer J Clin 41:264–278, 1991.

Office of Occupational Medicine, Occupational Safety and Health Administration: Work practice guidelines for personnel dealing with cytotoxic (antineoplastic) drugs, OSHA Instruction Pub 8-1.1, Washington, DC, 1986, US Department of Labor.

Oncology Nursing Society: Cancer chemotherapy guidelines: recommendations for the management of vesicant extravasation, hypersensitivity, and anaphylaxis, module IV, Pittsburgh, 1992, Oncology Nursing Society.

Oncology Nursing Society: Safe handling of cytotoxic drugs: independent study module, Pittsburgh, 1989, Oncology Nursing Society.

Ratain MJ: Therapeutic relevance of pharmacokinetics and pharmacodynamics, Semin Oncol 19(Suppl 11): 8–13, 1992

Waksvik H, Klepp O, and Brogge: Chromosome analyses of nurses handling cytostatic agents, Cancer Treat Rep 65:607–610, 1981.

Weiss GR: Clinical oncology, Norwalk, Connecticut, 1993, Appleton & Lange.

Chapter 5

❖ *Biotherapy*

Debra Wujcik

After deoxyribonucleic acid (DNA) was identified in 1953 and studied in the laboratory, researchers began to explore how to manipulate it. This led to the development of recombinant DNA technology in the 1980s. *Recombinant* refers to the recombination of sequences from different DNA molecules into a new strand. In the laboratory, a gene for a particular protein is selected and extracted. It is then inserted into a strand of DNA from another organism such as a bacterium, which then becomes a "protein factory" that continues to produce protein identical to the original molecule (Jaramilla, 1992). Through this process a desired protein such as the biological agent interferon can be produced in large quantities in the laboratory, even though it may be scarce in nature. This ability has resulted in the development of many new biological tools to treat patients with cancer.

The technological advances of the 1980s brought the use of immune-system regulating agents back to the forefront. *Biological response modifiers* (BRMs) are agents or approaches that use mechanisms of action involving the patient's own biological responses. A list of BRMs and possible side effects are shown in Table 5-1. *Biotherapy* is the use of agents that affect biological responses or that are produced from biological (living) sources.

❖ *Mechanism of Action*

Biotherapy agents have several different and sometimes overlapping mechanisms of action (Figure 5-1) (Wujcik, 1993). All BRMs affect the cells of the immune system in some way. Some agents affect the host's immune function. Some such as tumor necrosis factor have direct activity against the tumor. Other agents do not have an anticancer effect but express biological effects that support the patient undergoing cancer treatment. Still other agents interfere with the transformation of normal cells into malignant cells or the ability of the tumor to metastasize (Borden and Sondel, 1990; Dutcher, 1992).

Table 5-1   Side Effects of Biological Response Modifiers

Agent	Alteration in hematological lab values	Alteration in mental status	Anaphylaxis	Anorexia	Bone pain	Bronchospasm	Capillary leak syndrome	Chills	Desquamation	Diarrhea	Edema, peripheral	Edema, pulmonary	Fever	Fluid retention	Flushing	Headache	Hives	Hypotension	Liver enzymes	Mucositis	Myalgias	Nausea	Pruritis	Rash	Tachycardia	Weight loss	Weight gain	Other Side Effects
Interferon-α and -β	+	O	R	+	O	R	R	+	R	O	R	R	+	R	O	+	R	O	+	R	+	O	O	O	O	+	R	Fever dissipates after first week
Interferon-γ	+	O	R	+	O	R	R	+	R	O	R	R	+	R	O	+	R	+	+	R	+	O	O	O	O	+	R	Fever higher and more persistent
GM-CSF**	+	O	R	O	O	R	O	O*	R	O	R	R	+	R	O	O	O	O†	R	R	O	O	O	O	O	O	O	Erythema at injection site
G-CSF**	+	R	R	O	O	R	R	R	R	R	R	R	R	R	O	O	R	R	O	O	R	R	R	O	R	O	R	
Monoclonal antibodies	O	R	O	O	R	O	R	O	R	R	R	R	O	O	O	O	O	O	O	R	R	R	R	O	R	O	R	Side effects depend on what is attached
Tumor necrosis factor	+	O	R	+	R	R	R	+	R	O	R	R	+	R	R	+	R	O	O	R	+	O	O	R	O	+	R	Severe rigors
Interleukin-2	+	O	R	+	R	R	+	+	O	+	+	O	+	+	+	+	R	+	+	O	+	+	+	+	+	+	+	Weight gain during treatment and weight loss (occurs over time due to decrease in appetite)

*Dose-dependent; as dose increases, chills are more regularly seen preceding fever.
**GM-CSF = Granulocyte-macrophage colony-stimulating factor; G-CSF = granulocyte colony-stimulating factor
†Patients may exhibit 10–20 mm decreases in systolic blood pressure; however, symptomatic hypotension is generally seen at higher doses given intravenously.
+ = Common; O = Occasional; R = Rare
Reprinted with permission from Rumsey KA and Rieger PT, editors: Biological response modifiers: a self-instructional manual for health professionals, Chicago, 1992, Precept Press.

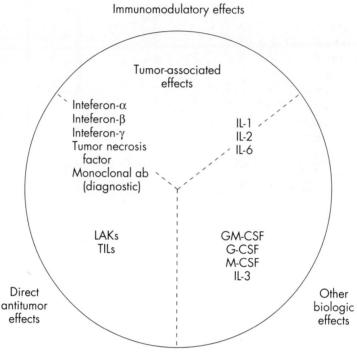

Fig. 5-1. Mechanism of action of biotherapy drugs. Reprinted with permission from Wujcik D: An odyssey into biologic therapy, Oncol Nurs Forum 20:879–997, 1993.

There are two main groups of biotherapy agents: cytokines and antibodies. Although many agents in these groups are being evaluated in clinical studies, only a few have been approved by the Food and Drug Administration (FDA) for clinical use. However, the rapid development of these agents will result in the clinical use of many more in the near future.

❖ *Cytokines*

A cytokine is one of a number of complicated proteins that regulate cells. These proteins are produced by activated cells of the immune system that govern the functioning of the immune system and that affect the actions of other cells. Cell biologists have identified more than 25 cytokines. Earlier researchers thought these cells were produced by lymphocytes and thus were named *lymphokines*. Other cells are produced by monocytes and are called *monokines*. *Cytokine* is the broader name that includes all of these chemical messengers (Rumsey and Rieger, 1992). Cytokines have multiple functions, some of which overlap, whereas others conflict. Often a ripple effect occurs; when one cytokine is produced, it stimulates several others.

Natural cytokines occur in limited quantities, but the development of recombinant or synthetic cytokines has allowed the production of large enough quantities for researchers to study the effects of cytokines on tumors in large numbers of patients. The most widely used cytokines are interferons (IFN), interleukins (IL), hematopoietic growth factors (HGF), and tumor necrosis factor (TNF).

Interferons

Interferons are the model of discovery and development for all other biotherapy agents. Natural IFN is the body's first line of defense against viruses (Isaacs and Lindenmen, 1957). Lymphocytes produce interferons in response to stimulation by a virus. Interferons have a variety of actions, including both antiviral and antitumor effects.

Classification
Two types of IFN have been identified: Type I and Type II. *Type I IFN* includes alpha (α) and beta (β) varieties. Each of these binds to the same receptor on an infected cell. *Type II,* or gamma (γ) IFN, binds to a separate cell surface receptor (Figlin, 1989). A number of white blood cells (B-cells, T-cells, null cells, and macrophages) produce IFN-α after being exposed to antigens such as viruses, foreign cells, or tumor cells. Fibroblasts exposed to viruses or foreign nucleic acids produce IFN-β. IFN-γ is produced by T-lymphocytes that have been stimulated by antigens or by another cytokine, interleukin-2.

Mechanism of Action
In cancer, IFNs work by slowing cell replication. The normal cell cycle is prolonged as protein synthesis and DNA production are inhibited. IFNs can also stimulate a host immune response by enhancing the activity of natural killer (NK) cells. Other proteins are released when IFN is produced, causing side effects such as fever and chills. Although the exact mechanism of action of IFN is not known, it seems clear that the action varies with changes in dosage and depends on the disease being treated (Dutcher, 1992).

Administration Issues
IFN is administered in a variety of dosages and by different routes to treat indications such as those shown in Table 5-2. Side effects and pharmacologic action are clearly dose dependent (Moldawer and Figlin, 1995). The most frequent acute side effects include fever, chills, malaise, headache, and anorexia. Nausea, vomiting, and diarrhea can also be acute but occur less frequently. Chronic fatigue and weight loss tend to be the most problematic side effects because they can interfere with continued therapy. Many side effects can be controlled by giving acetaminophen before the administration of IFN therapy. However, if severe chronic fatigue sets in, a reduction of the dose of IFN may be required.

Table 5-2   Dosages, Routes, and Indications of Interferon

Generic Name	Indication	Dose	Route
Interferon-alfa-b	Hairy-cell leukemia	2 MIU/m² 3x/wk	SC/IM
	Chondyloma acuminata	10 MIU/1 cc 3x/wk Inject 0.1 cc per lesion 3x/wk for 3 wks	Intralesional
	Hepatitis B	30–35 MIU/wk as 5 MIU/day or 10 MIU 3x/wk for 16 wks	SC/IM
	Hepatitis non-A, non-B/C	3 MIU 3x/wk	SC/IM
Interferon-alfa-2a	Hairy-cell leukemia	3 MIU q d for 16–24 wks	SC/IM
	Kaposi's sarcoma	36 MIU q d 3x/wk for 10–12 wks	SC/IM
Interferon-alfa-n3	Condyloma acuminata	250,000 IU/wart 2x/wk for up to 8 wks	Intralesional
Interferon-gamma-1b	Chronic granulomatous disease	1.5 MIU/m² 3x/wk	SC
Interferon-beta-1b	Multiple sclerosis	8 MIU q 48 hours	SC

M = Million; I = International; U = Units; SC = Subcutaneous; IM = Intramuscular; q = Every; d = Day

Patients receiving higher dosages of IFN may experience more severe side effects such as hypotension, tachycardia, somnolence, confusion, and peripheral neuropathies. These patients require more intense monitoring with frequent assessment by the health care team.

Clinical Applications

There are multiple clinical uses for IFN in cancer care and with other viral diseases. Clinical trials with malignant diseases such as renal cell carcinoma, malignant melanoma, colon cancer, and lymphoma are under way. There are many studies evaluating combinations of IFN with cytotoxic chemotherapy or with other biologic agents (Dutcher, 1992). IFN is currently used with 5-fluorouracil, cisplatin, doxorubicin, cyclophosphamide, and vincristine to treat a variety of tumors. In addition, some oncologists combine IFN-α with interleukin-2, IFN-γ, or monoclonal antibodies to treat malignant melanoma or renal cell cancer.

Interleukins

The term *interleukin* (IL) describes molecules that send signals between leukocytes. More simply, ILs are chemical messengers. The ILs can produce an effect in the same cell that produced the IL, in nearby cells, and occasionally in distant cells. At this time, biochemists have identified 12 interleukins, which they numbered in the order of discovery. Each IL may have both an action unique to itself and an action shared by one or more of the other ILs. Interleukin-2 (IL-2) is the only FDA-approved IL, to date, although IL-1, IL-3, IL-4, and IL-6 are currently being evaluated in human trials.

Interleukin-2 (IL-2)

IL-2 was first described in 1976 as a lymphokine secreted by helper T-lymphocytes that had been activated (stimulated) by an antigen. Subsequent studies proved that IL-2 is produced when T-cells recognize foreign antigens.

MECHANISM OF ACTION.   IL-2 prompts the growth and maturation of more T-lymphocytes and activates NK cells and monocytes (Boldt and Ellis, 1993). Two subsets of cells that are produced in response to IL-2 stimulation are lymphokine-activated killer (LAK) cells and tumor-infiltrating lymphocytes (TILs) (Grimm, 1993). After stimulation by IL-2, lymphocytes become highly cytotoxic and transform into LAK cells. These LAK cells and TILs kill tumor cells directly. However, TILs found in tumors are 100 times more active than LAK cells (Siegel and Puri, 1991; Batchelor, 1992).

ADMINISTRATION ISSUES.   IL-2 has multiple side effects, depending on the dose, but they usually resolve once the drug is discontinued. Low-dose therapy (up to 18 million IU/day) is well tolerated as an outpatient therapy, whereas high-dose therapy (600,000 IU/kg every 8 hours) requires intense monitoring. Cardiovascular toxicity with capillary-leak syndrome is common at high dosages and may require intensive-care monitoring (Sargent and Shelton, 1990).

CLINICAL APPLICATIONS.   The FDA approved recombinant IL-2, or aldesleukin, for treatment of renal cell carcinoma in May 1992, and current studies of IL-2 focus on the treatment of malignant melanoma, colon and breast cancer, and lymphoma. IL-2 can be administered in an intravenous bolus, by continuous infusion, or by subcutaneous injection, and in combination with LAK cells, IFN, and a variety of chemotherapeutic agents as well (Sharp, 1995).

Interleukin-1 (IL-1)

IL-1 influences cells involved in immunity, wound healing, the inflammatory response, and hematopoiesis (Dinarello and Wolff, 1993). IL-1 can modify some of the toxicity seen with IL-2 therapy (Dutcher, 1992). Activated monocytes and macrophages release IL-1, which stimulates release of neutrophils. In addition, increased muscle breakdown occurs, causing the release of amino acids for formation of new proteins (such as immunoglobulin, B-lymphocytes, and T-cell activation) (Kuby, 1992).

IL-1 has shown antitumor activity in several end-stage malignancies. In addition, preclinical studies have shown that IL-1 can stimulate production of hematopoietic growth factors (HGFs), granulocyte-macrophage colony-stimulating factor, monocyte colony-stimulating factor, and IL-6, which accelerate the recovery of neutrophils and platelets after chemotherapy and radiation therapy, and which protect the marrow if given before treatment (Castelli et al., 1988). IL-1 is the only interleukin that clinically demonstrates such an effect on platelet recovery after chemotherapy (Smith et al., 1993; Vadhan Raj et al., 1994).

The toxic side effects of IL-1 include fever, chills, rigor, flulike syndrome, tachycardia, nausea, vomiting, headache, myalgia, hypotension, and erythema at the injection site (Smith et al., 1992).

Interleukin-3 (IL-3)

IL-3 is technically an interleuken but functions more like a hematopoietic growth factor (HGF). IL-3 will be discussed later in this chapter (see p. 82).

Interleukin-4 (IL-4)

IL-4 is a B-cell regulator produced by activated T-lymphocytes. In vitro, IL-4 stimulates the growth of resting B-cells, increases production of immunoglobulin, and seems to stimulate certain T-lymphocytes. This cytokine also functions like an HGF and may stimulate growth or maturation of mast cells.

IL-4 has been administered to patients with a variety of tumors by intravenous bolus, continuous infusion, or subcutaneous injection. The most common side effects observed in clinical trials are fever, headache, nausea, vomiting, diarrhea, anorexia, fatigue, capillary-leak syndrome, weight gain, dyspnea, and nasal congestion (Sharp, 1995).

Taylor, Grogan, and Salmon (1990) conducted clinical trials combining IL-4 with IL-2. Results show that IL-4 inhibits IL-2 activity when given simultaneously but that the combination acts synergistically when the IL-4 is given sequentially 2 to 4 days after the IL-2.

Interleukin-6 (IL-6)

IL-6 promotes communication between cells of the bone marrow and the immune system. IL-6 is produced by IL-1 and tumor necrosis factor. There is evidence that IL-6 may have several actions: stimulation of platelet production, stimulation of a growth factor for myeloma cells, and destruction of malignant breast cancer and leukemia cells (Dutcher, 1992; Niewig, 1992).

Hematopoietic Growth Factors

Hematopoietic growth factors (HGFs) are chemical messengers in the hematopoietic cascade. More specifically, they are hormonelike proteins produced in the body that regulate the proliferation (reproduction) and differentiation (maturation) of blood cells. HGFs were formerly called colony-stimulating factors (CSFs) because each one seemed to produce a specific colony of cells. The four classic CSFs are granulocyte-CSF, granulocyte-macrophage-CSF, erythropoietin, and interleukin-3. Because they are now considered part of a larger family of blood cell regulators, they are called HGFs (Wujcik, 1995).

Classification

HGFs are classified as multilineage (affecting several different cell lineages) or lineage-restricted (affecting only one lineage). They bind to specific receptors on the surface of the cell membrane, and each HGF receptor appears to accept only one type of HGF in the same way that a specific key fits only one lock. However, receptors for more than one type of CSF may be available.

Mechanism of Action

The direct activity of a specific HGF begins with the binding of the HGF to the cell-surface receptor. The HGF protein and receptor are then taken into the cell.

This complex gives instructions to the cell either to divide to produce more cells or to mature into a fully functional cell. The remaining cell-surface receptors specific for the HGF are inactivated.

Some multilineage HGFs also initiate indirect actions. That is, other cytokines such as tumor necrosis factor or IL-2 may be produced as well. These additional cytokines cause more side effects.

Clinical Applications

Table 5-3 shows the current clinical indications for HGFs, along with their treatment dosages and routes of administration. For patients receiving myelosuppressive chemotherapy, a common problem is a low count of white blood cells (WBC). HGFs can shorten the length and decrease the severity of the nadir (period of low WBC) (Crawford et al., 1991; Herrmann et al., 1990). HGFs can hasten engraftment of bone marrow cells for patients undergoing bone marrow transplantation (Nemunaitis et al., 1988; Taylor et al., 1989). HGFs are used in peripheral stem cell transplantation to control the timing and volume of marrow cell release to ensure an adequate collection of the peripheral cells (Sheridan et al., 1990).

HGFs play a unique role in differentiation therapy for myelodysplastic disorders. In this disease, the cells do not mature to a fully functional state, and there is cellular arrest along the cell line. The HGFs can restimulate the maturation process (Demetri and Antman, 1992; Thompson et al., 1989).

HGFs are also given to patients with acute leukemia before chemotherapy. The goal of this approach is to recruit a maximum number of cells into the active cell cycle, where the chemotherapy is most effective in killing tumor cells (Buchner et al., 1991; Ohno, Tomonoaga, and Kogayashi, 1990).

Table 5-3   Dosages, Routes, and Indications of Hematopoietic Growth Factors

Generic Name	Indication	Dose	Route
Filgrastim	Chemotherapy-associated neutropenia in patients with nonmyeloid malignancy	5 mcg/kg/d for 14 d	SC
	Patients with prolonged myelosuppression after bone marrow transplant		
Sargramostim	Autologous bone marrow transplant	250 mcg/kg/d for 21 d	IV
Epoetin alfa	Anemia in patients with dialysis-dependent end-stage renal disease	50–100 U/kg 3x/wk	IV
	Anemia in cancer patients on chemotherapy	150 U/kg 3x/wk	SC/IV
	Anemia in AZT-treated HIV-infected patients	100 U/kg 3x/wk for 8 wks	SC/IV

U = Units; SC = Subcutaneous; IV = Intravenous

Approved HGFs

There are three HGFs currently approved by the FDA for clinical use. They are granulocyte-CSF (G-CSF), granulocyte-macrophage-CSF (GM-CSF), and erythropoietin (EPO).

Granulocyte-CSF (G-CSF) is a lineage-restricted HGF that stimulates neutrophil production and maturation. It promotes the functional activity of mature cells, including enhanced phagocytosis and cellular metabolism, increased antibody-dependent killing, and increased antigen processing (Crosier and Clark, 1992; Wujcik, 1993).

Recombinant G-CSF, filgrastim, was approved in 1991 for treating patients with nonmyeloid malignancy who receive myelosuppressive chemotherapy. Filgrastim reduces the severity and length of myelosuppression (lower blood counts) after chemotherapy. This may prevent infection, allowing the patient to tolerate higher doses of chemotherapy. G-CSF is usually well tolerated; bone pain is the most common side effect. Monitoring of the patient begins with a baseline complete blood count (CBC) and platelet count, which are then repeated twice weekly.

Granulocyte-macrophage colony-stimulating factor (GM-CSF) is a multilineage HGF that stimulates proliferation and differentiation of multiple cell lines, specifically, neutrophils, eosinophils, and macrophages. Like G-CSF, GM-GSF can enhance the functional activity of mature neutrophils, macrophages, and eosinophils (Demetri and Antman, 1992).

Recombinant GM-CSF, sargramostim, approved by the FDA in 1991, accelerates myeloid recovery in selected patients undergoing autologous bone marrow transplantation for non–Hodgkin's lymphoma, Hodgkin's disease, and acute lymphocytic leukemia. GM-CSF can cause diarrhea, rash, and malaise. Patient monitoring begins with a baseline CBC, followed twice weekly with a CBC, a differential cell count, a platelet count, and a reticulocyte count.

Recombinant GM-CSF can be produced in yeast, bacteria, or mammalian cells (Wujcik, 1995). Sargramostim is produced in yeast and seems to be most like natural GM-CSF. Molgrastim is produced in *Escherichia coli* bacteria and is currently under investigation.

Erythropoietin (EPO) is an HGF that selectively acts on the early erythroid cells to stimulate maturation of red blood cells (Spivak, 1989). EPO was first used in transfusion-dependent patients with chronic renal failure on dialysis and in patients with HIV infection receiving myelosuppressive therapy. Recently clinicians have begun to use EPO in the treatment of anemia due to cancer or cancer therapy as well. An increase in hematocrit is expected 2 to 6 weeks after beginning therapy.

Investigational HGFs

Investigators are actively studying several HGFs in humans. These include interleukin-3 (IL-3), a protein called PIXY 321, macrophage-CSF (M-CSF), and stem cell factor (SCF).

Interleukin-3 has been called the multi-CSF because it acts on many immature cells within the hematopoietic cascade. IL-3 stimulates the production of neutrophils, erythrocytes, and megakaryocytes (Holzer, Seipelt, and Ganser, 1993), and it is synergistic with GM-CSF, G-CSF, and EPO. Other actions include the potentiation of IL-2, which then stimulates macrophages to produce IL-1, TNF, and IFN-γ, thereby causing a wide range of side effects.

PIXY 321 is a protein formed by combining IL-3 and GM-CSF. The combination has more effectiveness than either HGF alone. PIXY 321 is being studied in clinical trials at this time (Vadhan-Raj et al., 1993; Vadhan-Raj, 1994).

Macrophage-CSF (M-CSF) acts on both progenitor cells and mature cells to stimulate the production and activation of macrophages. It is produced by fibroblasts, monocytes, and macrophages and then stimulates other macrophages, increasing antibody-dependent cellular cytotoxicity. M-CSF is being studied in the treatment of invasive fungal infections, myelodysplasia, and melanoma (Nemunaitis et al., 1993; Weiner et al., 1993).

Stem cell factor (SCF), also known as mast cell factor, kit ligand, and steel factor, is an HGF that acts at the earliest level of the hematopoietic cascade (Bernstein and Kufe, 1992). In the laboratory, SCF stimulates the cell groups to grow larger and to have an increased number of cells when compared to those stimulated by IL-3 or GM-CSF. Also in the laboratory, when cell colonies are exposed to SCF alone, there is no growth, but in combination with IL-3, G-CSF, or GM-CSF, synergism occurs and the number and size of colonies increase.

SCF has several possible clinical uses. Researchers have proposed that the use of SCF would decrease the dosages required of other HGFs. SCF may also help restore bone marrow function more quickly after bone marrow transplantation or stimulate production of all blood cells from one marrow stem cell.

Tumor Necrosis Factor

Tumor necrosis factor (TNF) is a monokine that stimulates IL-1, IL-6, GM-CSF, and G-CSF production. TNF damages the blood supply of cancer cells while protecting normal cells. The exact mechanism of action is not clear. However, like the other cytokines, TNF binds to cell-surface antigens and then is taken into the cell (Frei and Spriggs, 1989).

Tumor necrosis factor is administered both locally to the tumor and intravenously. The side effects of TNF appear similar to those associated with IFNs and IL-2. Flulike syndrome with fever, chills, rigors, and headaches is common (Jassak, 1993). Side effects are dose-dependent and resolve quickly after the TNF is discontinued.

❖ Monoclonal Antibodies

Antibody therapy utilizes the normal functions of the immune system to treat cancer. If an antibody is made that responds to a specific antigen on a cell, therapy can be delivered directly to the cell. Kohler and Milstein developed this technique of hybridoma technology in 1975 (Milstein, 1980). In this process, tumor cells and normal lymphocytes are joined together. The resulting cells produce the same immunoglobulin as the parent cells and are called *monoclonal antibodies* (MoAbs).

Classification

Monoclonal antibodies can be used alone or in combination with other therapies (Jassak, 1993). Pure MoAbs are called *unconjugated* and are usually obtained from mice. *Immunoconjugates* are MoAbs combined with toxins such as ricin or diph-theria toxin, chemotherapeutic agents, or radioisotopes such as iodine to deliver the therapy directly to the target cell.

Mechanism of Action

Antibodies to a specific cancer are produced from a single cell line, or clone. These are directed against specific antigen markers on the cell surface. The MoAb binds to target antigens by identifying the antigen carried on the surface of a specific type of tumor cell. The MoAb then signals other cells to destroy the tumor by phagocytosis.

MoAbs are bound to a toxic agent such as a chemotherapeutic agent, a radioac-tive isotope, or another BRM in the laboratory (Dutcher, 1992). The MoAb is then injected into the patient, allowing delivery of the agent directly to tumor cells. Although the concept of monoclonal antibody therapy is promising, in reality there are problems with the technology. Normal cell antigens can also react to the MoAb. To be useful, the MoAb must recognize antigens present on the tumor only.

Clinical Applications

The FDA approved one MoAb (OncoScint) in 1992 for clinical use as an imaging agent to diagnose colorectal or ovarian cancer. A MoAb specific for the tumor is tagged with a radioisotope. When injected into the patient, the MoAb seeks out and binds to cancer cells. A gamma camera detects the radioactive substance and pinpoints the location and extent of the disease.

Other clinical uses for MoAbs include the diagnosis and histopathological clas-sification of hematologic malignancies, the imaging of tumor masses when radioiso-topes are attached, and the targeting of radiation therapy, chemotherapy, and biotherapy. In bone marrow transplantation, MoAbs purge the bone marrow of residual diseases, and they remove T-lymphocytes to decrease graft-versus-host dis-ease (Dillman, 1990).

❖ Nursing Considerations

Nurses must understand the mechanism of action and potential side effects of bio-therapy, whether utilized as a single therapy or in combination with other cancer treatment modalities. As in all aspects of oncology nursing, the nurse provides infor-mation and coaching to the patient and family to prevent or minimize side effects produced by the therapy.

Unit III provides an in-depth description of nursing assessment and nursing management of side effects. They are usually related to the dose of the agent and are said to be dose-dependent. However, unlike chemotherapy, the dose-dependent side effects of biotherapy are not cumulative, and there is not a maximum dose beyond which the patient no longer can receive therapy (Rieger, 1995). Side effects usually occur at the time of therapy, but they can also occur later in the therapy. Although side effects are generally reversible once therapy is discontinued, the impact on the patient's quality of life is not so easily reversed (Brophy and Sharp, 1991).

Fatigue

Patients receiving BRMs describe being drowsy and tired, having a lack of energy, and feeling weak and listless (Robinson and Posner, 1992). The sequelae of extreme fatigue are decreased appetite, an inability to perform the activities of daily living, decreased concentration, and a decreased sex drive. In some instances, patients may refuse to continue biotherapy due to the extreme fatigue.

Flulike Symptoms

Flulike symptoms of biotherapy include fever, chills, malaise, myalgia, and fatigue. The symptoms develop within hours of administration and may be decreased by administering BRMs later in the day or evening rather than in the morning (Janson et al., 1989).

Cardiopulmonary Effects

Cardiopulmonary effects are frequently associated with high doses of IL-2 and TNF. A variety of cardiac arrhythmias, such as sinus and ventricular tachycardia, premature ventricular contractions, atrial fibrillation, and heart block, can occur. These arrhythmias usually resolve without intervention.

Hypotension can occur any time during treatment with IL-2 and TNF due to capillary leak syndrome. This is a shift of intravascular fluid into interstitial space (Shelton and Sargent, 1990). Because of the risk of hypotension and fluid shifts with intermediate- and high-dose therapy, patients are often hospitalized. A weight gain ≥5% of pretreatment weight is considered a toxic side effect requiring aggressive management (Lotze and Rosenberg, 1991). A shift of fluid into the lungs easily develops into pulmonary complications.

Gastrointestinal Disorders

Gastrointestinal disorders such as nausea, vomiting, and diarrhea are most often associated with IL-2. Weight loss of 5% to 10% of body weight or greater is considered serious and warrants intervention with enteral feedings (Mayer et al., 1984). Stomatitis is also common with IL-2. Patients describe feeling as if the mucous membranes have been scalded by a hot drink.

Renal Toxicity

Renal toxicity evidenced by oliguria, anuria, proteinuria, and increased creatinine (Cr) and BUN is associated with IL-2 and IFNs. Results of a Cr test greater than 4.0 g/24 hours by the end of a 5-day infusion of IL-2 is not uncommon, although the Cr level usually returns rapidly to baseline at the conclusion of treatment (Hynes et al., 1990).

Mental Changes

Treatment with IL-2 and IFN can produce significant mental changes. Patients may experience a range of difficulties that include haziness, difficulty concentrating, mood changes, cognitive dysfunction, expressive aphasia, seizures, paranoia, and full-blown psychosis (Shelton and Sargent, 1990).

Integumentary Changes

Skin changes have been noted with the use of IL-2 and some HGFs, notably, GM-CSF. Patients may experience a mild erythema, causing a maculopapular rash. Diffuse erythema can cause a burning sensation and pruritus (Niewig, 1992). Inflammation at injection sites is common. Although the inflammatory response usually clears quickly, there can be residual nodules under the skin for several months, especially with IL-2 given subcutaneously.

❖ Summary

Biotherapy is the use of agents that affect biological responses or that are produced from biological (living) sources. There are many different biological agents under study in cancer care—some that demonstrate direct antitumor activity, some that show an ability to modify the immune response, and some that produce a desired biological response.

The nursing care of the patient receiving biotherapy is challenging and complex. Each of the biotherapy agents has unique actions and side effects. In general, side effects are dose-dependent and resolve after the therapy is discontinued.

❖ References

Batchelor D: International perspectives on the present and future use of interleukin-2 therapy, Oncol Nurs Forum 19:182–211, 1992.

Bernstein SH and Kufe DW: Future of basic/clinical hematopoiesis research in the era of hematopoietic growth factor availability, Semin Oncol 19:441–448, 1992.

Boldt D and Ellis T: Biologic effects of interleukin-2 administration on the immune system. In Atkins M and Mier J, editors: Therapeutic applications of interleukin-2, New York, 1993, Marcel Dekker, pp. 73–91.

Borden EC and Sondel PM: Lymphokines and cytokines as cancer treatment: immunotherapy realized, Cancer 65:800–814, 1990.

Brophy L and Sharp E: Physical symptoms of combination biotherapy: a quality of life issue, Oncol Nurs Forum 18:25–30, 1991.

Buchner T, Hidemann W, Koenigsmann M, Zuhlsdorf M, Wormann B, Boeckmann A, Greire EA, Inning G, Maschmeyer G, and Ludwig WD: Recombinant human granulocyte-macrophage colony-stimulating factor after chemotherapy in patients with acute myeloid leukemia at higher age or after relapse, Blood 78:1190–1197, 1991.

Castelli MP, Black PL, Schneider M, Pennington R, Abe F, and Talmadge JE: Protective, restorative, and therapeutic properties of recombinant human IL-1 in rodent models. J Immunol 140:3830–3837, 1988.

Crawford J, Ozer H, Stoller R, Johnson D, Lyman G, Tabbara T, Kris M, Grous J, Picozzi V, and Rausch G: Reduction by granulocyte colony-stimulating factor of fever and neutropenia induced by chemotherapy in patients with small-cell lung cancer, N Eng J Med 325: 164–170, 1991.

Crosier PS and Clark SC: Basic biology of the hematopoietic growth factors, Semin Oncol 19:349–361, 1992

Demetri GD and Antman KH: Granulocyte-macrophage colony-stimulating factor (GM-CSF): pre-clinical and clinical investigations, Semin Oncol 19:362–385, 1992.

Dillman RO: Rationale for combining chemotherapy and biotherapy in the treatment of cancer, Molec Bioth 2:201–207, 1990.

Dinarello C and Wolff S: Mechanisms of disease: the role of interleukin-1 in disease. N Eng J Med 328:106–116, 1993.

Dutcher JP: Future directions in biologic therapy of cancer. Hospital Formulary 27:694–707, 1992.

Farrell M: The challenge of adult respiratory syndrome during interleukin-2 therapy. Oncol Nurs Forum 19:475–480, 1992.

Figlin RA: Biotherapy in clinical practice, Semin Hemat 26(suppl) 3:15–24, 1989.

Frei E and Spriggs D: Tumor necrosis factor: still a promising agent. J Clin Oncol 7:291–294, 1989.

Grimm E: Properties of IL-2-activated lymphocytes. In Atkins M and Mier J, editors: Therapeutic applications of interleukin-2, New York, 1993, Marcel Dekker, pp. 27–38.

Herrmann F, Schulz G, Wieser M, Kolbe K, Nicolay U, Moack M, Lindemann A, and Martelsmann R: Effect of GM-CSF in neutropenia and related morbidity induced by myelotoxic chemotherapy, Amer J Med 88:619–624, 1990.

Holzer D, Seipelt G, and Ganser A: Interleukin-3 alone and in combination with GM-CSF in the treatment of patients with neoplastic disease, Semin Hemat 28(suppl 2):17–24, 1993.

Hynes M, Bournes L, Brish A, Cuppernall G, Hanzelin J, Ramming K, and Pitler LR: Managing side effects associated with IL-2 therapy, Oncol Nurs Forum, 17:963–964, 1990.

Isaacs A and Lindenmen J: Virus interference: I, the interferon. Proc Royal Soc London. Series B: Biological Sciences 147:258–267, 1957.

Janson CH, Tehrani M, Wigzell H, and Mellstedt M: Rational use of biological response modifiers in hematological malignancies—a review of treatment with interferon, cytotoxic cells, and antibodies, Leuk Res 13:1039–1046, 1989.

Jaramilla JP: Biotechnology overview, Pharm & Therap 17:1372–1377, 1992.

Jassak P: Biotherapy. In Groenwald SL, Frogge MH, Goodman M, and Yarbro CH, editors: Cancer nursing: principles and practice, ed 3, Boston, 1993, Jones & Bartlett, pp. 366–392.

Kuby J: Cytokines. In Kuby J, editor: Immunology, New York, 1992, WH Freeman, pp. 245–270.

Lotze M and Rosenberg S: Interleukin-2: clinical applications. In DeVita V, Hellman S, and Rosenberg S, editors: Biologic therapy of cancer, Philadelphia, 1991, JB Lippincott Co, pp. 159–177.

Mayer D, Hetrick K, Riggs C, and Sherwin S: Weight loss in patients receiving recombinant leukocyte-A interferon (IFNrA): a brief report, Cancer Nurs 7:53–56, 1984.

Milstein C: Monoclonal antibodies, Sci Amer 243:66–74, 1980.

Moldawer NP and Figlin RA: The interferons. In Rieger PT, editor: Biotherapy: a comprehensive overview, Boston, 1995, Jones & Bartlett, pp. 69–92.

Nemunaitis J, Meyers J, Buckner C, Branco JC, Groves E, Higans CS, Shulman J, Storb R, Hansen F, Applebaum FR, and Singer JW: Phase I/II trial of recombinant human monocyte colony-stimulating factor (M-CSF) in patients with invasive fungal infections, Proc Am Soc Clin Oncol 12:159, 1993 (abstract).

Nemunaitis J, Singer JW, Buckner CD, Hill R, Storb R, Thomas ED, and Applebaum FR: Use of recombinant human granulocyte-macrophage colony-stimulating factor in autologous marrow transplantation for lymphoid malignancies, Blood 72:834–836, 1988.

Nieweg R: Interleukins in cancer therapy. Proceedings of the Seventh International Conference on Cancer Care, Middlesex, England, 1992, Scatari Projects Limited, pp. 12–16.

Ohno R, Tomonoaga M, Kogayashi T: Effect of G-CSF after intensive induction therapy in relapsed or refractory acute leukemia, N Eng J Med 323:871–877, 1990.

Rieger PT: Patient management. In Rieger PT, editor: Biotherapy: a comprehensive overview, Boston, 1995, Jones & Bartlett, pp. 495–555.

Robinson KD and Posner JS: Patterns of self-care needs and interventions related to biologic response modifier therapy: fatigue as a model, Sem Oncol Nurs 8:17–22, 1992.

Rumsey KA and Rieger PT, editors: Biological response modifiers: a self-instructional manual for health professionals, Chicago, 1992, Precept Press.

Sargent CA and Shelton BN: Cardiotoxicities of interleukin-2 (IL-2): the nursing challenge, Oncol Nurs Forum 17:964, 1990.

Sharp E: The interleukins. In Rieger PT, editor: Biotherapy: a comprehensive overview, Boston, 1995, Jones & Bartlett, pp. 242–279.

Shelton BN and Sargent CA: Neurologic toxicity management with BRMs, Oncol Nurs Forum 17:964–965, 1990.

Sheridan WP, Juttner C, Szer J, Begley G, DeLuca E, Rowlings PA, McGrath K, Vincent M, Morstyne G, and Fox RM: Granulocyte colony-stimulating factor (G-CSF) in peripheral blood stem cell (PBSC) and bone marrow (BM) transplantation, Blood 76:2251, 1990 (abstract).

Siegel JP and Puri RK: Interleukin-2 toxicity, J Clin Oncol 9:694–704, 1991.

Smith JW, Urba WJ, Curti BD, Elwood LJ, Steis RG, Janik JE, Sharfman WH, Miller LL, Genton RG, and Conlon KC: The toxic and hematologic effects of interleukin-1 alpha administered in a phase I trial to patients with advanced malignancies, J Clin Oncol 10:1141–1152, 1992.

Smith JW, Longo DL, Alvord WG, Janik JE, Sharfman WH, Glause BL, Curti BD, Creekmore SP, Holmlund JT, and Fenton RG: The effects of treatment with interleukin-1α on platelet recovery after high-dose carboplatin, N Eng J Med 328:756–761, 1993.

Spivak JL: Erythropoietin, Blood Reviews 3:130–135, 1989.

Taylor KM, Jagannath S, Spitzer G, Spinolo JA, Tucker DL, Fogel B, Cabanillas FT, Hagemeister FB, and Souza LM: Recombinant human granulocyte colony-stimulating factor hastens granulocyte recovery after high-dose chemotherapy and autologous bone marrow transplantation in Hodgkin's disease, J Clin Oncol 7:1791–1799, 1989.

Taylor CW, Grogan TM, and Salmon SF: Effects of interleukin-4 on the in vitro growth of human lymphoid and plasma cell neoplasms, Blood 75:1114–1118, 1990.

Thompson JA, Lee DJ, Kidd P, Rillun E, Kaufmann J, Bonnem EM, and Fefer A: Subcutaneous granulocyte-macrophage colony-stimulating factor in patients with myelodysplastic syndrome: toxicity, pharmacokinetics and hematological effects, J Clin Oncol 7:629–637, 1989.

Vadhan-Raj S: PIXY 321 (GM-CSF/IL-3 fusion protein): biology and early clinical development, Stem Cells 12:253–261, 1994.

Vadhan-Raj S, Kudelka A, Garrison L, Gano J, Edwards CL, Freedman RS, and Kavanagh JJ: Effects of interleukin-1α on carboplatinum-induced thrombocytopenia in patients with recurrent ovarian cancer, J Clin Oncol 12:707–714, 1994.

Vadhan-Raj S, Papadoupoulos N, Burgess M, Patel S, Linke K, Plager C, Hayes C, Arcenas A, Kudelka A, Williams D, Garrison R, and Benjamin R: Optimization of dose and schedule of PIXY 321 (GM-CSF/IL-3 fusion protein) to attenuate chemotherapy (CT)-induced multilineage myelosuppression in patients with sarcoma, Proc Amer Soc Clin Oncol 12:470, 1993 (abstract).

Weiner LM, Li W, Catalano RB, Kaye J, Padavic K, and Alpaugh K: Phase I trial of recombinant macrophage colony-stimulating factor (M-CSF) and recombinant gamma-interferon (γ-IFN): peripheral blood mononuclear phagocyte proliferation and differentiation, Proc Amer Soc Clin Oncol 12:291, 1993 (abstract).

Wujcik D: An odyssey into biologic therapy, Oncol Nurs Forum 20:879–997, 1993.

Wujcik D: Hematopoietic growth factors. In Rieger PT, editor: Biotherapy: a comprehensive overview, Boston, 1995, Jones & Bartlett, pp. 113–124.

Chapter *6*

❖ *Bone Marrow Transplantation*

Debra Wujcik

In cancer treatment, bone marrow transplantation (BMT) is used to replace stem cells in a person whose bone marrow is diseased or deficient, as in cases of leukemia or aplastic anemia, or to "rescue" a patient after high doses of chemotherapy and radiation are given to destroy marrow stem cells, as in cases of a solid tumor such as breast cancer.

Stem cells are the least mature cells found in the bone marrow. They are described as *pluripotent* because they have the potential to mature into any of the blood cells—white blood cells, red blood cells, or platelets. Stem cells for BMT are *autologous* (obtained from self) or *allogeneic* (obtained from another person who is a Human Leukocyte Antigen (HLA) match). The type of BMT selected depends on the disorder being treated and the availability of donor marrow.

❖ *Types of Bone Marrow Transplantation*

Allogeneic

Allogeneic BMT is used to treat both malignant and nonmalignant disorders. Allogeneic bone marrow can be obtained from an identical twin (synergeneic BMT), an HLA-matched related donor, or an HLA-matched unrelated donor (MUD).

Autologous

Autologous transplants, performed only to treat malignant disease, are used to rescue the bone marrow after high doses of chemotherapy and/or radiation damage (Crouch and Ross, 1994). If the disease involves hematopoietic tissue, as in cases of leukemia or lymphoma, the marrow is harvested when the person is in complete remission (i.e., when there is no evidence of disease). If the oncologist is concerned that microscopic disease may persist, the marrow is purged with chemotherapeutic drugs or the immune system is stimulated with monoclonal antibodies to rid the marrow of disease (Santos, 1984).

Peripheral Blood Stem Cells

Peripheral blood can provide stem cells in the form of progenitor cells (Crouch and Ross, 1994). Progenitor cells are hematopoietic cells that have matured to the point of commitment to the lymphoid or the myeloid cell line. The progenitor cells are used for peripheral blood stem cell (PBSC) transplantation, also called peripheral blood progenitor cell (PBPC) transplantation. Peripheral blood stem cells are harvested by pheresis and used alone or in combination with autologous bone marrow. For patients unable to undergo anesthesia for an autologous bone marrow harvest, PBSC transplantation provides another treatment option.

Malignancies Treated with Bone Marrow Transplantation

Standard Treatment

Bone marrow transplantation is considered the standard treatment for certain diseases at specific stages (Buchsel, 1990). Hematologic disorders such as acute lymphocytic leukemia (ALL), acute myelogenous leukemia (AML), and chronic myelogenous leukemia (CML) are treated with allogeneic or autologous BMT (Bortin, Horowitz, and Rimm, 1992). Patients with ALL undergo BMT after the cancer is in first remission or early relapse (when a small number of malignant cells are detected in the bone marrow). It is unclear whether BMT in the first remission of ALL is a treatment superior to chemotherapy given alone. However, some patients who have negative features in the prognosis of their cancers, such as high leukocyte count at diagnosis or certain chromosomal abnormalities, benefit from BMT during first remission (Barrett et al., 1989; Bortin and Horowitz, 1990). Patients in second or subsequent remission or those given a transplant during late relapse have a significant survival advantage (20%) over those treated with chemotherapy alone, especially patients younger than 25 (Bortin and Horowitz, 1990).

The use of BMT in persons with AML in first remission is controversial. Persons younger than 25 years of age appear to survive the high-dose chemotherapy intensification phase of standard AML treatment, whereas those older than 40 do better with BMT. Persons age 30 to 40 experience equivalent results (Forman and Blume, 1990).

BMT is the preferred treatment for persons with CML, because it offers the only hope for cure (Thomas and Clift, 1989). The natural course of this disease is divided into a chronic stage and a terminal phase. Because there are few signs and symptoms in the chronic phase, CML is usually diagnosed during a routine physical exam. The chronic phase lasts from 30 to 60 months, then the disease transforms into a more aggressive condition. The terminal phase is marked by an accelerated stage and a blastic stage in which immature stem cells are released into the peripheral blood. The optimum time for BMT is during the chronic phase of the disease. BMT is less successful in the accelerated phase and is poorly tolerated during the blastic phase (Horowitz and Bortin, 1990).

Autologous BMT is used in patients who do not have a suitable donor. There is less toxicty with autologous BMT because the host and the donor are the same person. However, there is a higher relapse rate after autologous BMT. Autologous BMT has been effective in patients with solid tumors such as breast cancer, testicular cancers, and neuroblastoma (Antman, 1992; Frei, 1992; Keating, 1992).

❖ *Transplant Process*

Bone Marrow Donor

Donor Selection

The selection of the donor for allogeneic BMT is determined by the compatibility of tissue between the potential donor and the recipient (the patient). A histocompatibility system is used to determine a suitable match. Six human leukocyte antigen (HLA) groups located on the sixth chromosome have been identified: HLA-A, HLA-B, HLA-C, HLA-DR, HLA-DQ, and HLA-DP. These groups include more than 90 antigens, which form more than 26 million combinations (Welte, 1994). These determine the unique HLA type of each individual. Currently, labs use HLA-A, HLA-B, and HLA-DR antigens from both the donor and the recipient blood samples to determine compatibility. A "match" occurs when four or more of the antigens are alike. A perfect match is six of six antigens (Weinberg, 1991).

Approximately 30% to 40% of patients who need BMT have a matched sibling donor. Partial matches, that is, four or five out of six antigens, may be found within the extended family. When a suitable donor cannot be found, the health care team frequently initiates a search for an HLA-matched unrelated donor through the National Marrow Donor Program (NMDP) (Beatty and Anasetti, 1990). The NMDP was established in 1987 and consists of donor centers, transplant centers, and collection centers (Welte, 1994). Donor centers recruit and educate volunteer donors. Transplant centers care for patients who receive high-dose therapy followed by BMT. Collection centers harvest marrow from a donor for a matched, unrelated person having BMT. In addition, there is a centralized computer file of HLA-typed donors from regional donor registries affiliated with blood centers in the United States and abroad (McCullough et al., 1989).

The same criteria for matching apply to both unrelated and related donors. Once selected, potential donors receive education, counseling, and an extensive physical examination. The donors must understand that if they withdraw after the recipient's conditioning therapy has begun, the recipient will die because the immune system is destroyed.

Harvesting

The bone marrow is obtained or "harvested" from the donor in the same manner for both allogeneic and autologous BMT (Buckner et al., 1984; Wallerstein and Deisseroth, 1993). The procedure is done in the operating room under spinal or general anesthesia. In the operating room, the patient is prepped on each posterior iliac crest and multiple aspirations are performed. The volume of marrow obtained equals 10 ml/kg body weight of the recipient, usually between 400 and 600 ml.

The marrow is placed in heparinized tissue-culture medium and filtered several times to remove fat and bone particles. For autologous BMT, it is then prepared for the freezing process or, for allogeneic BMT, immediate administration. If the marrow is obtained from a matched, unrelated donor located at a different center, the harvest, processing, and transport of the viable stem cells have to be coordinated so the recipient gets them in a timely manner.

Collecting peripheral blood stem cells is called *apheresis,* or simply *pheresis* (Jassak and Riley, 1994). The stem cells are obtained when the patient's blood is circulated through a cell separator, which culls the stem cells and returns the plasma and red blood cells to the patient. The outpatient procedure requires 2 to 4 hours per harvest, and it may require between 3 and 7 procedures to obtain the quantity of stem cells necessary for transplantation.

Postoperative Care

For 12 to 24 hours after surgery, the staff needs to assess a donor of allogeneic marrow for fluid imbalance and anemia. Occasionally autologous red blood cells may need to be given to the donor. Oral narcotics usually relieve any discomfort, and the donor can be discharged the next day (Ruggiero, 1988).

Conditioning Therapy

Conditioning therapy is given to the recipient to remove any remaining malignant cells before performing either allogeneic or autologous BMT. In addition, for allogeneic BMT, the bone marrow must be depleted to allow room for new cells to grow, and the immune system must be destroyed to decrease the risk of rejection of the new cells (the *graft*) (Wujcik and Downs, 1992).

The type of conditioning is related to the underlying disease. Protocols for BMT conditioning vary in length and feature different combinations of therapies. Chemotherapy and radiation are given on days preceding the transplant, identified as minus days. The bone marrow is infused on day 0. A sample protocol for allogeneic BMT is shown in Table 6-1.

Table 6-1   Typical Protocol for Allogeneic Bone Marrow Transplantation

Treatment Day	Therapy
−7	Etoposide by continuous infusion
−6	Cyclophosphamide
−5	Cyclophosphamide
−4	Cyclophosphamide
−3	Total body irradiation
−2	Total body irradiation
−1	Total body irradiation
0	Bone marrow infusion (transplantation)
+1	Nadir phase
+2	Nadir phase
+3	Nadir phase

Chemotherapy

High-dose chemotherapy is used to prepare the patient to receive the bone marrow. Commonly used drugs are cyclophosphamide, etoposide, cytarabine, busulfan, and carmustine (Franco and Gould, 1994). Each of these drugs produces severe side effects such as nausea, vomiting, stomatitis, and diarrhea. Because a goal of therapy is to empty the marrow of stem cells, the patient experiences a predictable period of myelosuppression that continues until engraftment (Wujcik, 1993a) (Figure 6-1). *Engraftment* occurs when the stem cells begin to grow and mature and is evidenced by a rising white blood cell count.

Radiation Therapy

Total body irradiation (TBI) is given to eradicate malignant cells in the central nervous system and sanctuary sites such as the gonads and the skin (Yee and McGuire, 1985). Patients receive multiple treatments in divided doses to maximize the cell-kill effect and to decrease toxicity to vital organs such as the lungs and the kidneys.

Nausea, vomiting, and diarrhea are the most immediate side effects produced by TBI. These should resolve in about 5 days after the completion of conditioning therapy. Other side effects are fever, parotid tenderness, decreased salivation, and the temporary loss of taste or a change in taste perception. Early skin changes include

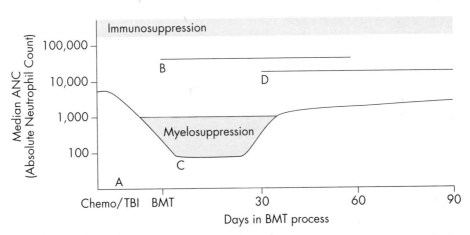

Fig. 6-1. Infection risk and prophylaxis in patients undergoing bone marrow transplantation (BMT). **A,** High-dose chemotherapy and total body irradiation (TBI) are administered to prepare the patient for BMT. **B,** Immunosuppression to prevent graft-versus-host disease is accomplished by administering cyclosporin and methotrexate. Prophylactic antibiotics given to the patient to decrease colonization. **C,** During a period of severe myelosuppression, empiric antibiotic therapy is initiated with the first fever. **D,** As the stem cells engraft and peripheral counts recover, prophylaxis for *Pneumocystis carinii* is added. Although the risk of bacterial infection diminishes by the third and fourth month after BMT, continued immunosuppression keeps the patient at risk for fungal, viral, and other infections. From Wujcik D: Infection control in oncology patients, Nurs Clin North Am 28:647, 1993. Reprinted with permission.

erythema and tenderness, which worsen up to 2 weeks after radiation. Hyperpigmentation continues for 2 to 3 weeks after BMT (Dreifke and DeMeyer, 1992).

Marrow Transplantation

Allogeneic BMT

An allogeneic transplant is administered at the bedside similar to a blood transfusion (Wujcik and Downs, 1992). The marrow is unfiltered to prevent loss of stem cells. The patient is monitored for signs and symptoms of reaction to the transfusion, which may include shortness of breath, back pain, and general discomfort. If the donor and the recipient are ABO-incompatible even though they are HLA matched, the usual treatment is to remove all red blood cells from the donor marrow to decrease the incidence of transfusion reaction. Benadryl and epinephrine should be kept available to administer in the event of a reaction.

Autologous BMT

Autologous marrow is administered by rapid infusion or by intravenous bolus. The marrow is brought to the patient-care area in a frozen state and thawed in a warm-water bath. Adding a preservative, dimethyl sulfoxide (DMSO), prevents lysis of blood cells during the thawing procedure. Excretion of DMSO through the lungs causes the patient's breath to have a garlic smell and the patient to experience sudden nausea and vomiting. The vomiting clears rapidly, but the odor and nausea may continue for 36 hours. Other side effects include cough, tachypnea, and dyspnea, due to microemboli passing though the lungs. Fever may occur after the transplant because of pyrogens released from lysed white blood cells. The thawing process also causes red blood cell lysis, which in turn causes *hemoglobulinuria* or dark red or amber urine for approximately 24 hours after the infusion.

❖ Nursing Considerations

The focus of nursing care varies, depending on the time after transplant and the expected complications. Acute problems that commonly occur during the first 100 days after transplantation include acute graft-versus-host disease (GVHD), infection, bleeding, and venoocclusive disease (VOD). Chronic problems occur after the first 100 days following transplantation, usually after the patient has been discharged from the hospital and sometimes after the patient has returned to the care of the referring physician.

Acute Problems

Acute Graft-versus-Host Disease

Graft-versus-host disease (GVHD) is a major complication of allogeneic BMT that occurs at the time of bone marrow engraftment (20 to 30 days after transplantation). GVHD develops when immunologically active cells are infused into an immunologically incompetent host (McDonald et al., 1986a; Wujcik, Ballard, and Camp-Sorrell, 1994). The new T-lymphocytes from the graft (the new cells) attack the host tissue in the patient.

The incidence of acute GVHD ranges from 40% to 50% of all allogeneic BMT patients (Bortin and Horowitz, 1990; Weisdorf et al., 1990). Although there are some reports of GVHD following autologous transplantation (Hood et al., 1987), for the most part GVHD is associated with allogeneic BMT. Acute GVHD causes 8% of BMT deaths (Spruce, 1983).

PATHOPHYSIOLOGY.   Acute GVHD is caused by donor T-lymphocytes attacking the epithelium of the skin, the gut, and the liver in the BMT recipient. Once the lymphocytes are recognized as foreign to the recipient's immune system, multiple cytokines are released, which causes cell necrosis and death (Wujcik, Ballard, and Camp-Sorrell, 1994). The risk factors for developing acute GVHD include age, sex of the donor, histoincompatibility, and number of blood transfusions. Acute GVHD is especially associated with chronic myelogenous leukemia and acute lymphocytic leukemia (Wujcik, Ballard, and Camp-Sorrell, 1994).

Skin manifestations are usually the first sign of acute GVHD; a maculopapular rash on the trunk, palms, soles, and ears with characteristic blanching. The rash may progress to generalized erythroderma, blister formation, and desquamation (Press, 1987). To differentiate skin symptoms of GVHD from a drug reaction, a biopsy is performed (Sale and Shulman, 1984).

GVHD of the gut involves degeneration of the mucosal lining of the GI tract, which the patient experiences as profuse diarrhea with accompanying nausea, vomiting, and abdominal cramping (Sullivan et al., 1984). The diagnosis is occasionally confirmed with rectal biopsy but the GI tract disturbance with skin changes confirms the clinical diagnosis.

GVHD of the liver involves degeneration of the liver mucosa and small bile ducts and is evidenced by increased bilirubin, serum glutamic oxaloacetic transaminase (SGOT), and alkaline phosphatase. Signs and symptoms include jaundice, hepatomegaly, right-upper-quadrant pain, and ascites (Ford and Ballard, 1988). Because these symptoms are similar to those of VOD, the nurse must refer to the amount of time after BMT to differentiate the symptoms.

MANAGEMENT OF GVHD.   Prevention of GVHD takes several routes. All blood products are irradiated to inactive T-lymphocytes (Anderson and Weinstein, 1990). Cyclosporin A (CSA) is given beginning the day before transplant (day −1). This drug acts selectively on T-lymphocytes, preventing the production of sensitized T-cells without disturbing the recovering function of B-lymphocytes, macrophages, and granulocytes.

Cyclosporin A has multiple side effects, including nephrotoxicity, hypertension, hepatotoxicity, gastrointestinal disturbances, and neurologic alterations (Wingard, 1990). BUN, creatinine, and potassium levels should be monitored diligently and CSA dosages modified accordingly. Red blood cell recovery may be delayed by CSA. Cyclosporin A is given alone or with methotrexate, an antimetabolite chemotherapeutic agent, to slow the growth of T-lymphocytes. Another method to prevent GVHD involves depleting the donor marrow of T-cells before transplantation.

Acute GVHD is treated primarily with corticosteroids (e.g., prednisone). Antithymocyte globulin (ATG) also is used to modulate T-lymphocyte function (Weisdorf et al., 1990).

Nursing care of patients with skin reactions should focus on comfort and infection prevention (Wujcik, Ballard, and Camp-Sorrell, 1994). Inspecting the skin and paying attention to complaints of itching or discomfort become crucial around the time of engraftment. Bathwater oils and lotions can decrease pruritus. Pigskin or a hydrogel dressing can provide protection (Caudell and Schauer, 1989; Buchsel and Kelleher, 1989). Skin debridement in a whirlpool may be necessary to minimize infection and to promote healing. Special air-flow beds increase patient comfort by decreasing friction with the skin.

When the GI tract is affected by acute GVHD, the patient may have several liters of diarrhea per day. Accordingly, fluid and electrolyte levels should be monitored closely and replaced as needed. Nutritional support becomes a big challenge. Meticulous personal hygiene is required, and sitz baths may soothe irritated skin. Because mucosal sloughing can occur, all stools should be measured and assessed for occult blood (Buchsel and Kelleher, 1989; Ford and Eisenberg, 1990).

Infection

During the first 100 days after transplantation, there are two phases when the patient faces risk of infection from specific organisms. The first phase occurs immediately after BMT or preengraftment, and the second phase occurs in midrecovery or early postengraftment. A third phase, during late recovery or late postengraftment, occurs after 100 days (Caudell and Whedon 1991; Wingard, 1990).

PREENGRAFTMENT INFECTION.   Preengraftment infection occurs during the first month after BMT when the patient is neutropenic and susceptible to bacterial infections from both gram-negative and gram-positive organisms. *Neutropenia* is defined as an absolute neutrophil count of less than 500 cells/m^2. A predictable period of neutropenia of about 30 days follows conditioning therapy until new white blood cells are produced and released into the bloodstream (Figure 6-1).

The usual signs and symptoms of infection, such as swelling, redness, and pus, are often absent because the neutropenic patient does not produce an adequate inflammatory response (Sickels, Greene, and Wiernik, 1975). Fever is usually the first and often the only sign of infection.

Conditioning therapy alters the physical barriers against infection. The direct effects of chemotherapeutic drugs and TBI cause breaks in the integrity of the oral and gastrointestinal (GI) mucosa, providing avenues for normal flora such as bacteria, fungi, and viruses to invade the bloodstream. Neutropenic enterocolitis, an inflammation of the small intestine or colon, can be life threatening (Smith and Van-Gulick, 1992).

The herpes simplex virus (HSV) generally causes most viral infections during this period (Zaia, 1990). Because 90% of patients whose blood tests prove positive for HSV prior to BMT develop active infections after the transplantation, acyclovir is given as a prophylaxis beginning the day before BMT.

POSTENGRAFTMENT INFECTION.   Postengraftment infection occurs after the transplanted stem cells become established in the bone marrow and mature cells begin appearing in the peripheral circulation. A patient who has had an allogeneic BMT may develop mild to severe GVHD at this time. The usual treatment for

GVHD, steroids and increased dosages of cyclosporin A (CSA), causes severe loss of cellular immunity and allows infection to occur.

Cytomegalovirus (CMV) infection is the major problem during this phase and, second to GVHD, is the most common cause of death following BMT. CMV infections occur as hepatitis, retinitis, enteritis, pneumonitis, or prolonged myelosuppression (Meyers et al., 1988). CMV is transmitted by blood products or the donor marrow, or it occurs as a reactivation of latent CMV in the patient. Prophylactic treatment for CMV infection includes acyclovir and weekly intravenous administration of immunoglobulins. In addition, CMV-negative blood products are given to the patient who is CMV-negative and has a CMV-negative donor.

A newer strategy to prevent CMV infection is to identify patients whose tests reveal the presence of the virus. Weekly cultures to detect CMV are obtained beginning at the time of marrow engraftment. Gancyclovir, a new antiviral agent, is recommended as prophylaxis for patients whose blood, urine, and sputum cultures indicate the increasing presence of CMV (Wingard, 1990).

Pneumocystis carinii pneumonia occurred frequently in the early years of BMT, but this infectious problem is now almost completely avoided by initiating treatment with trimethoprim-sulfamethaxazole (TMX) at the time of engraftment. Unfortunately, the drug cannot be started earlier because of its myelosuppression activity (Wingard, 1990). Patients allergic to TMX receive aerosolized pentamidine instead.

MANAGEMENT OF INFECTION. It is critical for the BMT nurse to assess for signs and symptoms of endotoxic shock caused by gram-negative bacilli. Those symptoms include hyperthermia or hypothermia, chills, tachypnea and tachycardia, hypotension, cold-and-clammy extremities, cyanosis, oliguria, and a decreased level of consciousness (Barry, 1989). If the BMT unit does not have cardiac-monitoring and critical care capabilities, the patient may be moved to the intensive-care setting for hemodynamic monitoring and the administration of vasoactive medications.

Bleeding
During the first 3 to 4 weeks after transplantation, the patient is at high risk for hemorrhage because there is no platelet production. Patients must receive platelet transfusions until their marrow produces sufficient megakaryocytes to prevent life-threatening bleeding.

The most common site for bleeding is the nose, although bleeding in the mouth frequently occurs simultaneously. Topical adrenaline or cocaine can be used to control severe nasal and oral bleeding. A prolonged nose bleed may require nasal packing. The nursing staff must frequently assess the patient's airway for patency during a bleeding episode (Caudell and Whedon, 1991; Ford and Ballard, 1988).

Spontaneous intracranial bleeding can occur if the platelet count falls below 20,000/mm^3. The nurse should diligently observe the patient for signs and symptoms of increased intracranial bleeding, such as headache, blurred vision, and pupil changes (Caudell and Whedon, 1991; Ford and Ballard, 1988).

MANAGEMENT OF BLEEDING. Complete blood counts must be determined daily during the period following transplantation. The hematocrit should be kept above 25% by means of packed red blood cell (RBC) transfusion. In general, platelets should be maintained at a concentration of 20,000/mm³ by means of platelet transfusions, unless the patient shows evidence of bleeding. For all invasive procedures, the platelet count should be kept above 50,000/mm³ (Ford and Ballard, 1988; Caudell and Whedon, 1991). Random-donor platelets are administered, unless the patient becomes *refractory*, that is, if there is no rise in platelet count after platelet transfusion. In that case, the patient receives single-donor pheresis products. All blood products should also be irradiated to prevent the possibility of GVHD from transfused T-lymphocytes (Caudell and Whedon, 1991; Ford and Ballard, 1988). Leukocyte-removing filters are used to avoid transfusion reactions.

Venoocclusive Disease

Venoocclusive disease (VOD) is an acute complication that occurs in the period following BMT. It results from vascular damage in the liver from the combination of chemotherapy and radiation therapy. VOD may occur in up to 50% of patients undergoing allogeneic BMT; the mortality rate ranges from 7% to 50% (McDonald et al., 1985; Rollins, 1986; Wujcik, Ballard, and Camp-Sorrell, 1994).

VOD is associated with increased age, malignancy other than acute lymphocytic lymphoma, and a history of hepatitis before BMT. Patients with elevated SGOT before BMT have 3.4 times greater incidence of VOD. VOD seems to occur less in patients undergoing autologous transplantation.

MANAGEMENT OF VOD.   Supportive treatment of VOD focuses on maximum renal and hepatic blood flow and minimal extracircular fluid accumulation (Wujcik, Ballard, and Camp-Sorrell, 1994). Sodium intake is restricted and plasma expanders such as albumin are given to maintain intravascular volume to limit ascites development (Rollins, 1986; McDonald, 1986a and 1986b).

Third spacing of fluid (accumulation outside the arteriovenous system) can be minimized by restricting fluid intake. This allows better renal blood flow, decreases congestion in the lungs and the brain, and improves patient comfort (Wujcik, Ballard, and Camp-Sorrell, 1994).

Treatment with lactulose reduces ammonia production in the intestines and the serum. Protein-sparing parenteral nutrient solutions provide proteins through animo acids. Aldactone may be given to inhibit sodium and water retention. Its effectiveness is inhibited by variations in oral absorption and by delays in response. Mucositis, nausea, and vomiting affect patient compliance, and oral absorption is questionable when there is toxicity in the gastrointestinal tract.

Current research in this area focuses on removing fibrin and clots that obstruct hepatic circulation. Several days of tissue plasminogen activator administered intravenously, followed by heparin therapy, has provided some improvement to patients with severe VOD (Bearman et al., 1992).

Chronic Problems

Chronic Graft-versus-Host Disease

The most frequently seen late complication related to allogeneic transplant is chronic GVHD occurring in 30% to 40% of all long-term survivors of BMT. The risk factors for chronic GVHD include previous acute GVHD and increasing age (Wingard, 1989). Although chronic GVHD usually develops about 3 months after BMT, this complication has been reported to occur up to 2 years later (Deeg, 1990). Patients experience opportunistic infections, nutritional deficits, abnormal pigmentation and hardening of the skin, and joint contractures.

Late Postengraftment Infection

The patient's humoral and cellular immunity continue to be severely deficient during late recovery or the postengraftment period. The gradual recovery of normal immunity takes several months. If chronic GVHD occurs, recovery is much slower, due to the immune response to GVHD and the treatment with cyclosporin A and steroids (Wingard, 1990). The patient is at risk for encapsulated organisms, especially *Streptococcus pneumoniae* and *Herpes zoster* (Feld, 1989). In addition, infection with *Varicella zoster* occurs in approximately 40% to 50% of patients by the end of the first year after BMT (Wujcik and Downs, 1992). Prompt treatment is required to avoid fatal disseminated disease.

Cataracts

Approximately 50% of BMT patients develop cataracts. The incidence is associated with total body irradiation and decreases with the use of fractionated or divided doses. Patients are advised to report any visual changes. Lifelong regular eye evaluations are recommended (Nims, 1991).

Other Complications

Other late complications may be related to the conditioning therapy. Late pulmonary complications include interstitial pneumonia and restrictive and obstructive disease. Endocrine dysfunction and infertility are also common concerns.

❖ Summary

Bone marrow transplantation is a critical component of multimodal therapy. The use of marrow stem cells allows lethal doses of multimodal treatments to be given. For example, in some solid tumors, such as breast cancer, surgical intervention is followed by high-dose chemotherapy and rescue with peripheral blood stem cells. Continued research will enhance this modality as a safe, effective method of treatment for specific malignant and nonmalignant conditions.

❖ References

Anasetti C, Doney KC, Storb R, Meyers JD, Farewell VT, Buchner CD, Applebaum FR, Sullivan KM, Clift RA, and Deeg HJ: Marrow transplantation for severe aplastic anemia. Long-term outcome in fifty "untransfused" patients, Ann Intern Med 104:461–466, 1986.

Anderson KC and Weinstein HJ: Transfusion-associated graft-versus-host-disease, N Eng J Med 323:315–321, 1990.

Antman KH: Dose-intensive therapy in breast cancer. In Armitage JO and Antman KH, editors: High-dose cancer therapy: pharmacology, hematopoietins, stem cells, Baltimore, 1992, Williams & Wilkins, pp. 701–718.

Barrett AJ, Horowitz M, Gale RP, Biggs JC, Camotta BM, Diche KA, Gluckman E, Good RA, Herzig RH, and Lee MB: Marrow transplantation for acute lymphoblastic leukemia: factors affecting relapse and survival, Blood 74:862–871, 1989.

Barry SA: Septic shock: Special needs of patients with cancer, Oncol Nurs Forum, 16:31–35, 1989.

Bearman SI, Shuhart MC, Hinds MS, and McDonald GB: Recombinant human tissue plasminogen activator for the treatment of established severe venoocclusive disease of the liver after bone marrow transplantation, Blood 80:2458–2462, 1992.

Beatty PG and Anasetti C: Marrow transplantation from donors other than HLA identical siblings, Hematol Oncol Clin North Am 4:677–688, 1990.

Bortin M and Horowitz M: Current status of bone marrow transplantation. In Teraski P, editor: Clinical transplants, Los Angeles, 1990, UCLA Tissue Typing Laboratory, pp. 93–101.

Bortin M, Horowitz M, and Rimm A: Increasing utilization of allogeneic bone marrow transplantation, Ann Intern Med 116:505–512, 1992.

Buchsel PC: Bone marrow transplantation. In Groenwald SL, Frogge MH, Goodman M, and Yarbro CH, editors: Cancer nursing: principles and practice, ed 3, Boston, 1990, Jones & Bartlett, pp. 307–337.

Buchsel PC and Kelleher J: Bone marrow transplantation, Nurs Clin North Am 24:907–939, 1989.

Buckner CD, Clift RA, Sanders JE, Stewart P, Bensinger W, Doney KC, Sullivan KM, Witherspoon RP, Deeg NJ, and Applebaum FR: Marrow harvesting from normal donors, Blood 64:630–634, 1984.

Caudell KA and Schauer V: A dressing used for GVHD skin desquamation, Oncol Nurs Forum 16:726, 1989.

Caudell KA and Whedon MB: Hematologic complications. In Whedon MB, editor: Bone marrow transplantation: principles, practice, and nursing insights, Boston, 1991, Jones & Bartlett, pp. 135–159.

Crouch MA and Ross JA: Current concepts in autologous bone marrow transplantation, Semin Oncol Nurs 10:12–19, 1994.

Deeg HJ: Delayed complications and long-term effects after bone marrow transplantation, Hematol Oncol Clin North Am 4:641–657, 1990.

Dreifke L and DeMeyer E: Information guide for patients receiving total body irradiation before bone marrow transplantation, Cancer Nurs 15:206–210, 1992.

Feld R: The compromised host, Eur J Cancer Clin Oncol 25:S1–S7, 1989.

Ford R and Ballard B: Acute complications after bone marrow transplantation, Semin Oncol Nurs 4:15–22, 1988.

Ford R and Eisenberg S: Bone marrow transplant: recent advances and nursing implications, Nurs Clin North Am 25:405–423, 1990.

Forman SJ and Blume KG: Allogeneic bone marrow transplantation for acute leukemia, Hematol Oncol Clin North Am 4:517–533, 1990.

Franco T and Gould DA: Allogeneic bone marrow transplantation, Semin Oncol Nurs 10:3–11, 1994.

Frei E: Pharmacologic strategies for high-dose chemotherapy. In Armitage JO and Antman KH, editors: High-dose cancer therapy: pharmacology, hematopoietins, stem cells. Baltimore, 1992, Williams & Wilkins, pp. 3–13.

Hood AF, Vogelsang GB, Black LP, Farmer ER, and Santos GW: Acute graft versus host disease: development following autologous and syngeneic bone marrow transplantation, Arch Dermatol 123:745–750, 1987.

Horowitz M and Bortin M: Current status of allogeneic bone marrow transplantation. In Teraski P, editor: Clinical transplants, Los Angeles, 1990, UCLA Tissue Typing Laboratory, pp. 41–52.

Jassak PF and Riley MG: Autologous stem cell transplant, Cancer Prac 2:141–145, 1994.

Keating A: Autologous bone marrow transplantation. In Armitage JO and Antman KH, editors: High-dose cancer therapy: pharmacology, hematopoietins, stem cells. Baltimore, 1992, Williams & Wilkins, pp. 162–181.

McCullough J, Hansen JA, Perkins H, Stroncek D, and Bartsch J: The national marrow donor program: how it works, accomplishments to date, Oncol 3:63–68, 1989.

McDonald GB, Sharma P, Matthews DE, Shulman JM, and Thomas ED: The clinical course of 53 patients with venoocclusive disease of the liver after marrow transplantation, Transplantation 39:603–608, 1985.

McDonald GB, Shulman HM, Sullivan KM, and Spencer GD: Intestinal and hepatic complications of human bone marrow transplantation, Part I, Gastroenterology 90:460–477, 1986a.

McDonald GB, Shulman HM, Sullivan KM, and Spencer GD: Intestinal and hepatic complications of human bone marrow transplantation, Part II, Gastroenterology 90:770–784, 1986b.

Meyers JD, Reed ED, Shepp DJ, Thornquist M, Dandiker DS, Vicary CA, Flournoy N, Kirk LE, Kersey JH, and Thomas ED: Acyclovir for prevention of cytomegalovirus infection and disease after allogeneic marrow transplantation, N Eng J Med 318:70–75, 1988.

Nims JW: Survivorship and rehabilitation. In Whedon MB, editor: Bone marrow transplantation: principles, practice, and nursing insights, Boston, 1991, Jones & Bartlett, pp. 334–335.

Press OW: Bone marrow transplant complications. In Pereya LH, editor: Complications of organ transplantation, New York, 1987, Marcel Dekker, pp. 339–342.

Rollins BJ: Hepatic veno-occlusive disease, Am J Med 81:297–306, 1986.

Ruggiero MR: The donor in bone marrow transplantation, Semin Oncol Nurs 4:9–14, 1988.

Sale GE and Shulman HM: Pathology of other organs. In Sale GE and Shulman HM, editors: The pathology of bone marrow transplantation, New York, 1984, Masson, pp. 192–198.

Santos GW: Bone marrow transplantation in leukemia: current status, Cancer 54 (suppl 11):273–274, 1984.

Sickels EA, Greene EH, and Wiernik PH: Clinical presentation of infection in granulocytopenic patients, Arch Intern Med 135:715–719, 1975.

Smith LJ and VanGulick J: Management of neutropenic enterocolitis in the patient with cancer, Oncol Nurs Forum 19:1337–1344, 1992.

Spruce WE: Bone marrow transplantation: major problems and future directions, Am J Pediatr Hematol Oncol 5:301–306, 1983.

Sullivan KM, Deeg JD, Sanders JE, Shulman JM, Witherspoon RP, Doney K, Applebaum FR, Schubert MM, Stewart P, and Springmeyer S: Late complications after marrow transplant, Semin Hematol 21:53–63, 1984.

Thomas ED and Clift RA: Indications for marrow transplantation in chronic myelogenous leukemia, Blood 73:861–864, 1989.

Wallerstein RO and Deisseroth AB: Bone marrow dysfunction in the cancer patient. In DiVita VT, Hellman S, and Rosenberg SA, editors: Cancer: principles and practice of oncology, ed 4, Philadelphia, 1993, JB Lippincott Co, pp. 2462–2475.

Weinberg PA: The human leukocyte antigen (HLA) system, the search for a matching donor, national marrow donor program development, and marrow donor issues. In Whedon MB, editor: Bone marrow transplantation: principles, practice, and nursing insights, Boston, 1991, Jones & Bartlett, pp. 105–131.

Weisdorf D, Hakke R, Blazar B, Miller W, McGrave P, Ramsey N, Kersey J, and Filopovick B: Treatment of moderate/severe acute graft-versus-host disease after allogeneic bone marrow transplantation: an analysis of clinical risk features and outcome, Blood 75:1024–1030, 1990.

Welte K: Matched unrelated transplants, Semin Oncol Nurs 10:20–27, 1994.

Wingard JR: Advances in the management of infectious complications after bone marrow transplantation, Bone Marrow Transplant 6:371–383, 1990.

Wujcik D: Infection control in oncology patients, Nurs Clin North Am 28:639–650, 1993a.

Wujcik D, Ballard B, and Camp-Sorrell D: Selected complications of allogeneic bone marrow transplantation, Semin Oncol Nurs 10:28–41, 1994.

Wujcik D and Downs S: Bone marrow transplantation, Crit Care Nurs Clin North Am 4:149–166, 1992.

Yee GC and McGuire TR: Allogeneic bone marrow transplantation in the treatment of hematologic diseases, Clin Pharm 4:149–160, 1985.

Zaia JA: Viral infections associated with bone marrow transplantation, Hematol Oncol Clin North Am 4:603–623, 1990.

Chapter 7

❖ *Clinical Trials*

Ann Marie Dose

A clinical trial is an experiment designed to evaluate the potential value of a specific therapy in human subjects (Jenkins and Hubbard, 1991). The goal of cancer clinical trials is to improve the efficacy of treatment while minimizing toxicity and improving quality of life (Cheson, 1991).

Oncology clinical research has greatly increased in the last 25 years. The National Cancer Act, passed in 1971, mandated the National Cancer Institute (NCI) to conduct research to decrease the incidence of and the mortality and morbidity from cancer. To this end the NCI established formal training programs in oncology and a comprehensive information-dissemination program. In addition, new treatment and research facilities were constructed. In 1973, the NCI designated comprehensive cancer centers as nationally recognized centers for cancer practice, research, and education. Box 7-1 lists elements of an NCI Designated Comprehensive Cancer Center.

❖ *Development and Implementation of Clinical Trials*

Protocol Development

A protocol is a document that identifies the objectives of the clinical trial and the specific procedures needed to accomplish those objectives (Cassidy and Macfarlane, 1991). Components in most protocols include the objectives or goal of the clinical trial; a background section citing the rationale for the trial; patient selection criteria or eligibility criteria, which define the sample; a schema or schematic design of the flow of the protocol; a treatment plan; dosage adjustments; toxicity evaluation criteria; information about the drugs being used; parameters for monitoring patients; criteria to evaluate response to treatment; statistical considerations; data analysis; and criteria for terminating clinical trials. As part of the protocol package, references are cited and the patient consent form and copies of the data submission forms are included (Melink and Whitacre, 1991).

Box 7-1 Essential Programmatic Elements of a National Cancer Institute–Designated Comprehensive Cancer Center

◆ Basic laboratory research
◆ A linkage between basic and clinical research
◆ Clinical research
◆ High-priority clinical trials research
◆ Cancer prevention and control research
◆ Education and training of biomedical researchers and health care professionals
◆ Public information services
◆ Community services and outreach activities

From National Cancer Institute: Guidelines: NCI-Designated Comprehensive Cancer Center, Washington, DC, 1992, National Institutes of Health, Department of Health and Human Services.

The objectives of a clinical trial usually support one primary goal, and all study components are designed to answer this primary question. The goal of most treatment protocols is to improve a standard therapy, as measured by how well the tumor responds to treatment (*response rate*), how long a patient is free of cancer symptoms (*disease-free survival*), and overall survival. Secondary goals may include evaluation of treatment toxicities and improvement in the patient's quality of life (Melink and Whitacre, 1991).

The background section of the protocol provides a description of previous research that led the investigator to the present clinical trial with a rationale to conduct the clinical trial. Patient selection criteria help define the clinical trial population and eligibility requirements for participation. Examples of eligibility criteria include histologic or pathologic evidence of the particular cancer under study, prior treatment, age, performance status, and baseline laboratory tests. Patients with poor health status are generally ineligible as subjects of clinical trials because they may confound results of the study by adding existing comorbidity factors to treatment evaluation or assessment of side effects. Eligibility criteria must be broad enough to allow adequate numbers of subjects to generalize the results but narrow enough so there are common elements among subjects (Melink and Whitacre, 1991).

In a randomized trial, neither the investigator nor the patient chooses the treatment. To avoid introducing bias, a computer makes the "choice." This may include stratification factors, which determine patient characteristics to allow equal distribution in all treatment groups (e.g., whether a mastectomy or lumpectomy was performed to treat breast cancer). In addition, descriptive factors may also be assessed to provide additional information about the participants (e.g., their histologic tumor grade or what type of therapy they previously have had).

The methodology section of the protocol includes specifications for the treatment regimens, a schedule for patient follow-up during and after treatment, and the tests required for monitoring follow-up. These need to be adequate to ensure patient safety but not so rigorous or costly that they affect patient accrual and compliance with study guidelines (Melink and Whitacre, 1991). A *schema,* or visual graph of the study flow, can be helpful (Figure 7-1).

Study Approval Process

Clinical trials are conducted by National Cancer Institute–sponsored cooperative groups, cancer centers, and pharmaceutical companies. A protocol chairperson assumes administrative responsibility for the clinical trial from beginning to end. This includes writing the study, often in collaboration with other investigators; meeting all approval requirements; monitoring the progress of the study, including the promptness and accuracy of data collection procedures; and analyzing, reporting, and publishing study results. The chair makes any amendments needed during the course of the study and obtains approval from the local Institutional Review Board (IRB) and the sponsoring agency. Because numerous protocols are multiinstitutional in nature, each institution also has a principal investigator. This individual is responsible for the study at that particular institution and is required to follow the protocol precisely, reporting any variations immediately to the chair (Cassidy and Macfarlane, 1991).

After the study is written, it needs to be reviewed by many individuals and approved by committees on a specific disease (e.g., breast or colon cancer) or modality (e.g., radiation, medical, or surgical oncology) and by individual institutions. The NCI reviews protocols if they involve investigational drugs or will accrue more than 100 patients (Cheson, 1991).

Protocol Implementation

Within many institutions, ongoing systems and procedures are in place to implement clinical trials, whereas in other institutions new trials are addressed on a case-by-case basis. Clinical trials involving new agents, novel methods of drug delivery, multidisciplinary collaboration, or multimodal treatment require that issues of responsibilility for what, where, when, and how be addressed. The ability of the staff to conduct the trial also needs to be assessed; staff education programs may be necessary. Anticipating patient education needs and addressing these needs enhances the outcome for the patient and the clinical trial. For example, a patient who understands the expected side effects, reports them, and is helped to manage them is less likely to drop out of a clinical trial (Wheeler, 1991).

Quality control begins during the development of the clinical trial, when reviewers check the feasibility of different methods of conducting the trial, the expected outcomes, and the protection of the subjects. All data must be monitored and corrective actions taken, if needed. This includes, for example, ensuring that the consent form has both the patient's and the investigator's signatures and the date of study entry. All treatment and follow-up data need to be recorded on study report forms or flow sheets. These are then sent to a central data office, where accuracy, completeness, and compliance with study guidelines are checked in a timely manner. The principal investigator or study chair in turn checks these forms regularly to evaluate the progress of the study and to identify any problems. The investigator or chair notes any protocol deviations and notifies the appropriate health care personnel. For example, adverse drug reactions (ADRs) are reported

RADIATION THERAPY ONCOLOGY GROUP

RTOG 91-11
ECOG R 9111
SWOG 9201

Phase III Trial to Preserve the Larynx: Induction Chemotherapy and Radiation Therapy versus Concomitant Chemotherapy and Radiation Therapy versus Radiation Therapy

SCHEMA

S T R A T I F Y

Location:
1. Glottic
2. Supraglottic

T Stage:
1. T_2
2. T_3, fixed cord
3. T_3, no cord fixation

N Stage
1. N_0, N_1
2. N_2, N_3

R A N D O M I Z E

CDDP/5-FU
CR,PR × 1 cycle → RT*

CDDP/5-FU
Arm 1: × 2 cycles

NR   Surgery → RT*

Arm 2: Radiation therapy* + CDDP

Arm 3: Radiation therapy*

Chemotherapy

Arm 1: Cisplatin 100 mg/m^2 over 20–30 minutes followed by 5-FU 1 gm/m^2/24 hours by continuous infusion over 120 hours. Administered × 3, three weeks apart.

Arm 2: Cisplatin 100 mg/m^2 over 20–30 minutes administered on days 1, 22, and 43 of RT.

*Radiation Therapy

Arms 1, 2 and 3: 70 Gy total dose, 2.0 Gy 5 days a week for 7 weeks.
Treatment for Arm 1 will begin 3 weeks after the start of the third chemo cycle or 2–3 weeks after surgery as applicable.

Eligibility
- Stages III and IV (excluding T_1 or T_4) squamous cell cancer of the glottic and supraglottic larynx as assessed by CT scan and clinical evaluation.
- Resectable disease requiring total laryngectomy
- No prior surgery, chemotherapy, or radiation therapy
- KPS ≥ 60
- WBC ≥ 3500, platelets ≥ 100,000, creatinine clearance ≥ 50 ml/ min
- No distant metastases
- No synchronous primary

Required Sample Size: 546

Key:

CDDP	=	Cisplatin		
5-FU	=	5-Fluorouracil		
RT	=	Radiation therapy		
CR	=	Complete response		

PR	=	Partial response
NR	=	No response
KPS	=	Karnofosky Performance Scale

Fig. 7-1. Schema example.

initially by telephone within 24 hours of the event, with a specified number of days allowed for written notification, to alert others of potential toxicities or problems with the agent being studied. The chair also visits each institution participating in the study at specific time intervals to audit records and practices. In addition, some of the cooperative groups may require review of radiographic films and pathology slides (Melink and Whitacre, 1991).

❖ Phases of Clinical Trials

Clinical trials are designated as phase I, phase II, or phase III, with the increasing numbers representing progressively closer steps toward becoming standard treatment.

Phase I Trial

In a phase I trial, an agent is often being used in humans for the first time. If their cancers are advanced and no other effective treatment exists, patients may be placed in phase I trials. The primary goal of phase I trials is to determine the maximum tolerated dose of a new drug or drug combination or a new way to deliver treatment, or the highest dose possible without serious toxicities. The secondary goal is to evaluate toxicities quantitatively and qualitatively. In phase I trials, pharmacologic data, including drug absorption, distribution, metabolism, and excretion, are collected through frequent blood and urine samples.

The starting dose is usually one tenth of the maximum tolerated dose in mice in preclinical studies. Usually three to five patients are treated at each dose level and are evaluated before dosages are escalated. Dosage escalations are determined either by pharmacologic data or by a preset percentage (e.g., increasing the previous dose by one half). If dosage levels are nearing the maximum tolerated dose, often six or more patients are evaluated to support and define the maximum tolerated dose better.

A phase I trial is completed when the maximum tolerated dose has been reached and the schedule of drug administration has been established. Shrinkage of the tumor or other objective response is not necessary because it is not a goal of the study (Jenkins and Hubbard, 1991; Melink and Whitacre, 1991).

Phase II Trial

Phase II trials are designed to determine the activity of a new drug for specific cancers. Patients have measurable disease, relatively normal organ function as measured by blood studies, reasonable life expectancy, and adequate nutritional status. Selection of which tumor types to explore in phase II trials can be based either on pharmacologic data or on evidence of antitumor activity from phase I studies.

Eligibility criteria for phase II trials are usually more stringent than for phase I trials. There are clear study objectives, regular evaluations of toxicities, and objective measurements of disease, such as tumor size. Drug schedules are checked often and closely, and dosages are adjusted based on toxicities; cumulative and delayed toxicities are evaluated as well. Tumor measurements by laboratory and radiographic studies are done at regular intervals. The number of study subjects needed is statistically predetermined (Jenkins and Hubbard, 1991; Melink and Whitacre, 1991).

Phase III Trial

Phase III trials are randomized trials that compare two or more treatments for efficacy and toxicity. Often this will compare a new regimen with standard treatment. The new treatment may consist of a single drug, a combination of drugs, or multimodal treatment.

Multiple institutions often participate in these trials because large numbers of patients—sometimes several hundred to several thousand—are needed to answer study questions. Protocols are clear so that all patients are treated equally in such areas as toxicity assessment, evaluation of treatment effectiveness, patient care management, and leaving the study early. Patients may discontinue participation in a study early because of significant side effects, a lack of response by the tumor to treatment, or tumor progression.

Occasionally phase III trials consist of *double-blind* randomized studies in which neither the participant nor the physician knows which treatment is given until the study ends (usually 5 or more years after treatment is stopped in order to allow for follow-up). With double-blind, *placebo-controlled*, randomized design, some patients receive a placebo and some receive the actual treatment. If medically necessary—for example, if the patient becomes pregnant—the code can be broken. Recently quality-of-life assessment has been added as an additional end point in clinical trials (Jenkins and Hubbard, 1991; Melink and Whitacre, 1991). If length of life is extended through treatment but patients suffer numerous side effects, the treatment may not be determined to be beneficial.

❖ Cooperative Groups

Cooperative groups participate in a multiinstitutional, multidisciplinary effort to conduct oncology clinical trials. Group members consist of academic institutions and cancer-treatment centers. Several of these groups are listed in Table 7-1. These groups are financially supported by the NCI and conduct small pilot studies as well as large phase III trials. Five goals of the cooperative-group research program include the following:

- ◆ To increase survival rates and improve the quality of life for cancer patients
- ◆ To conduct basic research regarding biology, pathology, epidemiology, and supportive care related to cancer-treatment trials
- ◆ To serve as a research basis for cancer-control research, which is sponsored by the Division of Cancer Prevention and Control (DCPC)
- ◆ To study various statistical methods used in clinical trials
- ◆ To conduct nursing research (Cheson, 1991)

The Cancer Therapy Evaluation Program (CTEP) within the Division of Cancer Treatment (DCT) at the NCI is responsible for interacting with and monitoring all cooperative groups. The groups compete for funds distributed by the CTEP. A site-visit team reviews the cooperative group every 2 to 4 years. The team consists of medical, surgical, and radiation oncologists, pathologists, statisticians,

Table 7-1   Clinical Trials Cooperative Groups Funded by the National Cancer
Institute

Name of Group	Population Served	Comments
Children's Cancer Group (CCG)	Pediatric	Multidisciplinary
Pediatric Oncology Group	Pediatric	Multidisciplinary
National Wilms' Tumor Study Group	Pediatric	Disease-specific
Intergroup Rhabdomyosarcoma Study (IRS)	Pediatric	Disease-specific
Cancer and Leukemia Group B (CALGB)	Adult	Multidisciplinary
Eastern Cooperative Oncology Group (ECOG)	Adult	Multidisciplinary
North Central Cancer Treatment Group (NCCTG)	Adult	Multidisciplinary
Southwest Oncology Group (SWOG)	Adult	Multidisciplinary
European Organization for Research on Treatment of Cancer (EORTC)	Adult	Multidisciplinary
Radiation Therapy Oncology Group (RTOG)	Adult	Radiation-specific
National Surgical Adjuvant Breast and Bowel Project (NSABP)	Adult	Disease-specific
Brain Tumor Cooperative Group (BTCG)	Adult	Disease-specific
Gynecologic Oncology Group (GOG)	Adult	Disease-specific

From Cheson B: Clinical trials programs, Semin Oncol Nurs 7:235–242, 1991.

data managers, and nurses. It examines any improvements or corrections made to previously identified deficiencies in scientific quality, explores the significance and importance of the scientific questions the group has studied, evaluates accrual to studies, and notes future plans (Cheson, 1991).

The Community Group Outreach Program (CGOP), sponsored by the DCT, links community-based physicians with one cooperative group. This program allows patients to be registered by the community institution affiliated with a member institution of a cooperative group. The Community Clinical Oncology Program (CCOP), established in 1983 and sponsored by the DCPC, is also designed to bring clinical trials to the community. Community physicians and institutions can link with numerous cooperative groups and cancer centers. To maintain membership, the institutions need to accrue a certain number of "CCOP credits" per year (50 for cancer treatment and 50 for cancer-control research) (Cheson, 1991; Jenkins and Hubbard, 1991; Meili, 1991).

Community institutions range in size from large urban teaching hospitals to small community hospitals or physician groups. Some have specialized oncology units; some operate out of general medical surgical units. Usually phase II and phase III trials are conducted in the community, but phase I trials are conducted only in large cancer centers (Meili, 1991).

The institutional principal investigator is responsible for preparing for routine audits. The purpose of these audits is to verify that participating institutions have met the protocol requirements and that treatment results are accurately reported. Patient charts are compared with all data submitted to assure accuracy. There must be verification that the Institutional Review Board has approved the study, reviewed each study annually, and included any amendments made by the study group. Finally, all investigational drugs distributed to the institution by the investigation group have to be accounted for, and appropriate records must be made available to the audit team. Audits can be very helpful in improving practice and procedures for institutions and for cooperative groups as a whole. Occasionally, disciplinary action needs to be taken. This may be a letter of warning, or it may eventually lead to the disqualification of investigators (Cassidy and Macfarlane, 1991).

❖ Ethical Issues

The goal of clinical practice is to provide the best options at the time for the individual patient. Clinical research, on the other hand, is designed to test hypotheses, answer questions, and contribute to knowledge pertaining to a particular treatment for a large number of patients (Grady, 1991). If an individual patient benefits from clinical research, that is an ancillary gain. Engelhardt (1988) contends that because knowledge is applied so rapidly and because clinical trials are a rigorous way to test new knowledge, clinical trials benefit both society as a whole and individual patients.

Ethical Principles

Numerous ethical principles must be upheld in the conduct of clinical trials. *Nonmaleficence,* or the principle of doing no harm, is a basic element in clinical trials. Cancer patients in particular are vulnerable because their situation may be viewed as life-threatening with seemingly few options. Some will grasp at anything to help themselves; other patients, especially those entering phase I trials, realize that nothing may benefit them directly but are willing to contribute to scientific knowledge to help future patients (Grady, 1991; Melink and Whitacre, 1991). *Beneficence* takes the principle of nonmaleficence one step further and includes acts of kindness and charity. *Respect for persons* includes both respect for individuals' autonomy, or their right to make their own decisions, and protection of those unable to make their own decisions. The principle of *justice* seeks equal distribution of benefits and burdens for individuals. Within clinical trials, risks must be reasonable and weighed against potential benefits. With the uncertainties associated with clinical trials, risk/benefit ratios are at best estimations of potential future events.

For clinical research to be ethically justified, the following rules need to be satisfied:

- ◆ The research design must generate a high level of useful knowledge.
- ◆ Proposed benefits should outweigh potential risks.
- ◆ Subjects must be treated fairly.
- ◆ Subjects must give consent that is informed.
- ◆ Subjects' privacy and confidentiality rights must be protected (Beauchamp and Childress, 1983).

The principles of autonomy and respect for persons are evident in the informed-consent process. Justice is practiced when there is fair selection of subjects. The randomization process helps reduce bias in subject selection to some extent (Grady, 1991).

Informed Consent

Informed consent includes both the consent form and the process. As part of the process, the investigator should provide information to the subject, the subject should comprehend it, and the subject should participate voluntarily. Participants are given both a verbal and written explanation of the study, according to their level of understanding and learning abilities. Children and teenagers are to be included in this process as well, even if they cannot legally sign the consent form. The patient and family must be given an opportunity to consider whether to participate in the clinical trial without coercion or persuasion. Federal law mandates that each subject needs to be informed in a manner the subject understands and to have an IRB-approved consent form signed and dated before participation in a clinical trial. Ethically, consent should be a shared decision based on mutual respect between participants and health care personnel and not just the signing of a form. Legally, subjects cannot be treated without their consent. As a condition throughout the study, patients also should understand that they can terminate the study at any time without compromising future care (Grady, 1991; Melink and Whitacre, 1991). Box 7-2 reviews the components of informed consent.

❖ Nursing Roles in Clinical Trials

Various levels and types of nursing expertise are needed for the development, implementation, and evaluation of clinical trials. Some roles include clinician, researcher, data manager, and educator, or a combination.

Clinician

The clinician, as primary caregiver, provides individualized care and promotes continuity of care for patients in clinical trials (Melink and Whitacre, 1991). The primary

---

Box 7-2 Components of Informed Consent

As part of the process of informed consent, the patient should be given the following:

- ◆ A statement regarding:
  - ◆ The experimental nature of the study
  - ◆ The purpose of the study
  - ◆ Any drugs, treatments, or procedures that are experimental
  - ◆ The expected duration of participation
- ◆ A description of potential risks and benefits
- ◆ A disclosure of treatment alternatives to study participation
- ◆ A description of how confidentiality will be maintained
- ◆ A description of availability and components of any compensation or medical treatments if undesirable results occur
- ◆ The names and numbers of persons to contact for answers to questions
- ◆ A statement that participation is voluntary and that future care will not be compromised if the study is refused or discontinued at any future point in time

functions of assessment, planning, intervention, and evaluation continue, regardless of the nurse's participation in a clinical trial. However, the nurse needs to follow the study protocol guidelines, whether or not the procedures follow the institution's standard practice.

Clinical trials require collaboration with other colleagues: with pharmacists in procuring and administering new investigational agents or with basic scientists in conducting pharmacologic studies with phase I trials, for example. Caregivers must ensure continuity of care for their patients as they move from one setting to another and, for those in multimodal treatment, from one type of treatment to another.

Patients with cancer are particularly vulnerable to false hopes and may be willing to try anything to treat their disease. The nurse, therefore, acts as patient advocate, especially in facilitating the informed-consent process. The nurse assists patients to define their own goals for entering the clinical trial and to review them periodically, mindful that patients have the right to withdraw from the study at any time. Although this may not benefit the study, it protects patients' rights. Patients who question remaining in the study may need help with physical or emotional needs that they feel are not being met. The nurse should assess the situation and interact appropriately.

The number of protocols used by an institution can vary from a few to 100 or more, depending on the number of cooperative groups affiliated with the institution. The staff must refer to the protocol document for specifics regarding admixture of drugs, order of agents given (if there are multiple drugs), the route of administration, and whether the drugs are to be infused or pushed with a syringe. All chemotherapy orders need to be double-checked to avoid errors in calculating the dosage, which are usually based on kilograms of body weight or body surface area.

Patients are assessed frequently for treatment toxicities. This includes not only toxicities from investigational agents but from commercial drugs. Nurses need good observation skills, good communication skills, and assertiveness. They need to distinguish between expected toxicities and symptoms associated with cancer. Documentation is vital to clinical trials. Nurses translate detailed descriptions of patient symptoms into toxicity-grading scales (see Chapter 1, Tables 1-4 through 1-6). Instead of simply stating that a patient reported moderate diarrhea, for example, it is more helpful to document that a patient reports having seven watery stools per day as compared to two semisoft stools per day before protocol entry. Accurate descriptions of patient symptoms help plan necessary modifications to dosage levels and enable health care professionals to evaluate toxicity objectively (Cassidy and Macfarlane, 1991; Meili, 1991).

The nurse can facilitate continuity of care by arranging follow-up appointments and by double-checking that appropriate tests are ordered. Nurses may be involved with conducting pharmacokinetic studies for phase I trials or ensuring that they are done at appropriate times.

Patients need to understand the reasons for frequent checkups and evaluations. If patients are not able to keep appointments, it is helpful to have a logbook of all phone calls and to document in the chart the reasons that patients give for missing appointments. This may provide additional data or a rationale for decision making. It is helpful to keep the name and phone number of the patient's local physician for additional information if the patient does not return to the treatment center (Cassidy and Macfarlane, 1991). If the treatment center is not the patient's primary health care institution, the nurse can send a message to the nurse who will follow the patient at home. This includes the home institution nurse as a part of the clinical trial team and makes him or her more apt to report any late effects to the protocol team.

Research Nurse

The role of the research nurse often combines clinical and data management responsibilities, plus some staff education. In many cases, the research nurse is a protocol case manager who facilitates and coordinates patient care from entry into the study through long-term follow-up. Research nurses often facilitate the informed-consent process and assist the patient and staff through all protocol requirements, ensuring that the guidelines are met and that pertinent data are gathered (McEvoy, Cannon, and MacDermott, 1991; Meili, 1991; Wheeler, 1991).

Data Manager

The data manager is responsible for data collection and for handling and reporting all the research information. The data manager is not necessarily a nurse, but a nurse playing this role brings knowledge of health care as well as clinical experience. The data manager has knowledge of general and specific oncology anatomy and terminology, cancer staging procedures, the approval and review process, and audit procedures.

The duties of the data manager include monitoring patient accrual, abstracting and entering data, assuring data quality and validity, and managing computer systems. Key data elements include patient demographics, disease information, history and physical exam findings, staging, treatment specifics, and follow-up notations. Sometimes the data manager designs forms; at other times the forms are provided by the sponsor or cooperative group. Data managers need to be self-motivated, well organized, detail-oriented, comfortable with paper work, and analytical, because they may be the first to notice trends, protocol violations, or unusual toxicities (Cassidy, 1993).

Educator

Before a clinical trial starts, the impact on existing resources, the locations where patients will be seen (inpatient, clinic, or physician offices), nursing staffing, and nursing roles and responsibilities must be determined. A systematic approach can help smoothly incorporate study requirements into existing policies regarding staff and resources.

Every institution participating in the trials must provide education on informed consent, treatment administration, treatment toxicities, and documentation. Nurses need to identify their feelings about research and to weigh the practice and ethical issues carefully. Those nurses who feel uneasy should discuss their concerns with a trusted member of the clinical trials team.

The staff needs to be familiar with the protocols and to have the protocol requirements close at hand for reference. For example, the treatment units could make notebooks available that arrange the active protocols by disease site and protocol number. Institutions can also make abstracts of protocols, consisting of one-page, abbreviated summaries of pertinent information such as eligibility criteria, the protocol schema, drug administration, expected toxicities, and dosage modifications. Pertinent portions of the protocol can be photocopied and attached to the patient chart. The protocol and any disease-specific information can be taught through nursing education programs or individualized instruction. Fact sheets containing the name of the drugs or the modality used in treatment and the names and phone numbers of the principal investigator, the protocol chair, and other important contact people have proven useful (Cassidy and Macfarlane, 1991; Meili, 1991).

The staff also needs to be proficient in procedures; for example, techniques of administering chemotherapy. Whenever there are new methods of drug administration or new technologies, nurses need information on the procedures involved; for example, intraperitoneal therapy using an implanted pump or a peripherally inserted central catheter (PICC). Orientation of new employees should include administration of new investigational drugs, understanding the research process, learning assessment skills to monitor patients, and discussion of ethical issues (Wheeler, 1991).

Patients and families often feel anxious about unproven treatments and need to deal with feelings of "being a guinea pig." Patients respond well to education about clinical trials and the informed consent process (Wheeler, 1991). Goals for patients under protocol are not much different from those of patients not in clinical trails. As clinical trials move into the community and outpatient settings, patient education becomes even more of a challenge because of time limitations (Johansen, Mayer, and Hoover, 1991: Meili, 1991).

The Onocology Nursing Society's standards for educating patients and families about cancer can be helpful in designing patient education programs pertaining to clinical trials (Oncology Nursing Society, 1995). The NCI video "Patient to Patient: Clinical Trials and You" is a good resource for patients considering clinical trials. The NCI also has a brochure for patients entitled "What are Clinical Trials All About?" In addition, a video about clinical trials is available for professionals. The NCI information is available free by calling 1-800-4-CANCER.

Researcher

Nurses are competent collaborators in clinical research and leaders in study implementation, improving quality within the research process, exploring cost-effective methods of conducting clinical trials, and promoting timely completion of studies. Nurses also lend their unique perspective to clinical trials, particularly their focus on symptom management (Guy, 1991; McEvoy, Cannon, and MacDermott, 1991).

The requirements of cancer research play to the strengths of good nursing research, including such priorities as disease prevention, identifying and minimizing risks, symptom management, and patient comfort. Nursing researchers can be leaders in this area by incorporating their skills in continuity of care into the job. They can also conduct the long-term follow-up needed for many of these studies (Guy, 1991).

Ferrell and Cohen (1991) proposed the concept of *companion studies.* Nursing research questions—such as questions about the management or prevention of stomatitis—can be addressed simultaneously with a medical study, in a "piggyback" fashion. Both studies benefit from joint subject recruitment, data collection, logistics management, and study analysis. Companion studies promote interdisciplinary collaboration (Ferrell and Cohen, 1991).

Potential research areas for companion studies include the following:

♦ Cancer control, including prevention, early detection, or compliance
♦ Treatment effects or symptom management, including pain, nausea, fatigue, mucositis, and quality of life
♦ Rehabilitation, including survivorship issues, recovery from treatment or surgery, and follow-up issues
♦ Assessment of instrumentation, including development and testing of nursing instruments, or measuring individual responses to interventions

❖ Issues and Obstacles with Clinical Trials

Numerous issues continue to make clinical trials a challenging endeavor. Some of the issues include patient accrual, the changing health care environment, the costs, and various barriers between patients, physicians, and nurses.

Patient access to clinical trials remains low, hampering patient accrual, which in turn postpones completion of the study. Large numbers of patients are eligible to participate, but few actually enter clinical trials for a variety of reasons. It has been suggested that fewer than 20% of all eligible adult patients enroll in clinical trials, whereas more than 80% of all pediatric patients do. It is not clear why there is this disparity between adult and pediatric accrual rates. However, the high-priority clinical trials program established in 1988 should ease this problem somewhat (Cheson, 1991; Johansen, Mayer, and Hoover, 1991).

The changing health care environment and associated costs continue to shape clinical trials programs. Since diagnosis related groups (DRGs) were implemented in 1983 for Medicare patients, a large shift has occurred from inpatient to outpatient treatment. Various health care professionals have attempted to establish day hospitals to support cancer research initiatives in the face of shrinking research budgets (Sands et al., 1993). Third-party payers also affect the delivery of cancer care because they approve fewer hospitalizations, pay for fewer tests, and pay more attention to drug costs. With more than 85% of clinical research being conducted in the community, advanced technologies such as autologous bone marrow transplant are being shifted to larger group practices and sites designated by third-party payers (Guy, 1991; McCabe, 1992).

Some patients have been denied payment by insurance companies for new investigational drugs and "off-label" use of chemotherapy. It was found that three of the eight most commonly used chemotherapy drugs were used for indications not listed in the package inserts but in keeping with the literature and recent research findings. Labeling this as experimental treatment, insurance companies deny payment (Mortenson, 1988). In 1990 the National Commission to Review Current Procedures for Approval of New Drugs for Cancer and AIDS (Lasagna Committee) concluded that Medicare, Medicaid, and private insurers should pay for all investigational and commercial drugs given off-label if verified in the medical literature or in an authoritative medical compendium; for example, the American Hospital Pharmacy Service Drug Information (Guy, 1991).

Physicians may have concerns about clinical trials interfering with the patient-doctor relationship and may feel uncertain about study outcomes. Patients may feel uncomfortable with the randomization process, and it may be difficult to obtain informed consent. The time and logistical difficulties involved in following study requirements can also be barriers. Nurses can foster collaboration and work toward joint decision making (Johansen, Mayer, and Hoover, 1991).

Obstacles can occur within the health care setting as well. Some factors that may affect patient participation include patients' lack of interest in research or disapproval of research; the inconveniences associated with research; fear, anxiety, or denial; patients' unwillingness to accept randomization; or family influences. To overcome these kinds of obstacles, nurses can educate patients and the public about clinical trials, they can address feelings that may accompany decision making, and they can include the family and significant others in discussions of clinical trials, allow them to express their concerns, and gain their support (Johansen, Mayer, and Hoover, 1991).

❖ *Summary*

The future of oncology nursing practice is affected by scientific and technological advances and changes in the nursing profession (Miaskowski, 1990). Nurses continue to be recognized for their collaborative efforts in research. Nurses are vital to the clinical trial process and frequently are the ones to foster continuity of care in multimodal therapy. The current body of knowledge about cancer is a direct result of clinical trials conducted in the past. The future of oncology practice depends on today's carefully designed, thoughtfully conducted, and critically analyzed clinical trials.

❖ *References*

Beauchamp T and Childress J: Principles of biomedical ethics, ed 2, New York, 1983, Oxford University Press.

Cassidy J and Macfarlane DK: The role of the nurse in clinical cancer research, Cancer Nurs 14:124–131, 1991.

Cassidy T: The role of the data manager in clinical cancer research: an opportunity for nurses, Cancer Nurs 16:131–138, 1993.

Cheson B: Clinical trials programs, Semin Oncol Nurs 7:235–242, 1991.

Engelhardt HT: Diagnosing well and treating prudently: randomized clinical trials and the problem of knowing truly. In Spiker S, Alon A, deVries A, and Engelhardt HT, editors: The use of human beings in research, Norwell, Massachusetts, 1988, Klumer Academie, pp. 123–141.

Ferrell BR and Cohen MZ: Companion studies, Semin Oncol Nurs 7:252–259, 1991.

Grady C: Ethical issues in clinical trials, Semin Oncol Nurs 7:286–296, 1991.

Guy J: New challenges for nurses in clinical trials, Semin Oncol Nurs 7:297–303, 1991.

Jenkins J and Hubbard S: History of clinical trials, Semin Oncol Nurs 7:228–234, 1991.

Johansen MA, Mayer DK, and Hoover HC: Obstacles to implementing cancer clinical trials, Semin Oncol Nurs 7:260–267, 1991.

McCabe M: Reimbursement of biotherapy: present status, future directions and perspectives of the hospital-based oncology nurse, Semin Oncol Nurs 8(suppl 1):3–7, 1992.

McEvoy MD, Cannon L, and MacDermott ML: The professional role for nurses in clinical trials, Semin Oncol Nurs 7:268–274, 1991.

Meili L: The community hospital perspective of clinical trials and the role of the nurse educator, Semin Oncol Nurs 7:280–287, 1991.

Melink TJ and Whitacre MY: Planning and implementing clinical trials, Semin Oncol Nurs 7:243–251, 1991.

Miaskowski C: The future of oncology nursing: a historical perspective, Nurs Clin N Am 25:461–473, 1990.

Mortenson LC: Audit indicates many uses of combination therapy are unlabeled, J Cancer Prog Mgmt 3:21–25, 1988.

National Cancer Institute: Guidelines: NCI-Designated Comprehensive Cancer Center, Washington, DC, 1992, National Cancer Institute, National Institutes of Health, Department of Health and Human Services.

Oncology Nursing Society: Standards of oncology education: patient/family and public, Pittsburgh, 1995, Oncology Nursing Society.

Sands D, Galassi A, Chisholm L, Diamond E, Caubo K, and Jenkins J: A cancer day hospital: an alternative approach to caring for patients in clinical trials, Oncol Nurs Forum 20:787–793, 1993.

Wheeler V: Preparing nurses for clinical trials: the cancer center approach, Semin Oncol Nurs 7:275–279, 1991.

UNIT *II*

SITE-SPECIFIC CANCERS

Chapter 8

❖ Breast Cancer

Mary Mrozek-Orlowski

Major scientific advances since the 1960s have drastically changed the diagnosis and treatment of breast cancer. The most important change relates to advances in knowledge about the natural history of the disease and therefore its treatment. Unfortunately, the mortality rate of breast cancer has remained the same.

In the late 1800s, Halstead introduced the radical mastectomy. Halstead hypothesized that breast cancer spreads in a contiguous manner from the breast to the regional lymph nodes, then to distant sites (Halstead, 1907). However, Halstead's theory was not universally accepted. As early as 1924, Keynes (1937) implanted radium needles to treat breast cancer. Use of the modified radical mastectomy was first reported in the late 1940s (McWhirter, 1948; Patey and Dyson, 1948).

It was not until 1967 that an alternative hypothesis for the natural history or spread of breast cancer emerged (Fisher and Fisher, 1967). The Fishers and their colleagues proposed that breast cancer is a systemic disease and has the ability to metastasize from its inception (Fisher et al., 1985). Furthermore, they suggested that variations in local and regional therapy would be unlikely to change survival rates. This new hypothesis has guided the direction of breast cancer research since the 1970s. Today breast cancer is recognized as a systemic disease. The treatment of breast cancer is based on two major concepts: local-regional control and systemic control.

❖ Treatment

Today treatment of breast cancer is multimodal. Surgical oncologists, plastic surgeons, radiation oncologists, medical oncologists, nurses, social workers, pharmacists, and psychologists comprise the team dedicated to assisting women in choosing treatment options, beginning with local-regional control of the disease. This usually includes making a decision between having a mastectomy or having conservative surgery followed by radiation. Both options include an axillary node dissection for staging purposes (see Patient Education Guidelines on p. 120 and Nursing Care for Patients with Axillary Lymph Node Dissection on p. 121). Consultations with a plastic surgeon and a radiation oncologist are included in the planning process to discuss options about reconstructive surgery (if mastectomy is the choice) or

Patient Education Guidelines for

Patients with Axillary Lymph Node Dissection

♦ Numbness in the affected arm is common. Changes in sensation sometimes described as "arm falling asleep" can happen over time.
♦ Be cautious when shaving under your arm. Skin cuts may occur without your knowledge because of loss of sensation.
♦ Begin stretching exercises about 24 hours after surgery, but limit the exercises to those that do not involve the shoulder. More strenuous exercises may begin a week or so after surgery, once the drains are removed. Exercises are important to prevent shoulder stiffness.
♦ Avoid carrying heavy loads with the affected arm.
♦ Avoid having blood pressures taken, IVs placed, or injections in the affected arm.
♦ Report any redness or warmth in the affected arm to your doctor. These are signs of infection.
♦ Do not cut your cuticles; prevent dry skin by using hand cream.
♦ If your shoulder is still stiff and interferes with daily activities a month after surgery, consult with your doctor about the possibility of physical therapy. The exercises and massage may ease tightness in shoulder.

Permission granted to reproduce these guidelines for educational purposes only.

radiation therapy to the affected breast (if conservative surgery is the choice). It is important to stress that the entire breast needs treatment; that is, if conservative surgery is chosen, radiation therapy almost always follows.

Modified radical mastectomy (MRM) is generally preferred over conservative surgery if the lesion is larger than 4 cm in size (Levitt and Perez, 1987). If removal of the tumor will cause a significant decrease in the size of the affected breast, MRM will allow better cosmetic results. The acceptable cosmetic result, however, is a subjective concept that only women can define. *Multicentricity,* or tumors located in more than one area of the breast, is another indication for MRM (Rosen, Fracchia, and Urban, 1975). Some women prefer a mastectomy as an alternative to the time commitment required by radiation therapy.

Reconstruction

Reconstructive surgery has made MRM a more acceptable option. Initially, radical mastectomies prohibited reconstruction because of the aggressiveness of the surgery. Today implants, soft tissue flaps, and microsurgical techniques as well as a better understanding of breast cancer biology have made reconstruction a viable option. Reconstruction can occur immediately after mastectomy but may be delayed if adjuvant chemotherapy or radiation is immediately needed. There must be adequate time for healing and recovery from blood counts after radiation therapy and chemotherapy before reconstruction. The plastic surgeon should be involved in the decision-making process as early as possible because reconstructive surgery on irradiated skin can also delay healing.

Nursing Care of

The Patient with Axillary Lymph Node Dissection

Nursing Care	Rationale/Comments
◆ Ascertain from any patient with breast cancer which side is the treated side. Unless contraindicated, use the opposite side for a blood pressure measurement, drawing blood, placing IVs, or injections. If the patient is in the hospital, put up a sign saying "Avoid BP or venipuncture in_____arm."	◆ The skin is the first line of defense against infection. A break in the skin increases the risk of infection.
◆ If the arm from the treated side must be used (if there is bilateral breast cancer, if the untreated arm is in a cast, or if there is cellulitis of untreated arm, or an emergency), proceed with caution. Monitor the arm for redness, heat, and infection. Some institutions require a physician's order before using affected arm.	◆ A break in skin integrity increases the risk of infection.
◆ Teach lymph node dissection care to the patient. Stress that precautions need to be maintained throughout the patient's life.	◆ Lymphedema has occurred as late as 10 years after axillary node dissection.
◆ Begin limited exercises (involving only the wrist and elbow) after surgery; delay exercises involving the shoulder until drains are removed.	◆ Vigorous exercise begun too soon after surgery may increase seroma (fluid in lower axilla) development.
◆ For patients with lymphedema, consider physical therapy.	◆ May aid in lymph drainage from affected arm.

Several methods of breast reconstruction are available, including tissue expanders, implants, flap transfers, or a combination of these procedures. Tissue expanders are placed beneath the skin or skin and muscle and are gradually inflated by injecting saline solution into the expander. This can be done in the physician's office or in a clinic, or occasionally the patient and family learn the procedure. Expansion usually exceeds the size of the unaffected breast, so that when the placement of the permanent prosthesis takes place, an adequate amount of soft tissue cover exists to allow for a softer, pitotic breast. Once the desired expansion occurs, the expander is surgically removed and the permanent prosthesis is placed. Silicone implants, which may provide a softer, more cosmetically appealing effect, are available through clinical trials only.

Skin flaps can also be used for breast reconstruction when insufficient or poor-quality skin exists. This technique is also used when soft tissue is needed to augment the reconstruction. The latissimus dorsi flap often requires an additional implant because of its lack of soft tissue bulk. A transverse rectus abdominis flap (TRAM) is indicated for reconstruction when adequate abdominal skin and fat tissue exist; when the unaffected breast is large and tissue is needed for symmetry; or when patients do not desire prosthetic implants. Patients who smoke or are relatively obese are not candidates for TRAM flaps because these factors may compromise the blood supply, thus causing greater potential for flap loss.

The second stage of reconstruction deals with symmetry and creation of the areola-nipple complex. Many women need reduction of the contralateral breast to create symmetry with the reconstructed breast. The areola-nipple complex is created by first making a small incision and pulling a small amount of tissue through to create the nipple. This is followed by tattooing the areola. Tattooing requires practice to match coloring and artistry to create symmetry. Skin grafts from the labia and inner thigh for the areola and grafts from toe-tips or earlobes are additional methods for achieving the aesthetics desired.

Patient education (see Patient Education Guidelines for Care of the Reconstructed Breast [data from Harden and Girard, 1994; Hinojosa, 1991; and Walsh,

Patient Education Guidelines for

Care of the Reconstructed Breast

Preoperative Instructions
♦ The reconstructed breast will stabilize in size in approximately 3 months, but subtle changes may happen for as long as 18 months after surgery.
♦ No medications that interfere with clotting or blood flow (nonsteroidal antiinflammatory drugs or aspirin) may be taken either before or after surgery.
♦ Review upper-extremity range-of-motion exercises, deep breathing exercises, and, if TRAM-flap reconstruction is featured, leg exercises.

For All Types of Reconstruction
♦ You will have drains in place around the reconstruction. If they do not come out before you go home, the nurses will teach you how to empty them and keep track daily of the amount of drainage.
♦ You may shower when the sutures are removed. Until then, bathing is allowed as long as the incisions are kept dry.
♦ You will have discomfort after the surgery. Take your pain medication as directed.
♦ You will be instructed to begin upper-extremity range-of-motion exercises about 1 week after surgery. It is important to do these exercises to keep the muscles from becoming stiff.
♦ You may begin sexual activity once you are home. Do not place pressure on the reconstruction.
♦ Avoid heavy lifting for several weeks after surgery. Your surgeon will instruct you when you may begin lifting heavy objects (over 10 pounds).
♦ Take your antibiotics as instructed. Infection in the reconstruction may delay healing.
♦ Massage techniques to prevent scar tissue in the reconstruction will be demonstrated to you by your nurse or physician.

Permission granted to reproduce these guidelines for educational purposes only.

1991]) and nursing support are crucial for women considering reconstruction. Many women believe that the reconstructed breast will appear exactly like the unaffected breast, but there are structural differences between the reconstructed breast and the unaffected breast. Women may become frustrated with the length of time needed between surgeries. Photographs that depict both desirable and less-than-desirable results of reconstruction help women with decision making. Videos are available for the patient to view or she can be visited by an American Cancer Society Reach to Recovery volunteer who has had reconstructive surgery.

Surgery Followed by Radiation Therapy

Conservative surgery (lumpectomy, quadrantectomy, segmentectomy) combined with radiation for women with early-stage breast cancer is essentially equivalent to mastectomy for local-regional control (Clark et al., 1982; Findlay et al., 1986; Fisher et al., 1989; Veronesi et al., 1993). Conservative surgery preserves the breast and for many women helps maintain normalcy.

Radiation therapy usually follows conservative surgery within 2 to 4 weeks to allow healing at the surgical site. Radiation therapy is time-consuming because a small dose to the entire breast (Figure 8-1) is given daily over 5 to 6 weeks with an additional "boost" dose to the former tumor site given over 1 to 2 weeks. One way to reduce the time required for radiation therapy is to utilize radioactive implants for a portion of the treatment (Figure 8-2). Negative aspects of radioactive implants include the hospitalization required to receive the implants, the discomfort of placing the catheters, and the inactivity required when the implants are in place.

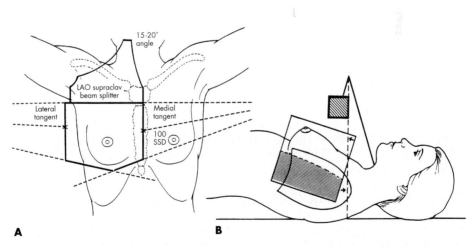

Fig. 8-1. External-beam radiation therapy of the breast. **A,** Inferior angulation of tangential beams eliminates divergence into supraclavicular field. **B,** Half-beam block splitting supraclavicular field eliminates divergence into tangential fields. After couch is rotated, the collimator must also be rotated (note arrows). Courtesy RR Kuske, MD, New Orleans.

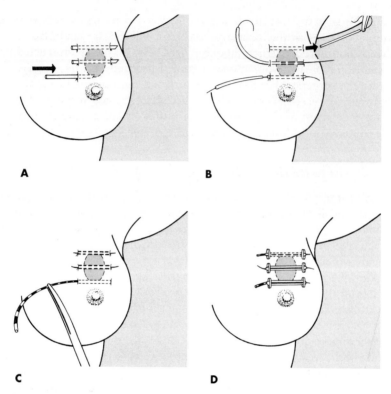

Fig. 8-2. Radiation implants. **A,** Placement of hollow needles. **B,** Replacement of hollow needles by plastic catheters. **C,** Loading of iridium sources. **D,** Interstitial implant in place with buttons to secure catheters. From Belcher AE: Cancer nursing, St. Louis, 1992, Mosby.

Surgery (or Surgery Followed by Radiation) Followed by Adjuvant Chemotherapy or Hormone Therapy

Adjuvant treatment follows definitive local-regional control of breast cancer. Traditionally, premenopausal women with large tumors (>2 cm) or any lymph node involvement have received chemotherapy. Postmenopausal women were offered tamoxifen. Women with negative axillary lymph nodes (no cancer found in the lymph nodes) were considered finished with treatment after surgery (and radiation if the surgery was conservative). After oncologists realized that breast cancer is a systemic disease, even at very early stages, systemic therapy was added to the treatment regimen, regardless of lymph node involvement.

Negative Axillary Lymph Nodes
In 1988 the National Cancer Institute (NCI) published a clinical alert stating that adjuvant hormone therapy or chemotherapy can positively affect the survival rate of some patients with stage I breast cancer (negative axillary lymph nodes) (National

Cancer Institute, 1988). Controversy continues about which women will benefit from adjuvant chemotherapy. Not only do the patient's chances of disease-free survival need to be considered but the quality of life as well. The decision to administer chemotherapy to a group of women who may not really need it (because many of them are already cured) is a difficult one. The determination of which women should receive adjuvant chemotherapy has relied heavily on profiles of the risk of relapse developed from studies of prognostic factors such as tumor size, axillary lymph node involvement, estrogen receptor status, tumor grade, and S-phase fraction. The National Institutes of Health Consensus Panel on Breast Cancer stated in 1990 that women with a tumor of less than 1 cm in diameter have less than a 10% chance of relapse within 10 years and should not be treated adjuvantly.

The first study of women with negative axillary lymph nodes receiving adjuvant chemotherapy randomized women who were node-negative and estrogen-receptor-negative to receive cyclophosphamide, methotrexate, and 5-fluorouracil (CMF) intravenously every 3 weeks for a total of 12 courses over 9 months versus a control group receiving no chemotherapy (Bonadonna, 1990). After 7 years, 85% of the treatment group was disease-free compared to only 42% of the control group.

The Intergroup Trial (Eastern Cooperative Oncology Group, Southwest Oncology Group, and the Cancer and Leukemia Group B) randomized premenopausal and postmenopausal women with node-negative breast cancer to chemotherapy or observation only (see the Research Highlight on p. 126). In this study 83% of the women who received treatment and 61% of the women who did not receive chemotherapy had disease-free survival.

Toxicities from CMF chemotherapy include mild to moderate nausea and vomiting, thinning hair, and neutropenia. Cystitis occurs rarely but is more often seen with dose-intensive cyclophosphamide. Nausea is more problematic with the use of oral as opposed to intravenous cyclophosphamide.

Methotrexate may exacerbate skin changes seen with radiation therapy (O'Rourke, 1987). Women receiving radiation therapy who have wet desquamation in the treatment field should be healed before receiving methotrexate. When chemotherapy is given concurrently with radiation therapy, the methotrexate may be omitted.

Doxorubicin is another chemotherapy agent given to women with breast cancer. Radiation recall (recurrence of skin changes in the radiation field, as well as other soft tissue damage that occurs during radiation) may be seen when doxorubicin is administered after a course of radiation therapy. Other side effects include nausea, vomiting, alopecia, and bone marrow depression.

Tamoxifen, despite its published benefits, remains controversial as a treatment for node-negative breast cancer. Several studies have shown that tamoxifen can reduce recurrence by 36% to 38% (Glick, 1991), and this benefit appears constant regardless of age, menopausal status, or duration of therapy. However, the Early Breast Cancer Trialists' Collaborative Group (1992) reviewed 28 trials and concluded that the effect of tamoxifen on early breast cancer was greater for postmenopausal women than for premenopausal women. The NIH Consensus Development Conference (1991) commented that benefits from tamoxifen in postmenopausal women clearly outweighed the risks, but long-term risks in premenopausal women are not clear. The

---

── *RESEARCH HIGHLIGHT* ──────────────────────────

Tourney DC, Eudey L, and Mansour EG: CMFP versus observation in high-risk node-negative breast cancer patients. Program of the NIH Consensus Development Conference on Early-Stage Breast Cancer, Washington, DC, 1990, National Institutes of Health, pp. 61–62.

Sample 425 patients with node-negative breast cancer.

Randomization After local surgery or surgery and radiation therapy, patients with any size tumor, with negative estrogen receptors, or with tumors equal to or greater than 3 cm in size with positive estrogen receptors were eligible. These women were randomized between observation and cyclophosphamide, methotrexate, fluorouracil, and prednisone chemotherapy. Patients with tumors less than 3 cm in size and positive estrogen receptors were registered for observation only.

Treatment Women received cyclophosphamide 100 mg/m² orally on days 1 to 14; methotrexate 40 mg/m² and fluorouracil 600 mg/m² on days 1 and 8, and prednisone 40 mg/m² on days 1 to 14. The cycle was repeated every 29 days, and treatment lasted for 6 cycles.

Results Of the patients in the chemotherapy arm, 83% experienced disease-free survival versus 61% of those in the observation arm. These results were significant regardless if the woman had negative or positive estrogen receptors, if the tumor was less than or greater than 3 cm, or if she was pre- or postmenopausal.

---

risk-benefit ratio for adjuvant tamoxifen in node-negative premenopausal breast cancer is not known and is being studied, although because of the long follow-up required, the results will not be available for years.

Toxicities include hot flashes, thrombophlebitis, and uterine cancer. Hot flashes are the most frequently reported side effect associated with tamoxifen. While not harmful, they can be uncomfortable and may interfere with the patient's quality of life. Thrombophlebitis is reported in approximately 1% of women taking tamoxifen. Uterine cancer is reported to be 0.3% (Nayfield et al., 1991) to 0.6% (Fisher et al., 1994). Researchers conclude that the risk of developing uterine cancer is less than the risk of breast cancer recurrence. Although these toxicities are rare, they need to be discussed with women before they take tamoxifen.

The benefits of taking tamoxifen include a 25% reduction in cardiovascular events (Rutquist and Mattsson, 1993) and possible prevention of bone loss.

Positive Axillary Lymph Nodes in Premenopausal Women
The history of adjuvant chemotherapy for node-positive breast cancer began in the 1970s. Clinical trials randomized women with positive lymph nodes to receive 12 cycles of CMF chemotherapy after surgical therapy or to surgical therapy alone (Bonadonna et al., 1985; Fisher, Fisher, and Redmond, 1986). These trials demonstrated improved overall survival after 10 years in the group receiving both

chemotherapy and surgery; however, this benefit was observed primarily in pre-menopausal women with three or less positive lymph nodes.

A subsequent trial randomized women to 6 or 12 cycles of CMF. Because no significant difference was found between these two groups, researchers conclude that 6 cycles of CMF is as effective as 12 cycles (Tancini et al., 1983). Six cycles of CMF have been established as the standard regimen for many years (Early Breast Cancer Trialists' Collaborative Group, 1992).

The dosage-intensity and the percentage of planned chemotherapy received are concepts that may additionally affect survival. Bonadonna retrospectively found improved survival in patients who received higher percentages of intended doses (Bonadonna and Valagussa, 1981). The Cancer and Leukemia Group B (CALGB) study randomized women to 1 of 3 groups. All 3 groups received cyclophos-phamide, doxorubicin, and 5-fluorouracil; however, the total dose and length of treatment varied between groups. The total dose of chemotherapy received was equivalent in groups 1 and 2, although the intensity was higher in group 1. Group 3 received a lower total dose of chemotherapy as well as a lower intensity. Overall and disease-free survival was significantly improved for the higher-dose groups (1 and 2). Toxicity was related to dose intensity, with women in group 1 experiencing more neutropenia, thrombocytopenia, and stomatitis. Reports of nausea were sim-ilar for groups 1 and 2 (Wood et al., 1994). High-dose and dose-intensification chemotherapy are still investigational.

Positive Axillary Lymph Nodes in Postmenopausal Women

The benefit of adjuvant chemotherapy in postmenopausal women with node-posi-tive breast cancer is controversial. Bonadonna and colleagues showed only a 5-month improvement in relapse-free survival for postmenopausal women treated with CMF (Bonadonna et al., 1985). Reasons for this difference between pre- and postmenopausal women include the following:

◆ A difference in the biology of breast cancer in younger women, which makes cancer amenable to chemotherapy. This concept is theoretical and has to be supported by clinical trials.
◆ Dose intensity may be compromised in older patients because of medical conditions that require dose adjustment.
◆ The use of overall survival as an end point for clinical trials. Alternate causes of death need to be considered when analyzing data in this population.

The addition of tamoxifen to chemotherapy in postmenopausal women with positive lymph nodes has improved disease-free survival versus taking tamoxifen only (Goldhirsch and Gelber, 1987).

Neoadjuvant Chemotherapy Followed by Surgery

Neoadjuvant chemotherapy, or chemotherapy given before surgery, is used for women diagnosed with locally advanced breast cancer. Tumors that are large and fixed to the chest wall but not metastatic beyond the axillary lymph nodes may respond to neoadjuvant chemotherapy. Mastectomy may then be successfully performed. Depending on the woman's age and overall health, she may then receive radiation to the chest wall, further chemotherapy, or autologous bone marrow transplantation.

Neoadjuvant Chemotherapy Followed by Radiation

When breast cancer has locally advanced beyond the axillary lymph nodes—that is, into the mediastinum or the internal mammary nodes, or through the chest wall—surgery may not be feasible. Cases such as these are treated with chemotherapy and radiation. Chemotherapy may be given for several courses, followed by radiation, followed by several more courses of chemotherapy. Tamoxifen may be used if appropriate.

Autologous Bone Marrow Transplantation

Initially, women who had relapsed with metastatic disease entered ABMT trials and had a 70% response rate. However, the responses were not long-lasting and toxicities from the ABMT were significant. Prolonged neutropenia and thrombocytopenia were the major complications. Fungal infections occurred as a result of broad-spectrum antibiotics given to prevent or treat bacterial infections. Nausea and vomiting were also problematic (Stadtmauer, 1991). Current trials are evaluating ABMT in women with earlier stages of breast cancer, untreated locally advanced breast cancer, and inflammatory breast cancer.

❖ Nursing Management

Possible side effects from multimodal therapy for breast cancer include bone marrow depression, nausea, vomiting, alopecia, lymphedema, rib fracture, brachial plexopathy, pneumonitis, radiation recall, and secondary malignancies. Possible Side Effects from Multimodal Therapy in Breast Cancer are listed on page 129. Nursing management of treatment side effects is discussed in Unit III. Issues specific to the treatment of breast cancer are discussed here.

Breast cancer is a disease that affects a woman and her family more than just physically. Treatment choices that a woman needs to make are psychologically distressing. Levy and colleagues found that women who could choose between breast conservation or mastectomy experienced more psychological discomfort than women who participated in a clinical trial that randomized them to one procedure or the other (Levy et al., 1989). Today women are not only asked to choose between surgical options but are also asked to make choices about adjuvant chemotherapy. Nurses have a role to play in the education of women making these treatment decisions. Nurses need to stress that choosing the right treatment options may depend equally on a person's lifestyle and on the psychological and physical issues. For instance, a woman may choose mastectomy over conservative surgery followed by radiation therapy because the long drive to a center that offers radiation may not be feasible.

Possible Side Effects from Multimodal Therapy in Breast Cancer

Multimodal Treatment	Enhanced Possible Side Effects
Surgery followed by adjuvant chemotherapy:	
Cyclophosphamide, methotrexate, 5-fluorouracil	No enhanced side effects
Cyclophosphamide, methotrexate, 5-fluorouracil, vincristine, prednisone	
Cyclophosphamide, doxorubicin, 5-fluorouracil	
Tamoxifen	
Paclitaxel	
Cyclophosphamide, doxorubicin	
Doxorubicin	
Axillary node dissection or modified radical mastectomy followed by radiation therapy to the axilla	Increased risk of lymphedema in affected arm
Conservative surgery followed by radiation therapy followed by adjuvant chemotherapy	
Cyclophosphamide, methotrexate, 5-fluorouracil	Increased risk of rib fracture; increased photosensitivity in radiated field; increased risk of brachial plexopathy; increased risk of pneumonitis
Cyclophosphamide, methotrexate, 5-fluorouracil, vincristine, prednisone	
Cyclophosphamide, doxorubicin, 5-fluorouracil	Radiation recall dermatitis
Doxorubicin, cyclophosphamide	
Doxorubicin	
Paclitaxel	
Neoadjuvant chemotherapy followed by radiation therapy with or without surgery	
Cyclophosphamide, doxorubicin, 5-fluorouracil	Increased photosensitivity in irradiated field
Doxorubicin, cyclophosphamide	No enhanced side effects
Doxorubicin	
Paclitaxel	
Neoadjuvant chemotherapy followed by surgery	No enhanced side effects

Data taken from Larsen et al., 1986; Olsen et al., 1993; Pierce et al., 1992; Recht et al., 1986; Shenkier and Gelmon, 1994; Townsend, Abston, and Fish, 1985.

Women who choose breast reconstruction need reassurance that they are entitled to want to be "whole" and that they are not giving in to vanity by wanting the breast reconstructed. Women who choose reconstruction because of the inconvenience of dealing with a breast prosthesis also need to have their decision supported. Patient Education Guidelines for Care of the Reconstructed Breast are discussed on page 122.

Lymphedema is not as common today as it used to be, but it can still be debilitating. Lymphedema increases the risk of infection in the affected arm. As the swelling in the arm increases, a woman becomes self-conscious of the size difference in her arms. Jewelry may need to be removed, rings enlarged, or sleeve size altered.

Pain may derive from surgery, from skin desquamation related to radiation, from progressive disease, or from postmastectomy pain syndrome (PMPS). PMPS is a lesser known syndrome related to the entrapment of the intercostobrachial nerve following mastectomy. PMPS is usually described as a burning, hyperesthetic, and painful numbing of the upper arm and chest wall. Treatment of this is similar to the treatment of other neurologic pain syndromes. Antiinflammatory drugs, antidepressants, anticonvulsants, and neuroleptics all play a role in the treatment of PMPS.

Another toxicity associated with treatment of breast cancer is brachial plexopathy. It is described as numbness, paresthesia, and possibly motor dysfunction in median and ulnar nerve distributions of the affected arm and hand. The incidence of brachial plexopathy is 1.2%. When combined with chemotherapy, the incidence increases (Pierce et al., 1992).

Weight gain is commonly observed in women receiving adjuvant treatment for breast cancer. The etiology is unclear. One study reported a weight gain of greater than 10 pounds for women over a period of 15 months (Knobf et al., 1983). The weight gain can increase psychological distress.

Women experiencing premature menopause because of hormone treatment or chemotherapy may suffer hot flashes, vaginal dryness, and mood swings. Although not life-threatening, hot flashes interfere with sleep. Sleep loss can exacerbate other symptoms and coping problems in an already difficult situation.

❖ Summary

Nurses caring for women with breast cancer are faced with new challenges, especially in making decisions regarding treatment options. Toxicity patterns change when the sequence of agents changes. The severity of toxicities correlates with the intensity of the dose. Breast cancer treatment is generally conducted in an ambulatory setting, so that coordination of time-intensive therapies and outpatient or home toxicity management are important components of the nurse's role.

❖ References

Belcher AE: Cancer nursing, St. Louis, 1992, Mosby.

Bonadonna G: Milan adjuvant chemotherapy trial for node negative breast cancer patients. Program of the NIH Consensus Development Conference on Early Stage Breast Cancer, 1990.

Bonadonna G and Valagussa P: Dose-response effect of adjuvant chemotherapy in breast cancer, N Eng J Med 304:10–15, 1981.

Bonadonna G, Valagussa P, Rossi A, Brambilla C, Zametti M, and Veronesi U: Ten-year experience with CMF-based adjuvant chemotherapy in resectable breast cancer, Br Canc Res Treat 5:95–115, 1985.

Clark RM, Wilkinson RH, Mahoney LJ, Reid JG, and MacDonald WD: Breast cancer: a 21-year experience with conservative surgery and radiation, Int J Radiat Oncol Biol Phys 8:967–979, 1982.

Early Breast Cancer Trialists' Collaborative Group: Systemic treatment of early breast cancer by hormonal, cytotoxic, or immune therapy, Lancet 339:1–15, 1992.

Findlay P, Lippman M, Danforth D, McDonald H, d'Angelo T, Gorrell C, Gerber L, Reichert C, and Schain W: A randomized trial comparing mastectomy to radiotherapy in the treatment of stage I–II breast cancer: a preliminary report, Proc Am Soc Clin Oncol 5:63, 1986 (abstract).

Fisher B, Bauer M, Margolese R, Poisson R, Pilch Y, Redmond C, Fisher E, Wolmark N, Deutsch M, Montague E, Saffer E, Wickham L, Lerner H, Glass A, Shibta H, Deckers P, Ketchum A, Oishi R, and Russell I: Five-year results of a randomized clinical trial comparing total mastectomy and segmental mastectomy with or without radiation in the treatment of breast cancer, N Eng J Med 312:665–673, 1985.

Fisher B, Constantino JP, Redmond CK, Fisher ER, Wickerham DL, and Cronin WM: Endometrial cancer in tamoxifen-treated breast cancer patients: findings from the National Surgical Adjuvant Breast and Bowel Project (NSABP) B-14, J Nat Canc Inst 86:527–537, 1994.

Fisher B, Fisher E, and Redmond C: Ten-year results from the NSABP clinical trial evaluating the use of L-phenylalanine mustard (L-PAM) in the management of primary breast cancer, J Clin Oncol 4:929–941, 1986.

Fisher B and Fisher ER: The barrier function of the lymph node to tumor cells and erythrocytes. II. Normal nodes, Cancer 20:1907–1913, 1967.

Fisher B, Redmond C, Poisson R, Margolese R, Wolmark N, Wickerham L, Fisher E, Deutsch M, Caplan R, Pileh Y, Glass A, Shibata H, Lerner H, Terez S, and Sidorovich L: Eight-year results of a randomized clinical trial comparing total mastectomy and lumpectomy with or without irradiation in the treatment of breast cancer, N Eng J Med 320:822–828, 1989.

Fornander T, Rutquist LE, Sjobert HE, Blomquist L, Mattsson A, and Glas U: Long-term adjuvant tamoxifen in early breast cancer: effect on bone mineral density in postmenopausal women, J Clin Oncol 8:1019–1024, 1990.

Glick J: Adjuvant therapy for node-negative breast cancer. In Fowble B, Goodman RL, Glick JH, and Rosato EF, editors: Breast cancer treatment: a comprehensive guide to management, St. Louis, 1991, Mosby, pp. 243–264.

Goldhirsch A and Gelber RD: Adjuvant therapy for breast cancer: the Ludwig Breast Cancer Trials 1987. In Salmon SE, editor: Adjuvant therapy for cancer V, Orlando, 1987, Grune & Stratton, pp. 297–309.

Halstead WS: The results of radical operations for the cure of carcinoma of the breast, Ann Surg 46:1–85, 1907.

Harden JT and Girard N: Breast reconstruction using an innovative flap procedure, AORN J 60:184–192, 1994.

Hinojosa R: Breast reconstruction through tissue expansion, Plastic Surg Nurs 11(2):52–57, 1991.

Keynes G: Conservative treatment of cancer of the breast, Brit Med J 2:643, 1937.

Knobf MK, Mullen JC, Xistris D, and Moritz DA: Weight gain in women with breast cancer receiving adjuvant chemotherapy, Oncol Nurs Forum 10(2):28–33, 1983.

Larson D, Weinstein M, Goldberg I, Silver B, Recht A, Cady B, Silen W, and Harris JR: Edema of the arm as a function of the extent of axillary surgery in patients with stage I–II carcimona of the breast treated with primary radiotherapy, Int J Radiat Oncol Biol Phys 12:1575–1581, 1986.

Levitt SH and Perez CA: Breast cancer. In Perez CA and Brady LW, editors: Principles and practice of radiation oncology, Philadelphia, 1987, JB Lippincott Co, pp. 730–792.

Levy SM, Herberman RB, Lee JK, Lippman ME, and d'Angelo T: Breast conservation versus mastectomy: distress sequelae as a function of choice, J Clin Oncol 7:366–375, 1989.

McGuire WL, Tandon AK, Allred DC, Chamness GC, and Clark GM: How to use prognostic factors in axillary node-negative breast cancer patients, J Nat Canc Inst 82:1006–1015, 1990.

McWhirter R: The value of simple mastectomy and radiotherapy in the treatment of cancer of the breast, Brit J Radiol 21:599–610, 1948.

National Cancer Institute: Clincal Alert, Bethesda, Maryland, 1988, The Institute.

National Institutes of Health: Consensus development conference statement: treatment of early stage breast cancer, JAMA 265:391–394, 1991.

Nayfield SG, Karp JE, Ford LG, Dorr A, and Kramer BS: Potential role of tamoxifen in prevention of breast cancer, J Nat Canc Inst 83:1450–1459, 1991.

Olsen NK, Pfeiffer P, Johannsen L, Schroder H, and Carsten R: Radiation-induced brachial plexopathy: neurological follow-up in 161 recurrence-free breast cancer patients, Int J Radiat Oncol Biol Phys 26:43–49, 1993.

O'Rourke ME: Enhanced cutaneous effects in combined modality therapy, Oncol Nurs Forum 14(6):31–35, 1987.

Patey DH and Dyson WH: The prognosis of carcinoma of the breast in relation to the type of operation performed, Brit J Canc 2:7–13, 1948.

Pierce SM, Recht A, Lingos TI, Abner A, Vicini F, Silver B, Herzog A, and Harris JR: Long-term radiation complications following conservative surgery (CS) and radiation therapy (RT) in patients with early stage breast cancer, Int J Radiat Oncol Biol Phys 23:915–923, 1992.

Recht A, Connolly J, Schnitt S, Cady B, Love S, Osteen R, Patterson B, Shirley R, Silen W, Come S, Henderson IC, Silver B, and Harris J: Conservative surgery and radiation therapy for early breast cancer: results, controversies, and unsolved problems, Semin Oncol 13:434–449, 1986.

Rosen PP, Fracchia AA, and Urban JA: "Residual" mammary carcinoma after simulated partial mastectomy, Cancer 35:739–745, 1975.

Rutquist LD and Mattsson A, for the Stockholm Breast Cancer Study Group: Cardiac and thromboembolic morbidity among postmenopausal women with early-stage breast cancer in a randomized trial of adjuvant tamoxifen, J Nat Canc Inst 85:1398–1406, 1993.

Shenkier T and Gelmon K: Paclitaxel and radiation-recall dermatitis, J Clin Oncol 12:439, 1994 (letter).

Stadtmauer EA: Bone marrow transplantation for breast cancer. In Fowble B, Goodman RL, Glick JH, and Rosato EF, editors: Breast cancer treatment: a comprehensive guide to management, St. Louis, 1991, Mosby, pp. 498–506.

Tancini G, Bonadonna G, Valagussa P, Marchini S, and Veronesi U: Adjuvant CMF in breast cancer: comparative 5-year results of 12 versus 6 cycles, J Clin Oncol 1:2–10, 1983.

Tourney DC, Eudey L, and Mansour EG: CMFP versus observation in high-risk node-negative breast cancer patients. Program of the National Institutes of Health Consensus Development Conference on early-stage breast cancer, Washington, DC, 1990, pp. 61–62.

Townsend CM Jr, Abston S, and Fish JC: Surgical adjuvant treatment of locally advanced breast cancer, Ann Surg 201:604–610, 1985.

Veronesi U, Luini A, Del Vechhio M, Greco M, Galimberti V, Merson M, Rilke F, Sacchini V, Saccozzi R, Savio T, Zucall R, Zurrida S, and Salvadori B: Radiotherapy after breast-preserving surgery in women with localized cancer of the breast, N Eng J Med 328:1587–1591, 1993.

Walsh K: Breast reconstruction using the latissimus dorsi flap, Plastic Surg Nurs 11(2):43–50, 1991.

Wood W, Budman D, Korzun A, Cooper MR, Younger J, Hart R, Moore A, Ellerton J, Norton L, Ferree C, Ballow A, Frei E, and Henderson IC: Dose and dose intensity of adjuvant chemotherapy for stage II, node-positive breast carcinoma, N Eng J Med 330:1253–1259, 1994.

Chapter 9

❖ *Lung Cancer*

Marcia C. Liebman

Approximately 170,000 cases of lung cancer are diagnosed in the United States each year. The incidence has been steadily increasing and, for both men and women, lung cancer is now the leading cause of cancer deaths (Wingo, Tong, and Bolden, 1995).

Considerable changes in the approach to lung cancer have evolved over the last two decades. Redefinition of stages and more accurate staging techniques have better defined the extent of disease. The use of combinations of drugs, as well as combinations of treatment modalities, has modestly increased survival rates. Of the 191 current clinical trials for lung cancer treatment listed by the National Cancer Institute (1994), 74 involve multimodal treatment.

❖ *Treatment*

Surgery, radiation therapy, and chemotherapy have been used in various combinations for the treatment of lung cancer. Biotherapy is still used only investigationally as a treatment modality, although it is gaining popularity as a supportive therapy in the form of colony-stimulating factors (Astoul et al., 1994; Demitri, 1993; Sikov et al., 1994). Treatment also depends on the classification of lung cancer.

Operability depends on pulmonary function, comorbid disease, tumor involvement of vital structures, ability to remove all of the gross tumor, and metastatic disease (Elias, 1993). In the 1950s and 1960s, in an attempt to decrease tumor bulk and to make tumors operable, preoperative radiation therapy was given. Early trials failed to show the benefit of preoperative radiation therapy over surgery alone, and postoperative healing was complicated by skin changes caused by the radiation (Payne, 1991). Radiation creates vascular changes that affect the delivery of nutrients and oxygen to the irradiated skin and therefore delays healing (Sitton, 1992). In further attempts to improve the outcome, chemotherapy was given either before radiation therapy or concurrently with radiation (Albain et al., 1990; Bonomi, 1986). The combination of chemotherapy and radiation therapy was associated with improved survival rates, leading to more attempts to use combinations of treatment modalities to decrease tumor bulk and prolong survival (Albain, 1993).

133

Today thoracic radiation therapy (TRT) is typically delivered in daily fractional doses of 1.8 to 2.0 Gy over a 5- to 6-week period to give a total dose of 50 to 60 Gy. The actual dose and area to be irradiated, called a *port* (Figure 9-1), are carefully calculated. Patient Education Guidelines for Thoracic Radiation Therapy are presented on the opposite page.

TRT can also be given in split courses (two courses separated by 2 to 3 weeks "rest") in order to allow shrinkage and reoxygenation of the tumor (poorly oxygenated areas have reduced radiation sensitivity) and time for normal tissue to heal. Because each course of radiation therapy is shorter, larger daily doses can be given

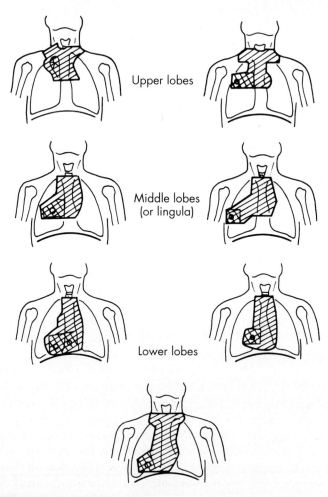

Fig. 9-1.   Radiation therapy fields. Examples of portals used for irradiation of non-oat cell carcinoma of the lung, depending on the anatomical location of the primary tumor. The tumor and grossly enlarged lymph nodes are treated to higher doses (cross-hatched pattern). From Emanmi B and Perez CA: Lung. In Perez CA and Brady LW, editors: Principles and practice of radiation oncology, ed 2, Philadelphia, 1992, JB Lippincott Co.

Patient Education Guidelines for

Thoracic Radiation Therapy with Concomitant Chemotherapy of Cyclophosphamide, Doxorubicin, and Cisplatin

GI Effects

♦ Expect to experience difficulty swallowing, sore throat, substernal pain, and possibly indigestion or nausea about 2 weeks after starting treatment.

♦ Take 1 teaspoon of "radiation mixture" as needed, not to exceed 8 doses a day. The most common recipe for the mixture is equal amounts of 2% viscous xylocaine, elixir of diphenhydramine, and Maalox or other antacid. May cause dry mouth, drowsiness, and possibly high blood pressure and fast heart beat.

♦ Use milk, antacids, sour cream, yogurt, or cottage cheese every 2 to 4 hours to promote healing and comfort.

♦ Use a straw for liquids and soft foods.

♦ Eat puddings, jello, ice cream, milkshakes, and eggnog. Dunk bread in milk or cocoa.

♦ Avoid spicy foods, hot foods, citrus fruits or drinks, and hard foods such as crackers or nuts. Avoid alcohol.

♦ Eat foods that are cold, cool, or at room temperature.

♦ Report pain that interferes with your ability to drink fluids to your nurse. Tell your nurse if you think you are not getting enough fluids.

♦ Take antinausea medication if needed 1 to 2 hours before your treatment. Repeat in 6 hours and again in 12 hours. Try to sleep after your treatment.

Bladder Effects

♦ You will need to keep your bladder as empty as possible. Unless contraindicated, drink 12 8-ounce glasses of fluid a day. Empty your bladder every 2 hours when you are awake and every 4 hours when you are in bed. If you cannot drink enough fluids, call your nurse or doctor.

♦ Your urine will turn red for a day or two after you receive doxorubicin. This is not blood but the color of the drug. If you feel any burning when urinating, have trouble starting to urinate, or are unable to empty your bladder, call your nurse or doctor.

Hematologic Effects

♦ You may feel fatigued and be at an increased risk for infection. A daily nap may help. Avoid people who have colds or are sick. Call your doctor if your temperature is more than 100°F.

Pulmonary Effects

♦ Report to your nurse any temperature, chills, dry hacking cough, or shortness of breath, even up to 6 months after completion of treatment.

♦ If pneumonitis has occurred, use a humidifier and, unless contraindicated, drink 12 8-ounce glasses of fluid a day.

♦ Use a cough suppressant if coughing is fatiguing or interferes with sleep.

♦ Avoid smoking or being in the same room as someone who is smoking.

♦ Practice deep breathing with pursed-lip expiration at least 4 times per hour.

Skin Effects

♦ Do not wash off purple marks outlining treatment area.

♦ Avoid tight-fitting clothing, such as bras, in the treatment field.

♦ Wear cotton clothing over the treatment field.

Continued

♦ Use baby detergent on clothing worn over the treatment area.
♦ Protect the skin from sun exposure, both during and after completion of treatment.
♦ Avoid heat to the skin: hot water bottles, heating pads, hot shower water.
♦ Avoid swimming in salt water or in chlorinated pools.
♦ Avoid the use of soaps, lotions, or powders in the treatment area. If lotion is needed for dry skin, consult the radiation nurse or physician about specific products to use. Cornstarch can be used as a powder substitute, if necessary.
♦ Do not rub the treatment area with a washcloth when bathing. Instead, splash water over the area or squeeze the water out of the washcloth and let it dribble over the area. In the shower, if the direct spray of water is painful, stand with your back to the shower and allow the water to dribble over your shoulder.
♦ Check the skin daily for signs of breakdown or infection.
♦ You will lose your hair from the chemotherapy. After all your chemotherapy is completed, however, your hair will grow back. You may want to wear scarves, wigs, or hats until it does.

Neurologic Effects
♦ If you have ringing in your ears or feel tingling in your feet or hands, let your nurse know before you receive any more chemotherapy.

Permission granted to reproduce these guidelines for educational purposes only.

without an increase in acute side effects. However, this practice has been questioned by some practitioners because the rest period also gives the tumor time to grow.

Recently thoracic radiation therapy has been given as *hyperfractionation,* in which more than one dose is given per day and each dose is less than the normal daily dose, but the total of the two or three doses given daily is greater than the normal daily dose, and the total dose prescribed is reached in fewer treatment days than usual. The hypothesis supporting hyperfractionation is that tumors have a slower repair rate than normal tissue (Aisner and Belani, 1993), and that hyperfractionation decreases the time for regeneration of the tumor cells between treatments (Shaw et al., 1993; Taylor et al., 1994). Theoretically, normal tissue is able to regenerate between treatments but tumor cells are not. It is also thought that this keeps late side effects to a minimum because each dose given is lower than the usual dose (Ginsberg, Kris, and Armstrong, 1993).

Radiation therapy is similar in all types of lung cancer treatment, whereas variations among the lung cancers require a variety of surgical techniques and chemotherapy. For treatment purposes, because they behave in similar ways, epidermoid, adenocarcinoma, and large-cell lung cancers are grouped together as non-small-cell lung cancer (NSCLC). Small-cell lung cancer (SCLC) has a more aggressive clinical behavior and is therefore categorized separately (Ginsberg, Kris, and Armstrong, 1993; Holmes, Livingston, and Turrisi, 1993).

Non-Small-Cell Lung Cancer

Surgery continues to be the most effective modality in early-stage (I and II) NSCLC (Belani, 1993). Surgical procedures include pneumonectomy, lobectomy,

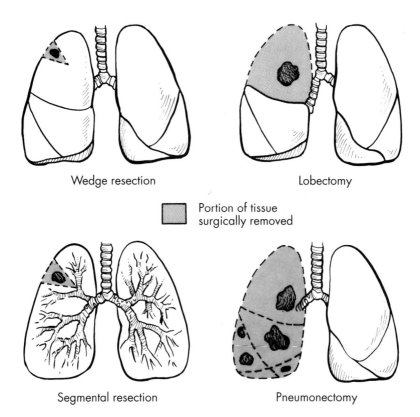

Wedge resection

Lobectomy

Portion of tissue surgically removed

Segmental resection

Pneumonectomy

Fig. 9-2. Surgical options. From Cronen SN: Nursing care of clients with lower airway disorders. In Black JM and Matassarin-Jacobs E: Luckmann and Sorensen's medical-surgical nursing: a psychophysiologic approach, ed 4, Philadelphia, 1993, WB Saunders Co.

segmental resection, or wedge resection (Figure 9-2). A *pneumonectomy* is the removal of an entire lung; a *lobectomy* is the removal of part of the lung, allowing for conservation of functional lung tissue. A *segmental resection* removes a segment of the lung, and a *wedge resection* removes a small section (smaller than a segment) of the lung.

However, approximately 55% of all NSCLCs are inoperable at the time of diagnosis (Albain, 1993; Klasterly and Sculier, 1986), and 75% to 80% of all NSCLC patients have distant metastasis at the time of diagnosis (Hazuka and Turrisi, 1993). Radiation therapy is given instead of surgery when the tumor is inoperable, and varying chemotherapy combinations are used when the patient has disease outside the radiation field.

Surgery Followed by Adjuvant Chemotherapy
Because curative surgery for stages I and II NSCLC often fails (Green, 1993; Ludwig Lung Cancer Study Group, 1987), a few studies have used adjuvant chemotherapy to attempt to improve survival. Niiranen et al. (1992) found an improved survival

rate when giving postoperative chemotherapy, but the improvement was not seen in subsequent clinical trials in stages I and II (Holmes, 1993). At present, outside of clinical trials, the standard treatment for operable stage I and II NSCLC is surgery alone, with the possible addition of radiation therapy to the hilar lymph nodes.

Neoadjuvant Chemotherapy Followed by Surgery With or Without Radiation Therapy
Stage III NSCLC has been the subject of many clinical trials because these patients are more likely to have distant microscopic metastasis and are therefore more likely to benefit from systemic treatment. Although adjuvant therapy has improved control of disease, results have been disappointing (Ginsberg, 1993). Neoadjuvant chemotherapy is used in an attempt to shrink the tumor before surgery to limit the amount of surgery needed or to make a tumor operable and to improve the patient's chances of survival. The rationale behind giving systemic therapy first is to decrease the chance of the tumor spreading outside the surgical or radiation therapy field by treating micrometastasis that may have already occurred (Sause, 1994). Pisters et al. (1993) and Elias et al. (1994) gave preoperative chemotherapy to stage IIIA NSCLC patients. The Pisters group gave mitomycin, vincristine, and cisplatin (MVP), whereas Elias et al. gave cyclophosphamide, doxorubicin, and cisplatin (CAP). Both studies noted an improvement in survival when compared to the survival rate after standard treatment. Rosell et al. (1994), also studying stage IIIA NSCLC patients, compared the results of surgery followed by radiation therapy to the results of chemotherapy (mitomycin, ifosfamide, and platinum) given before the surgery and radiation therapy, and they found an improved response rate in the group that received the preoperative chemotherapy (see the Research Highlight on p. 139).

Neoadjuvant Chemotherapy Followed by Radiation Therapy
Neoadjuvant chemotherapy is given before radiation therapy for the same reasons it is given before surgery. Radiation therapy is given instead of, or in addition to, surgery when the tumor is inoperable. Studying patients with stage III NSCLC, Dillman et al. (1990) compared neoadjuvant chemotherapy (cisplatin and vinblastine) before radiation therapy to radiation therapy alone. The chemoradiotherapy group had twice the number of long-term survivors as did the radiation-therapy-only group.

Surgery Followed by Adjuvant Concomitant Radiochemotherapy
Recently, investigators have started giving chemotherapy at the same time as radiation therapy. The Lung Cancer Study Group (LCSG) compared surgery followed by split-course radiation therapy (2 weeks of radiation, followed by 3 to 4 weeks of rest, followed by 2 more weeks of radiation) to surgery followed by the same radiation therapy given concurrently with chemotherapy (CAP) (LCSG, 1988). A statistically significant difference favored the group that received the chemotherapy.

Neoadjuvant Concomitant Radiochemotherapy Followed by Surgery
Combining the rationale of concomitant radiochemotherapy with the rationale of neoadjuvant treatment, Pincus et al. (1988) attempted to improve the outcome for stage III NSCLC patients by giving concomitant radiochemotherapy (cyclophosphamide, etoposide, and 5-fluorouracil) before surgery. Again, the group that received the treatment under study showed marked improvement when compared

---
| RESEARCH HIGHLIGHT |

Rosell R, Gomez-Codina J, Camps C, Maestre J, Padille J, Canto A, Mate JL, and Roig J: A randomized trial comparing preoperative chemotherapy plus surgery with surgery alone in patients with non-small-cell lung cancer, New Eng J Med 330:153–158, 1994.

Study Patient received either surgery followed by radiation therapy (50 Gy to the mediastinum over 5 to 6 weeks) or mitomycin 6 mg/m², ifosfamide 3 g/m², and cis-platin 50 mg/m² every 21 days for three cycles before receiving the surgery and radi-ation therapy.

Sample 60 patients with stage IIIA NSCLC at three hospitals in Spain.

Study Aim To clarify the role of preoperative chemotherapy in stage IIIA NSCLC.

Findings Median survival for the surgery-radiation-therapy group was 8 months and for the chemotherapy-surgery-radiotherapy group 26 months.

Discussion Side effects included mild bone marrow depression, mild nausea and vomiting, and alopecia. This study demonstrates a role for neoadjuvant chemotherapy

---

to the group that received the standard sequential treatment of surgery followed by radiation therapy and then chemotherapy.

Neoadjuvant Concomitant Radiochemotherapy Followed by Surgery Followed by Adjuvant Concomitant Radiochemotherapy

Strauss et al. (1992a) gave very aggressive treatment, consisting of concomitant radiochemotherapy (cyclophosphamide, vincristine, and 5-fluorouracil) both before and after surgery, to stage IIIA NSCLC patients. They found a high rate of patients who ultimately became disease-free, but they also had a high rate of treatment-related morbidity and mortality.

Concomitant Radiochemotherapy

Umsawasdi et al. (1988) gave two courses of chemotherapy (CAP) alone, followed by radiation therapy given concurrently with low doses of the same chemotherapy in an effort to improve survival in inoperable stage I to stage III NSCLC patients. Schaake-Koning et al. (1990) also treated inoperable stage I to stage III NSCLC patients, and they gave patients split-course radiation or the same radiation con-currently with weekly cisplatin, or the same radiation concurrently with daily cis-platin (the same dose as the weekly dose, but broken down into daily increments). Both chemotherapy groups had better 1-year survival rates than the radiation-ther-apy-alone groups; the group with daily chemotherapy had the best 2-year survival rate. Toxicities, however, were severe.

Reboul et al. (1994) also treated inoperable stage I to stage III NSCLC patients, but, unlike Schaake-Koning et al., the chemotherapy was given over a 5-day, 24-hour continuous infusion. Survival was comparable to that of Schaake-Koning et al.'s chemotherapy groups.

Concomitant Radiochemotherapy with Hyperfractionation Radiation Therapy
Shaw et al. (1993) and Taylor et al. (1994) gave twice-a-day radiation (doses separated by 4 to 6 hours) to stage III NSCLC patients. Both groups gave patients chemotherapy (etoposide and cisplatin [EP]) concurrently with radiation therapy. In the Shaw group, 1- and 2-year survival rates were 74% and 51%, respectively. In the Taylor group of potentially operable patients, the 3-year survival rate was 39%, and in the potentially nonoperable group it was 18%. Cox et al. (1993) warn, however, that treatment interruptions because of acute side effects are more frequent and last longer when giving hyperfractionated doses such as Shaw and Taylor had done, and that ultimately hyperfractionation may decrease long-term survival.

Surgery Followed by Adjuvant Biotherapy
In an LCSG clinical trial of 130 stage II and stage III NSCLC patients, after surgery half received chemotherapy (CAP) and half received one dose of intrapleural bacillus *Calmette-Guerin* (BCG) and oral levamisole for a total of 18 months. The biotherapy group showed no improvement over the expected survival rate (Holmes, 1993). Reviews of other biotherapy agents have demonstrated little efficacy. The literature on biotherapy, however, leaves hope that it may play a future role in the treatment of lung cancer (Ardizzoni et al., 1994; Fishbein, 1993; Lissoni et al., 1994; Vokes et al., 1994).

Today there is no "best" way to treat NSCLC. Currently, unless enrolled in a clinical trial, a patient with stage I or stage II NSCLC will not have more than surgery, except if the tumor is inoperable. For stage III, some combination of chemotherapy and radiation therapy, with or without surgery will probably be the treatment choice. Currently treatment for stage III NSCLC is controversial, because there is no standard (Haraf et al., 1992; Strauss et al., 1992b). Stage IV NSCLC is usually treated symptomatically with radiation therapy or chemotherapy, if treatment is given at all. If surgery is used for any stage NSCLC, the type of procedure (pneumonectomy, lobectomy, segmental resection, or wedge resection) depends on the size and location of the tumor. If radiation therapy is used, it is generally given in single daily doses 5 days a week for 5 to 6 weeks, although variations do occur.

Small-Cell Lung Cancer

If left untreated, the median survival time of SCLC is 5 to 12 weeks (Siefter and Ihde, 1988). Because SCLC grows so rapidly, rather than following the TNM staging system, SCLC is staged as limited disease or extensive disease, with limited disease defined as follows: "The tumor is limited to one hemithorax and can be encompassed in a single radiotherapy port" (Bunn et al., 1977, p. 335).

Surgery can be used as an adjuvant modality to debulk the tumor or to remove residual disease after chemotherapy in an effort to decrease significantly the probability of local recurrence (Mentzer, Reilly, and Sugarbaker, 1993). More often, however, radiation therapy is used for debulking, because the tumor is usually inoperable. Poor survival rates after local therapy have emphasized the need for systemic treatment (Haraf et al., 1992; Turrisi, 1994); local recurrence after systemic therapy indicates the need for local treatment, because current chemotherapy regimens appear unable to control totally areas of bulky tumor (Bunn et al., 1987; Hazuka and Turrisi, 1993; Siefter and Ihde, 1988).

The timing of radiation therapy is controversial and is still being studied in clinical trials (Turrisi, 1994). Radiation therapy is probably most effective when given concurrently with chemotherapy (Bunn et al., 1987; Haraf et al., 1992; McCracken et al., 1990) and early in the course of chemotherapy before cells resistant to chemotherapy metastasize (Murray et al., 1993). Interruption of chemotherapy to give thoracic radiation therapy (TRT) (the sandwich technique) is less effective (Kies et al., 1987; Nou, Brodin, and Bergh, 1988), although more effective than if giving TRT after chemotherapy (Cook, Miller, and Bunn, 1993). Perez et al. (1984) demonstrated the effectiveness of "nearly simultaneous" radiation therapy and chemotherapy (also known as *alternating therapy*) by giving radiation on days of the chemotherapy cycle when no drugs were given and not allowing for delay of subsequent chemotherapy. This was done in an effort to decrease the acute toxicity seen when giving concomitant radiochemotherapy and appears to achieve that goal without compromising effectiveness (Arrigada et al., 1990). Currently TRT is given only to patients with limited SCLC. Outside of clinical trials, chest radiation is inappropriate in extensive disease other than for palliation of symptoms (Siefter and Ihde, 1988).

Although cyclophosphamide, doxorubicin (Adriamycin), and vincristine (CAV) had been the standard chemotherapy regimen in the past, etoposide and cisplatin (Platinol) (EP) have been used with increasing frequency. EP is more suitable when the patient is given concurrent TRT because it has a less damaging effect on the hematologic system (Johnson, 1993), decreasing the severity of esophagitis and causing less pulmonary toxicity (Cook, Miller, and Bunn, 1993; Turrisi, 1993). Because the majority of patients responding well to initial treatment will relapse with drug-resistant disease, some clinicians are giving alternating courses of CAV and EP in order to decrease drug resistance (Cook, Miller, and Bunn, 1993; Ihde, Pass, and Glatstein, 1993). Chemotherapy is usually given in four to six cycles (repeated four to six times).

Although much of the research occurs in the laboratory, the role of biotherapy in the treatment of small-cell lung cancers is being explored with optimism (Beck, Kane, and Bunn, 1988; Mattson et al., 1994). A phase II study is now being conducted in which patients with SCLC receive a monoclonal antibody following chemotherapy in an attempt to treat residual disease (Lynch, 1993). Also under investigation are systemic anticoagulation for use in the treatment of SCLC (Aisner et al., 1992; Lebeau et al., 1994; Meehan et al., 1994) and autologous bone marrow transplant after initial treatment for early SCLC (Elias et al., 1993). Most people, however, would not be eligible for the rigorous transplant regimen because of comorbidities, especially those with a history of smoking.

❖ Prophylactic Cranial Irradiation

Because most chemotherapeutic agents do not cross the blood-brain barrier (Abner, 1993b), the brain is the most common site of distant metastasis in both NSCLC and SCLC (Siefter and Ihde, 1988). Prophylactic cranial irradiation (PCI), however, is controversial. Relapse to the brain after PCI is frequent because PCI does not prevent metastasis; the metastasis can occur after the brain has been irradiated (Ihde, Pass, and Glatstein, 1993). PCI does not increase survival, and it can cause neurologic changes. Only those who have completely responded to initial treatment are candidates for PCI (Rose, 1991). Other patients are closely monitored for symptoms of brain metastasis.

❖ *Nursing Management*

Multimodal therapy leads to increased side effects, because each modality brings its own complications as well as benefits. The more aggressive and complex the treatment, the more severe the side effects. The trend today is toward more aggressive chemotherapy and radiation therapy and less aggressive surgery, with nurses supporting patients through treatment complications. Side effects from multimodality treatment can be complicated by disease-related symptoms, disease progression, or aging.

Side effects of multimodal therapy for lung cancer include infection, fatigue, bleeding, nausea, vomiting, diarrhea, cachexia, esophagitis, esophageal fibrosis, severe weight loss, alopecia, dyspnea, pneumonitis, pulmonary fibrosis, delayed wound healing, cardiomyopathy, radiation recall, persistent abnormalities in bone marrow with the possibility of developing leukemia, CNS toxicity, second primary cancers, and death (Crossen et al., 1994; Wagner, 1993). Most of these are discussed in Unit III. Possible Side Effects from Multimodal Therapy in Lung Cancer are shown on page 143. Specifics that relate only to lung cancer will be discussed here.

Postoperative Care

After lung surgery, patients may be on a ventilator for a brief period of time. This is discontinued as soon as possible to decrease pressure on the surgical site. After extubation, coughing and deep breathing are encouraged to prevent atelectasis and pneumonia. Analgesics are given to control incisional pain and to allow the patient to cough and breathe deeply. Chest tubes are usually in place for 3 to 4 days after a lobectomy to allow drainage of air or fluid within the pleural cavity so that the remaining lobe(s) can expand as fully as possible. After a pneumonectomy, chest tubes will either be absent or clamped to prevent fluid drainage and to allow the empty side of the chest to fill up with fluid to keep the remaining lung from shifting across the mediastinum. The chest tube may lead to a drainage bottle (or bottles) or a disposable, closed drainage system. In both cases, a water seal is used to prevent air from getting into the pleural cavity. All tubing connections and the entry site at the chest wall should be airtight for the same reason. If the tube has been inserted for air removal, it is usually placed in the anterior chest on the midclavicular line at the second or third intercostal space, and the patient should remain in semihigh to high Fowler's position. If the tube has been inserted for fluid removal, it is usually placed on the mediaxillary line at the fourth to sixth intercostal space, and the patient should be kept in high Fowler's position. The reason for the differences in tube placement and patient position is that air rises to the highest point in the chest, whereas fluid goes to the lowest point. After a lobectomy, two tubes

Possible Side Effects from Multimodal Therapy in Lung Cancer

Multimodal Treatment	Possible Enhanced Side Effects
Thoracic surgery followed by adjuvant chemotherapy	
Cyclophosphamide, doxorubicin, cisplatin	No enhanced side effects
Neoadjuvant chemotherapy followed by thoracic surgery followed by radiation therapy	
Cyclophosphamide, doxorubicin, cisplatin	Severe esophagitis, pneumonitis, cardiomyopathy
Mitomycin, vincristine, cisplatin	Severe esophagitis, pneumonitis
Etoposide, cisplatin	No enhanced side effects
Thoracic surgery followed by adjuvant concomitant thoracic radiochemotherapy	
Cyclophosphamide, doxorubicin, cisplatin	Severe esophagitis, cardiomyopathy, pneumonitis
Neoadjuvant concomitant thoracic radiochemotherapy followed by thoracic surgery	
Cisplatin, etoposide, 5-fluorouracil	Delayed wound healing, cardiomyopathy, severe esophagitis
Etoposide, cisplatin	Delayed wound healing, severe esophagitis, pneumonitis, adult respiratory distress syndrome
Mitomycin, vincristine, cisplatin Cyclophosphamide, doxorubicin, cisplatin	No enhanced side effects
Neoadjuvant concomitant thoracic radiochemotherapy followed by surgery followed by radiochemotherapy	Delayed wound healing, severe esophagitis, cardiomyopathy, pneumonitis
Concomitant thoracic radiochemotherapy	
Cyclophosphamide, doxorubicin, cisplatin	Severe esophagitis, cardiomyopathy, pneumonitis
Etoposide, cisplatin	Severe esophagitis, pneumonitis, adult respiratory distress syndrome
Cisplatin	No enhanced side effects
Cisplatin, etoposide, 5-fluorouracil	Severe esophagitis, pneumonitis, adult respiratory distress syndrome, cardiomyopathy

Data taken from Dorr and Von Hoff, 1994; Haraf et al., 1992; Komaki and Cox, 1994; Mah et al., 1994; Robben, Pippas, and Moore, 1993; Rubin, 1984; Schaake-Koning et al., 1990; Tucker et al., 1994; Weidmann, Teipel, and Niederle, 1994.

are usually used, one anterior and one posterior. The tube(s) may or may not need to be sutured in place; the most important thing is that dressing changes be done carefully and only if necessary (i.e., wetness, soiling, suspected infection at the insertion site, the loss of airtight seal). The dressing consists of a petroleum gauze wrapped around the tube at the insertion site, covered by a drain sponge, which is covered in turn by an airtight adhesive bandage.

The bottle or chamber (if using a disposable, closed-drainage systems such as a Pleur-evac) closest to the patient's chest tube serves as a collection chamber, and the bottle or chamber next to it contains a water seal to prevent air from entering the pleural space through the collection chamber. If suction is needed, a third bottle or chamber can be used as a suction control chamber.

The tube in the water-seal chamber should be submerged under 2 cm of sterile water or saline to prevent air from entering the system. If suction is ordered, the control chamber should have 15 to 20 cm water (as ordered by the physician) to prevent more than 15 to 20 cm of negative pressure being exerted on the pleura. The suction-control bottle or chamber needs to bubble continuously (not vigorously) in order to maintain the expected degree of suction. Nursing Care of the Patient with a Chest Tube is outlined on page 145.

Pulmonary Toxicity

Most patients with lung cancer have a long history of smoking cigarettes and have suffered secondary lung damage as well (Holmes, Livingston, and Turrisi, 1993). They do not tolerate the pulmonary side effects of treatment very well. Worsening pulmonary symptoms can be caused by the treatment or by progression of the disease. If the treatment is effective, productive coughing might increase; material trapped behind the tumor can be expectorated as the tumor shrinks. Because the lung is very sensitive to radiation, treatment also causes pulmonary damage. Bleomycin, mitomycin, lomustine, methotrexate, and the alkalating agents compound the lung damage caused by radiation and increase the incidence of pneumonitis (Komaki and Cox, 1994). Mah et al. (1994) found that concurrent radiochemotherapy appeared to decrease the lungs' tolerance of TRT, especially when doxorubicin or 5-fluorouracil was used.

It is important to stress to patients and their families that smoking cessation, even after diagnosis, will benefit the patient. Smoking is a factor in prognosis and in the occurrence of a second primary cancer (Brown, 1993; Richardson et al., 1993). Nicotine has been reported to increase energy expenditure and can be another factor in the weight loss commonly seen in lung cancer patients during treatment (Brown, 1993). In addition, smoking irritates the tissue lining the lungs and the upper respiratory tract; smoking cessation eliminates that irritation, allowing tissues to regenerate. This may help to improve respiration and to decrease treatment side effects.

Superior Vena Cava Obstruction

Superior vena cava obstruction (SVCO) is not a side effect of therapy but is related to the pathology of lung cancer and can be seen in patients with lung cancer at any time during the course of illness. It deserves mention here because

Nursing Care of

The Patient with a Chest Tube

Nursing Care	Rationale/Comments

◆ Assess patient's respiratory status every 2–4 hours
  ◆ Vital signs
  ◆ Color of lips and nailbeds
  ◆ Presence and quality of breath sounds
  ◆ Arterial blood gases as ordered
  ◆ Chest X ray as ordered
  ◆ Ascertain if patient's anxiety is due to fear or hypoxia
	◆ Will indicate if there is a problem with the chest tube, among other things. Fluctuations in the water level in the water-seal bottle or chamber of 5–10 cm with normal breathing are common. Shallow breathing causes very slight fluctuation. Atelectasis or retained secretions are indicated by large fluctuations, because the patient is working harder to breathe. If suction is used, fluctuations do not occur.

◆ Assess type of drainage
  ◆ Quality
  ◆ Color
  ◆ Characteristics
	◆ Pneumothorax usually drains 10–20 cc/hr of serosanguineous to serous fluid; hemothorax usually drains 50–100 cc/hr bloody to serosanguineous fluid.

◆ Maintain patency of chest tube
  ◆ Keep drainage system below patient's chest
  ◆ Check chest tube for kinks or fluid accumulation within the tube
  ◆ Mark level of drainage on drainage-collection system at the end of each shift and more frequently if there is greater than 100 cc/hr drainage. Record on I & O sheet
	◆ Drains by gravity. If tubing is kinked or patient is lying on it, there will be no fluctuations with breathing. Decreased drainage can also indicate obstruction of flow. Stripping (milking) the tubing is controversial and should not be done unless it is within hospital policy and the physician specifically orders it. Stripping causes increased pressure on the pleural space and can cause tissue damage or lung entrapment in the chest tube eyelets (Duncan and Erickson, 1982). Increased drainage can result from a change in the patient's position but, if it continues, may indicate hemorrhage.

◆ Provide pulmonary toilet every 2 hours
  ◆ Supply patient with small pillow for splinting
  ◆ Have patient turn, cough, and breathe deep every 2 hours
  ◆ Provide humidity and fluids as ordered
	◆ Prevents atelectasis. A pillow at the incision site helps the patient feel more secure when coughing and breathing deeply. Humidity and fluids help liquefy secretions.

◆ Assess for air leaks	◆ Bubbling should be seen in the water-seal bottle or chamber. However, if suction is used, bubbling in the water-seal chamber will stop. If it continues, there is an air leak between the pleural space and the water seal. Make sure all connections are tight. If bubbling still

Continued

Nursing Care	Rationale/Comments
◆ Assess for air leaks—cont'd	continues, momentarily clamp the chest tube, beginning close to the chest and working down to the collection bottle. When the bubbling stops, the leak is located between the current clamp position and the preceding clamp position.
◆ Prevent and monitor for infection ◆ Daily white blood cell count ◆ Vital signs every 2–4 hours ◆ Maintain sterility of drainage system ◆ Observe for changes in amount or character of sputum	◆ There is high risk of infection because of the chest tube insertion site.
◆ Assess and medicate for pain	◆ Some differences in opinion exist about pain medication. While adequate pain medication will enable the patient to cough and breathe deeply, thereby helping to prevent atelectasis, some pain medications decrease the respiration rate. Careful dose titration and nursing assessment is needed to medicate patients adequately without compromising their respiration.
◆ Provide patient and family education	◆ The more that patients and their families understand, the less anxious and more cooperative they will be.

early diagnosis and intervention of SVCO depends many times on good nursing-assessment skills.

The superior vena cava (SVC) is the major drainage system for blood returning to the heart from the upper extremities, upper thorax, head, and neck. The SVC lies within the mediastinum, surrounded by lymph nodes. It is thin-walled and has low venous pressure, making it very susceptible to compression. The syndrome of SVC obstruction (SVCO) occurs when there is a complete or partial obstruction of the SVC, caused by compression of the tumor on the mediastinum, compression of mediastinal lymph nodes on the SVC, or thrombosis (a clot) within the SVC (Abner, 1993a). SVCO is associated with lung cancer about 80% of the time.

The most common symptoms of SVCO are dyspnea and swelling of the face and upper extremities, many times with distension of the jugular veins. Cough, chest pain, orthopnea, difficulty swallowing, cyanosis, hoarseness, headache, somnolence, and lethargy are less common. The onset of symptoms may be gradual or rapid. Symptoms can be enhanced by lying down and therefore may be more prominent in the morning but gradually lessen as the day progresses (Liebman, 1992). Acute onset of symptoms is deemed a medical emergency.

Symptoms often improve when treated by elevating the head of the bed, positioning the patient with arms supported on pillows, and administering oxygen. Chemotherapy or radiation therapy may be given to shrink the tumor.

❖ *Summary*

Comparing the results of clinical trials can be difficult because of the variability of criteria used to select patients and to measure results. This leaves the clinician with a lot of unanswered questions about the best way to care for patients. Therapies can be concurrent or sequential. The main drawback of concurrent therapy is the toxicity and the possibility that the dose of the chemotherapy may have to be reduced, possibly compromising the patient's ability to conquer disseminated disease (Belani, 1993), or radiation therapy will have to be interrupted because of toxicities of treatment, compromising the patient's ability to fight local disease (Cox et al., 1993). More information is needed to find a balance between maximum dose and acceptable toxicity (Elias, 1993).

Treatments are becoming more toxic as physicians give more aggressive therapy. The nurse's role is to anticipate patient problems and to initiate early, if not prophylactic, interventions to prevent or minimize complications of therapy. The nurse can help the patient and family by preparing them and guiding them down the long road ahead.

❖ *References*

Abner A: Approach to the patient who presents with superior vena cava obstruction, Chest 103:394s–397s, 1993a.

Abner A: Prophylactic cranial irradiation in the treatment of small-cell carcinoma of the lung, Chest 103:445s–448s, 1993b.

Aisner J and Belani CA: Lung cancer: recent changes and expectations of improvements, Semin Oncol 20:383–393, 1993.

Aisner J, Goutsou M, Maurer LH, Cooper R, Chahinian P, Carey R, Skarin A, Slawson R, Perry MC, and Green MR: Intensive combination chemotherapy, concurrent chest irradiation, and warfarin for the treatment of limited-disease small-cell lung cancer: a Cancer and Leukemia Group B pilot study, J Clin Oncol 10:1230–1236, 1992.

Albain KS: Induction therapy followed by definitive local control for stage III non-small-cell lung cancer: a review, with a focus on recent trimodality, Chest 103:43s–50s, 1993.

Albain KS, Crowley JJ, LeBlanc M, and Livingston RB: Determinants of improved outcome in small-cell lung cancer: an analysis of the 2,580-patient Southwest Oncology Group data base, J Clin Oncol 8:1563–1574, 1990.

Ardizzoni A, Bonavia M, Viale M, Baldini E, Mereu C, Verna A, Ferrini S, Conquegrana A, Molinart S, Mariani G, Roest GJ, Sharenbert J, Patmer PA, Rosso R, Ropolo F, and Raso C: Biological and clinical effects of continuous infusion interleukin-2 in patients with non-small cell lung cancer, Cancer 73:1353–1360, 1994.

Arrigada R, LeChevalier T, Ruffie P, Baldeyrou P, DeCremoux H, Martin M, Cerrina ML, Pallae-Cosset B, Tarayre M, and Sancho-Garnier H: Alternating radiotherapy and chemotherapy in 173 consecutive patients with limited small cell lung cancer, Int J Radiat Oncol Biol Phys 19:1135–1138, 1990.

Astoul P, Bertault-Peres P, Durand A, Catalin J, Vagnal F, and Boutin C: Pharmacokinetics of intrapleural recombinant interleukin-2 in immunotherapy for malignant pleural effusion, Cancer 73:308–313, 1994.

Beck LK, Kane MA, and Bunn PA Jr: Innovative and future approaches to small cell lung cancer treatment, Semin Oncol 15:300–314, 1988.

Belani CP: Multimodality management of regionally advanced non-small-cell lung cancer, Semin Oncol 20:302–314, 1993.

Bonomi P: Brief overview of combination chemotherapy in non-small cell lung cancer, Semin Oncol 13:89–94, 1986.

Brown JK: Gender, age, usual weight, and tobacco use as predictors of weight loss in patients with lung cancer, Oncol Nurs Forum 20:466–472, 1993.

Bunn PA Jr, Cohen MH, Ihde D, Fossieck BE, Matthews MJ, and Minna JD: Advances in small-cell bronchogenic carcinoma, Canc Treat Rep 61:2333–2342, 1977.

Bunn PA Jr, Lichter AS, Makuch RW, Cohen MH, Veach SR, Matthews MJ, Anderson AJ, Edison M, Glatstein E, Minna JD, and Ihde DC: Chemotherapy alone or chemotherapy with chest radiation therapy in limited stage small-cell lung cancer, Ann Int Med 106:655–662, 1987.

Cook RM, Miller YE, and Bunn PA: Small cell lung cancer: etiology, biology, clinical features, staging, and treatment, Cur Prob Canc 17:69–144, 1993.

Cox JD, Pakak TF, Asbell S, Russell AH, Pederson J, Byhardt RW, Emami B, and Roach M III: Interruptions of high-dose radiation therapy decrease long-term survival of favorable patients with unresectable non-small cell carcinoma of the lung: analysis of 1244 cases from 3 Radiation Therapy Oncology Group (RTOG) trials, Int J Radiat Oncol Biol Phys 27:493–498, 1993.

Crossen JR, Garwood D, Glatstein E, and Neuwelt EA: Neurobehavioral sequelae of cranial irradiation in adults: a review of radiation-induced encephalopathy, J Clin Oncol 12:627–642, 1994.

Demitri GD: Impact of hematopoietic growth factors on the management of small-cell lung cancer, Chest 103:427s–432s, 1993.

Dillman RO, Seagren SL, Propert KJ, Guerra J, Eaton WL, Perry MC, Carey RW, Frei E III, and Green MR: A randomized trial of induction chemotherapy plus high-dose radiation versus radiation alone in stage III non-small-cell lung cancer, N Eng J Med 323:940–945, 1990.

Dorr RT and Von Hoff DD: Cancer chemotherapy handbook, ed 2, Norwalk, Connecticut, 1994, Appleton & Lange.

Duncan C and Erickson R: Pressures associated with chest tube stripping, Heart and Lung 11:166–171, 1982.

Elias A: Chemotherapy and radiotherapy for regionally advanced non-small-cell lung cancer, Chest 103:362s–366s, 1993.

Elias AD, Ayash L, Skarin AT, Wheeler C, Schwartz G, Mazanet R, Tepler J, Schnipper L, Frei E III, and Antman KH: High-dose combined alkylating agent therapy with autologous stem cell support and chest radiotherapy for limited small-cell lung cancer, Chest 103:433s–435s, 1993.

Elias AD, Skarin AT, Gonin R, Oliynyk P, Stomper PC, O'Hara C, Socinski MA, Sheldon T, Maggs P, and Frei E III: Neoadjuvant treatment of stage IIIA non-small cell lung cancer, Am J Clin Oncol 17(1):26–36, 1994.

Fishbein GE: Immunotherapy of lung cancer, Semin Oncol 20:351–359, 1993.

Ginsberg RJ: Multimodality therapy for stage IIIA (N_2) lung cancer: an overview, Chest 103:356s–359s, 1993.

Ginsberg RJ, Kris MG, and Armstrong JG: Non-small cell lung cancer. In DeVita VT Jr, Hellman S, and Rosenberg SA, editors: Cancer: principles and practice of oncology, ed 4, Philadelphia, 1993, JB Lippincott Co, pp. 673–723.

Green MR: New adjuvant strategies for the management of resectable non-small-cell lung cancer, Chest 103:352s–355s, 1993.

Haraf DJ, Devine S, Ihde DC, and Vokes EE: The evolving role of systemic therapy in carcinoma of the lung, Semin Oncol 19(suppl 11):72–87, 1992.

Hazuka MB and Turrisi AJ III: The evolving role of radiation therapy in the treatment of locally advanced lung cancer, Semin Oncol 20:173–184, 1993.

Holmes EC: Postoperative chemotherapy for non-small-cell lung cancer, Chest 103:30s–34s, 1993.

Holmes EC, Livingston R, and Turrisi A III: Neoplasms of the thorax. In Holland JR, Frei E III, Bast RC Jr, Kufe DW, Morton DL, and Weichselbaum RR, editors: Cancer medicine, ed 3, Philadelphia, 1993, Lea & Febiger, pp. 1285–1337.

Ihde DC, Pass HI, and Glatstein EJ: Small cell lung cancer. In DeVita VT Jr, Hellman S, and Rosenberg SA, editors: Cancer: principles and practice of oncology, ed 4, Philadelphia, 1993, JB Lippincott, pp. 723–758.

Johnson DJ: Recent developments in chemotherapy treatment of small-cell lung cancer, Semin Oncol 20:315–325, 1993.

Kies MS, Mira JG, Crowley JJ, Chen TT, Pazdur R, Grozea PN, Rivkin SE, Coltman CA Jr, Ward JH, and Livingston RB: Multimodal therapy for limited small-cell lung cancer: a randomized study of induction combination chemotherapy with or without thoracic radiation in complete responders; and with wide-field versus reduced-field radiation in partial responders: a Southwest Oncology Group study, J Clin Oncol 5:592–600, 1987.

Klasterly J and Sculier JP: Nonsurgical combined modality therapies in non-small cell lung cancer, Chest 89:289s–294s, 1986.

Komaki R and Cox JD: The lung and thymus. In Cox JD, editor: Moss's radiation oncology, ed 7, St. Louis, 1994, Mosby, pp. 320–351.

Lebeau B, Chastang C, Brechot J, Capron F, Dautzenberg B, Delaisements C, Mornet M, Brun J, Hurdebourcq J, and Lamarie E: Subcutaneous heparin treatment increases survival in small-cell lung cancer, Cancer 74:38–45, 1994.

Liebman MC: Overview of cancer care. In Burke MB, editor: Oncology nursing homecare handbook, Boston, 1992, Jones & Bartlett, pp. 9–30.

Lissoni P, Meregalli S, Paolorossi F, Fossati V, Frigerio F, Tancini G, Andizzoit A, and Barni S: A randomized study of immunotherapy with low-dose IL-2 plus melatonin vs. chemotherapy with cisplatin and VP-16 as a first-line therapy in advanced nonsmall cell lung cancer, Proc Am Soc Clin Oncol 13:325, 1994 (abstract).

Ludwig Lung Cancer Study Group: Patterns of failure in patients with resected stage I and II non-small-cell carcinoma of the lung, Ann Surg 205(1):67–71, 1987.

Lung Cancer Study Group: The benefit of adjuvant treatment for resected locally advanced non-small-cell lung cancer, J Clin Oncol 6:9–17, 1988.

Lynch TJ: Immunotoxin therapy of small-cell lung cancer, Chest 103:436s–439s, 1993.

Mah K, Keane TJ, Van Dyk J, Braban LE, Poon PY, and Hao Y: Quantitative effect of combined chemotherapy and fractionated radiotherapy on the incidence of radiation-induced lung damage: a prospective clinical study, Int J Radiat Oncol Biol Phys 28:563–574, 1994.

Mattson K, Niiranen A, Pyrhonen S, Maasilta P, Kajanti M, and Cantell K: Interferon maintenance therapy for small cell lung cancer: long-term survival, Proc Am Soc Clin Oncol 13:333, 1994 (abstract).

McCracken JD, Janki LM, Crowley JJ, Taylor SA, Shankir Giri PG, Weiss GB, Gordon W Jr, Baker LH, Mansouri A, and Kuebler JP: Concurrent chemotherapy/radiotherapy for limited small-cell lung carcinoma: a Southwest Oncology Group study, J Clin Oncol 8:892–898, 1990.

Meehan KR, Zacharski LR, Maurer LH, Memoli VA, Rousseau SM, and Henkin J: Mechanism of urokinase therapy in small-cell carcinoma of the lung, Proc Am Soc Clin Oncol 13:341, 1994 (abstract).

Mentzer SJ, Reilly JJ, and Sugarbaker DT: Surgical resection in the management of small-cell carcinoma of the lung, Chest 103:349s–351s, 1993.

Murray N, Coy P, Pater JL, Hodson I, Arnold A, Zee BC, Payne D, Kostashuk EC, Evans WK, Dixon P, Sadura A, Feld R, Levitt M, Wierzbicki R, Ayoub J, Maroun JA, and Wilson KS: Importance of timing for thoracic irradiation in the combined modality treatment of limited-stage small-cell lung cancer, J Clin Oncol 11:336–344, 1993.

National Cancer Institute: Current clinical trials: oncology 1(1):1-167–1-177, 1994.

Niiranen A, Niitamo-Korhonen S, Douri M, Assendelft A, Mattson K, and Pyrhonen S: Adjuvant chemotherapy after radical surgery for non-small-cell lung cancer: a randomized study, J Clin Oncol, 10:1927–1932, 1992.

Nou E, Brodin O, and Bergh J: A randomized study of radiation treatment in small cell bronchial carcinoma treated with two types of four-drug chemotherapy regimens, Cancer 62:1079–1090, 1988.

Payne DG: Pre-operative radiation therapy in non-small cell cancer of the lung, Lung Cancer 7:47–56, 1991.

Perez CA, Einhorn L, Oldham RK, Greco FA, Cohen HJ, Silberman H, Krauss S, Hornback N, Comas F, Omura G, Salter M, Keller JW, McLaren J, Kellermeyer R, Storaasli H, Birch R, and Dandy M: Randomized trial of radiotherapy to the thorax in limited small-cell carcinoma of the lung treated with multiagent chemotherapy and elective brain irradiation: a preliminary report, J Clin Oncol 2:1200–1208, 1984.

Pincus M, Reddy S, Lee MS, Bonomi P, Taylor S IV, Rowland K, Faber LP, Warren W, Kittle CF, and Hendrickson FR: Preoperative combined modality therapy for stage III non-small cell lung carcinoma, Int J Radiat Oncol Biol Phys 15:189–195, 1988.

Pisters KMW, Kris MG, Gralla RJ, Zaman MB, Heelan RT, and Martini N: Pathologic complete response in advanced non-small-cell lung cancer following preoperative chemotherapy: implications for the design of future non-small-cell lung cancer combined modality trials, J Clin Oncol 11:1757–1763, 1993.

Reboul F, Vincent P, Chauvet B, Brewer Y, Felix-Faure C, Taulelle M, and Shrieve DC: Radiation therapy with concomitant continuous infusion cisplatin for unresectable non-small-cell lung carcinoma, Int J Radiat Oncol Biol Phys 28:1251–1256, 1994.

Richardson GE, Tucker MA, Venzon DJ, Linnoila RI, Phelps R, Phares JC, Edison M, Ihde DC, and Johnson BE: Smoking cessation after successful treatment of small cell lung cancer associated with fewer smoking-related secondary primary cancers, Ann Intern Med 119:383–390, 1993.

Robben NC, Pippas AW, and Moore JO: The syndrome of 5-fluorouracil cardiotoxicity: an elusive cardiopathy, Cancer 71:493–509, 1993.

Rose LJ: Neoadjuvant and adjuvant therapy on non-small cell lung cancer, Semin Oncol 18:536–542, 1991.

Rosell R, Gomez-Codina J, Camps C, Maestre J, Padille J, Canto A, Mate JL, Le S, and Roig J: A randomized trial comparing preoperative chemotherapy plus surgery with surgery alone in patients with non-small-cell lung cancer, N Eng J Med 330:153–158, 1994.

Rubin P: Late effects of chemotherapy and radiation therapy: a new hypothesis, Int J Radiat Oncol Biol Phys 10:5–34, 1984.

Sause WT: Principles of combining radiation therapy and surgery. In Cox JD, editor: Moss's radiation oncology, ed 7, St. Louis, 1994, Mosby, pp. 67–78.

Schaake-Koning C, Maat B, van Houtte P, van den Bogaert W, Dalesio O, Kirkpatrick A, and Bartelink H: Radiotherapy combined with low-dose cis-dimmine dichlorplatinum (II) (CDDP) in inoperable nonmetastatic non-small cell lung cancer (NSCLC): a randomized three arm phase II study of the EORTC Lung Cancer and Radiotherapy Cooperative Groups, Int J Radiat Oncol Biol Phys 19:967–972, 1990.

Shaw EG, McGinnis WL, Jett JR, Su JQ, Frank AR, Mailliard JA, Engel RE, Wiesenfiel M, and Rowland KM Jr: Pilot study of accelerated hyperfractionated thoracic radiation therapy plus concomitant etoposide and cisplatin chemotherapy in patients with unresectable stage III non-small cell carcinoma of the lung, J Nat Canc Inst 85:321–323, 1993.

Siefter EJ and Ihde DC: Therapy of small cell lung cancer: a perspective on two decades of clinical research, Semin Oncol 15:278–299, 1988.

Sikov WM, Akerley W, Browne M, and Rosmarin A: Dose escalation of carboplatin with cisplatin and etoposide with filgrastin (G-CSF) for advanced non-small cell lung cancer, Proc Am Soc Clin Oncol 13:341, 1994 (abstract).

Sitton E: Early and late radiation-induced skin alterations. Part I: mechanisms of skin changes, Oncol Nurs Forum 19:801–807, 1992.

Strauss GM, Herndon JE, Sherman DD, Mathisen DJ, Carew RW, Choi NC, Rege VB, Modeas C, and Green MR: Neoadjuvant chemotherapy and radiotherapy followed by surgery in stage IIIA non-small-cell carcinoma of the lung: report of a Cancer and Leukemia Group B phase II study, J Clin Oncol 10:1237–1244, 1992a.

Strauss GM, Lander MP, Elias AD, Skarin AT, and Sugarbaker DJ: Multimodality treatment of stage IIIA non-small cell lung carcinoma: a critical review of the literature and strategies for future research,. J Clin Oncol 10:829–838, 1992b.

Taylor MA, Reddy S, Lee M, Bonomi P, Taylor SG IV, Kaplan E, Faber PL, Warren W, and Hendrickson FR: Combined modality treatment using BID radiation for locally advanced non-small cell lung carcinoma, Cancer 73:2599–2606, 1994.

Turrisi AT: Principles of combined radiation therapy and chemotherapy. In Cox JD, editor: Moss's radiation oncology, ed 7, St. Louis, 1994, Mosby, pp. 79–95.

Turrisi AT III: Innovations in multimodality therapy for lung cancer: combined modality management of limited small-cell lung cancer, Chest 103:56s–59s, 1993.

Umsawasdi T, Valdivieso M, Barkley HT Jr, Chen T, Booser DJ, Chiuten DF, Dhingra HM, Murphy WK, and Carr DT: Combined chemoradiotherapy in limited-disease, inoperable non-small cell lung cancer, Int J Radiat Oncol Biol Phys 14:43–48, 1988.

Vokes E, Hochster H, Lotze M, Foglin R, and Rybak U: Recombinant human interleukin 4 (IL-4) SCH 39400 in non-small cell lung cancer (NSCLC): results of a phase II investigation, Proc Am Soc Clin Oncol 13:334, 1994 (abstract).

Wagner H Jr: Rational integration of radiation and chemotherapy in patients with unresectable stage IIIA or IIIB NSCLC: results from the Lung Cancer Study Group, Eastern Cooperative Oncology Group, and Radiation Therapy Oncology Group, Chest 103:35s–42s, 1993.

Weidmann B, Teipel A, and Niederle N: The syndrome of 5-fluorouracil cardiotoxicity: an elusive cardiopathy, Cancer 73:2001–2002, 1994 (letter).

Wingo PA, Tong T, and Bolden S: Cancer statistics, CA Cancer J Clin, 45:8–30, 1995.

Chapter 10

❖ *Lower Gastrointestinal Cancers*

Patricia A. Spencer-Cisek

Cancers of the lower gastrointestinal (GI) tract include those of the colon, rectum, and anus. There were approximately 138,200 cases of colorectal cancer diagnosed in 1995 (American Cancer Society, 1995). Of those, 100,000 occurred in the colon. An estimated 45,500 individuals died of colorectal cancer in that same year (American Cancer Society, 1995). Tumors of the anal region account for less than 4% of all lower-GI-tract tumors. The overall 5-year survival rate of 50% for colorectal cancers has remained constant for decades, although encouraging statistics report a decline in mortality from colorectal cancer of 30% in females and 7% in males over the last 30 years (American Cancer Society, 1994). New approaches to multimodal therapy are being investigated to improve on the survival rates for this disease.

❖ *Treatment of Colon Cancer*

Surgery

Surgery is the primary curative treatment for individuals with cancer of the large bowel and rectum. About 80% of individuals with colon cancer can successfully undergo complete resection of the primary tumor (Vaughn and Haller, 1993). Of that group, approximately 50% have a significant risk of recurrence.

Colorectal surgery requires wide resection of the primary tumor, removal of the mesentery and all lymph node groups at risk for spread, ligation of major vessels, and en bloc removal of all involved adjacent organs (Abcarian, 1992; Beart, 1991). Aggressive surgery aimed at obtaining negative margins (disease-free area around the removed tumor) improves the length of survival regardless of tumor stage (Peloquin, 1988). The exact surgical procedure varies depending on the location of the

152

tumor, extent of disease, and the surgeon's preference. Table 10-1 lists surgical procedures for tumors at various locations.

The need for permanent ostomy formation has significantly decreased as surgical techniques have been modified. Occasionally, left-sided or obstructing tumors may require a two-step Hartmann procedure in which the tumor is resected to form a temporary end-colostomy. Subsequent surgery is performed to reconnect the bowel.

Surgery Followed by Adjuvant Chemotherapy

More than 25 years ago, 5-fluorouracil (5-FU) was found to be effective on colorectal cancers. About 20% of patients treated with 5-FU have some response, although the treatment does not demonstrably improve survival rates when compared with historical controls. These poor outcomes led to multiple studies with combination regimens dating back to the 1970s.

Leucovorin (calcium leucovorin or folinic acid) acts as a modulator that enhances the cytotoxicity of 5-FU (Vaughn and Haller, 1993). The combination of 5-FU and leucovorin has a significant impact on both disease-free survival and overall 3-year survival rates among persons with stage IV cancer (Wolmark et al., 1993), but its use as adjuvant therapy in stage I to stage III is still under investigation.

Table 10-1   Surgical Procedures in the Treatment of Colorectal Cancers

Tumor Location	Procedure
Colon Tumors	
Cecum Ascending colon	Right hemicolectomy; en bloc resection; regional lymphadenectomy (remove terminal ilium, cecum, right half of transverse colon, and mescocolon)
Splenic flexure Descending colon Sigmoid colon	Subtotal colectomy (remove distal transverse colon, descending colon, sigmoid colon, and mesocolon)
Young age with history of adenomas	Total colectomy with ileosigmoidal anastomosis
History of ulcerative colitis or familial polyposis	Total proctocolectomy
Rectal Tumors Upper to mid rectum (>10 cm from anal verge)	Lower anterior resection (LAR) with reanastomosis if adequate margins (at least 2 cm distal)
Mid rectum (7–11 cm)	Controversial: LAR with spincter-sparing vs. abdominal perineal resection
Mid to lower rectum	Abdominal perineal resection (APR)
Early rectal (superficial invading wall only, well differentiated, <3 cm lesion)	Wide local excision or electrocoagulation
Recurrent/advanced	Pelvic exenteration

Surgery Followed by Adjuvant Concomitant Chemobiotherapy

Levamisole is a biotherapeutic agent that has been shown to enhance the immune response in normal hosts and to restore the immune response when deficient (Renoux, 1980). The North Central Cancer Treatment Group (NCCTG) utilized levamisole with 5-FU as an adjuvant treatment for patients with colorectal cancer. Individuals with stage III disease who received 5-FU and levamisole experienced a significant increase in disease-free survival (DFS) rates with a small increase in overall survival. Levamisole alone has not been shown to be effective (Laurie et al., 1989).

Moertel and colleagues (1990) randomized patients with stage II and stage III cancer to surgery alone, to surgery with levamisole, or to surgery with 5-FU and levamisole. There was a 41% decrease in the recurrence rate and a 31% decrease in the 5-year death rate among those patients with stage III cancer treated with surgery followed by 5-FU and levamisole.

Based on data from this study, the 5-FU–levamisole regimen was deemed the standard of care for individuals with stage III colon cancer at the NIH Consensus Conference on Adjuvant Therapy in 1990. The consensus statement recommended initiating the regimen within 6 weeks after surgery with a 5-FU 450 mg/m² IV bolus daily for 5 days followed by 3 weeks rest and 450 mg/m² on a weekly basis for 1 year. The levamisole is administered as 150 mg by mouth 3 days a week every other week for 1 year (Laurie et al., 1989). Table 10-2 shows the current NIH consensus recommendations for treatment of colorectal cancers.

Interferon-alpha (IFN-α) has been demonstrated to enhance the effect of 5-FU in vitro through what appears to be biochemical modulation rather than an immunologic enhancement (Sinicrope and Sugarman, 1994). Wadler et al. (1989) published data reporting a 76% response rate with the combination of 5-FU and INF-α in patients with advanced colon cancer, although the toxicities were significant. Those results have yet to be replicated in other studies (Pazdur et al., 1990; Kemeny et al., 1990; Wadler et al., 1991). The National Surgical Adjuvant Breast and Bowel Project (NSABP) has an ongoing adjuvant trial using the combination

Table 10-2   Adjuvant Therapy Recommendations According to Stage for Cancer of the Colon and Rectum

| | *Treatment Regimen* | |
Stage	*Colon Cancer*	*Rectal Cancer*
I (Duke's A/B1)	Surgery alone	Surgery alone
II (Duke's B2–3)	Surgery alone	Surgery followed by concomitant chemoradiotherapy (5-FU and radiation)
III (Duke's C)	Surgery followed by concomitant chemobiotherapy (5-FU and levamisole)	Surgery followed by concomitant chemoradiotherapy (5-FU and radiation)

From National Institutes of Health: Adjuvant therapy for patients with colon and rectal cancer. NIH Consensus Development Conference Statement, Washington, DC, 1990, National Institutes of Health.

of 5-FU and levamisole with and without IFN-α for stage II and stage III colon cancers.

Controversy surrounds the use of adjuvant, autologous, tumor-cell vaccine therapy in which tumor cells are mixed with Bacillus Calmette-Guerin (BCG) and reinjected into the patient. Hoover et al. (1993) reported impressive results, but analysis has met criticism from other investigators (Moertel, 1993). There is currently a clinical trial evaluating the combination 5-FU and levamisole with and without the autologous tumor-cell vaccine.

Surgery Followed by Adjuvant Radiation Therapy

The use of adjuvant radiation therapy for colon tumors above the rectosigmoid area has not been definitively endorsed. When studied, high local failure rates and low survival rates were seen (Cohen, Minsky, and Schilsky, 1993). For this reason, large-scale randomized studies that would be required to confirm these results have not been undertaken.

Surgery Followed by Concomitant Chemoradiotherapy

In a current study by the North Central Cancer Treatment Group (NCCTG), 5-FU and levamisole with or without radiation therapy is administered postoperatively to individuals at high risk of local recurrence (Sinicrope and Sugarman, 1994). In this study, the radiation is targeted at a specific site, not the whole abdomen.

❖ Treatment of Rectal Cancer

Individuals with rectal cancers demonstrate a higher risk of local-regional recurrence than persons with colon tumors (Papillon, 1994). Therefore adjuvant therapy of surgically resected rectal cancer must address the potential for both local and systemic relapse (National Institutes of Health, 1990). Improvements in preoperative staging techniques have dramatically changed the treatment course of rectal cancer, allowing for cure to be achieved while preserving the anal sphincter (Billingham, 1992; Frykholm, Glimelius, and Pahlman, 1993; Landry et al., 1993; Rich, 1988).

Surgery

Approximately one in seven patients with rectal cancer will require a permanent colostomy (DeCosse and Cennerazzo, 1992). In tumors of the upper third of the rectum, an anterior resection or lower-anterior resection (LAR) with reanastomosis is performed. The development of sphincter-sparing techniques utilizing coloanal anastomosis and new stapling devices have greatly improved the management of tumors located in the mid-rectum (6 to 11 cm from the anal verge) (Figure 10-1). Abdominal perineal resection (APR) is necessary if the tumor has invaded the pelvic or anal musculature. Low-lying rectal tumors in early stages may also be treated successfully with local therapy and radiation as an alternative to APR, avoiding permanent colostomy and potential impotence.

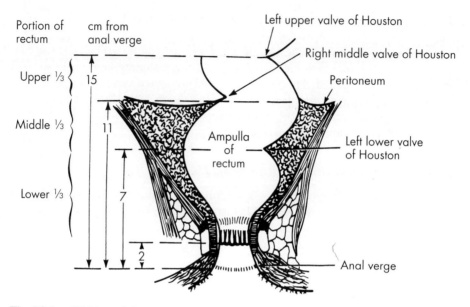

Fig. 10-1. Division of the rectum into upper, middle, and lower thirds. From Cohen AM, Minsky BD, and Friedman MA: Rectal cancer. In DeVita VT, Hellman S, and Rosenberg SA, editors: Cancer: principles and practice of oncology, ed 4, Philadelphia, 1993, JB Lippincott Co.

Surgery Followed by Adjuvant Radiation Therapy

In the past, low-lying rectal cancers, even in early stages, were treated by APR. Currently several options for local therapy include electrocoagulation (the clotting of tissue by means of a high-frequency electric current), fulguration (essential destruction by electronic current), and local excision (Rich, 1988). In a review of the literature by Rich (1988), the local recurrence rates for these modalities ranged from 8% to 39% for local excision and from 4% to 66% for electrocoagulation or fulguration. In two studies where postoperative radiation therapy was added to the local procedure (Rich et al., 1985; Rich, 1988), results improved. In the second study, 15 patients were treated with local procedures followed by external-beam radiation at a median dose of 53 Gy. The local control rate was 93% at a median follow-up period of 48 months. The one local recurrence was successfully treated by APR.

In reviews by Schilsky and Brochman (1992); Cummings (1992); and Cohen, Minsky, and Friedman (1993), the results of postoperative radiation on improvements in survival have not been substantiated in randomized trials. In one NSABP study, less local failure was demonstrated in the group receiving adjuvant radiation therapy than in the group receiving surgery alone (16% versus 25%) (Fisher et al., 1988). Poulter (1992) points out advantages to postoperative radiation therapy, including the ability to place a mesh or sling in the abdomen to protect the small intestine and the use of clips to highlight the location of the tumor bed. Because these results have not been overwhelmingly positive, however, postoperative adjuvant radiation therapy alone is not justified.

Neoadjuvant Radiation Therapy Followed by Surgery

Among the studies of neoadjuvant (preoperative) radiation therapy, a Stockholm study showed that the local recurrence rate after radiation therapy and surgery decreased significantly to 11% as compared to a rate of 25% after surgery alone (Stockholm Rectal Cancer Study Group, 1990). In the Veterans Administration Study reported by Higgins et al. (1986), no significant difference was demonstrated. Gerard et al. (1988) reported on the European Organization for Research on the Treatment of Cancer (EORTC) study that demonstrated a 15% local recurrence rate for combination therapy as compared to a rate of 30% for surgery alone. The occurrence of distant metastases was equivalent in both groups. The study recommendations included a minimum preoperative dose of radiation of 40 Gy over 4 weeks.

According to Cohen, Minsky, and Friedman (1993), the studies utilizing neoadjuvant radiation are difficult to interpret. In a review of eight randomized studies, the following problems were identified:

◆ The radiation doses employed were less than the 45 Gy recognized as therapeutic
◆ The recommended interval for tissue recovery of 4 to 6 weeks before surgery was not adhered to
◆ All of the studies used the AP/PA technique, which is suboptimal because it results in maximum small bowel exposure.

The recommended technique for this location involves the use of multiple fields, with the patient in a prone position on an open tabletop to exclude the bowel from the radiation field (Rich, Terry, and Meistrich, 1994) (Figure 10-2).

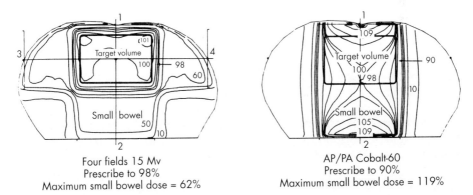

Four fields 15 Mv
Prescribe to 98%
Maximum small bowel dose = 62%

AP/PA Cobalt-60
Prescribe to 90%
Maximum small bowel dose = 119%

Fig. 10-2. Isodose distribution of a four-field technique compared with AP/PA cobalt-60 in a patient receiving radiation therapy for rectal cancer. The patient is prone, and the distribution is through the center of the field. From Cohen AM, Minsky BD, and Friedman MA: Rectal cancer. In DeVita VT, Hellman S, and Rosenberg SA, editors: Cancer: principles and practice of oncology, ed 4, Philadelphia, 1993, JB Lippincott Co.

Radiation Therapy Followed by Surgery Followed by Radiation Therapy: the Sandwich Technique

In more advanced rectal tumors, radiation therapy has been studied as a preoperative or a postoperative treatment and as both, when given before and after surgery using the "sandwich" technique. Patient Education Guidelines for Radiation Therapy to the Colon or Rectum appear on page 159.

In sandwich-technique radiation therapy, a low dose (5–15 Gy) is administered preoperatively to decrease tumor seeding, followed by an additional 41 Gy postoperatively for stage III tumors. Using this technique, Cohen, Minsky, and Friedman (1993) report local failure rates ranging from 0% to 13% and 3- to 5-year survival rates ranging from 78% to 82%. Frykholm, Glimelius, and Pahlman (1993) reported a decrease in local-regional recurrence of 50% with adequate radiation dosing, but little survival advantage. Cohen and his group (1993) caution against misinterpretation of the results because they are preliminary. The use of sandwich-technique radiation therapy on rectal cancer is also affected by the success of concomitant therapy such as chemoradiotherapy.

Surgery Followed by Adjuvant Concomitant Chemoradiotherapy

Advances in the multimodal treatment of rectal cancer are exciting. Two recent randomized studies using chemoradiotherapy have demonstrated a decrease in local recurrence and improved overall survival rates (Peacock, Keller, and Ashbury, 1993). The landmark study by the Gastrointestinal Tumor Study Group (GITSG) compared (1) adjuvant concomitant chemoradiotherapy to (2) adjuvant radiation therapy of 40 to 58 Gy, (3) adjuvant concomitant chemotherapy with 5-FU and semustine, and (4) surgery alone. The 7-year survival rate in the concomitant chemoradiotherapy arm was 58% compared with 34% for surgery alone (GITSG, 1986). The NCCTG, the Mayo Clinic, and Duke University collaborated on a study comparing the results of postoperative radiation therapy of 50 Gy to the results of concurrent treatment with radiation, 5-FU, and semustine. This study demonstrated similar results: a reduction in recurrence rate of 34% and a decrease in mortality rate of 29% in the chemoradiotherapy arm.

In 1990, those participating in the NIH Consensus Conference on Adjuvant Therapy for Colon and Rectal Cancer analyzed data from multiple studies and concluded that there was a survival advantage to using 5-FU and semustine in combination with local radiation therapy as compared to radiation therapy alone in the adjuvant setting. Concurrent chemotherapy, when started within 6 weeks of surgery, yielded a local failure rate one half that of adjuvant radiation therapy used alone. Because of the risk of leukemia development with semustine, the conference panel stopped short of recommending 5-FU and semustine outside of an organized clinical trial. They did, however, endorse the use of 5-FU with radiation therapy for adjuvant treatment.

Many in the GITSG questioned the need to include semustine in the treatment because of its leukemogenic potential. This was evaluated in a subsequent GITSG study. Participants were randomized to radiation therapy combined with

Patient Education Guidelines for

Radiation Therapy to the Colon or Rectum

You will be receiving radiation therapy to your colon or rectal area. This may cause side effects that you can help to control.

You may have nausea. To help, you can do the following:
◆ Try not to eat a full meal for 4 hours before treatment.
◆ Snack on crackers or bland food before and after your treatment.
◆ Ask your nurse about ways to help relax before treatment.
◆ If nausea occurs tell your doctor or nurse, and you can get medicine to help.

Your bowel is affected by the radiation and many people will have diarrhea. If this happens, try the following:
◆ Drink a lot of fluids to prevent dehydration.
◆ Avoid alcohol, coffee, milk, spicy or fried foods, fresh fruits, vegetables, and food high in fiber (bran).
◆ Try eating bananas, rice, dry toast, jello, broth, applesauce, mashed potatoes, apple juice, and weak tea.

You may have skin changes within the treatment area. To help care for your skin you should do the following:
◆ Do not remove the treatment marks that the therapist puts on your skin. If they fade the radiation therapist will redo them.
◆ Use a mild soap to clean the area. Rinse well and gently pat the area dry. Do not scrub.
◆ Use gentle detergent to wash your clothes. Rough clothing may irritate your skin.
◆ Cotton underwear should be worn.
◆ Women should not wear pantyhose.
◆ Do not expose your skin to the sun.
◆ Avoid hot and cold temperatures from such things as: heating pads, hot baths or showers, saunas, and ice packs.
◆ Do not use creams or powder on the skin in the treatment area unless ordered by your doctor.
◆ If your skin is irritated let your nurse or doctor know right away.
◆ Do not shave the hair in the treatment area.
◆ Do not use tape or a Band-Aid in the treatment area.

If you are getting radiation to your rectum your skin in that area may have what looks like a bad diaper rash. It may be very sore and drain fluid.
◆ Keep the area clean by using plain water to rinse after going to the bathroom.
◆ You can soak in a tub or sitz bath two or three times a day.
◆ If you have diarrhea use the ideas above. Let your doctor or nurse know; they may want you to have medicine to help.
◆ If your skin is sore let the nurse or doctor know. There may be medicine that will help to heal it.
◆ Do not use enemas, suppositories, or any other thing in your rectum during or after radiation until approved by your doctor.

Women may have vaginal dryness from the radiation. Do not douche. Vaginal lubricants can be used during intercourse to decrease dryness.

Men can have a change in desire or other effects from the treatment, including impotence.

If you have other concerns regarding sexual activity please talk to your nurse or doctor.

5-FU followed by 5-FU and semustine or to radiation with 5-FU alone. After follow-up for close to 6 years, the combination of radiation therapy and 5-FU appears to be as effective without semustine (GITSG, 1990).

There are still questions regarding the optimal schedule and dosages for adjuvant therapy. Findley and Cunningham (1993) and Ajani and Rich (1993) conclude that standard practice for stage II and stage III is chemoradiotherapy. They each anticipate studies to continue using radiation therapy with a chemosensitizer in addition to adjuvant chemotherapy, with 5-FU and levamisole as the standard treatment.

❖ Treatment of Advanced Disease in Colorectal Cancers

Surgery Followed by Adjuvant Hepatic Arterial Infusion Chemotherapy

Multiple approaches have been attempted to treat the individual with advanced or recurrent colorectal cancer. The liver is the most common site of metastases. Surgical resection of isolated liver metastases results in a 5-year survival rate of 20% (Steele and Ravikumar, 1989). Systemic chemotherapy with 5-FU and leucovorin has a 20% response rate (Vaughn and Haller, 1993). Hepatic arterial infusion (HAI) of various agents, either alone or as an adjunct to liver resection, is being investigated. The goal of hepatic artery infusion is to increase drug concentration while decreasing systemic toxicity (Curley et al., 1993; Mayer, 1992). In a pilot study by Kemeny et al. (1993), 21 individuals with metastatic disease to the liver were evaluated. Eight had resections of their liver lesions and subsequently were treated with both HAI floxuridine and systemic 5-FU with leucovorin. An overall response rate of 56% was reported; among the eight individuals treated with both surgery and chemotherapy none showed any evidence of disease after 23 months. There was significant toxicity in the form of diarrhea and chemical hepatitis. In previous studies reviewed by Mayer (1992), initial improvement in the disease was demonstrated, but there was substantial toxicity with minimal improvement to overall survival. Vaughn and Haller (1993) cite similar conclusions. This area remains controversial.

Chemoradiotherapy and Surgery in Advanced Disease

Minsky et al. (1992 and 1993) reported positive results from the use of multimodal therapy with advanced colorectal cancer. In a study of 20 initially unresectable patients treated with preoperative radiation combined with 5-FU and high-dose leucovorin, 90% became resectable. Six patients also received intraoperative radiation therapy. All were subsequently treated with 5-FU and leucovorin postoperatively. Based on this study, a subsequent study with higher doses of 5-FU is ongoing. Papillon (1994) recommends a single course of low-dose 5-FU and leucovorin for 5 days commencing with day 1 of radiation therapy, giving 40 Gy over 4 weeks. Cummings (1992) and Poulter (1992) also report benefits to chemoradiotherapy in advanced disease.

Intraoperative Radiation Therapy in Advanced Rectal Cancer

Intraoperative radiation therapy (IORT) is undergoing investigation for both recurrent and advanced rectal carcinoma. Its success appears to be related to the amount of residual disease at the time of treatment. Because the radiation is given directly to the tumor during surgery, acute side effects have not been a major difficulty. There have been reports of peripheral neuropathies and necrosis of soft tissue or bone within the treatment field (Lanciano et al., 1993; Willett et al., 1991).

Concomitant Radiochemobiotherapy in Advanced Rectal Cancer

Based on the success of chemobiotherapy and radiation therapy for stage III rectal cancer, Moertel and colleagues (1994) studied the concomitant use of radiation therapy, chemotherapy, and biotherapy in unresectable, residual, or recurrent gastrointestinal cancers (see the Research Highlight on p. 162). Response rates were favorable; additional studies are currently under way.

❖ Treatment of Anal Cancer

Anal cancers are rare and account for less than 4% of cancers of the lower gastrointestinal tract in the United States. A long lag time often occurs between initiation of symptoms and diagnosis, because the cancer is often associated with benign conditions such as hemorrhoids or fissures (Coffey, Gunderson, and McDonald, 1993).

Surgery

The management of anal carcinoma depends on the exact location of the primary tumor. Lesions of the anal margin (perineal lesions) can be managed conservatively by local excision and have excellent outcomes. Anal-canal lesions that are smaller than 2 cm in size, superficial, and positioned below the dentate line can also be treated with local excision.

Concomitant Chemoradiotherapy

In the past, stage II anal cancer required an APR for adequate control, but the advent of multimodal therapy has improved treatment significantly. After Nigro published a multimodal regimen in 1974, treatment changed dramatically. On the first day of treatment, Nigro gave mitomycin-C 15 mg/m^2 and started a continuous infusion of 5-FU 1000 mg/m^2 per day to run for 96 hours. Radiation therapy of 2 Gy per day was given to the primary tumor, the pelvic lymph nodes, and the inguinal lymph nodes, and was continued for a total dose of 30 Gy (about 2 weeks). Four weeks after the patient started treatment, the 4-day 5-FU infusion was repeated. Multiple other studies have confirmed the success of concomitant treatment with 5-FU, mitomycin-C, and radiation therapy (Cho et al., 1991; Coffey, Gunderson, and McDonald, 1993; Miller, Quan, and Thaler, 1991; Quan, 1992; Tanum et al., 1991).

RESEARCH HIGHLIGHT

Moertel et al.: Early evaluation of combined fluorouracil and leucovorin as a radiation enhancer for locally unresectable, residual, or recurrent gastrointestinal carcinoma, J Clin Oncol 12:21–27, 1994.

Study Patients were given various doses of radiation therapy over a 5- to 6-week period while also receiving 5-fluorouracil 400 mg/m² IV bolus and leucovorin 20 mg/m² IV bolus for 3, 4, or 5 days on the first and fifth week of radiation. All patients received 5-fluorouracil 425 mg/m² IV bolus and leucovorin 20 mg/m² IV bolus for 4 days on the fourth and ninth weeks after completion of radiation.

Sample Forty patients with cancers of the stomach, pancreas, or large bowel with unresectable, residual, or recurrent local tumor at least 4 weeks but no longer than 8 weeks after biopsy or surgery, with oral nutrition of at least 1200 calories daily, no or minimal nausea and vomiting, and an ECOG performance score of 0 or 1.

Study aim To determine the maximum tolerated toxicity of concomitant radiochemo-biotherapy, using radiation therapy to the upper abdomen or pelvis (depending on the location of the tumor), combined with 5-fluorouracil and leucovorin.

Findings Almost all patients had leukopenia, which was more severe in the patients receiving upper abdominal radiation and in patients after the second course of chemotherapy. There was one nonfatal episode of sepsis due to leukopenia. Nausea and vomiting were experienced mostly by patients who received upper abdominal radiation; only one patient withdrew from the study because of intolerable nausea and vomiting. Almost half of all the patients experienced diarrhea, including 7 of the 10 who received pelvic radiation. Four of the 10 patients treated with pelvic radiation developed mild to moderate dermatitis of the perineum. Stomatitis occurred infrequently, but 90% of patients who received upper abdomen radiation experienced a median of 4.0 kg weight loss.

Two patients with pancreatic cancer had gastrointestinal hemorrhage; one patient with rectal cancer had a period of bowel obstruction; one patient died from aspiration pneumonitis due to repeated vomiting; one patient died from pulmonary embolus; and one died from sepsis not associated with leukopenia.

Discussion Although this was a study to assess patient tolerance to concomitant radiation therapy, chemotherapy, and biotherapy, improvement in survival was also demonstrated. The median survival times for patients with pancreatic and rectal-sigmoid cancers were 13 months and 31 months, respectively. Two patients with rectal cancer, two with gastric cancer, and one with pancreatic cancer had no evidence of disease 38 to 50 months after the onset of therapy.

It appears that three-modality treatment in these difficult cancers increases the survival rate with mild to moderate side effects. This was a phase I study to assess toxicity; phase II and phase III studies to assess effects on the disease are forthcoming.

The need for APR has been eliminated in about 80% of cases (Coffey, Gunderson, and McDonald, 1993). In the series reported by Cho et al. (1991) of 20 patients treated with the Nigro regimen, 17 achieved complete response. Two of three individuals who experienced local recurrence were treated with salvage chemoradiotherapy regimens that again prevented the need for APR.

❖ Nursing Management

Basic preoperative nursing care for all lower GI surgical procedures includes patient education regarding the anticipated procedures, the role of coughing and deep breathing, the need for nasogastric decompression, use of the Foley catheter, and the potential impact on the individual's life-style if an APR or colostomy formation are necessary. All individuals must undergo preparation of the bowel to decrease the risk of infection. This includes preoperative cathartics, enemas, and antibiotic prophylaxis.

The nursing plan of care must be individualized for each patient, based on the kind of surgery to be performed and the factors determining the risk of developing complications. For example, an individual who smokes may require more aggressive pulmonary management to prevent development of pneumonia. When the colostomy formation is planned, whether temporary or permanent, an enterostomal therapy nurse, or someone trained in those skills, should meet with the patient before the surgery to provide information and select the best site for the stoma. Nursing Care of the Patient Undergoing Bowel Resection is presented on page 164.

The implications for nursing are great. In order to begin adjuvant therapy in a timely manner, it is imperative that the recovery from surgery proceed smoothly and without complications. Treatment delays due to slow recovery can potentially affect the patient's survival. Therefore patients must be educated so they participate to the fullest in treatment planning and care.

Before undergoing therapy, the patient must have a baseline assessment of nutrition status, skin integrity, and bowel pattern. The common chemotherapy regimens, which use 5-FU with leucovorin or levamisole, cisplatin, or mitomycin-C, all have the potential to cause nausea, vomiting, taste alterations, mucositis, and diarrhea, which directly affect the individual's nutritional status. Possible Side Effects from Multimodal Therapy in Lower Gastrointestinal Cancers are listed on page 168. Concurrent treatment of the lower gastrointestinal tract by 5-FU and radiation may cause severe diarrhea, possibly leading to perianal skin breakdown, poor nutrition, and fecal incontinence.

Complications associated with multimodal therapy must be prevented or minimized to obtain the optimum benefit and to avoid delays in further treatment. The majority of these therapies are performed on an outpatient basis: the importance of collaboration among health care team members to provide support and education to the patient and family cannot be overstressed. Self-care strategies and early recognition of complications are key to the success of multimodal therapy.

❖ Summary

Advances in the treatment of lower gastrointestinal cancers focus on the use of multimodal therapy. With the exception of stage I colon tumors or very superficial rectal lesions, multimodal therapy is the standard of care in the 1990s. Adjuvant and neoadjuvant chemotherapy and radiation therapy play increasingly important roles in the treatment of lower gastrointestinal cancer. As current studies yield results, there may be further modifications to avoid the radical surgeries of the past.

Nursing Care of

The Patient Undergoing Bowel Resection

Nursing Care	Rationale/Comments
Preoperative	
At preoperative visit	
◆ Teach bowel preparation	
◆ Low-residue, liquid diet	◆ Decrease fecal material in bowel
◆ Antibiotic prophylaxis (usually oral sulfonamides neomycin and/or cephalexin)	◆ Decrease bowel flora to lower risk of infection
◆ Enema administration	◆ Cleanse the bowel to facilitate as clean a procedure as possible
◆ Teach regarding proposed surgery and expected course of recovery	◆ Be aware of surgeon's style and typical orders; prepare appropriately
◆ Anticipation of a stay in the ICU	
◆ Prevention of complications: *Pulmonary*—cough and deep breathe, incentive spirometer *Thrombus*—compression boots, exercises, heparin *Bowel*—NG drainage, diet progression *Fluid balance*—Foley catheter, IV hydration *Transfusion*—potential	◆ Adjust teaching to individual's risk factors with emphasis on areas of most concern
◆ Anticipated surgical incision	◆ If APR is planned, patient needs to know about both abdominal and perineal wounds
◆ Anticipated length of procedure	◆ Prepare family members
◆ Anticipated length of stay	◆ Share case management plan as appropriate to setting
◆ Teach if colostomy formation is anticipated	
◆ Type of colostomy—temporary or permanent	◆ If temporary, a Hartmann's pouch may be formed with a single ostomy. In some cases a loop or double-barrel ostomy may be formed. These look different, and the patient should be prepared in order to facilitate coping
◆ Explore feelings regarding the procedure—anticipatory grieving	
◆ Location of ostomy regarding type of output	◆ Ileostomy: liquid Transverse: semisolid Descending: solid
◆ Mark stoma location	◆ An enterostomal therapy nurse, or nurse trained in the care of ostomies, should mark the stoma location after discussion with the physician. Placement is critical to the successful management
◆ The stoma should ideally be placed at least 2" away from the waist, leg folds, or belt line. Scars, bony prominences, and skinfolds should be avoided	

Nursing Care	Rationale/Comments

- Mark the location with the patient in several different positions: lying, sitting, standing, and bending
- Accurate positioning will facilitate ease of care, allow greater flexibility with clothing choices, and, most importantly, decrease the risk of complications, i.e., skin irritation

- Mark within the borders of the rectus abdominus muscle
- Muscle assists in preventing retraction, or herniation

Postoperative
- Basic nursing interventions are similar to any abdominal surgery: vital signs, strict intake and output, nasogastric tube decompression, pulmonary toilet, wound care. Particular emphasis will be placed on the complications associated with specific procedures.
- Assess for complications
  - Abdomen: pain, rigidity, rebound tenderness, peritonitis
    Bowel sounds (BS)

    - Anastomatic leak: peritonitis, pain, abscess (increased risk if s/p neoadjuvant radiation)
    - Bowel obstruction: to BS-hypoactive or high-pitched tinkling, nausea, vomiting, abdominal pain or distention, decrease in output, constipation

  - Infection: increased WBC with left shift (increased bands)
    Sepsis

    - Intraabdominal abscess: recurrent or persistent fever >38°C more than 72 hours postoperative
    - Wound: erythema, edema, tenderness at site, foul smelling, purulent drainage
    - Change in respiratory status: r/o pneumonia
    - Urine: color, dysuria, r/o UTI
    - Staphylococcal enteritis: diarrhea, sepsis

  - Genitourinary injury
  - Fluid and electrolyte balance

    - Oliguria, anuria, urine in wound
    - Monitor for excess loss through wound, fistula, or ostomy
    - Monitor electrolytes, strict I and O, weights daily
    - IV hydration, nutrition support as necessary.

  - Perineal wound

    - After APR the perineal wound may be left to close by secondary intention. This will require extensive care by the patient or support person
    - Assess for sign and symptoms of infection
    - Prevent contamination from ostomy output

  - Abdominal wound: assess for complications, i.e., infection, bleeding, dehiscence.
  - Pain management
- Management of colostomy
  - Stoma
    Color

    - Follow standards of acute pain management

    - Should be pink and moist. Dusky gray or black are signs of hypoxia

    Position

    - Assess for retraction, prolapse, stricture (narrowing), or peristomal hernia

Continued

Nursing Care	Rationale/Comments
◆ Care of stoma Protect peristomal skin	◆ Choose a pouch system that is appropriate for the location, size of stoma, manual dexterity, and cost ◆ Assess skin with each change of appliance for signs of irritation, erosion, infection, or fistula formation ◆ Change appliance at the first sign of leakage; discourage unnecessary changes that would irritate skin ◆ Empty pouch when full, prevent dislodgment.
Measure size with each change initially	◆ Stoma has considerable edema post-operatively. Measure with each change in first 6 weeks, then monthly to ensure proper fit
Opening should be ⅛" larger than base of stoma with sufficient adhesive to obtain an adequate seal Apply effective skin barrier Cleanse pouch on routine basis	◆ Proper fit will protect peristomal skin and avoid trauma to the tissue. Too tight a fit could cause edema or stenosis ◆ Use paste as necessary for adequate seal
◆ Psychosocial adjustment Assess for stages of adjustment	◆ Provide opportunities to discuss feelings ◆ Stages of adjustment to an ostomy have been identified by Watson (1985) as (1) shock, (2) defensive retreat, (3) acknowledgment, and (4) adaptation
Support will be required Individuals will adapt at their own pace. Learning to care for the stoma will not successfully occur until the individual has reached the acknowledgment stage Provide step-by-step written instructions Encourage the patient to begin by watching only	◆ Arrange visit from ostomy association Beginning the process preoperatively may help to facilitate adaptation. With short hospital stays successful adaptation will require follow-up support as an outpatient or at home ◆ This will facilitate self-care; the individual can proceed at their own pace ◆ Once comfortable, encourage the patient to take control over emptying the appliance. The next step is to have the patient assist in appliance changes
Encourage participation of support person	◆ Most individuals will be able to perform self-care. The preparation of a support person, if acceptable to the patient, can facilitate the transition to home
Note behaviors of withdrawal, nonparticipation, or increased dependency	◆ Excessive difficulty with adjustment may require a referral for support and coping strategies

Nursing Care	Rationale/Comments

◆ Long-term management
  Nutrition: foods can affect ostomy
  output
    Flatus: soda, beer, beans,
    onions, fish, cabbage, highly
    seasoned foods
    Odor: onions, cabbage, fish,
    eggs, beans
  Caution: prunes, dates, bananas,
  strawberries
 	
  Increase amount of yogurt,
  buttermilk consumed
	◆ Changes in diet can create problems with
	  the function and management of the ostomy
	  (odor, gas)
	
	◆ Anything that changes the consistency of
	  stool needs to be evaluated on an individual
	  basis

◆ Sigmoidostomy: due to consistency
  of stool, patient can have "continent"
  ostomy. Teach irrigation techniques,
  and set up regular schedule
	◆ Individuals will vary in their desire to
	  perform regular irrigations. Some prefer
	  regulation with diet alone

◆ Sexual dysfunction after APR
  Discuss the implications of procedure
  preoperatively. Explore alternatives,
  e.g., penile implants
  Focus on intimacy and provide
  information and support
 	
  Recommend lubricants to females.
  Multiple choices available over
  the counter
	◆ An ostomy by itself can affect self-image
	  and sexual function. If APR is performed,
	  the majority of men will be impotent
	
	◆ ACS publications on sexuality in male and
	  female versions are a good resource. Use
	  as a basis for discussion
	◆ Postoperatively the length of the vagina may
	  be altered. A perineal wound can take a
	  lengthy time to heal. Avoid Vaseline (because
	  it dries the skin). Dryness and irritation may
	  be exacerbated by multimodal therapy:
	  ovarian failure with radiation therapy and/or
	  chemotherapy, perineal skin irritation with
	  radiation

Possible Side Effects from Multimodal Therapy in

Lower Gastrointestinal Cancers

Multimodal Treatment	*Possible Enhanced Side Effects*
Colon	
Surgery followed by adjuvant chemotherapy	
5-Fluorouracil	No enchanced side effects
5-Fluorouracil, leucovorin	
5-Fluorouracil, vincristine, semustine	
Surgery followed by adjuvant concomitant chemobiotherapy	
5-Fluorouracil, levamisole	Neutropenia, diarrhea
5-Fluorouracil, interferon	Stomatitis, fatigue
Surgery followed by adjuvant radiochemotherapy	
5-Fluorouracil	Small-bowel obstruction, nausea and vomiting, severe diarrhea, enteritis, fibrosis, perineal tissue breakdown, photosensitivity
Surgery followed by adjuvant concomitant chemobiotherapy with targeted radiation therapy	
5-Fluorouracil, levamisole	Neutropenia, diarrhea, fibrosis, anastomotic leak, fistula formation
Surgery followed by adjuvant hepatic arterial chemotherapy infusion	
Floxuridine	No enchanced side effects
Concomitant chemobiotherapy	
5-Fluorouracil, interferon	Stomatitis, fatigue
5-Fluorouracil, levamisole	Neutropenia, diarrhea
Rectal	
Surgery followed by adjuvant radiation therapy	Stricture, perianal skin excoriation, rectal oozing, diarrhea
Neoadjuvant radiation therapy followed by surgery	Diarrhea, delayed wound healing
Radiation therapy followed by surgery followed by radiation therapy	Diarrhea, delayed wound healing
Surgery followed by adjuvant concomitant chemoradiotherapy	
5-Fluorouracil	Diarrhea
5-Fluorouracil, leucovorin	Fatigue, stomatitis, diarrhea, nausea
5-Fluorouracil, semustine	Tenesmus, erythema dermatitis, enteritis, stomatitis, leukemia

Data taken from Cho, 1993; Cohen, Minsky, and Schilsky, 1993b; Curley et al., 1993; Hampton, 1993; Hoebler and Irwin, 1992; Lanciano et al., 1993; Minsky et al., 1992; Moertel, 1992; Willett et al., 1991; Wolmark et al., 1993.

Multimodal Treatment	Possible Enhanced Side Effects
Surgery followed by adjuvant hepatic arterial chemotherapy infusion	No enchanced side effects
Neoadjuvant concomitant chemoradiotherapy followed by surgery	Diarrhea, delayed wound healing
Intraoperative radiation therapy	Delayed wound healing, infection, bleeding, fistula formation
Anal	
Concomitant chemoradiotherapy 5-Fluorouracil, mitomycin-C	Diarrhea, proctitis, perineal excoriation, bone marrow depression, cystitis, ilius, fibrosis
Concomitant chemoradiotherapy followed by surgery	Diarrhea, proctitis, perineal excoriation, bone marrow depression, cystitis, ilius, fibrosis, delayed wound healing

❖ *References*

Abcarian H: Operative treatment of colorectal cancer, Cancer 70:29–35, 1992.

Ajani JA and Rich TA: Colon and rectum. In John MJ, Flam M, Legha S, and Phillips T, editors: Chemoradiation: an integrated approach to cancer treatment, Philadelphia, 1993, Lea & Febiger, pp. 330–336.

American Cancer Society: Cancer facts and figures, Atlanta, 1994, American Cancer Society.

American Cancer Society: Cancer facts and figures, Atlanta, 1995, American Cancer Society.

Beart RW: Colorectal cancer. In Holleb AI, Fink DJ, and Murphy GP, editors: Textbook of clinical oncology, Atlanta, 1991, American Cancer Society, pp. 213–218.

Billingham R: Conservative treatment of rectal cancer: extending the indications, Cancer 70:1355–1363, 1992.

Cho CC, Taylor CW, Padmanabhan A, Arnold M, Aguilar P, Meesig D, Hartman R, Khanduja KS, Rahman SM, and Stewart WR: Squamous-cell cancer of the anal canal: management with combined chemoradiation therapy, Dis Colon Rectum 34:675–768, 1991.

Coffey RJ, Gunderson LL, and McDonald JS: Neoplasms of the anus. In Calabresi P and Schein PS, editors: Medical oncology: basic principles and clinical management of cancer, ed 2, New York, 1993, McGraw Hill, Inc, pp. 783–793.

Cohen AM, Minsky BD, and Friedman MA: Rectal cancer. In DeVita VT, Hellman S, and Rosenberg SA, editors: Cancer: principles and practice of oncology, Philadelphia, 1993, JB Lippincott Co, pp. 978–1005.

Cohen AM, Minsky BD, and Schilsky RL: Colon cancer. In Devita VT, Hellman S, and Rosenberg SA, editors: Cancer: principles and practice of oncology, Philadelphia, 1993, JB Lippincott Co, pp. 929–977.

Cummings B: Adjuvant radiation therapy of colorectal cancer, Cancer 70:1372–1383, 1992.

Curley SA, Roh MS, Chase JL, and Hohn DC: Adjuvant hepatic arterial infusion chemotherapy after curative resection of colorectal liver metastases, Am J Surg 166:743–748, 1993.

DeCosse JJ and Cennerazzo W: Treatment options for the patient with colorectal cancer, Cancer 70:1342–1345, 1992.

Findley M and Cunningham D: Current advances in the treatment of gastrointestinal malignancy, Crit Rev Oncol Hematol 14:127–152, 1993.

Fisher B, Wolmark N, Rockette H, Redmond C, Deutsch M, Wickerham DL, Fisher ER, Caplan R, Jones J, and Lerner H: Postoperative adjuvant chemotherapy or radiation for rectal cancer: Results from NSABP protocol R-01, J Nat Cancer Inst 80:21–29, 1988.

Frykholm GJ, Glimelius B, and Pahlman L: Preoperative and postoperative irradiation in adenocarcinoma of the rectum: final treatment results of a randomized trial and an evaluation of late secondary effects, Dis Colon Rectum 36:564–572, 1993.

Gastrointestinal Tumor Study Group (GITSG): Radiation therapy and 5-fluorouracil (5-FU) with or without methyl-CCNU for the treatment of patients with surgically adjuvant adenocarcinoma of the rectum, Proc Am Soc Clin Oncol 9:106, 1990 (abstract).

Gastrointestinal Tumor Study Group (GITSG): Survival after postoperative combination treatment of rectal cancer, N Eng J Med 315:1294–1295, 1986.

Gerard A, Buyse M, Norlinger B, Loyque J, Pene F, Kemp FP, Bosset JF, Gignoup M, Arnaud JP, and Desaiv C: Preoperative radiotherapy as adjuvant treatment in rectal cancer, Ann Surg 208:606–614, 1988.

Hampton B: Gastrointestinal cancer: colon, rectum, and anus. In Groenwald SL, Frogge MH, Goodman M, and Yarbro C, editors: Cancer nursing: principles and practice, ed 3, Boston, 1993, Jones & Bartlett Publishers, pp. 1044–1064.

Higgins GA, Humphrey EW, Dwight RW, Roswit B, Lee LE Jr, and Keehn RJ: Preoperative radiation therapy and surgery for cancer of the rectum: Veterans Administration Surgical Oncology Group Trial II, Cancer 58:352–359, 1986.

Hoebler L and Irwin MM: Gastrointestinal tract cancer: current knowledge, medical treatment, and nursing management, Oncol Nurs Forum 19:1403–1415, 1992.

Hoover HC, Brandhorst JS, Paters LC, Surdyke MJ, Takeshita Y, Madariaga J, Munez LR, and Hanna MG Jr: Adjuvant active specific immunotherapy for human colorectal cancer: 6.5 year median follow-up of phase III prospective randomized trial, J Clin Oncol 11:390–399, 1993.

Kemeny N, Conti JA, Sigurdson E, Cohen A, Seiter K, Linder R, Niedzwiecki D, Botet J, Chapman D, Costa P, and Budd A: A pilot study of hepatic arterial infusion of floxuridine compared with systemic 5-FU and leucovorin, Cancer 71:1967–1971, 1993.

Kemeny N, Younes A, Seiter K, Kelsen D, Sammarco P, Adams L, Derby S, Murray P, and Houston C: Interferon-alpha-2a and 5-fluorouracil for advanced colorectal carcinoma: assessment of activity and toxicity, Cancer 66:2470–2475, 1990.

Lanciano RM, Calkins AR, Wolkov HB, Buzydlowski J, Noyes RD, Sause W, Nelson D, Willett C, Owens JC, and Hanks GM: A phase I/II study of intraoperative radiotherapy in advanced unresectable or recurrent carcinoma of the rectum: a Radiation Therapy Oncology Group (RTOG) study, J Surg Onc 53:20–29, 1993.

Landry J, Koretz MJ, Wood WD, Bahri S, Smith RG, Costa M, Daneker GW, York MR, Sarma PR, and Lynn M: Preoperative irradiation and fluorouracil chemotherapy for locally advanced rectosigmoid carcinoma: phase I-II study, Radiology 188:423–426, 1993.

Laurie JA, Moertel CG, Fleming TR, Wieand HS, Leigh JE, Rubin J, McCormack GW, Gerstner JB, Krook JE, and Malliard J: Surgical adjuvant therapy of large bowel carcinoma: an evaluation of levamisole and the combination of levamisole and fluorouracil, J Clin Oncol 7:1447–1456, 1989.

Mayer RJ: Chemotherapy for metastatic colorectal cancer, Cancer 70:1414–1424, 1992.

Miller T, Quan SHQ, and Thaler W: Treatment of squamous cell carcinoma of the anal canal, Cancer 67:2038–2041, 1991.

Minsky BD, Cohen AM, Kemeny N, Enker WE, Kelson DP, Saltz L, and Frankel J: The efficacy of preoperative 5-FU, high-dose leucovorin and sequential radiation therapy for unresectable rectal cancer, Cancer 71:3486–3492, 1993.

Minsky BD, Cohen AM, Kemeny N, Enker WE, Kelson DP, Reichman B, Saltz L, Sigurdson E, and Frankel J: Enhancement of radiation-induced downstaging of rectal cancer by fluorouracil and high-dose leucovorin chemotherapy, J Clin Oncol 10:79–84, 1992.

Moertel CG: Accomplishments in surgical adjuvant therapy for large bowel cancer, Cancer 70:1364–1371, 1992.

Moertel CG: Vaccine adjuvant therapy for colorectal cancer: very dramatic or ho-hum, J Clin Oncol 11:385–386, 1993.

Moertel CG, Fleming TR, McDonald JS, Haller DG, Laurie JA, Goodman PJ, Unglerleider JS, Emeson WA, Tormey DC, and Glick JH: Levamisole and fluorouracil for adjuvant therapy of resected colon carcinoma, N Eng J Med 322:352–358, 1990.

Moertel CG, Gunderson LL, Maillard JA, McKenna PJ, Martenson JA Jr, Burch PA, and Cha SS, for the North Central Cancer Treatment Group: Early evaluation of combined fluorouracil and leucovorin as a radiation enhancer for locally unresectable, residual, or recurrent gastrointestinal carcinoma, J Clin Oncol 12:21–27, 1994.

National Institutes of Health: Adjuvant therapy for patients with colon and rectum cancer, NIH Consensus Development Conference Statement 8(4), 1990.

Papillon J: Surgical adjuvant therapy for rectal cancer: present options, Dis Colon Rectum 37:144–148, 1994.

Pazdur R, Ajani A, Patt Y, Winn R, Jackson D, Shepard B, Du Brow R, Campos L, Quaraishi M, and Faintuck J: Phase II study of fluorouracil and recombinant interferon-alpha-2a in previously untreated advanced carcinoma, J Clin Oncol, 8:2027–2031, 1990.

Peacock JL, Keller JW, and Ashbury RF: Alimentary cancer. In Rubin P, McDonald S, and Qazi R, editors: Clinical oncology: a multidisciplinary approach for physicians and students, ed 7, New York, 1993, WB Saunders Co, pp. 557–596.

Peloquin AB: Cancer of the colon and rectum: comparison of the results of three groups of surgeons using different techniques, Can J Surg 16:28–34, 1988.

Poulter CA: Radiation therapy for advanced colorectal cancer, Cancer 70:1434–1437, 1992.

Quan SH: Anal cancers: squamous and melanoma, Cancer 70:1384–1387, 1992.

Renoux G: The general immunopharmacology of levamisole, Drugs 19:89–99, 1980.

Rich TA: Radiotherapy for early rectal cancer. In Levin B, editor: Gastrointestinal cancer: current approach to diagnosis and treatment, Austin, 1988, UT Press, pp. 1364–1371.

Rich TA, Terry NH, and Meistrich WL: Chemoradiotherapy for anal and rectal carcinomas, CA Bull 46:322–325, 1994.

Rich TA, Weiss DR, Mies C, Fitzgerald TJ, and Chaffey JT: Sphincter preservation in patients with low rectal cancer treated with radiation with or without local excision or fulguration, Radiol 156:527–531, 1985.

Schilsky RL and Brochman DG: Adjuvant chemotherapy and radiation therapy in colorectal cancer, PPO Updates 6(3):1–11, 1992.

Sinicrope FA and Sugarman SM: Adjuvant therapy for colon carcinoma: current status and future directions, Cancer Bull 46:344–351, 1994.

Steele G and Ravikumar TS: Resection of hepatic metastases from colorectal cancer: biological perspective, Ann Surg 210:127–138, 1989.

Stockholm Rectal Cancer Study Group: Preoperative short-term radiation therapy in operable rectal cancer, Cancer 66:49–55, 1990.

Tanum G, Tviet K, Kadsen KO, and Hauer-Jensen M: Chemotherapy and radiation therapy for anal carcinoma: survival and late morbidity, Cancer 67:2462–2466, 1991.

Vaughn DJ and Haller DG: Nonsurgical management of recurrent colorectal cancer, Cancer 71:4278–4292, 1993.

Wadler S, Lembersky B, Atkins M, Kirkwood J, and Petrelli N: Phase II trial of fluorouracil and recombinant interferon-alpha-2a in previously untreated advanced colorectal cancer: an Eastern Cooperative Oncology Group (ECOG) study, J Clin Oncol 9:1806–1810, 1991.

Wadler N, Schwartz EI, Goldman M, Lyver A, Rader M, Zimmerman M, Itri L, Weinberg V, and Wiernik PH: Fluorouracil and recombinant alpha-2a interferon: an active regimen against advanced colorectal carcinoma, J Clin Oncol 7:1769–1775, 1989.

Watson PG: Meeting the needs of the patient undergoing ostomy surgery, J Enterostomal Therapy 12:121–124, 1985.

Willett CG, Shellito PC, Tepper JE, Eliseo R, Convery K, and Wood W: Intraoperative electron beam radiation therapy for recurrent locally advanced rectal or rectosigmoid carcinoma, Cancer 67:1504–1508, 1991.

Wolmark N, Rockett H, Fisher B, Wickerham DL, Redmond C, Fisher ER, Jones J, Mamounas Ed, Ore L, and Petrelli NJ: The benefit of leucovorin-modulated fluorouracil as postoperative adjuvant therapy for primary colon cancer: results from National Surgical Adjuvant Breast and Bowel Project protocol C-03, J Clin Oncol 11:1879–1887, 1993.

Chapter 11

❖ *Upper Gastrointestinal Cancers*

Patricia A. Spencer-Cisek

Cancers of the upper gastrointestinal tract include cancers of the esophagus, stomach, and pancreas. Although these tumors are very distinct in their presentation, treatment, and outcome, they unfortunately have one common thread: a poor prognosis. The development of new multimodal therapies offers hope of increased survival.

❖ *Cancer of the Esophagus*

Approximately 12,000 individuals were diagnosed with cancer of the esophagus in 1995, with an estimated 10,900 deaths that same year (American Cancer Society, 1995). Despite improvements in therapy and the fact that over two thirds of patients present with localized diseases, less than 20% are alive 2 years after diagnosis (Wilke et al., 1994). The 5-year survival rate is only 10%. Many researchers believe that subclinical metastatic disease is a common occurrence at the time of diagnosis (John and Flam, 1993; Leichman and Israel, 1993; Roth et al., 1993).

Treatment

Although the long-term survival rate from esophageal cancer remains low, multimodal therapies have started to improve disease outcome. Clinical trials to determine the optimal regimen, sequence, chemotherapeutic agent, form of radiation therapy, and type of surgical procedure are ongoing (Wilke et al., 1993).

Surgery
Surgery is the initial strategy in the treatment of early-stage cancer of the esophagus; however, fewer than 20% of patients qualify as candidates for definitive surgery (John and Flam, 1993). The remainder have metastatic disease at the time they undergo resection.

Candidates for curative surgery should have a resectable stage I or stage II tumor without evidence of penetration into adjacent structures, metastatic disease, or serious concurrent illness. The surgical procedure selected depends on the tumor location, the availability of viable tissue for reanastamosis, and the surgeon preference. There are four standard approaches: Ivor-Lewis esophagogastrectomy, radical en bloc esophagectomy, total thoracic esophagectomy, or transhiatal esophagectomy (Roth et al., 1993) (Figure 11-1). Table 11-1 describes these approaches.

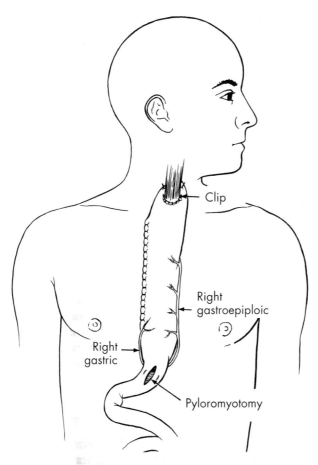

Fig. 11-1. Position of the stomach after esophagectomy. The stomach may be placed in a posterior mediastinal route or a retrosternal route. A posterior mediastinal position provides a shorter distance and may provide for better emptying after eating. The stomach is tacked to the prevertebral fascia. A pyloromyotomy or pyloroplasty is created to prevent gastric stasis and to enhance gastric emptying. The pyloromyotomy and the cervical anastomosis are marked with metal clips to enhance localization in postoperative radiographic studies. The proximal third of the clavicle and the lateral portion of the manubrium and first rib may be resected to increase the diameter of the thoracic inlet for a retrosternal conduit. From Roth JA, Putnam JB Jr, Lichter AS, and Forastiere AA: Cancer of the esophagus. In DeVita VT, Hellman S, and Rosenberg SA, editors: Cancer: principles and practice of oncology, ed 4, Philadelphia, 1993, JB Lippincott Co.

Table 11-1 Surgical Procedures in Upper Gastrointestinal Cancers

Type of Cancer	Procedure	Description	Key Points*
Esophageal	Ivor-Lewis esophagectomy (for tumor in upper to middle third)	Right thoracotomy and laparotomy. Pull up stomach with intrathoracic anastomosis.	This is standard approach. Stomach is used unless patient earlier had gastric surgery or other problem, then colon is used.
	Radical en bloc esophagectomy (for tumor in lower esophagus and cardia)	Laparotomy with resection of the thoracic esophagus, mediastinal lymph nodes, stomach, spleen, and celiac and thoracic nodes. Colon is used to replace esophagus: bowel interposition with intrathoracic anastomoses.	Not often used. Higher rate of difficulty with colonic interposition.
	Total thoracic esophagectomy	Thoracotomy, laparotomy, and neck exploration with resection of head of left clavicle. Cervical (retrosternal) anastomosis using stomach.	Aspiration a high risk in all procedures.
	Transhiatal esophagectomy (for any tumor, but preferred for cervical or thoracic inlet locations)	Neck exploration to mobilize and remove esophagus. Laparotomy with cervical anastomosis using stomach.	
Gastric	Total gastrectomy (for lesion in midsection)	Stomach is removed en bloc with mesentery and nodes. Esophagus anastomosed with jejunum. Laparotomy with or without thoracotomy.	Higher mortality rate. Infection, anastomatic leak, bleeding, pneumonia and aspiration are problems.
	Subtotal gastrectomy Two types:	En bloc removal of large part of stomach with greater and lesser omentum, with or without spleen, with or without distal pancreas.	Dumping syndrome: B vitamin deficiency, nausea, vomiting, weight loss, anastomotic leak, steatorrhea.
	Bilroth I	Anastomosis: gastroduodenostomy (stomach to duodenum)	Less aggressive, better tolerated if patient is debilitated. Leaves more residual tumor.
	Bilroth II	Anastomosis: gastrojejunostomy (stomach to jejunum; close duodenum)	75% of stomach removed and less chance of residual tumor.

Pancreatic	Pancreatoduodenectomy (Whipple procedure; for small tumor in head)	Remove head of pancreas, distal stomach, gallbladder, bile duct, entire duodenum, and first part of jejunum. Anastomosis (all with jejunum): Choledochojejunostomy (duct) Pancreaticojejunostomy (pancreas) Gastrojejunostomy (stomach)	May decrease problems with diabetes and malabsorption. Residual tumor possibly left. Pancreaticojejunostomy may not hold.
	Total pancreatectomy (for large tumor bulk)	Entire pancreas, duodenum, distal stomach, bile duct, gallbladder, spleen, and parapancreatic nodes. Anastomosis: Choledochojejunostomy Gastrojejunostomy	Brittle diabetes and malabsorption problems result. Less chance residual tumor remains. No pancreatico-jejunostomy.
	Regional pancreatectomy (if portal vein involved)	All organs as in total pancreatectomy plus celiac and mesenteric nodes. Anastomosis: Choledochojejunostomy Gastrojejunostomy Portal vein	Remove all regional nodes. No pancreaticojejunostomy. Very complex surgery. Brittle diabetes and malabsorption result. Portal vein anastomosis may not hold.
	Distal pancreatectomy (for tumor in tail or body)	Distal pancreas and spleen. No anastomosis.	Decrease risk of diabetes and malabsorption. May leave residual tumor.

* All procedures have risk of respiratory compromise, anastomotic leaks, and infections.

Data from Alexander, Kelson, and Tepper, 1993; Beazley and Cohn, 1991; Brennen, Kinsella, and Casper, 1993; Ellis, Levitan, and Lo, 1991; Frogge, 1993; Lawrence, 1991; and Roth et al., 1993.

Radiation Therapy

In a review of the literature, Earlam and Cunha-Melo (1980) concluded that there is no significant survival difference between surgery and radiation therapy, but that treatment-related mortality is higher with surgery.

Neoadjuvant Radiation Therapy Followed by Surgery

In John and Flam's review (1993), they discuss data from a study by Akakura and colleagues (1970). The resectability rate of esophageal tumors increased from 20% to 65% with the use of preoperative radiation therapy. An attempt to increase the radiation dose to 40 Gy over 7 to 10 days (Launois et al., 1981) or 66 Gy over 6 to 7 weeks (Doggett, Guernsey, and Bagshaw, 1970) resulted in a 25% to 33% operative mortality rate with increased morbidity. When treatment with 20 Gy over 4 to 5 days (Nakayama and Kinoshita, 1974) was compared with 40 Gy over 4 weeks (van Andel et al., 1979) the survival benefit was marginal. Morrison et al. (1991) reported a 5-year actuarial survival rate of 24% to 29% with preoperative therapy using hyperfractionated radiation therapy. Patients who received radiation therapy twice daily received a median dose of 33 Gy over a median of 14 days. Patients who received radiation therapy thrice daily received a median dose of 45 Gy over a median of 22 days. Severe toxicities caused treatment delays.

Chemotherapy

Despite the addition of radiation therapy to surgery, 75% to 85% of individuals diagnosed with cancer of the esophagus in the late 1970s and 1980s died within 1 year of diagnosis (John and Flam, 1993). Initially, single-agent chemotherapy with mitomycin-C, vindesine, cisplatin, or other agents resulted in tumor response rates of 20% to 30%. Combination chemotherapy regimens increased the response rates to 50% to 60% for individuals with regional esophageal disease.

Neoadjuvant Chemotherapy Followed by Surgery

Neoadjuvant chemotherapy regimens have increased survival rates for patients with esophageal cancer. John and Flam (1993) report that a preoperative regimen utilizing two to three cycles of a cisplatin-based combination resulted in 80% resectability, 5% operative mortality, and 5% pathological complete response. Several of the studies then utilized postoperative radiation therapy.

The Radiation Therapy Oncology Group (RTOG) is currently accruing patients to a randomized study comparing surgery alone to neoadjuvant and adjuvant chemotherapy with cisplatin and 5-fluorouracil (5-FU).

Neoadjuvant Concomitant Radiochemotherapy Followed by Surgery

In 1981, Steiger et al. reported on the use of 5-FU with mitomycin-C or with cisplatin for two courses concurrent with 30 Gy of radiation followed by esophagectomy. They reported a 2-year survival rate of 30% in both combined-modality arms.

A variety of other researchers have replicated the results of that study. The majority have evaluated 5-FU and cisplatin with concomitant radiation therapy. The chemotherapy was subsequently repeated for one additional course. Esophagectomy, performed approximately 3 weeks later, succeeded in 55% to 100% of cases, depending on the study. In select cases, additional radiation of 20 to 50 Gy was directed at positive surgical margins (John and Flam, 1993).

John and Flam (1993) also analyzed 9 studies, in which 394 patients treated in this manner survived a median period of 16 months. A mean of 21% had no evidence of disease at the time of surgery. The 1-year survival rate was 51%, whereas the 2-year rate was 31% (John and Flam, 1993).

Concomitant Radiochemotherapy

In advanced disease the combination of chemotherapy and radiation therapy has been effective. Byfield et al. (1980) used 5-FU 20 mg/m^2 per day continuous infusion for 5 days with concurrent radiation therapy. They reported an 83% response rate. Lokich, Shea, and Chaffey (1987) reported using 5-FU 300 mg/m^2 per day continuous infusion for 5 days for weeks 1 to 6 followed by radiation therapy in 13 patients. Patients received between 44 Gy and 69 Gy. The 1-year survival rate was 73%, and at 3 years, 22%. With the addition of chemotherapy, the improvement in dysphagia was rapid and sustained. Coia et al. (1993) also reported an improvement in dysphagia with combined therapy. Of 120 patients, 88% had an initial improvement in their swallowing ability within a median of 2 weeks. Those with distal tumors had earlier and more frequent initial improvement than those with tumors in the upper third of the esophagus. Of 25 treated with curative intent, the benign stricture rate was 12%. Among those with advanced disease, 91% had initial improvement, and in 67% of patients the local response lasted until death from systemic disease. A multimodal study by Adelstein et al. (1994) is highlighted on page 178.

Concomitant Chemobiotherapy

In a recent study by Ilson et al. (1994) the combination of 5-FU, cisplatin, and alpha-interferon (IFN-α) showed a significant impact. This has prompted the initiation of phase III trial of 5-FU, cisplatin, and IFN-α.

Nursing Management

Side effects from multimodal therapy of esophageal cancer include bone marrow depression, nausea, vomiting, esophagitis, weight loss, dehydration, bronchorrhea, development of esophageal-tracheal fistula, and pneumonitis. Enhanced side effects from using combinations of modalities are shown in the box on page 179. Treatment of these side effects is discussed in Unit III. Side effects specific to esophageal cancer treatments are discussed here.

The role of the nurse in the care of these individuals is essential to the early recognition of side effects and prompt initiation of treatment. Pulmonary toxicity is potentially the most life-threatening complication from combination therapy. The lung tissue is damaged by the effects of radiation and of mitomycin-C. During surgery, the forced oxygen with high tension may exacerbate the damage. This can lead to adult respiratory distress syndrome (ARDS) exhibited by progressive dyspnea with pulmonary infiltrates on X rays, both within and outside the radiation field (Seydel et al., 1987). Nursing care includes the frequent assessment of patient respiratory status and the early notification of the medical team if alterations become apparent. The use of oxygen, immediate evaluation by chest X ray, and arterial blood gas determination should be anticipated.

RESEARCH HIGHLIGHT

Adelstein DJ, Rice TW, Tefft M, Koka A, Kirby TJ, Tuason LJ, Taylor ME, and Van Kirk MA: Concurrent chemotherapy and hyperfractionated radiotherapy followed by surgical resection for esophageal carcinoma, Proc Am Soc Clin Oncol 13:206, 1994 (abstract).

Study All patients received concomitant chemoradiotherapy followed by surgical resection. Patients with residual tumors at the time of surgery also received additional postoperative chemoradiotherapy. The regimen consisted of chemotherapy (cisplatin 20 mg/m² and 5-FU 1000 mg/m² both continuous infusion for 4 days) with concurrent hyperfractionated radiation therapy (1.5 Gy bid for 8 days [24 Gy]). Following a 3-week break, the same course of radiation therapy was given for 7 days to reach a total of 45 Gy (from the two courses). After a break, all patients then underwent restaging and surgical resection. Patients with residual tumors at the time of surgery were treated with one postoperative course of chemotherapy with an additional 8 days of radiation therapy (24 Gy).

Sample The study included 26 patients with esophageal cancer: 13 with squamous cell carcinoma, 13 with adenocarcinoma. Pretreatment staging: 1 in stage I; 9 in stage II; 11 in stage III; 2 in stage IV.

Study aim To clarify the role of neoadjuvant concurrent chemotherapy combined with hyperfractionated radiation therapy in the treatment of esophageal cancer.

Findings At the time of surgical resection, a 69% overall response rate and 31% complete response rate were determined by pathological evaluation. The projected 2-year disease-free survival rate is 72%, with a projected 2-year overall survival rate of 64%. This regimen has significant toxicity, including nausea (69%), increased dysphagia (88%), neutropenia (42% with an absolute granulocyte count below 1000), thrombocytopenia (19% with platelet counts <50,000), and transient nephrotoxicity (12%). There were no preoperative deaths related to the therapy. Four patients died perioperatively (two with cirrhosis), and delayed recovery time in six patients prevented postoperative therapy.

Discussion Despite the toxicities, investigators were encouraged with the treatment response and planned to add additional patients to the study.

Bronchorrhea commonly occurs after esophagectomy and can lead to pulmonary compromise. Careful attention to preoperative pulmonary preparation is imperative. Patients should refrain from smoking at least 2 weeks before surgery. An incentive spirometer to facilitate deep breathing is used before and after surgery. Perioperative antibiotics and antiembolism prophylaxis also play important roles in improving the outcomes of surgery.

Another complication is the 5% to 10% incidence of esophageal-tracheal fistula, which develops from tumor destruction and from the combined use of radiation and chemotherapy. This can then lead to aspiration; any individual who develops a cough associated with swallowing should be evaluated immediately. If a fistula is present, jejunostomy feeding is recommended. The fistula may heal in some cases without medical intervention. Nursing care of a patient with a fistula is presented on page 181.

Dysphagia from the tumor and side effects of the combination therapy frequently impair the patient's nutritional status in the preoperative period. Impaired

Possible Side Effects from Multimodal Therapy in Upper Gastrointestinal Cancers

Multimodal Treatment	Possible Enhanced Side Effects
Esophageal Cancer	
Neoadjuvant radiation therapy followed by surgery	Delayed wound healing, esophageal-tracheal fistula, anastomotic leak, anastomotic stricture
Neoadjuvant chemotherapy followed by surgery	
5-Fluorouracil, cisplatin	Delayed wound healing
Neoadjuvant chemotherapy followed by surgery followed by radiation therapy	
5-Fluorouracil, mitomycin-C	Severe esophagitis, pneumonitis, esophageal-tracheal fistula, delayed wound healing, adult respiratory distress syndrome, bone marrow depression
5-Fluorouracil, cisplatin	Severe esophagitis, delayed wound healing, esophageal-tracheal fistula, bone marrow depression
Neoadjuvant concomitant chemoradiation therapy followed by surgery	
5-Fluorouracil, mitomycin-C	Delayed wound healing, esophageal-tracheal fistula, anastomotic leak, anastomotic stricture, severe esophagitis, adult respiratory distress syndrome, pneumonitis
5-Fluorouracil, cisplatin	Delayed wound healing, esophageal-tracheal fistula, anastomotic leak, anastomotic stricture, severe esophagitis, nausea and vomiting, dehydration
Concomitant chemoradiotherapy	
5-Fluorouracil, mitomycin-C	Severe esophagitis, pneumonitis, adult respiratory distress syndrome, esophageal-tracheal fistula, nausea and vomiting, severe mucositis, bone marrow depression, dehydration
5-Fluorouracil, cisplatin	Severe esophagitis, nausea and vomiting, esophageal-tracheal fistula, severe mucositis
Concomitant chemobiotherapy	
5-Fluorouracil, cisplatin, interferon	No enhanced side effects

Data taken from Alexander, Kelson, and Tepper, 1993; Brennan, Kinsella, and Casper, 1993; Bukowski et al., 1980; Frogge, 1993; Gunderson et al., 1987; Hoebler and Irwin, 1992; John and Flam, 1993; Kelson et al., 1991; Rich and Ajani, 1993; Roth et al., 1993.

Continued

Multimodal Treatment	Possible Enhanced Side Effects
Chemotherapy followed by radiation therapy	Severe esophagitis, nausea and vomiting, esophageal-tracheal fistula, severe mucositis
Gastric Cancer	
Surgery followed by adjuvant chemo-therapy	
5-Fluorouracil, doxorubicin, mitomycin-C	No enhanced side effects
Etoposide, doxorubicin, cisplatin	
5-Fluorouracil, doxorubicin, methotrexate	
Surgery followed by adjuvant radiation therapy	No enhanced side effects
Surgery followed by concomitant chemoradiotherapy	
5-Fluorouracil, semustine	Diarrhea, nausea and vomiting, gastritis,
5-Fluorouracil	photosensitivity, bleeding, nutritional deficiency
Neoadjuvant radiation therapy followed by surgery	Delayed wound healing
Neoadjuvant chemotherapy followed by surgery	
Etoposide, 5-fluorouracil, cisplatin	Delayed wound healing, nutritional deficiency
Neoadjuvant chemobiotherapy followed by surgery	
5-Fluorouracil, cisplatin, interferon	Bone marrow depression, stomatitis, nutritional deficiency, delayed wound healing
Intraoperative radiation therapy	Delayed wound healing, abscess, fistula, anastomotic leak, infection, bleeding, fibrosis, obstruction
Pancreatic Cancer	
Surgery followed by radiation therapy	Anastomotic leak, delayed gastric emptying, malabsorption
Surgery followed by chemotherapy	
5-Fluorouracil, mitomycin-C, streptozocin	No enhanced side effects
5-Fluorouracil, leucovorin	
Concomitant chemoradiotherapy	
5-Fluorouracil	Diarrhea, photosensitivity, nausea and vomiting,
5-Fluorouracil, mitomycin-C	nutritional deficiency, bone marrow depression
Concomitant chemotherapy with intraoperative radiation therapy	
5-Fluorouracil	Delayed wound healing, nausea and vomiting, nutritional deficiency, fibrosis with pain, delayed gastric emptying

Nursing Care of

The Patient with an Esophageal-Tracheal Fistula

Nursing Care	Rationale/Comments
◆ Assess for cough, especially when the patient is eating or drinking. Alert the patient to the sensation of "going down the wrong pipe." Assess the lungs on frequent basis. Abnormal sounds may be due to fistula and/or aspiration	◆ In esophageal cancer a fistula can form due to tumor invasion or treatment by lysis of the tumor from either chemotherapy or radiation therapy. When both are used concurrently there may be an increased occurrence. These findings need immediate assessment by a limited barium swallow to identify a fistula and by a chest X ray to determine if there is aspiration
◆ If a fistula occurs, maintain NPO and provide nutritional support via enteral feeding	◆ Jejunostomy is the preferred feeding method to decrease risk of reflux and aspiration. An extended period of rest may help with healing
◆ Maintain head of bed at 30 to 45 degrees	◆ To prevent reflux

nutritional status, as demonstrated by a low albumin level, adversely affects wound healing and increases the potential for infection (Naini, Dickerson, and Brown, 1988). Patients often receive nutritional support before surgery through the enteral or parenteral routes. Esophagogastrectomy can also compromise nutritional intake, and the patient may use supplements for extended periods of time. Patient education guidelines are outlined on page 182.

❖ Gastric Cancer

In 1995 an estimated 22,800 individuals in the United States were diagnosed with gastric cancer, and there were 14,700 deaths related to this disease (American Cancer Society, 1995). The rate of gastric cancer has declined since the turn of the century, but a recent trend of increased incidence of tumors at the cardia is disturbing because of its poor prognosis (Blot et al., 1991).

Treatment

Surgery

Historically surgery was the primary treatment for gastric cancer, although only early-stage tumors were cured. Today surgery is still of primary importance. The location and size of the tumor determine the type and extent of the surgery. An esophagogastrectomy is recommended for lesions of the proximal cardia. Large margins of at least 6 cm of noncancerous tissue are required. For a large lesion in

Patient Education Guidelines for

Care after Esophagectomy

♦ *For Preventing Reflux*
  ◆ Eat sitting up and do not lie down for at least 30 minutes after eating or drinking
  ◆ Raise head of bed using wedges and pillows at home
  ◆ Avoid bending over and lifting; squatting will decrease stress on abdomen

♦ *For Discomfort*
  ◆ Report throat pain to your doctor or physician
  ◆ Use antacids as ordered by your physician

♦ *For Fullness when Eating*
  ◆ Your stomach is now smaller and you may feel full after eating a small amount; eat small meals, often
  ◆ Avoid fatty foods
  ◆ Use high-calorie, high-protein supplements

♦ *For Difficulty in Swallowing*
  ◆ You may have a problem with narrowing in the area of surgery, especially if you had radiation too; report any problems with swallowing to your physician or nurse.

♦ *For Colon Interposition (if part of your bowel was used to replace your esophagus)*
  ◆ The speech therapist will meet with you to help you swallow
  ◆ Sit up straight when eating
  ◆ Solids may be easier to swallow than liquids
  ◆ Take small bites; swallow several times for each bite

♦ *For Foul-Smelling Breath*
  ◆ You may notice a change in the smell of your breath after surgery
  ◆ Clean your mouth every 2 hours by brushing your teeth and by using mouthwash (without alcohol to avoid drying)
  ◆ Avoid foods that cause you to belch
  ◆ Use mints and hard candy
  ◆ Take charcoal carbonate to decrease the odor
  ◆ Carry your mouth care supplies with you

Permission granted to reproduce these guidelines for educational purposes only.

the body of the stomach, a total gastrectomy is performed, and for smaller lesions, a subtotal gastrectomy. Refer to the specific procedures given in Table 11-1.

Radiation Therapy
Radiation therapy alone has not had a significant impact in the treatment of gastric cancer and is not recommended as a single modality for either primary therapy or palliation. However, researchers are investigating its use as an adjuvant treatment to combat the 50% to 80% rate of local-regional recurrence after gastric resection (Gunderson and Sosin, 1982). Figure 11-2 shows a possible radiation portal for the stomach. In Japan, where the incidence of this cancer is substantially higher than in the U.S., intraoperative (IORT) radiation therapy has been used. The delivery of 45 Gy

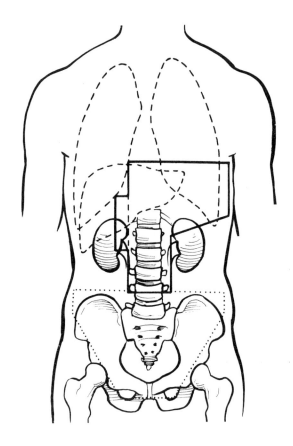

Fig. 11-2. Possible radiation portal for the stomach. Reprinted from Gunderson LL and Sosin H: Int J Radiat Oncol Biol Phys 8:1–11, 1982, with kind permission from Elsevier Science Ltd., The Boulevard, Langford Lane, Kidlington 0X5 1GB, UK.

during surgery resulted in a 27% increase in patient survival as compared to the survival rate when patients were treated with surgery alone (Abe and Takahashi, 1981).

Chemotherapy

Multiple studies have recently focused on a variety of chemotherapeutic agents in the treatment of gastric cancer. Single-agent therapy using 5-fluorouracil (5-FU), semustine, doxorubicin, or mitomycin-C resulted in tumor response rates between 18% and 30%. Combination therapy increased those rates to 30% to 40%. Mac-Donald et al. (1979) developed the combination of 5-FU, doxorubicin (Adriamycin) and mitomycin-C (known by the acronym FAM) that was used extensively in the 1980s. In 1989, Goldman and MacDonald reported on 400 patients treated in FAM trials who had an overall response rate of 33%. Various modifications of this regimen have been used without significant changes in outcome.

In recent years, a combination of etoposide, doxorubicin (Adriamycin) and cisplatin (platinum) (known by the acronym EAP) has been more widely studied. Preusser, Wilke, and Achterrath (1989) reported an overall response rate of 64% and a complete response rate of 20% with the EAP combination. In subsequent studies by several different groups, response rates ranged from 20% to 72%. Six percent of individuals obtained a complete response (Alexander, Kelsen, and Tepper,

1993). However, the regimen was not without difficulty, and treatment-related death rates were reported between 10% and 14% in the subsequent trials (Preusser, Wilke, Achterrath, 1989; Katz et al., 1989; Lerner, Steele, and Mayer, 1990; Taguchi, 1989).

Neoadjuvant Chemotherapy Followed by Surgery

Ajani, Ota, and Jackson (1991) administered etoposide, 5-fluorouracil, and cisplatin (platinum) (known by the acronym EFP) to 25 patients before and after surgery. Of those treated with neoadjuvant chemotherapy, 72% underwent resection. In a second study of 35 patients with proximal tumors who received neoadjuvant treatment, there was a 49% response, and 78% underwent curative resection (Ajani et al., 1990).

Surgery Followed by Adjuvant Chemoradiotherapy

Triple-modality treatment of gastric cancer is proving to be more successful than single- or dual-modality treatment, although the survival rates have not been dramatically affected as yet.

In 1982, the Gastrointestinal Tumor Study Group (GITSG) studied the use of adjuvant chemoradiotherapy for locally advanced gastric cancer. Participants underwent resection and were then treated with 5-FU and semustine alone, or with 5-FU and semustine followed by radiation to a dose of 50 Gy over 8 weeks with concomitant 5-FU. Those in the adjuvant chemoradiotherapy group had an actuarial survival rate of 25% after 2 years as compared to 10% in the group that received adjuvant chemotherapy alone. However, the adjuvant chemoradiotherapy group also experienced an increase in acute GI toxicity as compared to the adjuvant chemotherapy group.

Currently a high-priority study coordinated by the Southwest Oncology Group (SWOG) is investigating adjuvant chemoradiation therapy with 5-FU and leucovorin (folinic acid) (FA). The study compares the results of treatment with surgery alone to surgery followed within 48 days by 5-FU/FA, followed 4 weeks later by concomitant 5-FU/FA and 45 Gy over 5 weeks, followed 28 to 35 days later by two additional courses of 5-FU/FA scheduled 4 weeks apart (John and Flam, 1993).

Nursing Management

Whether an individual undergoes a total or a partial gastrectomy, the potential complications remain the same. Initially, the nurse watches for signs of an anastomotic leak or small bowel obstruction. Long-term complications are related to the loss of gastric surface area, loss of pyloric function, and parasympathetic innervation. *Dumping syndrome,* which occurs most frequently after a Bilroth I subtotal gastrectomy, is characterized by urgent diarrhea that occurs about 30 minutes after eating. Individuals also complain of weakness, dizziness, and palpitations.

When multimodal therapy is used, the GI toxicities can be substantial. For an individual prone to dumping syndrome, the treatment side effects of mucositis and diarrhea are compounded. Nutritional support is of utmost importance. In some treatment locations, the surgeon places a jejunostomy tube during a staging laparoscopy before therapy. This allows the individual to receive nutritional support during both neoadjuvant and adjuvant therapy. Patient Education Guidelines for Care After a Total or Partial Gastrectomy are presented below.

❖ *Cancer of the Pancreas*

As for other upper gastrointestinal malignancies, the long-term survival rates for patients with pancreatic cancer are poor. In 1995, the American Cancer Society predicted 24,000 cases of pancreatic cancer and 27,000 deaths.

Treatment

Surgery
Oncologists use several surgical interventions in the treatment of pancreatic cancer. At the time of diagnosis, only 20% of patients have disease confined to the pancreas and are therefore eligible for resection. The three types of procedures done to resect the primary tumor are a pancreatoduodenectomy (Whipple procedure), a total pancreatectomy, and a regional pancreatectomy (see Table 11-1). The total pancreatectomy causes problems of malabsorption and brittle diabetes. The regional pancreatectomy has high morbidity and mortality rates (Smalley and MacDonald, 1993).

Palliative surgery can substantially improve the quality of life for an individual with pancreatic cancer. Drainage devices can be placed to bypass biliary obstruction.

 Patient Education Guidelines for

Care After a Total or Partial Gastrectomy

♦ *For Anemia*
  ♦ When part of your stomach is removed your body does not get enough B vitamins
  ♦ You will need to get Vitamin B_{12} shots once a month

♦ *For Dumping Syndrome*   You may have a feeling of urgency to move your bowels about 30 minutes after eating. Some people also get weak and dizzy and may feel their heart beating fast. Here are several ways to help:
  ♦ Eat small meals frequently
  ♦ Avoid eating solids and liquids at same time
  ♦ Increase fat and protein in your diet
  ♦ Decrease carbohydrates in your diet
  ♦ Your physician may order medicine to slow the food down.

♦ *For Bezour Formation*
  ♦ To prevent food from becoming stuck in your throat, eat small amounts at a time and chew very well; avoid thick or stringy foods
  ♦ If something gets stuck, contact your physician or nurse

Permission granted to reproduce these guidelines for educational purposes only.

Symptoms of duodenal obstruction can be relieved with the use of a gastrostomy tube for drainage. A jejunostomy tube is often placed for nutritional support.

Radiation Therapy

Radiation therapy alone has not had a significant effect on this disease. When radiation therapy is used in combination with other therapies, the results improve. In several small studies, the use of neoadjuvant radiation therapy produced a small increase in survival rates, but according to Alexander, Kelsen, and Tepper (1993) the routine use of this combination is not warranted.

A variety of options currently under investigation include the administration of higher doses of radiation, changing the fractionation, concomitant chemotherapy, manipulation of the concomitant chemotherapy schedule, increasing the field of radiation, and combining more modalities.

Chemotherapy

Multiple single agents and combination chemotherapy regimens have been used with pancreatic cancer. The overall rate of success has been dismal, with most regimens except those based on 5-FU producing tumor responses of less than 20%. Evaluating the results of clinical trials can be problematical because the symptoms of disease progression are difficult to differentiate from side effects of chemotherapy.

Smalley and MacDonald (1993) reviewed 5 studies with a total of 143 patients and reported an overall response rate of 30%. Combination therapy with streptozocin, mitomycin-C, and 5-FU (known by the acronym SMF) was evaluated by the SWOG, who reported a 34% objective response rate compared with an 8% response rate in those treated with 5-FU and mitomycin-C alone. The overall median survival rate for both groups was the same (Bukowski et al., 1980). Ongoing studies are currently investigating the use of leucovorin with 5-FU and also evaluating new agents such as gemcitobene.

Concomitant Chemoradiotherapy

In 1981, the GITSG reported on a study comparing radiation therapy given alone to radiation therapy given with 5-FU. The radiation-alone arm was discontinued early, and the focus of the study became the evaluation of various doses of radiation given with 5-FU. A regimen combining 5-FU with 40 Gy of radiation resulted in a 23-week interval to disease progression with a median survival period of 36.5 weeks, and a regimen combining 5-FU with 60 Gy of radiation resulted in a 33.7-week interval to progression with a median survival period of 49.4 weeks.

The GITSG undertook a study of patients with unresectable local disease in which they compared treatment with SMF alone to treatment with SMF and concomitant 5-FU and radiation therapy. The combined-modality arm demonstrated a 1-year survival rate of 41% compared to a rate of 19% for the SMF-alone arm (Gastrointestinal Tumor Study Group, 1988).

In unresectable tumors intraoperative radiation therapy (IORT) with concomitant 5-FU has been studied. Gunderson and colleagues (1987) reported on a study of 49 patients with unresectable cancer who were treated with IORT to the tumor bed and with 5-FU. Though the doses of 5-FU differed between groups, all persons treated with the IORT had a local control rate of 85% after 1 year.

Neoadjuvant Concomitant Chemoradiotherapy Followed by Surgery

In patients with resectable tumors, several groups have investigated the use of multimodal therapy. In a small study by Weese et al. (1990), 14 patients received neoadjuvant therapy with 50 Gy of radiation therapy and concurrent 5-FU with mitomycin-C; 6 underwent curative resection. Of those 6, 5 remained disease-free from 4 to 40 months after surgery.

Surgery Followed by Adjuvant Chemoradiotherapy

An additional GITSG study to evaluate the use of adjuvant 5-FU with radiation therapy compared to the use of surgery alone was reported in 1985. The majority of participants underwent a pancreatoduodenectomy and were randomized to observation or to adjuvant therapy.

The adjuvant-therapy group received two courses of 20 Gy of radiation therapy with a 2-week break between courses. Each patient was administered 5-FU at 500 mg/m^2 for 3 days at the beginning of each course of radiation. The participants then continued with weekly doses of 5-FU for 2 years or until the disease progressed. Those treated with the multimodal therapy had a median survival period of 21 months compared to 11 months for those treated with surgery alone. The 2-year survival rate was 43% for the multimodal-therapy group compared with a rate of 18% for the surgery-alone group. Encouraged by these results, an additional 30 patients were added to the adjuvant-therapy group, and at 24 months the results were maintained. Alexander and colleagues (1993) caution against routine use of this therapy, citing similar outcomes and considerable variation in median survival rates in studies of treatment involving resection alone.

Nursing Management

In patients who undergo resection of a pancreatic tumor, skilled nursing assessment and intervention are essential. Immediate postoperative complications include hemorrhage, hypovolemia, hypotension, anastomotic leakage, infection, and fistula formation. Alterations in blood-glucose levels and nutritional deficiencies are common long-term problems. When chemotherapy and radiation therapy are given as adjuvant treatment, they can exacerbate complications.

In patients who have unresectable tumors and who are undergoing therapy with combination chemotherapy or chemoradiotherapy, close monitoring for complications related to therapy and disease progression are essential. Early recognition and management of symptoms hopefully minimize patient distress by controlling symptoms. Precise documentation will facilitate the investigation of new treatment methods.

❖ Summary

The statistics regarding survival of cancer of the upper gastrointestinal tract (esophagus, stomach, and pancreas) are dismal. However, the use of multimodal therapy improves survival rates.

When given multimodal therapy, this patient population can suffer substantial gastrointestinal toxicity. While investigators search for more effective multimodal treatment, nursing care must support the patients and their loved ones and focus on the quality of life for those who survive.

❖ References

Abe M and Takahashi M: Intra-operative radiotherapy: the Japanese experience, Int J Radiat Oncol Biol Phys 5:863–868, 1981.

Adelstein DJ, Rice TW, Tefft M, Koka A, Kirby TJ, Tuason LJ, Taylor ME, and Van Kirk MA: Concurrent chemotherapy and hyperfractionated radiotherapy followed by surgical resection for esophageal carcinoma, Proc Am Soc Clin Oncol 13:206, 1994 (abstract).

Ajani JA, Ota DM, and Jackson DE: Current strategies in the management of locoregional and metastatic gastric carcinoma, Cancer 56:260–265, 1991.

Ajani JA, Roth JA, Ryan B, McMurtrey M, Rich TA, Jackson DE, Abbruzzese JL, Levin B, DeCaro L, and Mountain C: Evaluation of pre- and postoperative chemotherapy for resectable adenocarcinoma of the esophagus for gastroesophageal junction, J Clin Oncol 8:1231–1238, 1990.

Akakura I, Nakamure Y, Kahegawa T, Nakayama R, Watanabe H, and Yamashita H: Surgery of carcimona of the esophagus with preoperative radiotherapy, Chest 56:47–57, 1970.

Alexander HR, Kelsen DP, and Tepper JE: Cancer of the stomach. In DeVita VT, Hellman S, and Rosenberg SA, editors: Cancer: principles and practice of oncology, ed 4, Philadelphia, 1993, JB Lippincott Co, pp. 818–848.

American Cancer Society: Cancer Facts and Figures, Atlanta, 1995, American Cancer Society.

Beazley RM and Cohn I Jr: Tumors of the pancreas, gall bladder, and extrahepatic ducts. In Holleb AI, Fink DJ, and Murphy GP, editors: Textbook of clinical oncology, Atlanta, 1991, American Cancer Society, pp. 219–236.

Blot WJ, Devesa SS, Kneller RW, and Fraemeni JF: Rising incidence of adenocarcinoma of the esophagus and gastric cardia, JAMA 265:1287–1289, 1991.

Brennen MF, Kinsella TJ, and Casper ES: Cancer of the pancreas. In DeVita VT, Hellman S, and Rosenberg SA, editors: Cancer: principles and practice of oncology, ed 4, Philadelphia, 1993, JB Lippincott Co, pp. 849–882.

Bukowski RM, Aberhalde RT, Hewlett JS, Weick JK, and Groppe CW Jr: Phase II trial of streptozocin, mitomycin-C, and fluorouracil in adenocarcimona of the pancreas, Cancer Clin Trials 3:321–324, 1980.

Byfield J, Barone R, Mendelsohn J, Frankel S, Quinol L, Sharp T, and Seagren S: Infusional 5-fluorouracil and x-ray therapy for nonresectable esophageal cancer, Cancer 45:703–708, 1980.

Coia LR, Saffen EM, Schultheiss TE, Martin EE, and Hanks GE: Swallowing function in patients with esophageal cancer treated with concurrent radiation and chemotherapy, Cancer 71:281–286, 1993.

Doggett RL, Guernsey JM, and Bagshaw MA: Combined radiation and surgical treatment of carcinoma of the thoracic esophagus, Rad Ther Oncol 5:147–152, 1970.

Earlam R and Cunha-Melo JR: Oesophageal squamous cell carcinoma: a critical review of radiotherapy, Br J Surg 67:457–461, 1980.

Ellis FH, Levitan N, and Lo TCM: Cancer of the esophagus. In Holleb AI, Fink DJ, and Murphy GP, editors: Textbook of clinical oncology, Atlanta, 1991, American Cancer Society, pp. 254–262.

Frogge MH: Gastrointestinal cancer: esophagus, stomach, liver, and pancreas. In Groenwald SL, Frogge MH, Goodman M, and Yarbro C, editors: Cancer nursing: principles and practice, ed 3, Boston, 1993, Jones & Bartlett, pp. 1004–1043.

Gastrointestinal Tumor Study Group: A comparison of combination chemotherapy and combined-modality therapy for locally advanced gastric carcinoma, Cancer 49:1771–1777, 1982.

Gastrointestinal Tumor Study Group: Treatment of locally unresectable carcinoma of the pancreas: comparison of combined-modality therapy (chemotherapy plus radiation therapy) to chemotherapy alone, J Natl Cancer Inst 80:751–755, 1988.

Goldman JJ and MacDonald JS: Chemotherapy of gastric cancer, Cancer Invest 7:39–52, 1989.

Gunderson LL, Martin JK, Kuols LK, Nagarney DM, Fieck JM, Wieand HS, Martinez A, O'Connell M, Earle JD, and McIlrath DC: Intraoperative and external-beam irradiation ±5-FU for locally advanced pancreatic cancer, Int J Radiat Oncol Biol Phys 13:319–320, 1987.

Gunderson LL and Sosin H: Adenocarcinoma of the stomach, areas of failure in a reoperation study, Int J Radiat Oncol Biol Phys 8:1–11, 1982.

Hoebler L and Irwin MM: Gastrointestinal tract cancer: current knowledge, medical treatment, and nursing management, Oncol Nurs Forum 19:1403–1415, 1992.

Ilson DH, Kelsen DP, Saltz L, Sirott MN, Keretzees R, and Dougherty JB: Alpha-interferon 5-fluorouracil and cisplatin in esophageal cancer: response in epidermoid carcinoma is significantly higher than in adenocarcinoma, Proc Ann Meet Am Soc Clin Oncol 13:194, 1994 (abstract).

John MJ and Flam MS: Esophagus. In John MJ, Legha S, and Phillips T, editors: Chemoradiation: an integrated approach to cancer treatment, Philadelphia, 1993, Lea & Febiger, pp. 285–301.

Katz A, Gansl R, Simon S, Gama-Rodrigues JJ, Waitzberg D, Bresciani C, and Pinotti HV: Phase II trial of VP-16, Adriamycin, and cisplatin in patients with advanced gastric cancer, Proc Am Soc Clin Oncol 8:89, 1989 (abstract).

Kelson D, Atiq O, Saltz L, Toomasi F, Trochanowski B, and Niedzwieck D: FAMTX (fluorouracil, methotrexate, adriamycin) is as effective and less toxic than EAP: a random assignment trial in gastric cancer, Proc Am Soc Clin Oncol 10:137, 1991 (abstract).

Launois B, Delarue D, Campion JP, and Kerbaol M: Preoperative radiotherapy for carcinoma of the esophagus, Surg Gynecol Obstet 153:690–692, 1981.

Lawrence W: Gastric neoplasms. In Holleb AI, Fink DJ, and Murphy GP, editors: Textbook of clinical oncology, Atlanta, 1991, American Cancer Society, pp. 245–253.

Leichman L and Israel V: Neoplasms of the esophagus. In Calabresi P and Schein PS, editors: Medical oncology: basic principles and clinical management of cancer, ed 2, New York, 1993, McGraw Hill Inc., pp. 649–667.

Lerner A, Steele GD, and Mayer RJ: Etoposide, doxorubicin, and cisplatin for advanced gastric adenocarcinoma: results of a phase II trial, Proc Am Soc Clin Oncol 9:103, 1990 (abstract).

Lokich JJ, Shea M, and Chaffey J: Sequential infusional radiation for tumors of the esophagus and gastrointestinal junction, Cancer 60:275–279, 1987.

MacDonald JS, Woolley PV, Smythe T, Ueno W, Hoth D, and Schein PS: 5-fluorouracil, Adriamycin, and mitomycin-C (FAM) combination chemotherapy in the treatment of advanced gastric cancer, Cancer 44:42–47, 1979.

Morrison WH, Rich TA, Quong G, McMurtrey MJ, and Peters LJ: Accelerated hyperfractionated preoperative radiation therapy for esophageal carcinoma, Proc 33rd Ann ASTRO Mtg 21(suppl):179, 1991 (abstract).

Naini AB, Dickerson JW, and Brown MM: Preoperative and postoperative levels of plasma protein and amino acid in esophageal and lung cancer patients, Cancer 62:355–360, 1988.

Nakayama K and Kinoshita Y: Surgical treatment combined with preoperative concentrated irradiation. JAMA 227:178–181, 1974.

Preusser P, Wilke H, and Achterrath W: Phase II study with the combination etoposide, doxorubicin, and cisplatin in advanced gastric cancer, J Clin Oncol 7:1310–1317, 1989.

Rich TA and Ajani JA: Stomach, pancreas, biliary system. In John MJ, Flam M, Legha S, and Phillips T, editors: Chemoradiation: an integrated approach to cancer treatment, Philadelphia, 1993, Lea & Febiger, pp. 303–314.

Roth JA, Putman JB Jr, Lichter AS, and Forastiere AA: Cancer of the esophagus. In DeVita VT, Hellman S, and Rosenberg SA, editors: Cancer: principles and practice of oncology, ed 4, Philadelphia, 1993, JB Lippincott Co, pp. 776–817.

Seydel HG, Leichman L, Byhardt R, Cooper J, Herskovic A, Libnock J, Pazdley R, Speyer J, and Tschan J: Preoperative radiation and chemotherapy for localized squamous cell carcinoma of the esophagus: a RTOG study, Int J Radiat Oncol Biol Phys 14:33–35, 1987.

Smalley SR and MacDonald JS: Pancreatic cancer. In Calabresi P and Schein PS, editors: Medical oncology: basic principles and clinical management of cancer, ed 2, New York, 1993, McGraw-Hill, Inc., pp. 691–706.

Steiger Z, Franklin R, Wilson R, Leichman L, Asfaw I, Vaishanpayan G, Rosenberg JC, Loh JJ, Dindogru A, Seydel H, Hoschner J, Miller P, Knechtges T, and Vaitkevicius V: Complete eradication of squamous cell carcinoma of the esophagus with combined chemotherapy and radiotherapy, Ann Surg 45:95–98, 1981.

Taguchi T: Combination chemotherapy with etoposide, adriamycin, cisplatin (EAP) for advanced gastric cancer, Proc Am Soc Clin Oncol 8:108, 1989 (abstract).

van Andel JG, Dees J, Dijkhius M, Fokkens W, van Houten H, de Jong PC, and van Woerkom-Eyken-boom WM: Carcinoma of the esophagus: results of treatment, Ann Surg 190:684–689, 1979.

Weese JL, Nussbaum ML, Paul AR, Engstrom PF, Solin LJ, Kowalyshyn MJ, and Hoffman JP: Increased resectability of locally advanced pancreatic and periampullary carcinoma with neoadjuvant chemoradiotherapy, Int J Pancreatology 7:177–185, 1990.

Wilke H, Fink U, Stahl M, Meyer HJ, and Seeber S: Neoadjuvant chemotherapy in esophageal cancer, Rev Oncol 3(1):3–4, 1993.

Wilke H, Siewert JR, Fink U, and Stahl M: Current status and future directions in the treatment of localized esophageal cancer, Ann Oncol 3(suppl 5):27–32, 1994.

Chapter 12

❖ *Genitourinary Cancers*

Jeanne Held-Warmkessel

Genitourinary malignancies (cancers of the prostate, bladder, kidney, and testicle) are common cancers. Frequently treatment for these diseases is multimodal. Over the past 10 years, the treatment of bladder cancer and testicular cancer has improved tremendously. Prostate cancer and renal cell cancer, however, continue to present treatment and management challenges.

❖ *Prostate Cancer*

Prostate cancer is the most commonly diagnosed cancer in American males and the second leading cause of male cancer-related deaths in the United States (Wingo, Tong, and Bolden, 1995). The incidence and the death rate from prostate cancer have increased over the past 20 years (Hanks, Myers, and Scardino, 1993).

Prostate cancer is classified by clinical importance. Clinically important cancers grow and spread, threatening the patient's life, whereas clinically unimportant cancers are indolent and not life threatening. A significant number of prostate cancers are clinically unimportant. The features that characterize these cancers include small size, well-differentiated grade, and a normal or slightly elevated level of prostate-specific antigen (PSA) (normal = 0–4 ng/ml). Clinically important cancers have a large tumor volume, moderate to poor grade, and an invasive pattern of growth, and the patient generally has an elevated PSA level (Scardino, Weaver, and Hudson, 1992).

Treatment

The treatment of early-stage prostate cancer is controversial. Even when tumor size and microscopic appearance are considered, it is not possible to determine whether a patient has a cancer that will become clinically significant or one that will remain indolent (Garnick, 1994).

191

Although typically a disease of older men, prostate cancer sometimes develops in patients as young as 40 or 50. These younger men will probably live long enough to develop metastatic disease. Also, because prostate cancer tends to be more aggressive in younger patients, these men might benefit from prostatectomy for early-stage disease (Garnick, 1994). It is not known if treatment of early-stage disease improves survival by preventing metastatic disease.

Given this information, some patients want treatment and some physicians encourage treatment. Traditionally therapy of stage A and stage B disease includes radical prostatectomy or radiation therapy, both with curative intent. Stage C tumors are usually too large for complete removal by prostatectomy and therefore radiation therapy is the preferred method for managing these tumors. In cases of widespread metastases, systemic therapy with antiandrogens or luteinizing-hormone-releasing-hormone (LHRH) analogues is required to block the effects of androgen on the prostate and metastatic sites.

Surgery Followed by Adjuvant Radiation Therapy
Radical prostatectomy with pelvic lymphadenectomy may result in an incompletely resected tumor, leaving the patient with a high risk of relapse. Radical prostatectomy is the removal of the entire prostate, prostatic capsule, seminal vesicles, and the bladder neck through an incision in the perineal or retropubic area. Complications include urinary or fecal incontinence, sexual dysfunction, infection, bleeding, and thromboembolism (Lind and Nakao, 1990). A tumor may involve the surgical margins of the specimen or the seminal vesicles. Radiation therapy may then be given to control residual disease. In a retrospective analysis of patients who underwent prostatectomy and limited pelvic lymphadenectomy, the addition of postoperative radiation therapy did not improve survival rates even though there was good tumor-bed control (Eisbruch et al., 1994). Side effects of postoperative radiation therapy include urinary and fecal incontinence, proctitis, cystitis, bladder neck stricture, and fistula formation. Given these side effects and the lack of evidence that radiation therapy improves survival rates, the decision to administer postoperative radiation therapy becomes a difficult one (Thompson et al., 1992). No randomized clinical trials have been done; the decision to give postoperative radiation therapy is not based on scientific evidence. Nonrandomized clinical trials of postoperative radiation therapy for bulky prostate cancer have been completed, but the number of patients in each study was small and complications such as incontinence were frequent, occurring in 16% to 40% of patients (Thompson et al., 1992). The Radiation Therapy Oncology Group (RTOG) is currently conducting a clinical trial to determine whether radiation therapy after radical prostatectomy with pelvic lymphadenectomy increases the rate of disease-free survival (see the Research Highlight on page 193).

Radiation Therapy Combined with Chemohormonal Therapy
Radiation therapy alone may not control bulky stage-C prostate tumors, and patients risk developing metastases (Green et al., 1984). Large tumors require higher doses of radiation to be well controlled (Sokol, 1980). However, higher doses of radiation also result in higher incidence of side effects (Hirshfield-Bartek, 1992). Doses of 45 to 50 Gy to the whole pelvis with a boost of 60 to 70 Gy to

| RESEARCH HIGHLIGHT |

Thompson I, Paradelo J, Miller G, Messing E, Martenson J, Schirrela R, Goldberg S, Porter A, Scrigley J, and Bard R. A phase III study of the treatment of pathologic stage C carcinoma of the prostate with adjuvant chemotherapy, RTOG 90-19, INT 0086, A research protocol, Philadelphia, 1992, Radiation Therapy Oncology Group.

Study Patients who undergo radical prostatectomy, including pelvic lymphadenectomy, are then randomized to receive postoperative adjuvant radiation therapy (60–64 Gy over 6 weeks) or no additional therapy.

Sample The study includes 538 patients with stage C adenocarcinoma of the prostate.

Study aim To determine the disease-free survival rates of patients who receive surgery and postoperative radiation therapy as compared to those who undergo surgery alone.

Findings This study continues as new patients are added.

Discussion This trial will help to define the role of adjuvant radiation therapy in patients who have undergone radical prostatectomy with pelvic lymphadenectomy for stage C adenocarcinoma of the prostate.

---

the prostate are required to manage prostate tumors (Hanks, Martz, and Diamond, 1988). Bulky stage-C tumors require doses of 71 to 79 Gy (Hanks, 1985).

Prostate cancer responds to androgen deprivation from orchiectomy, diethylstilbestrol (DES), luteinizing-hormone-releasing hormone (LHRH) analogue, and antiandrogens. There is often a dramatic reduction in tumor size because of the death of hormone-sensitive prostate cancer cells, or *cytoreduction* (Hanks, Myers, and Scardino, 1993). In a nonrandomized clinical trial, patients who received 3 mg DES for 2 months before, during, and up to 6 months after radiation therapy (65 to 67 Gy) for bulky prostate cancer had better local control of their tumors than patients who received radiation alone or radiation after failure of previous hormonal manipulation (Green et al., 1984).

A series of RTOG studies has evaluated the use of radiation and hormonal manipulation to improve local control and to reduce the incidence of metastases. DES or megestrol acetate given 2 months before and also concurrent with radiation therapy suppresses testosterone levels and improves local control of the tumor. Both drugs cause thromboembolic complications and fluid retention; DES also produces gynecomastia and more cardiovascular deaths than megestrol (Pilepich et al., 1993).

Hormonal manipulation with LHRH analogue produces fewer side effects than with DES or megestrol. The initial stimulation of cancer growth, or *flare,* that occurs with the initiation of LHRH drugs can be controlled with the concurrent administration of antiandrogens such as flutamide. The combination of these two drugs causes total androgen suppression. All hormonal agents cause impotence, decreased libido, and hot flashes (Taylor, 1991). In a randomized clinical trial, the LHRH agonist goserelin was given with flutamide 2 months before and during radiation therapy, and this was compared to radiation therapy alone. Estimated local control in the patients who received the hormone-radiation therapy was 84% compared to 71%

Nursing Care of

The Patient with a Radiation Implant

Nursing Care	Rationale/Comments
◆ Patient is placed in a single room	◆ To avoid radiation exposure to other patients and their visitors
◆ Visitation by pregnant women and children under 18 is prohibited	◆ To avoid radiation exposure to rapidly growing tissues
◆ Carefully plan patient care so that the nurse spends only 30 minutes (or time specified by the radiation safety officer) each shift in direct contact with the patient	◆ To avoid exposing the nurse to excess radiation
◆ When providing care, the nurse must stand behind the lead shield or stand at the foot or the head of the bed	◆ To avoid exposing the nurse to excess radiation
◆ The nurse may care for only one radiation-implant patient each shift	◆ To avoid exposing the nurse to excess radiation
◆ The nurse must always wear a radiation-monitoring badge	◆ To monitor the amount of exposure to radiation
◆ Keep all linens and dressings (packing, insertion devices, applicators, etc.) bagged and in the room until monitored by the radiation safety officer	◆ To avoid accidentally discarding radiation sources and subsequently exposing persons to radiation
◆ A lead container and pair of long forceps are to be kept in the room while the patient has an implant	◆ To place a dislodged source safely and in a safe location until the radiation safety officer and radiation therapy physician can examine the patient and replace the implant

Based on information from Black J and Matassarin-Jacobs E: Luckmann and Sorenson's medical-surgical nursing: a psychophysiologic approach, ed. 4, Philadelphia, 1993, WB Saunders Co; and from Held J, Osborne D, Volpe H, and Waldman A: Cancer of the prostate: treatment options and nursing implications, Oncol Nurs Forum 21:1517–1529, 1994.

in the patients who received only radiation; the estimated disease-free survival rate after 3 years was 61% for patients who received the hormone-radiation therapy compared to 43% for patients who received radiation alone (Pilepich et al., 1993). The continued administration of androgen-suppressing drugs after the completion of radiation therapy may contribute to continued disease-free status and survival (Hanks et al., 1992).

Prostate cancer is only minimally responsive to cytotoxic drug therapy. Estramustine, a combination drug consisting of estradiol bound chemically with nor-nitrogen mustard, is the most promising of the drugs studied. When given in oral doses of 140 mg three times daily with vinblastine in IV doses of 6 mg/m^2 weekly, it produced an overall response rate of 30% in men with progressive metastatic prostate cancer (Amato et al., 1991). In a randomized trial of patients after radiation therapy, estramustine was given in doses of 600 mg/m^2 orally daily for 2 years to one group, while another group received cyclophosphamide in IV doses of 1 gm/m^2 every 3 weeks for 2 years. The first group of patients experienced a median progression-free survival (PFS) period of 45.6 months compared to 38.7 months for the second group (Schmidt et al., 1993). In patients with lymph node involvement, PFS was still longer than treatment with radiation therapy only (37.3 months and 21.5 months, respectively). The results were similar for patients with extensive nodal disease (Schmidt et al., 1993). These results require confirmation in a phase III trial. The side effects of estramustine include nausea, vomiting, decreased libido, impotence, and cardiovascular and thromboembolic disorders (Fischer, Knobf, and Durivage, 1993).

Nursing Management

Many questions and controversies exist about current methods of prostate cancer management. Nurses must maintain up-to-date knowledge regarding these management controversies so that they can provide effective patient education, answer questions, and assist patients in making treatment-related decisions. Nursing management includes the assessment and management of disease and treatment-related complications, educating the patient and family about self-care measures, and participating in the prevention and early detection of prostate cancer (Held et al., 1994). Nursing diagnoses related to the care of patients receiving multimodal therapy for prostate cancer include altered sexual patterns, body-image disturbance, diarrhea, impaired skin integrity, bleeding, infection, fatigue, and altered patterns of elimination (Held et al., 1994). Possible Side Effects from Multimodal Therapy in Genitourinary Cancers are listed on page 196. These are discussed in Unit III.

❖ *Bladder Cancer*

Bladder cancer comprises approximately 4% of newly diagnosed cancers and is the fifth most common cause of cancer-related deaths in men over 75 years of age (Wingo, Tong, and Bolden, 1995). This is a highly treatable malignancy using multimodal therapy. Bladder cancers are multifocal, and for this reason their management can be difficult. After cancer has been eradicated in one section of the bladder, it can arise anew in a different section (Fair, Fuks, and Scher, 1993).

Treatment of Superficial Bladder Cancer

Removal of superficial bladder cancer with a resectoscope and fulguration is called a transurethral resection of a bladder tumor (TURBT) and controls approximately 80% of bladder cancers. However, TURBT controls only lesions that have been fulgurated (cauterized). For patients who suffer three or more recurrences of disease, additional therapy with intravesical drugs may be used. Other indications for intravesical therapy include incomplete resection of the tumor and risk of recurrence (Fair, Fuks, and Scher, 1993).

Possible Side Effects from Multimodal Therapy in **Genitourinary Cancers**

Multimodal Treatment	Possible Enhanced Side Effects
Bladder	
Neoadjuvant chemotherapy followed by cystectomy	
Cyclophosphamide, doxorubicin, cisplatin	No enhanced side effects
Methotrexate, vinblastine, cisplatin	Ileal conduit mucositis
Methotrexate, vinblastine, doxorubicin, cisplatin	
Methotrexate, doxorubicin, cyclophosphamide	
Methotrexate, vinblastine, mitoxantrone, carboplatin	
Neoadjuvant concomitant chemotherapy and radiation therapy followed by cystectomy	
Methotrexate, vinblastine, cisplatin	Bladder fibrosis, cystitis, diarrhea,
Methotrexate, vinblastine, doxorubicin, cisplatin	nausea and vomiting, bone marrow depression
Cisplatin	
Intraoperative radiation therapy and cystectomy	Delayed wound healing, infection, hemorrhage, fistula formation, obstruction
Neoadjuvant chemotherapy followed by cystectomy followed by concomitant chemotherapy and radiation therapy	
Methotrexate, cisplatin, vinblastine	Delayed wound healing, cystitis,
Methotrexate, vinblastine, doxorubicin, cisplatin	diarrhea, nausea and vomiting, bone marrow depression, bladder fibrosis, ileal conduit mucositis
Neoadjuvant chemotherapy followed by concomitant chemotherapy and radiation therapy	
Methotrexate, cisplatin, vinblastine	Cystitis, diarrhea, bone marrow
Methotrexate, vinblastine, doxorubicin, cisplatin	depression, bladder fibrosis
Cystectomy followed by adjuvant chemotherapy followed by radiation therapy	
Methotrexate, cisplatin, vinblastine	Diarrhea, bone marrow depression,
Methotrexate, vinblastine, doxorubicin, cisplatin	nausea and vomiting
Cystectomy followed by adjuvant chemotherapy	
Methotrexate, cisplatin, vinblastine	No enhanced side effects
Methotrexate, cisplatin, vinblastine, doxorubicin	

Data taken from Held et al., 1994; Held and Volpe, 1991; Loeher, 1992; Patterson and Reams, 1992; Rotman and Aziz, 1991.

Multimodal Treatment	Possible Enhanced Side Effects
Transurethral bladder resection followed by intravesical chemotherapy or biotherapy	
Thiotepa	Chemical cystitis
Mitomycin-C	
Doxorubicin	
Bacillus Calmette-Guerin (BCG)	
Interferon	
Neoadjuvant chemotherapy followed by radiation therapy followed by cystectomy	
Methotrexate, cisplatin, vinblastine	Bladder fibrosis, cystitis, diarrhea,
Methotrexate, cisplatin, vinblastine, doxorubicin	nausea, vomiting, bone marrow depression, delayed wound healing
Neoadjuvant chemotherapy followed by radiation therapy	
Methotrexate, cisplatin, vinblastine	Bladder fibrosis, cystitis, diarrhea,
Methotrexate, cisplatin, vinblastine, doxorubicin	nausea, vomiting, bone marrow depression
Prostate	
Radical prostatectomy followed by adjuvant radiation therapy	Cystitis, urinary or fecal incontinence, sexual dysfunction, fistula formation, scrotal edema, lymphedema of lower extremities, rectal stenosis
Radiation therapy followed by adjuvant chemo-hormonal therapy	
Hormonal manipulation	Sexual dysfunction, proctitis, cystitis,
Vinblastine and hormones	bone marrow depression
Cyclophosphamide and hormones	
Testicular	
Orchiectomy followed by adjuvant radiation therapy	Lymphedema if retroperitoneal lymph nodes are dissected
Orchiectomy followed by adjuvant chemotherapy	
Cisplatin, vinblastine, bleomycin	No enhanced side effects
Bleomycin, etoposide, cisplatin	
Vinblastine, cyclophosphamide, dactinomycin	
Ifosfamide, cisplatin, etoposide	
Carboplatin	
Neoadjuvant chemotherapy followed by orchiectomy	
Cisplatin, vinblstine, bleomycin	No enhanced side effects
Bleomycin, etoposide, cisplatin	
Vinblstine, cyclophosphamide, dactinomycin	
Ifosfamide, cisplatin, etoposide	
Carboplatin	

Continued

Multimodal Treatment	Possible Enhanced Side Effects
Kidney	
Chemotherapy with biotherapy	
Floxuridine, interferon-α	Elevations of liver enzymes,
Floxuridine, interleukin-2	cutaneous reactions
5-Fluorouracil, interferon-α	
5-Fluorouracil, interleukin-2	
Radical nephrectomy followed by biotherapy	
Interferon-α	No enhanced side effects
Interleukin-2	

Intravesical therapy involves instilling drugs into the empty bladder through a Foley or straight catheter. The drug dwells in the bladder for 2 hours. Intravesical therapy allows for direct contact between the drug and the urothelium and causes few systemic side effects (Fair, Fuks, and Scher, 1993). Drugs that have been used intravesically include the chemotherapeutic agents doxorubicin, thiotepa, and mitomycin-C and the biotherapeutic agents *Bacillus Calmette-Guerin* (BCG) and interferon-α-2b (Fleischmann and Goldberg, 1993; Lehmann et al., 1993; Witjes, Mulders, and Debruyne, 1994). BCG is as effective as any of the three chemotherapeutic agents in treating existing disease and for tumor prophylaxis (Fleischmann and Goldberg, 1993).

Treatment of Muscle-Invasive Bladder Cancer

The standard treatment of muscle-invasive bladder cancer includes radical cystectomy or radiation therapy. However, the 5-year survival rate of these patients is less than 50% and may be as low as 20% (Fair, Fuks, and Scher, 1993; Gospodarowicz and Warde, 1993; Miller, Torti, and Shipley, 1993). The addition of preoperative radiation therapy to radical cystectomy may not offer a survival advantage (Fair, Fuks, and Scher, 1993; Montie, Straffon, and Stewart, 1984).

Intravenous chemotherapy can effectively manage muscle-invasive bladder cancer, and the results of several clinical trials have led to the development of adjuvant and neoadjuvant protocols (Yagoda, 1987).

Surgery Followed by Adjuvant Chemotherapy

In a nonrandomized prospective clinical trial, postcystectomy patients were given IV cyclophosphamide (500 mg/m^2 on day 1), IV doxorubicin (50 mg/m^2 on day 1), and IV cisplatin (70 to 100 mg/m^2 on day 2) for a maximum of five cycles. The control arm consisted of patients who refused or were not offered chemotherapy. Patients who received chemotherapy had a survival advantage (Logothetis et al., 1988). These results need to be confirmed in a prospective randomized trial.

Concurrent Chemoradiotherapy

Radiation therapy has been combined with IV chemotherapy with the goal of bladder preservation, which may result in improved quality of life for the patient. A trial combining cisplatin and radiation therapy produced a 67% complete response rate with 64% actuarial survival at 3 years (Tester et al., 1993).

Neoadjuvant Chemotherapy Followed by Radiation Therapy
The preceding results led to nonrandomized RTOG trial 88-02 (Tester et al., 1991). Because the methotrexate, cisplatin, and vinblastine followed by pelvic radiation produced a 79% complete response rate, it was incorporated into RTOG bladder-preserving randomized trial 89-03 (Shipley et al., 1990). Figure 12-1 shows an example of radiation portals used in bladder-preserving protocols. Results from this last trial are pending. If trial 89-03 has a positive outcome, a prospective randomized trial comparing bladder-preserving therapy to radical cystectomy is needed. Until then, bladder-preserving therapy should be undertaken only in a clinical trial setting and cannot be considered standard therapy.

Nursing Management

The Possible Enhanced Side Effects from Multimodal Therapy are discussed on page 196. Patients eligible for bladder-preserving trials require an in-depth understanding of self-care management at home and the need to comply with all aspects of the trial in order to derive its full benefit. Bladder cancers that do not completely respond to bladder-preserving treatment will require removal by radical cystectomy. This outcome can be devastating to the patient. The patient needs nursing support to deal with this new crisis.

❖ Renal Cell Carcinoma

Renal cell carcinoma is uncommon in adults, comprising approximately only 2% of new malignancies (Davis, 1993; Linehan, Shipley, and Parkinson, 1993). The incidence of renal cell carcinoma has been slowly increasing (Couillard and White, 1993).

Treatment

Radical nephrectomy is the treatment of choice for local and regional renal cell carcinoma. The procedure involves ligation of the renal vessels and removal of the kidney, the adrenal gland, perirenal fat, the lymphatics, and Gerota's fascia (Couillard and White, 1993; Winter et al., 1990; Wood and Herr, 1989). The value of performing regional lymphadenectomy has not been demonstrated, and further research into this area is required (Couillard and White, 1993; Montie, 1989). Patients with bilateral renal tumors or patients with a solitary kidney may benefit from partial nephrectomy or enucleation of the tumor (Couillard and White, 1993; Wood and Herr, 1989). In the presence of metastatic disease, palliative nephrectomy may be performed to control pain, bleeding, or other distressing symptoms (Keller, Sahasrabudhe, and McCune, 1993).

The role of radiation therapy in treating renal cell carcinoma is limited to the palliation of metastasis to the bone and central nervous system and to the relief of pain (Keller, Sahasrabudhe, and McCune, 1993). Studies using adjuvant radiation therapy demonstrated no survival benefit (Forman, 1989), and postoperative radiation therapy was associated with significant morbidity and mortality (Kjaer et al., 1987).

Single-agent chemotherapy and combination chemotherapy both produce poor results (Yagoda, Petrylak, and Thompson, 1993). The multi-drug-resistant (MDR) gene is the most likely explanation for poor drug responsiveness (Fojo et

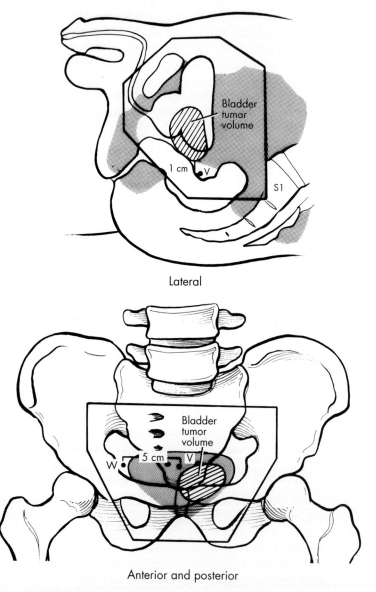

Fig. 12-1. Example of radiation portals used in bladder-preserving protocols. From Shipley W, Tester W, Donnelly B, and True L: A phase III trial to study the role of neoadjuvant MCV chemotherapy combined with transurethral surgery plus cisplatin with radiation therapy for the selective bladder presentation in patients with muscle-invading bladder cancer. RTOG 89-03, Philadelphia, 1990, Radiation Therapy Oncology Group. Used with permission.

al., 1987). Floxuridine (FUDR), administered by *circadian rhythm infusion* (administering chemotherapy at variable rates of infusion to decrease the incidence of side effects and to improve drug efficacy) may offer improved results. Floxuridine administered in daily doses of 0.25 mg/kg by circadian rhythm infusion into the hepatic artery produced responses in up to 16% of patients (Hrushesky et al., 1990; Yagoda, Petrylak, and Thompson, 1993). Giving 5-fluorouracil (5-FU) by continuous infusion produces responses in 7% to 9% of patients treated (Kish, Neefe, and Flannigan, 1991; Schulof et al., 1991). Continuous infusion FUDR for 14 days followed by continuous infusion vinblastine for 14 days produced a 27% partial response rate (Small et al., 1994). Clearly, more effective drugs need to be found to manage this disease.

Chemobiotherapy

Combining FUDR or 5-FU with biologic response modifiers such as interferon-alfa or interleukin-2 (IL-2) holds the most promise of effective results. Interferon-alfa produces responses in 14% of patients (Wirth, 1993). When interferon-alfa is given with FUDR or 5-FU, response rates increase to 35% and 27%, respectively (Yagoda, Petrylak, and Thompson, 1993). The side effects of interferon include flulike symptoms of fever, chills, rigors, and diaphoreses; fatigue; malaise; anorexia; muscle pain; arthralgia; headache; mild pancytopenia; mild elevations of liver enzymes; skin rash; and injection site reactions.

IL-2 has been administered in a variety of schedules and doses. Tumor response rates average 14% to 29% for IL-2 given by continuous infusion or by subcutaneous daily injection (Gore et al., 1994; Lissoni et al., 1994). IL-2 can produce capillary leak syndrome, hypotension, tachycardia, fluid weight gain, dyspnea, respiratory distress, elevated serum creatinine with oliguria, nausea, vomiting, diarrhea, disorientation, and flulike symptoms (Fischer, Knobf, and Durivage, 1993). When receiving IL-2, patients may require nursing care at the level of an intensive-care unit (Davis, 1993).

Trials combining IL-2 and interferon have not improved results over IL-2 alone, especially when high doses of IL-2 are used (Ravaud et al., 1994). When responses to IL-2 do occur, responses tend to range from 3 to 50 months (Linehan, Shipley, and Parkinson, 1993).

Surgery Followed by Biotherapy

Because nephrectomy produces the best response rates and biotherapy holds promise for the future management of renal cell carcinoma, a phase III trial is currently examining the role of nephrectomy and interferon in patients with a high risk of relapse (Sella, 1994).

Nursing Management

Care of a patient with renal cell carcinoma includes routine pre- and postoperative nursing care, management of patients receiving biotherapy, control of drug-related side effects, and education of the patient and family. Patient Education Guidelines

Patient Education Guidelines for

Care of a Nephrostomy Tube

♦ Wash around the nephrostomy tube each day with soap and water. Rinse well, pat dry, and apply a clean, dry dressing. Tape the tube to the skin to prevent it from falling out or being dislodged. The collection bag should be emptied when it is three-fourths filled or every 8 hours, whichever occurs first.

♦ As taught by your nurse, flush the tube with 10 ml of saline every day.

♦ Notify your physician if there is redness, pain, or drainage at the tube exit site, if the urine is cloudy or foul smelling, if there is blood in the urine, or if you have a fever over 100°F.

Permission granted to reproduce these guidelines for educational purposes only.

for Care of a Nephrostomy Tube are presented above. Possible enhanced side effects from multimodal therapy are listed on page 196 and discussed in detail in Unit III.

❖ Testicular Cancer

Testicular cancer is one of the most curable solid tumors that develop in young adult males. Developments in chemotherapy, tumor markers, radiation therapy, and surgery are responsible for the high rates of cure and long-term survival in these men. Testicular cancer is uncommon, but it is the most frequently occurring cancer in men 15 to 35 years of age (Brock et al., 1993; Richie, 1993; Einhorn, Richie, and Shipley, 1993).

Treatment of Nonseminomatous Germ Cell Tumors

After having a testicle removed through an inguinal incision, patients with stage I disease undergo either modified retroperitoneal lymph node dissection (RPLND) or monthly surveillance for the first year followed by bimonthly evaluations the second year and then two to four exams a year thereafter (Einhorn, Richie, and Shipley, 1993; Richie, 1993). Patients who have tumors that are 2.5 cm or larger, who have vascular or lymphatic invasion, or who have 50% less teratoma in their tumor are not good candidates for surveillance and should undergo RPLND (Fung et al., 1988). Stage I patients have a 96% cure rate with surgery alone. Those who relapse are treated with chemotherapy.

RPLND is indicated in patients with stage II disease. The disease will be controlled in more than half of the patients, especially in patients with nodal metastases less than 3 cm in diameter. Nodes larger than 3 cm indicate that chemotherapy may be necessary (Einhorn, Richie, and Shipley, 1993; Keller, Sahasrabudhe, and McCune, 1993; Richie, 1993). In the presence of large bulky nodes, chemotherapy can be administered first, followed by RPLND. Patients who relapse after RPLND can be treated with chemotherapy.

Cisplatin-based chemotherapy produces complete responses in 70% of patients with stage III disease. The BEP (bleomycin, etoposide, cisplatin [platinum]) regimen is commonly used and produces responses in 80% or more of patients. The treatment consists of cisplatin given in IV doses of 20 mg/m² per day for 5 days, etoposide given in IV doses of 100 mg/m² per day for 5 days, and bleomycin given in IV doses of 30 units per week. Each cycle is repeated every 3 weeks for a total of four cycles. Side effects and toxicities include sepsis, pulmonary fibrosis, small-bowel necrosis, myelosuppression, Raynaud's phenomenon, paresthesias, abdominal cramps, and myalgias. Patients with residual disease after chemotherapy benefit from surgical resection, which can then render them disease free. Three cycles of BEP can be given to patients with minimal to moderate bulk disease (Einhorn et al., 1989).

Several clinical trials are attempting to improve the 69% complete response rate to BEP seen in patients with advanced extent of disease. Doubling the dose of cisplatin to 40 mg/m² in the BEP regimen proved not more effective than the standard dose of BEP (Einhorn et al., 1990). A five-drug regimen (VIP/VB), consisting of etoposide (VP-16) (given as 75 mg/m² IV, days 1 to 5), ifosfamide (given as 1.2 gm/m² IV, days 1 to 5 with mesna), cisplatin (platinum) (given as 20 mg/m² IV, days 1 to 5, vinblastine (given as 0.18 mg/kg IV, day 1), and bleomycin (given as 30 units IV weekly), was given every 3 weeks for four cycles with hematopoietic growth factor support. Side effects included myelosuppression, infection, and pulmonary toxicity. After undergoing surgical resection with thoracotomy to remove residual mediastinal disease or RPLND or both, 67% of patients who had had advanced disease were disease free. This regimen is currently being investigated in a cooperative group trial at various sites (Blanke et al., 1994).

VAB-6 therapy (vinblastine 4 mg/m² IV on day 1, cyclophosphamide 600 mg/m² IV on day 1, dactinomycin [actinomycin-D] 1 mg/m² IV on day 1, bleomycin 30 units IV push followed by 20 units/m² IV continuous infusion over 72 hours on cycles 1 and 2, cisplatin 120 mg/m² on day 4) given for three cycles produces a 79% complete response rate. Toxicities and side effects include nausea, vomiting, alopecia, myelosuppression, nephrotoxicity, pulmonary fibrosis, ototoxicity, and color changes in hands (Bosl et al., 1986).

Etoposide given in IV doses of 100 mg/m² for days 1 to 5 and cisplatin (platinum) given in IV doses of 20 mg/m² for days 1 to 5 (the drug combination is known as EP) for four cycles was compared with VAB-6 given for three cycles when it was found that EP is useful in patients with refractory germ cell tumors (Bosl et al., 1985; Bosl et al., 1988). Complete responses occurred in 96% of patients treated with VAB-6 and in 93% of those treated with EP. Side effects with EP were more tolerable with less emesis, neutropenia, mucositis, and magnesium wasting and with no pulmonary toxicity. This regimen can be recommended for patients with small- to medium-size tumors.

Patients may relapse or progress after front-line therapy with PVB, BEP, VAB-6, or EP. If a patient has received vinblastine, then second-line therapy should contain etoposide and vice versa. Ifosfamide (given as 1.2 gm/m² IV for 5 days) may be used with cisplatin (given as 20 mg/m² IV for 5 days) plus etoposide (VP-16) (given as 75 mg/m² IV for 5 days) or vinblastine (given as 0.11 mg/kg

IV on days 1 and 2) (VIP) every 3 weeks for four cycles for second- or third-line therapy. This approach produces a response rate of 22% to 45% in previously treated patients (Lauer et al., 1987; Einhorn et al., 1992).

Autologous Bone Marrow Transplant

Giving etoposide and carboplatin in high doses to patients whose disease progressed while receiving cisplatin therapy or to patients with refractory testicular cancer produces modest results of 25% complete responses and 19% partial responses (Nichols et al., 1989). Patients are treated with etoposide (1200 mg/m²) and carboplatin (900 to 2000 mg/m²) followed by bone marrow transplantation. The associated toxicities include severe myelosuppression, fever, enterocolitis, stomatitis, nausea, vomiting, alopecia, hypomagnesemia, and elevated liver enzymes.

Treatment of Seminoma

The routine treatment of stage I seminoma testicular cancer after radical inguinal orchiectomy is radiation therapy. Doses of 25 to 35 Gy administered to the retroperitoneal lymph nodes over 3 to 4 weeks results in survival rates of 91% to 99% (Fung and Garnick, 1988). Radiation is also delivered to the ipsilateral external iliac nodes, the bilateral common iliac nodes, the paracaval nodes and the para-aortic nodes (Richie, 1993) and produces minimal side effects. Occasionally, patients are not given radiation therapy immediately after surgery; radiation is administered only if relapse occurs (Keller, Sahasrabudhe, and McCune, 1993). Figure 12-2 presents an example of radiation portals.

Patients with advanced seminoma (stage IIB to stage III) require treatment with cisplatin-based chemotherapeutic regimens similar to those used to treat non-seminomatous germ cell tumors. Loehrer et al. (1987) reported response rates of 61% to 88%. Single-agent carboplatin may also be useful in this patient population (Horwich et al., 1989), in which investigators observed a response rate of 80%. Treatment with carboplatin alone is being compared to treatment with the combination of cisplatin, etoposide, and ifosfamide (Clemm et al., 1991; Einhorn, Richie, and Shipley, 1993).

Nursing Management

Testicular cancer may have a profound effect on a man's physical and emotional well-being. Nursing management includes patient education, especially testicular self-exam in adolescent and young males, preoperative and postoperative nursing care, and management of chemotherapeutic and radiation therapy side effects.

Sterility is a concern in these patients because 80% of them are oligospermic before diagnosis (Loehrer, 1991). Because of testicular cancer's rapid growth, treatment needs to start quickly. Sperm banking takes time, and it may not be appropriate to delay treatment until adequate specimens have been obtained. Sperm counts improve in about 50% of patients in the first 2 years after treatment. Pregnancies have been possible for the female partners of about one third of men treated for testicular cancer. RPLND also affects sterility. Retrograde ejaculation occurs in all men who undergo a bilateral procedure. When the modified procedure is performed, antegrade ejaculation is preserved.

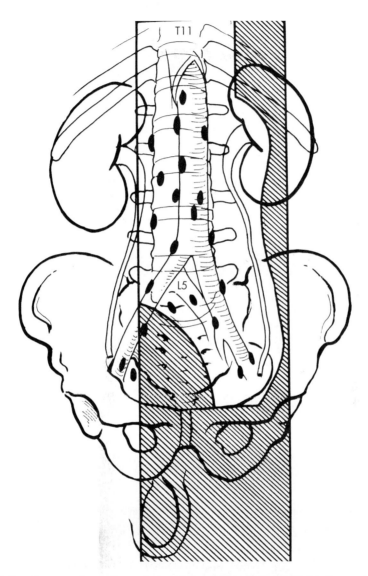

Fig. 12-2. Contoured anterior and posterior radiation treatment fields for men with clinical stage I or stage IIA left testicular cancer. The diagonally shaded area is an individually made, 8-cm-thick Ostalloy block (shield 2). Reprinted from Kubo H and Shipley W: Reduction of the scatter dose to the testicle outside the radiation treatment fields, Int J Radiat Oncol Biol Phys 8:1744–1745, copyright 1982, with kind permission from Elsevier Science Ltd. The Boulevard, Langford Lane, Kidlington 0X5 1GB, UK.

❖ Summary

Multimodal therapy has improved the survival rate in people with prostate, bladder, kidney, and testicular cancers, but randomized clinical trials are needed to improve the survival rate and to determine standard treatment regimens. Even when survival cannot be increased, extended disease-free intervals can improve a patient's quality of life. The nurse plays an important role in educating the patient about clinical trials and, if the opportunity arises, encouraging the patient to join a study to get sophisticated treatment and possibly to help a future patient.

❖ References

Amato R, Logothetis C, Dexeus F, Sella A, Kilbourne R, and Fitz K: Preliminary results of a phase II trial of estramustine and vinblastine for patients with progressive hormone refractory prostate carcinoma, Proc Am Soc Clin Oncol 32:186, 1991 (abstract).

Blanke C, Loehrer P, Einhorn L, Nichols C: A phase II study of VP-16 plus ifosfamide plus cisplatin plus vinblastine plus bleomycin (VIP/VB) with filgrastim for advanced-stage testicular cancer, Proc Am Soc Clin Oncol 13:234, 1994 (abstract).

Bosl G, Geller N, Bajorin D, Leitner S, Yagoda A, Golbey R, Scher H, Vogelzang N, Auman J, Carey R, Fair W, Herr H, Morse M, Sogani P, and Whitmore W: A randomized trial of etoposide + cisplatin versus vinblastine + bleomycin + cisplatin + cyclophosphamide + dactinomycin in patients with good prognosis germ cell tumors, J Clin Oncol 6:1231–1238, 1988.

Bosl G, Gluckman R, Geller N, Golbey R, Whitmore W, Herr H, Sogani P, Morse M, Martini N, Bains M, McCormack P: VAB-6: an effective chemotherapy regimen for patients with germ cell tumors, J Clin Oncol 4:1493–1499, 1986.

Bosl G, Yagoda A, Golbey R, Whitmore W, Herr H, Sogani P, Morse M, Vogelzang N, and MacDonald G: Role of etoposide-based chemotherapy in the treatment of patients with refractory or relapsing germ cell tumors, Am J Med 78:423–428, 1985.

Brock D, Fox S, Gosling G, Haney L, Kneebone P, Nagy C, Qualitza B: Testicular cancer, Semin Oncol Nurs 9:224–236, 1993.

Clemm C, Harenstein R, Mair W, Gerl A, and Willmanns W: VIP combination chemotherapy in bulky seminoma, Proc Am Soc Clin Oncol 10:178, 1991 (abstract).

Couillard D and White R: Surgery of renal cell carcinoma, Urol Clin No Am 20:263–275, 1993.

Davis M: Renal cell carcinoma, Semin Oncol Nurs 9:267–271, 1993.

Einhorn L, Richie J, and Shipley W: Cancer of the testis. In DeVita V, Hellman S, and Rosenberg S, editors: Cancer: principles and practice of oncology, ed 4, Philadelphia, 1993, JB Lippincott Co, pp. 1126–1151.

Einhorn L, Weathers T, Loehrer P, and Nichols C: Second-line chemotherapy with vinblastine, ifosfamide, and cisplatin after initial chemotherapy with cisplatin, VP-16, and bleomycin in disseminated germ cell tumors: long-term follow-up, Proc Am Soc Clin Oncol 11:196, 1992 (abstract).

Einhorn L, Williams S, Loehrer P, Birch R, Drasga R, Omura G, and Greco A: Evaluation of optimal duration of chemotherapy in favorable-prognosis disseminated germ cell tumors: a Southeastern Cancer Study Group protocol, J Clin Oncol 7:387–391, 1989.

Einhorn L, Williams S, Loehrer P, Crawford D, Wettlaufer J, Bartolucci A, and Schacter L: Phase III study of cisplatin dose intensity in advanced germ cell tumors: a Southeastern and Southwestern Oncology Group protocol, Proc Am Soc Clin Oncol 9:132, 1990 (abstract).

Eisbruch A, Perez C, Roessler E, and Lockett M: Adjuvant irradiation after prostatectomy for carcinoma of the prostate with positive surgical margins, Cancer 73:384–387, 1994.

Fair W, Fuks Z, and Scher H: Cancer of the bladder. In DeVita V, Hellman S, and Rosenberg S, editors: Cancer: principles and practice of oncology, ed 4, Philadelphia, 1993, JB Lippincott Co, pp. 1052–1072.

Fischer D, Knobf M, and Durivage H: The cancer chemotherapy handbook, ed 4, St. Louis, 1993, Mosby.

Fleischmann J and Goldberg G: Management of superficial transitional cell carcinoma of the bladder, Semin Urol 11:193–204, 1993.

Fojo A, Shen D, Mickley L, Pastan I, and Gottesman M: Intrinsic drug resistance in kidney cancers is associated with expression of human multidrug resistance gene, J Clin Oncol 5:1922–1927, 1987.

Forman J: The role of radiation therapy in the management of carcinoma of the kidney, Semin Urol 7:195–198, 1989.

Fung C and Garnick M: Clinical stage I carcinoma of the testis: a review, J Clin Oncol 6:734–750, 1988.

Fung C, Kalish L, Brodsky G, Richie J, and Garnick M: Stage I nonseminomatous germ cell testicular tumor: prediction of metastatic potential by primary histopathology, J Clin Oncol 6:1467–1473, 1988.

Garnick M: The dilemmas of prostate cancer, Scient Am 272(4):77–81, 1994.

Gore M, Galligioni E, Keen C, Sorio R, Loriaux E, Grobben H, and Franks C: The treatment of metatastatic renal cell carcinoma by continuous infusion of recombinant interleukin-2, Eur J Canc 30A(3):327–333, 1994.

Gospodarowicz M and Warde P: The role of radiation therapy in the management of transitional cell carcinoma of the bladder. Hematol Oncol Clin No Am 6:147–168, 1993.

Green N, Bodner H, Broth E, Chiang C, Garrett J, Goldstein A, Goldberg H, Gualtieri V, Gray R, Jaffe J, Kaplan R, Polse S, Ross S, Skaist L, Treible D, Vatz A, and Wallack H: Improved control of bulky prostate carcinoma with sequential estrogen and radiation therapy, Int J Radiat Oncol Biol Phys 10:971–976, 1984.

Hanks G: Optimizing the radiation treatment and outcome of prostate cancer, Int J Radiat Oncol Biol Phys 11:1235–1245, 1985.

Hanks GE, Martz KL, and Diamond JJ: The effects of dose on local control of prostate cancer, Int J Radiat Oncol Biol Phys 15:1299–1305, 1988.

Hanks GE, Myers C, and Scardino P: Cancer of the prostate. In DeVita V, Hellman S, and Rosenberg S, editors: Cancer: principles and practice of oncology, ed 4, Philadelphia, 1993, JB Lippincott Co, pp. 1073–1113.

Hanks G, Porter A, Lepor H, and Grignon D: A phase III trial of the use of long-term total androgen suppression following neoadjuvant hormonal cytoreduction and radiotherapy in locally advanced carcinoma of the prostate, RTOG 92-02: A research protocol, Philadelphia, 1992, Radiation Therapy Oncology Group.

Held J, Osborne D, Volpe H, and Waldman A: Cancer of the prostate: treatment options and nursing implications, Oncol Nurs Forum 21:1517–1529, 1994.

Hirschfield-Bartek J: Combined modality therapy. In Dow KH and Hilderley LJ, editors: Nursing care in radiation oncology, Philadelphia, 1992, WB Saunders Co, pp. 251–263.

Horwich A, Dearnaley D, Duchesne G, Williams M, Brada M, and Peckham M: Simple nontoxic treatment of advanced metastatic seminoma with carboplatin, J Clin Oncol 7:1150–1156, 1989.

Hrushesky W, von Roemeling R, Lanning R, and Rabatin J: Circadian-shaped infusions of floxuridine for progressive metastatic renal cell carcinoma, J Clin Oncol 8:1504–1513, 1990.

Keller J, Sahasrabudhe D, and McCune C: Urologic and male genital cancers. In Rubin P, McDonald S, and Quzi R, editors: Clinical oncology: a multidisciplinary approach for physicians and students, ed 7, Philadelphia, 1993, WB Saunders Co, pp. 419–453.

Kish J, Neefe J, and Flannigan R: Efficacy of low-dose continuous infusion of 5-fluorouracil in recurrent metastatic renal cell carcimona: a Southwest Oncology Group (SWOG) study, Proc Am Assoc Cancer Res 32:186, 1991 (abstract).

Kjaer M, Iversen P, Hvidt V, Brunn E, Skaarup P, Hansen J, and Fredericksen P: A randomized trial of postoperative radiotherapy versus observation in stage II and III renal adenocarcinoma, Scand J Urol Nephrol 21:285–289, 1987.

Lauer R, Roth B, Loehrer P, Einhorn L, and Williams S: Cisplatin and ifosfamide and either VP-16 or vinblastine (VIP) as third-line therapy for metastatic testicular cancer, Proc Am Soc Clin Oncol 6:99, 1987 (abstract).

Lehmann O, Blanco J, Trodler C, Santos R, Batagelj E, Wilson C, Torres A, and Santana J: Adjuvant intravesical interferon-alpha-2b vs interferon-alpha-2b and mitomycin-C in superficial bladder cancer, Proc Am Soc Clin Oncol 12:252, 1993 (abstract).

Lind J and Nakao S: Urologic and male genital cancers. In Groenwald S, Frogge M, Goodman M, and Yarbro C, editors: Cancer nursing: principles and practice, ed 2, Boston, 1990, Jones & Bartlett, pp. 1026–1073.

Linehan W, Shipley W, and Parkinson D: Cancer of the kidney and ureter. In DeVita V, Hellman S, and Rosenberg S, editors: Cancer: principles and practice of oncology, ed 4, Philadelphia, 1993, JB Lippincott Co, pp. 1023–1051.

Lissoni P, Barni S, Ardizzoia A, Crispino S, Paolorossi F, Andres M, Scardino E, and Tancini G: Prognostic factors of the clinical response to subcutaneous immunotherapy with interleukin-2 alone in patients with metastatic renal cell carcinoma, Oncol 51:59–62, 1994.

Loehrer P: Testicular cancer. In Carbone P and Brain M, editors: Current therapies in hematology/oncology, ed 4, Ontario, 1991, BC Decker Inc.

Loehrer P, Birch R, Williams S, Greco F, and Einhorn L: Chemotherapy of metastatic seminoma: the Southeastern Cancer Study Group experience, J Clin Oncol 5:1212–1220, 1987.

Logothetis C, Johnson D, Chong C, Dexeus F, Sella A, Ogden S, Smith T, Swanson D, Babaran R, Wishnow K, and von Eschenbach A: Adjuvant cyclophosphamide, doxorubicin, and cisplatin chemotherapy for bladder cancer: an update, J Clin Oncol 6:1590–1596, 1988.

Miller R, Torti F, and Shipley W: Bladder. In John M, Flam M, Legha S, and Phillips T, editors: Chemoradiation: an integrated approach to cancer treatment, Philadelphia, 1993, Lea & Febiger, pp. 384–399.

Montie J: Lymphadenectomy for renal cell carcinoma, Semin Urol 7:181–185, 1989.

Montie J, Straffon R, and Stewart B: Radical cystectomy with and without radiation therapy for carcinoma of the bladder, J Urol 131:477–482, 1984.

Nichols C, Tricot G, Williams S, vanBesien K, Loehrer P, Roth B, Akard L, Hoffman R, Goulet R, Wolff S, Giannone L, Greer J, Einhorn L, and Jansen J: Dose-intensive chemotherapy in refractory germ cell cancer—a phase I/II trial of high-dose carboplatin and etoposide with autologous bone marrow transplantation, J Clin Oncol 7:932–939, 1989.

Patterson WP and Reams GP: Renal toxicities of chemotherapy, Sem Oncol 19:521–528, 1992.

Pilepich M, Krall J, Al-Sarraf M, Roach M, Doggett R, Sause W, Lawton C, Abrams R, Rotman M, Rubin P, Shipley W, and Cox J: A phase III trial of androgen suppression before and during radiation therapy for locally advanced prostate carcinoma: preliminary report of RTOG 86-10, Int J Radiat Oncol Biol Phys 16:813–817, 1993.

Ravaud A, Negrier S, Cany L, Merrouche Y, LeGuillou M, Blay J, Clavel M, Gaston R, Oskam R, and Philip T: Subcutaneous low-dose recombinant interleukin-2 and alpha-interferon in patients with metastatic renal cell carcinoma, Br J Cancer 69:1111–1114, 1994.

Richie J: Detection and treatment of testicular cancer, CA Cancer J Clin 43:151–175, 1993.

Rotman M and Aziz H: Bladder Cancer. In Lokich JJ and Byfield JF: Combined modality cancer therapy: radiation and infusional chemotherapy, Chicago, 1991, Precept Press, Inc, pp. 199–208.

Scardino P, Weaver R, and Hudson M: Early detection of prostate cancer, Hum Pathol 23:211–223, 1992.

Schmidt J, Gibbons R, Murphy G, and Bartolucci A: Adjuvant treatment for localized prostate cancer following radical prostatectomy or definitive irradiation, Proc Am Soc Clin Oncol 12:230, 1993 (abstract).

Schulof R, Lokich J, Wampler G, Schulz J, and Ahlgren J: Phase II trial of protracted infusional 5-FU for metastatic renal cell carcinoma, Proc Am Soc Clin Oncol 10:170, 1991 (abstract).

Sella A: Phase III randomized trial of post-nephrectomy 5-FU/interferon A vs no adjuvant therapy in patients with renal cell carcinoma at high risk of relapse, Cur Clin Tri Oncol 1:442–443, 1994.

Shipley W, Tester W, Donnelly B, and True L: A phase III trial to study the role of neoadjuvant MCV chemotherapy combined with transurethral surgery plus cisplatin with radiation therapy for the selective bladder preservation in patients with muscle-invading bladder cancer. RTOG 89-03. A research protocol, Philadelphia, 1990, Radiation Therapy Oncology Group.

Small E, Frye J, Wilkinson M, Carroll P, Ernest M, and Stagg R: A phase I/II study of alternating constant-rate infusion of floxuridine with constant-rate infusion of vinblastine for the treatment of metastatic renal cell carcinoma, Cancer 73:2803–2807, 1994.

Sokol G: The rationale of combined-modality treatment of cancer. In Sokol G and Maickel R, editors: Radiation drug interactions in the treatment of cancer, New York, 1980, John Wiley & Sons.

Taylor R: Endocrine therapy for advanced stage D prostate cancer, Urol Nurs 11:22–26, 1991.

Tester W, Porter A, Asbell S, Coughlin C, Heaney J, Krall J, Martz K, Venner P, and Hammond E: Combined modality program with possible organ preservation for invasive bladder carcinoma: results of RTOG protocol 85–12, Int J Radiat Oncol Biol Phys 25:783–790, 1993.

Thompson I, Paradelo J, Miller G, Messing E, Martenson J, Schirrella R, Goldberg S, Porter A, Scrigley J, and Bard R: A phase III study of the treatment of pathologic stage C carcinoma of the prostate with adjuvant radiation therapy. RTOG 90-19, INT 0086. A research protocol, Philadelphia, 1992, Radiation Therapy Oncology Group.

Wingo PA, Tong T, and Bolden S: Cancer statistics, 1995, CA Cancer J Clin 45:8–30, 1995.

Winter P, Miersch W, Vogel J, and Jaeger N: On the necessity of adrenal extirpation combined with radical nephrectomy, J Urol 144:842–843, 1990.

Wirth M: Immunotherapy for metastatic renal cell carcinoma, Urol Clin No Am 20:283–295, 1993.

Witjes J, Mulders P, and Debruyne F: Intravesical therapy for superficial bladder cancer, Urol 43(2 supp):2–6, 1994.

Wood D and Herr H: The evolving role of surgery in the management of renal cell carcinoma, Semin Urol 7:172–180, 1989.

Yagoda A: Chemotherapy of urothelial tract tumors, Cancer 60:547–585, 1987.

Yagoda A, Petrylak D, and Thompson S: Cytotoxic chemotherapy for advanced renal cell carcinoma, Urol Clin No Am 20:303–321, 1993.

Chapter 13

❖ *Gynecologic Cancers*

Aurelie C. Cormier

Successful management of patients with gynecologic cancer is possible when their diseases are diagnosed in early stages. However, some patients with early-stage disease are at high risk of relapse, and others are diagnosed in advanced stages, especially those with ovarian cancer. These patients present challenges to treatment. Multimodal approaches have been developed to achieve greater local control of tumors, to prevent distant relapse, and to induce remissions in those with advanced disease. Although much has been learned about the treatment of these malignancies, more research is needed.

❖ *Ovarian Cancer*

Although ovarian cancer accounts for only 4% of all cancers in women in the U.S., it is the fourth leading cause of deaths from cancer. In 1995, about 26,600 women were diagnosed with the disease, and about 14,500 died (Wingo, Tong, and Bolden, 1995). Statistics also show that ovarian cancer is one of the major causes of death from cancer in women in most developed countries (Eriksson and Walczak, 1990).

Treatment

For early-stage tumors of moderate to well-differentiated proportions, surgery is the definitive treatment (Young et al., 1990). Standard surgery includes a total abdominal hysterectomy (TAH), bilateral salpingoophorectomy (BSO), omentectomy, multiple biopsies of lymph nodes, cytologic testing of any ascitic fluid, and optimal debulking of tumor masses (Cannistra, 1993; Hoskins, Perez, and Young, 1993).

Surgery Followed by Adjuvant Chemotherapy
Because the majority of patients have advanced disease at the time of diagnosis, adjuvant chemotherapy has been a mainstay of treatment for ovarian cancer. The

surgeon first attempts to debulk the tumor to less than 1 cm to offer better chances of long-term survival (Friedlander and Dembo, 1991; Richardson et al., 1985). For patients with no residual disease, the 5-year survival rate ranges from 50% to 70%, and for those with tumors greater than 2 cm in diameter, from 0% to 30% (Fuks, Rizel, and Biran, 1988).

Although 5% to 10% of women with advanced disease can be cured with single-agent adjuvant chemotherapy, most women show greater improvement from combination chemotherapy regimens after surgery (Dembo, 1985). Regimens based on cisplatin or carboplatin combined with other agents appear to provide the most benefits. Cisplatin with cyclophosphamide appears to be as effective as many of the other cisplatin regimens but with less toxicity.

Studies have shown that six cycles of adjuvant chemotherapy are the optimum number of cycles to achieve a response without increasing toxic effects (Cannistra, 1993; Ozols, 1991). For optimal results, cisplatin should be given in doses of 100 mg/m^2 (Kaye et al., 1992). Increasing the dose of cisplatin above this level only adds neurotoxicity without improving the survival rate (Ozols et al., 1992). The optimum dose of other drugs used in combination chemotherapy regimens is yet to be determined (Kaye et al., 1992; Levin, Simon, and Hryniuk, 1993).

Carboplatin can be substituted for cisplatin (Alberts et al., 1992; Swenerton et al., 1992). Patients receiving cisplatin have more neurotoxicity, renal toxicity, nausea, and vomiting, whereas those who receive carboplatin have more severe thrombocytopenia (see the Research Highlight on page 212).

Although postoperative chemotherapy has proven very effective in reducing the size of ovarian tumors, cure rates for women with ovarian cancer have not changed over time. Therefore researchers are studying newer drugs and treatments. Paclitaxel-based regimens are among the most promising, although paclitaxel causes severe neutropenia, elevated temperature, and hair loss (McGuire et al., 1993).

Surgery Followed by Adjuvant Chemotherapy Followed by Second-Look Surgery
and Intraperitoneal Chemotherapy
For most women, ovarian cancer spreads within the peritoneal cavity. Current clinical trials are studying postoperative adjuvant intravenous chemotherapy followed by second-look surgery to assess response and to debulk the tumor before administering intraperitoneal (IP) chemotherapy (Ozols et al., 1992). The peritoneum, like the blood-brain barrier, lowers the diffusion of substances across its surface. Intraperitoneal chemotherapy directly exposes the tumor to the drug and potentially improves overall tumor response and patient survival (Carney-Gersten, Moore, and Guiffre, 1990). Cisplatin, etoposide, and mitoxantrone can be instilled intraperitoneally as single agents, together with IV chemotherapy, or as IP combinations (Cannistra, 1993; Ozols, 1991). They are usually left within the peritoneal cavity for 4 hours while the patient changes position about every 15 minutes to distribute the drug evenly throughout the peritoneum. Some patients, however, develop adhesions secondary to their surgery and therefore have uneven distribution of the chemotherapy within the peritoneal cavity. Patients selected for IP chemotherapy include those who had high-grade or residual tumors less than $\frac{1}{2}$ cm in diameter in the peritoneal cavity (DiSaia and Creasman, 1993; Walczak and

---

┌─ *RESEARCH HIGHLIGHT* ┤ ────────────────────────────────

Alberts D, Green S, Hannigan E, O'toole R, Stock-Novack D, Anderson P, Surwit E, Malvyla Y, Nahhas W, and Jolles C: Improved therapeutic index of carboplatin plus cyclophosphamide versus cisplatin plus cyclophosphamide: final report by the Southwest Oncology Group of a phase III randomized trial in stages III and IV ovarian cancer, J Clin Oncol 10:706–717, 1992.

Study Patients who had surgery but still had residual tumors greater than 2 cm were randomized to receive adjuvant cisplatin (100 mg/m²) with cyclophosphamide for six cycles or adjuvant carboplatin (300 mg/m²) with cyclophosphamide for six cycles.

Sample There were 342 patients with stage III or stage IV ovarian cancer enrolled through the Southwest Oncology Group.

Study aim To compare the response of patients following surgery for advanced stage ovarian cancer to adjuvant cisplatin and cyclophosphamide and to adjuvant carboplatin and cyclophosphamide.

Findings The pathological response rates were similar in both treatment arms. The median survival period for patients in the cisplatin group was 17.4 months and in the carboplatin group 20 months. The cisplatin group suffered greater side effects compared to the carboplatin group.

Discussion Grade 2, 3, or 4 toxicities were greater in the cisplatin group as compared to the carboplatin group for nausea and vomiting (92% vs 80%), anemia (49% vs 33%) alopecia (26% vs 8%), renal toxicity (16% vs 2%), anorexia (8% vs 4%), hearing loss (7% vs 0%), and tinnitus (7% vs 1%). The carboplatin group had greater incidences of thrombocytopenia when compared to cisplatin (45% vs 17%). There were two treatment-related deaths in each group. Response rates and survival rates appear equivalent, although the carboplatin group had much fewer treatment-related toxic effects.

Klemm, 1993). Some studies have shown that 30% of women with minimal peritoneal involvement can experience a complete response using sequential IV and IP therapy with cisplatin (Young, Perez, and Hoskins, 1993).

Surgery Followed by Adjuvant Chemotherapy Followed by Second-Look Surgery
Followed by High-Dose Chemotherapy and Autologous Bone Marrow Transplantation
For patients with recurrent or persistent disease, researchers are investigating treatment with autologous bone marrow transplantation (ABMT). Ovarian cancer responds to chemotherapy in proportion to the dose administered. Shpall et al. (1990) therefore hypothesized that high-dose chemotherapy would produce better long-term remissions and potential cures. In a phase I trial, 11 patients with ovarian cancer who had previously been treated with surgery and standard chemotherapy were given high doses of carboplatin and ABMT. The tumors of 64% of patients responded to the treatment. Doses of carboplatin reached 2000 mg/m², and the toxic effects included transient bone marrow and hepatic and renal toxicity. Six patients developed hearing impairments; one was permanent. Although the numbers

are low, the trial demonstrated the effectiveness of carboplatin and ABMT for treating ovarian cancer (Shea et al., 1989).

In another study, 14 patients with advanced ovarian cancer had surgery followed by adjuvant cisplatin-based chemotherapy followed by second-look surgery plus high-dose melphalan and ABMT. Thirty-six percent of patients had no evidence of disease 30 to 60 months after initiation of ABMT. Toxic side effects included bone marrow depression, nausea, vomiting, mucositis, cytomegalovirus meningitis, and pneumonia (Dauplat et al., 1989).

Twelve patients with advanced ovarian cancer underwent a regimen similar to the preceding study except that they received high-dose cyclophosphamide and thiotepa intravenously along with intraperitoneal cisplatin followed by ABMT. Six of these patients had residual tumors greater than 3 cm in diameter after the second-look laparotomy. Three quarters of these patients responded to this regimen. However, the same percentage died within 9 months of treatment. In addition, there was a 25% treatment-related mortality rate. Complications included bone marrow depression with fatal fungal sepsis, nephrotoxicity, and hepatotoxicity. High-dose chemotherapy with ABMT may be more beneficial when the tumor burden is low (Shpall et al., 1990).

Surgery Followed by Adjuvant Radiation Therapy
The combination of surgery and adjuvant radiation therapy is beneficial and potentially curative in a select group of patients. The radiation therapy may be external-beam radiation or intraperitoneal radioisotopes.

Several important points are worth mentioning in regard to the use of radiation therapy with ovarian cancer. First, the residual tumor should be less than 2 cm in diameter. The 5- and 10-year survival rates were vastly better for those who had no residual disease compared to those who had residual tumors greater than 2 cm. The 5-year survival rates were 76% and 18%, respectively; the 10-year survival rates were 76% and 7%, respectively (Dembo, 1985). Second, the nature of ovarian cancer requires whole abdominopelvic radiation therapy for the treatment to make a difference in survival rates.

Figure 13-1 shows the treatment field for whole abdominopelvic irradiation. The pelvis itself receives a total dose of 45 to 50 Gy; to avoid toxic damage to the major organs, the upper abdomen receives 25 to 28 Gy. The kidneys are partially shielded with lead so that they do not receive more than 18 to 20 Gy of radiation (Dembo and Thomas, 1994).

Due to a lack of randomized clinical trials, no definitive statement can be made as to whether adjuvant radiation therapy is better than cisplatin-based adjuvant chemotherapy (Ozols et al., 1992). The literature suggests that adjuvant radiation therapy may have higher morbidity than chemotherapy. Although early side effects are mild and well tolerated, late side effects include bowel obstruction, basal pneumonitis, liver disease, and chronic bloating and diarrhea. The incidence of late side effects ranges from 1.4% to 14% (Dembo and Thomas, 1994).

The radioisotope chromic phosphate, infused intraperitoneally, has been used in patients with early disease. Side effects of treatment with IP chromic phosphate include abdominal pain, chemical and infectious peritonitis, and bowel obstruction.

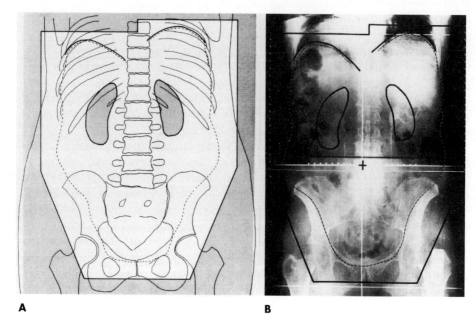

A   **B**

Fig. 13-1. Treatment field for whole abdominopelvic irradiation. **A,** Line drawing. **B,** Prone simulator radiograph example of whole abdominopelvic radiation field for ovarian cancer. Note the extension to the diaphragm and shielding of the kidneys. From Dembo A and Thomas G: The ovary. In Cox J, editor: Moss's radiation oncology: rationale, technique, results, ed 7, St. Louis, 1994, Mosby.

Surgery Followed by Adjuvant Chemotherapy with Radiation Therapy

One half of patients with ovarian cancer who have a good response to adjuvant cisplatin-based chemotherapy will later have a relapse. The prognosis for these patients is poor (Ozols et al., 1992). It has been hypothesized that the addition of radiation therapy to adjuvant chemotherapy enhances the patient's chances of survival. Complications include bowel obstruction, radiation enteritis, diarrhea, vomiting, bone marrow depression, and death (Fuks, Rizel, and Biran, 1988; Peters et al., 1986; Schray et al., 1988).

To reduce the morbidity associated with radiation therapy, Fein and associates split the daily dose in half and gave it twice a day (hyperfractionation). This reduced treatment-related complications compared to other studies using daily abdominopelvic radiation (Fein et al., 1994).

Other researchers found that patients tolerated the hyperfractionated treatment well; in one study 39% of 23 patients had no evidence of disease more than 1 year after radiation therapy (Kong et al., 1988).

Based on these studies, and because the toxic effects of treatment have an adverse effect on patients' quality of life, it is recommended that radiation therapy after adjuvant chemotherapy in the treatment of ovarian cancer be used in a select group of patients. Patients are selected who are disease-free at second-look laparotomy and who have a high histologic grade. A second group that may benefit are those with microscopic disease with low-grade histology at the time of second-look laparotomy (Dembo, 1985; Kong et al., 1988; Peters et al., 1986, Schray et al., 1988).

Chemoimmunotherapy or Radioimmunotherapy

Immunotherapy has been beneficial in the treatment of ovarian cancer when the tumor size is small and the biologic agent is given intraperitoneally (Hamilton, Ozols, and Longo, 1987; Walczak and Klemm, 1993). Several immunologic agents have been studied, including *Corynebacterium parvum* (*C. parvum*), *Bacillus Calmette-Guerin* (BCG), interferon (IFN), interleukin-2 (IL-2), lymphokine-activated killer cells (LAK), and monoclonal antibodies linked to drugs, toxins, or radioisotopes (Ozols et al., 1992).

Interferon may be one of the more promising biological agents in treating ovarian cancer. In some studies, when interferon was administered with chemotherapy, 50% of the women with small tumors had positive responses. Several researchers have reported that interferon enhances the effect of cisplatin, doxorubicin, vinblastine, and 5-fluorouracil (Boente, Berchuk, and Bast, 1992; Welander, 1987). In a phase II trial, interferon-α was administered intravenously and subcutaneously before a 2-hour intravenous infusion of doxorubicin. Of the 24 patients in the study, 29% had a complete or partial response from their tumors. Side effects were minimal, and the responses appeared better than those obtained when either agent was given alone (Welander, 1987). However, others have reported fatigue, anorexia, decreased weight, headaches, nausea, and vomiting as major side effects of IP interferon treatment (Carney-Gersten, Moore, and Guiffre, 1990).

Monoclonal antibodies have proven effective when linked to toxins and radioisotopes. Patients with persistent disease after chemotherapy and/or radiation therapy were given IP radioactive iodine monoclonal antibodies. Responses were inversely proportional to the size of the tumor, with the best responses seen in patients with tumors less than 2 cm. The initial response for patients with small tumors was 38%; however, only 16% of patients had no evidence of disease 3 years after treatment. Side effects included abdominal pain, fever, nausea, vomiting, diarrhea, peritonitis, and bone marrow depression (Epenetos et al., 1987). In another study, subjects received IP radioactive yttrium-90 monoclonal antibodies. Out of 14 patients, only 2 had a response. Side effects included abdominal pain, fever, and prolonged bone marrow depression due to absorption of the drug into the bone (Stewart et al., 1990).

Monoclonal antibodies have also been linked with *Ricin A* immunotoxin and *Pseudomonas* exotoxin. Further trials need to be designed to determine the potential benefits of this modality in treating ovarian cancer (Pai et al., 1991).

❖ Cervical Cancer

Ninety-five percent of cervical lesions begin at the squamocolumnar junction of the transformation zone (Mitchell, Sandella, and White, 1991). As the tumor grows, it can invade the entire cervix, paracervical or parametrial tissues, the vagina, the endometrium, the bladder, and the rectum.

Treatment

Cervical cancer, with its propensity to spread by direct extension, is treated mainly by surgery or radiation therapy alone. In treating early stages of disease, surgery or radiation therapy have equivalent results (DiSaia and Creasman, 1993; Hoskins, Perez, and Young, 1993; Thompson, 1990). For patients treated with radiation therapy, external-beam radiation is combined with intracavitary brachytherapy. In most patients with cervical cancer, external-beam radiation is limited to the pelvic area. In specific patients, the treatment area extends to the T10–T12 region of the spine to destroy any malignant cells in the para-aortic lymph nodes. Figure 13-2 shows the treatment area for patients receiving radiation to the pelvis and to the para-aortic lymph nodes. Intracavitary brachytherapy, usually administered after the external-beam treatment, can be delivered on an inpatient or outpatient basis (Dow, 1992). However, because of the effects to the vaginal mucosa, resulting in vaginal

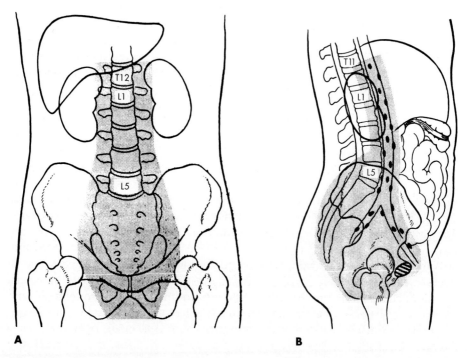

A **B**

Fig. 13-2. Example of extended-field radiation therapy for cervical cancer. **A,** Anterior and posterior portals. **B,** Lateral portals. Note that this field covers the para-aortic lymph nodes for patients determined to have lymph node involvement for those considered at high risk. From Russell A et al.: High-dose para-aortic lymph node irradiation for gynecologic cancer: technique, toxicity, and results, Int J Radiat Oncol Biol Phys 13:267–271, 1987.

stenosis, fibrosis, and dryness, radiation therapy is usually reserved for the elderly or for those who are medically compromised (Thompson, 1990).

In advanced disease, external-beam radiation combined with brachytherapy is the treatment of choice. If a woman has a malignancy that has involved the bowel or the bladder, radiation therapy can be given alone or pelvic exenteration can be performed (Million, Rutledge, and Fletcher, 1972; Perez et al., 1992). Depending on the area involved by the tumor, pelvic exenteration includes the removal of the pelvic organs plus the bladder (anterior pelvic exenteration) or the rectum (posterior pelvic exenteration) or both (total pelvic exenteration). It is done only if there is no evidence of metastasis or spread to the lymph nodes. Depending on the type of pelvic exenteration performed, patients may require an ileal conduit and/or colostomy. Vaginal reconstruction is an option for women.

Surgery Followed by Radiation Therapy
Hogan and colleagues (1982) reviewed the case histories of 50 patients who were at high risk of recurrence, some of whom were treated with radical hysterectomy followed by radiation therapy. The high-risk factors included involvement of the lymph nodes, surgical margins with residual malignancy, and spread of the tumor into the parametrial tissue. Of the 50 patients in the study, 24% developed complications from the combined-modality treatment: two incidences of cystitis, two of proctitis, one fistula, one bladder perforation, and one death due to renal failure as a result of radiation-induced ureteral stricture. There was a marginally significant difference in decreased local recurrence among those treated with adjuvant radiation; however, the rates of survival for both groups were equivalent. The lack of improvement in the survival rate for the group receiving radiation therapy may have been related to the presence of disease outside of the treatment field (Hogan et al., 1982).

Investigators also reviewed the cases of 38 patients after radical hysterectomy and adjuvant radiation therapy. At the time of hysterectomy these patients had lymph node involvement or positive (diseased) surgical margins. Most patients were treated with external-beam radiation, some patients received additional intracavitary brachytherapy, and a few received intracavitary brachytherapy alone. Of these patients, 15% developed small bowel obstruction or a fistula. Local recurrences were more likely to occur in those patients with disease in the paracervical area treated by brachytherapy alone. The researchers concluded that adjuvant radiation therapy administered after surgery can be used in high-risk patients, that patients with residual disease in the paracervical area require external-beam therapy and possibly additional intracavitary bracytherapy, and that those with residual disease in vaginal margins should receive external-beam therapy and possibly brachytherapy. However, although patients remain disease-free longer and the quality of their lives is improved, there is no difference in the rate of survival and the benefit of this multimodal therapy is not superior enough to consider it standard treatment (Hogan et al., 1982; Kim, Salter, and Shingleton, 1988).

Radiation Therapy Followed by Surgery
Preoperative radiation therapy has also been studied. This treatment regimen is usually reserved for patients who still have significant tumors after radiation therapy

alone or for patients with adenocarcinoma (Crook and Esche, 1994; Perez et al., 1992). Einhorn and colleagues analyzed the treatment results of 178 patients, the majority of whom received radiation therapy alone (external-beam radiation plus brachytherapy), and 74 of whom received radiation followed by surgery. Patients with early-stage cancer had a statistically significantly better 5-year survival outcome when treated by radiation followed by surgery (100%) compared to patients treated with radiation alone (81%). For those with advanced disease, there was no difference in outcomes between the two groups (Einhorn, Bygdeman, and Sjoberg, 1980). Current randomized trials are studying the results of adding hysterectomy to primary radiation therapy (Crook and Esche, 1994).

There have been higher complication rates with multimodal therapy, such as infection, deep-vein thrombosis, adhesions, and fistula formation. Complication rates range from 15% to 20% but may be reduced by giving moderate doses of brachytherapy, by using skilled surgical technique, and by disqualifying patients who have a history of pelvic inflammatory disease (Crook and Esche, 1994; Einhorn, Bygdeman, and Sjoberg, 1980; O'Quinn, Fletcher, and Wharton, 1980).

Intraoperative Radiation Therapy

Researchers have also studied intraoperative radiation therapy (IORT) to treat the tumor directly while minimizing the exposure of the surrounding area to radiation. Most patients receive external-beam radiation therapy and later, during a laparotomy, get a boost dose of IORT directly to the tumor. Although only a few nonrandomized studies have been done, this approach appears to offer some improvement in local control of the tumor. Complications have been minimal, although a few patients have experienced treatment-related side effects such as peripheral neuropathy, small-bowel obstruction, fistulas, ileus, and hemorrhage. So far, those who benefit the most from this multimodal treatment are patients with microscopic disease who receive IORT to a small treatment field (≤3 cm) (Delgado et al., 1984; Gunderson et al., 1982; Hicks et al., 1993).

Concomitant Chemoradiotherapy

Despite the excellent therapeutic effect that radiation and surgery have on cervical cancer, about one third of the women diagnosed with invasive cervical cancer will have a relapse of their disease within 2 years (Thompson, 1990). The main site where the disease recurs is the pelvis (Thomas et al., 1990). Clinical trials are focusing on enhancing the effects of radiation through concomitant chemoradiotherapy, neoadjuvant chemotherapy, and chemoimmunotherapy (Devine, Vokes, and Weichselbaum, 1991; John and Flam, 1993).

Concomitant chemoradiotherapy was developed to improve local control of the tumor. In some instances, the chemotherapy not only adds its effects to that of the radiation but enhances the tumor-killing effect of the radiation therapy by making the tumor more sensitive to radiation. Hydroxyurea, when given with radiation, increased the disease-free intervals for patients and their overall survival rates, whereas a placebo given with radiation did not (Stehman, 1992). The benefits of concomitant hydroxyurea and radiation therapy were also confirmed in a review of the literature by Maitra and Byfield (1991).

Smalley reported on the concomitant use of cisplatin with radiation. When the cisplatin was administered on a weekly basis, this regimen produced response rates that doubled those produced by radiation therapy alone (Smalley, 1990). Souhami, in a similar trial, found that the response rates were high (88%) but resulted in either rectal ulcers, rectovaginal fistulas, or small-bowel obstructions in 28% of patients (Souhami et al., 1993). Based on these studies, the Gynecologic Oncology Group currently has a study under way to compare the results of radiation therapy and hydroxyurea to the results of treatment with radiation therapy, cisplatin, and 5-fluorouracil (Grigsby, 1994).

Patients treated with a progressive schedule of pelvic radiation therapy and intracavitary brachytherapy concomitant with mitomycin-C and/or 5-fluorouracil had early complications, including mucositis, enteritis, neutropenia, and hemorrhage. Late complications were serious in 16% of patients and included fistula formation, hemorrhagic cystitis, gastrointestinal bleeding, bowel perforations, and three deaths. Mitomycin-C seemed to cause most of the bowel complications (Thomas et al., 1990). Researchers saw fewer complications in a similar study design that treated patients with cervical cancer with pelvic external-beam radiation, intracavitary brachytherapy, and concurrent mitomycin-C and cisplatin (Malviya et al., 1991).

Maruyama and colleagues studied 11 patients with advanced disease who received brachytherapy using radioactive californium-252 followed by concomitant chemoradiotherapy consisting of cisplatin and 5-FU during weeks 1, 4, and 10 of a 6-week course of external-beam radiation therapy. The external-beam radiation was given in a hyperfractionated method, twice a day. In 26 months of follow-up, there was 100% complete response. Treatments were well tolerated, although delayed complications included rectovaginal fistulas, proctitis, cystitis, and one treatment-related death. Survival outcomes are yet to be determined (Maruyama et al., 1994).

Neoadjuvant Chemotherapy Followed by Radiation Therapy and/or Surgery
Clinical trials with chemotherapy given by intraarterial infusion to the tumor bed before radiation therapy have not shown any survival benefit; however, patients had marked symptomatic relief of their pain, which improved their quality of life (John and Flam, 1993).

Panici and colleagues treated 75 women with neoadjuvant intravenous cisplatin, bleomycin, and methotrexate. Tumors in 62 patients (83%) responded, and these patients then were treated with radical hysterectomy with pelvic lymph node dissection and then additional chemotherapy or pelvic radiation therapy. Patients with cancers that did not respond to the neoadjuvant chemotherapy received radiation therapy only. Those responding to chemotherapy had better disease-free survival rates and overall survival rates (43% and 100%) compared to standard treatment (10% and 50%), and the response was inversely correlated to tumor size. Average follow-up time, however, was limited to 3 years (Panici et al., 1991). Similar results were obtained in a comparable study utilizing neoadjuvant intravenous bleomycin, vincristine, and cisplatin plus radiation therapy. Again, the response to chemotherapy was highly correlated to the response to radiation therapy (Kirsten et al., 1987).

In randomized clinical trials, neoadjuvant chemotherapy plus radiation therapy was compared to radiation therapy alone. Of four studies reported, three found no difference in survival rates between cisplatin-based chemotherapy plus radiation therapy and radiation therapy alone (Grigsby, 1994). One study using bleomycin, vincristine, cisplatin, and mitomycin-C found the chemotherapy arm to have higher mortality statistics directly related to treatment. Side effects included nausea, vomiting, diarrhea, photosensitivity, bone marrow depression, pulmonary toxicity, proctitis, cystitis, fistula formation, and vaginal stenosis (Souhami et al., 1991). Based on these data, investigation of the use of neoadjuvant chemotherapy continues.

Biotherapy and Radiation Therapy with or without Chemotherapy
More recently, the use of biological response modifiers has been tested against cervical cancer. In one study, 202 patients were randomized to receive external-beam radiation and brachytherapy plus a biological response modifier, LC9018, or to receive the same radiation therapy regimen alone. The patients who received LC9018 had increased disease-free intervals and 4-year survival rates compared to those who received radiation therapy alone (69.2% and 46.2%, respectively). Side effects of the biotherapy included fever, skin reaction at the injection site, and less-than-expected radiation-induced neutropenia (Okawa et al., 1993).

In another study, 26 patients with recurrent disease received intravenous concurrent cisplatin, 5-FU, and subcutaneous interferon over a 5-day period for four cycles. This regimen showed a modest benefit in that 34% of patients had a positive response to treatment; the duration of the response ranged from 3 to 34 months. Side effects included elevated temperature, headache, and malaise (de Leon et al., 1994). More clinical trials are needed for researchers to draw conclusions about the role of interferon in the treatment of cervical cancer.

❖ Endometrial Cancer

Mortality from endometrial (uterine) cancer, like cervical cancer, has decreased significantly in the last 50 years. The diagnosis of 75% to 80% of these tumors occurs during the menopausal and postmenopausal years when abnormal vaginal bleeding alerts the physician to the possibility of malignancy, and many of these tumors are therefore diagnosed in early stages (DiSaia and Creasman, 1993). Although endometrial cancer was diagnosed in approximately 32,800 women in 1995, the number of deaths was estimated to be proportionally low at 5,900 (Wingo, Tong, and Bolden, 1995).

Treatment

The primary treatment for endometrial cancer is a total abdominal hysterectomy (TAH) and a bilateral salpingoophorectomy (BSO). For patients with low-risk prognostic factors, no further treatment is required, although randomized clinical studies have been limited and there is a lack of general consensus on treatment. Multimodal therapy has seen limited use with this disease, partly because of the high number of cancers diagnosed in early stages of disease. It is vital to note, however, that patients with tumors diagnosed in later stages of endometrial cancer have mortality rates comparable to women with advanced-stage cervical cancer. Therefore, multimodal therapy may prove useful for treating advanced stages of endometrial cancer and needs to be studied within the context of randomized clinical trials (Hoskins, Perez, and Young, 1993; Maitra and Byfield, 1991).

Surgery Followed by Adjuvant Radiation Therapy

At present, primary surgery followed by adjuvant radiation therapy is the accepted sequence of multimodal therapy. Neoadjuvant radiation was often administered to patients in the past; however, based on current recommendations, surgery should precede radiation therapy except in certain situations (Creasman et al., 1987).

Patients found to benefit most from postoperative radiation therapy are those with prognostic indicators of metastatic spread or disease recurrence. High-risk factors include high-grade tumors, myometrial invasion, peritoneal involvement, cervical involvement, or the presence of disease in the pelvic or para-aortic lymph nodes (Eifel et al., 1983; Komaki, 1994).

Gibbons and colleagues treated 56 women with endometrial cancer at high risk of relapse with surgery plus adjuvant abdominopelvic radiation therapy. The 7-year disease-free survival rate varied by stage: stage I and stage II were 77%, stage III was 58%, and stage IV was 25%. Side effects included nausea, vomiting, diarrhea, bone marrow depression, chronic enteritis, and bowel obstruction (Gibbons et al., 1991). Radiation therapy has benefited patients by achieving better local control. Improvements in the rate of survival have yet to be determined (Park et al., 1992).

Stage II tumors with cervical involvement are uniquely different from other stages of endometrial cancer in that they usually require a radical hysterectomy rather than the standard total abdominal hysterectomy. A total abdominal hysterectomy includes excision of the uterus and the cervix, whereas a radical hysterectomy involves the same tissue plus the adnexa, paracervical and parametrial tissue, the upper part of the vagina, and the pelvic lymph nodes (Perez et al., 1985). These patients may receive external-beam pelvic radiation therapy, intravaginal brachytherapy, or both. The choice of treatment depends on the presence of disease in the lymph nodes, vaginal or parametrial involvement, extensive cervical involvement, or extensive myometrial invasion. Berman and Berek (1990) report that the addition of radiation to surgery in select groups of patients with higher risk-prognostic factors can decrease the chances of vaginal recurrence from 15% to 3%. The side effects of postoperative intravaginal brachytherapy include vaginal necrosis, cystitis, and fistula formation (Kucera, Vavara, and Weghaupt, 1990).

Patients with peritoneal involvement at high risk of relapse have been treated postoperatively with chromic phosphate administered intraperitoneally. In two separate studies of patients with peritoneal washings that tested positive for disease, IP chromic phosphate was found to increase the rate of disease-free survival. However, this therapy should not be combined with external-beam radiation therapy because it has been associated with a high risk of bowel complications such as chronic enteritis, fistula formation, short-bowel syndrome, and small-bowel obstruction (Heath et al., 1988; Soper et al., 1985). This method is not accepted as standard treatment (Hoskins, Perez, and Young, 1993).

Surgery Followed by Radiation Therapy Followed by Chemotherapy

Several randomized trials have looked at the addition of hormonal or cytotoxic chemotherapy to adjuvant radiation therapy in the treatment of endometrial cancer. Some researchers postulate that systemic therapy may reduce the incidence of distant metastases and increase overall survival. In a randomized trial by MacDonald and colleagues, 346 women who had received TAH and BSO plus pelvic irradiation with or without intravaginal brachytherapy were treated with provera or were given no further treatment. In 5 years of follow-up study, there was no significant difference in survival rates between the two treatments (MacDonald, Thorogood, and Mason, 1988).

In a clinical trial conducted by the Gynecologic Oncology Group, 181 patients who had a high risk of tumor recurrence were randomly selected after receiving postoperative adjuvant radiation therapy to receive doxorubicin every 3 weeks or to receive no further treatment. The overall 5-year survival rates for both groups were statistically equivalent (63% to 70%, respectively). In addition, chemotherapy did not appear to have a significant effect on distant metastases. The complications that arose were mainly due to toxic effects in the GI tract from the combination of surgery and radiation therapy. There were five treatment-related deaths, three in the doxorubicin arm and two in the no-further-treatment arm (Morrow et al., 1990). In patients with advanced or recurrent disease, progesterone, tamoxifen, and other chemotherapeutic agents palliate symptoms (Park et al., 1992).

❖ Nursing Management

Nursing care focuses on prevention and treatment of potential side effects. These commonly include bone marrow depression (which may result in hemorrhage or infection), nausea, vomiting, alopecia, diarrhea, weight loss, adhesions, bowel obstruction, fistula formation, delayed wound healing, and chronic enteritis. Side effects are discussed in detail in Unit III. Possible Side Effects from Multimodal Therapy in Gynecologic Cancers are listed on page 223. An example of nursing care for a patient receiving concomitant chemoradiotherapy is presented on page 226.

Sexual dysfunction and fertility are common concerns in this population. The vast majority of women will require a hysterectomy at the least, and a patient with ovarian cancer or a patient over 40 often will require a bilateral salpingoophorectomy as well. Issues of sexuality and reproduction will be discussed in detail in Chapter 24, Gonadal Toxicities.

A common nursing problem for patients with cervical and endometrial cancer undergoing combination surgery and radiation therapy or chemoradiotherapy is vaginal dryness, shortening, fibrosis, and stenosis, which can lead to altered sexual function and enjoyment (Jenkins, 1988). The incidence of vaginal alterations is sketchy, however, as Bruner and colleagues found in a search of the literature. They uncovered only 8 studies in the last 35 years related to vaginal changes secondary to treatment for cervical cancer and no studies of patients with endometrial cancer (Bruner et al., 1993). Patients report decreased sexual desire or frequency of intercourse and increased pain, dyspareunia, which can arise as a side effect of external-beam radiation or intracavitary brachytherapy in the pelvic area (Richards and Hiratzka, 1986). Yet this is not always the case. In fact, in one study some patients

Possible Side Effects from Multimodal Therapy in

Gynecologic Cancers

Multimodal Treatment	*Possible Enhanced Side Effects*

Ovarian Cancer

Surgery followed by adjuvant chemotherapy
  Carboplatin, cyclophosphamide
  Cyclophosphamide, cisplatin
  Carboplatin, ifosfamide, cisplatin
  Paclitaxel, cisplatin
  Paclitaxel, carboplatin

No enhanced side effects

Surgery followed by adjuvant abdominal/pelvic radiation therapy

Bowel obstruction, adhesions, fistula formation, diarrhea, basal pneumonitis, peritonitis

Surgery followed by adjuvant chemotherapy with abdominal/pelvic radiation therapy
  Doxorubicin, cyclophosphamide
  Cyclophosphamide, cisplatin, doxorubicin
  Altretamine, cisplatin, doxorubicin, cyclophosphamide
  Melphalan

Bowel obstruction, fistula formation, diarrhea, delayed wound healing, radiation enteritis, nephrotoxicity, cystitis

Surgery followed by adjuvant chemotherapy followed by second-look surgery followed by intraperitoneal chemotherapy
  Mitoxantrone (intraperitoneal)
  Cisplatin (intraperitoneal)
  Pacilitaxel (intravenous), cisplatin (intraperitoneal)
  Cyclophosphamide (intravenous), cisplatin (intraperitoneal)
  Cisplatin and etoposide (intraperitoneal)
  Systemic chemotherapy regimens as above

Bowel obstruction, adhesions

Surgery with adjuvant chemotherapy followed by second-look surgery followed by high-dose chemotherapy and autologous bone marrow transplantation
  Cisplatin-based regimen and high-dose carboplatin
  Doxorubicin, VM-26, 5-fluorouracil, cisplatin, cyclophosphamide, and high-dose melphalan
  Cisplatin-based regimen and high-dose thiotepa, cyclophosphamide, and cisplatin (intraperitoneal)

Nephrotoxicity, hepatotoxicity, bone marrow depression, diarrhea, nausea, and vomiting, delayed wound healing

Data taken from Bruner et al., 1993; Dauplat et al., 1989; Fuks, Rizel, and Bilan, 1988; Hogan et al., 1982; Jenkins, 1988; Kucera, Vavara, and Weghaupt, 1990; Peters et al., 1986; Schray et al., 1988; Stehman, 1992; Stewart et al., 1990; Thomas et al., 1990.

Continued

Multimodal Treatment	Possible Enhanced Side Effects

Chemobiotherapy
  Cisplatin-based regimen with monoclonal
    antibodies
	No enhanced side effects

Radiobiotherapy
  Radioactive-iodine-labeled monoclonal
    antibody
  Yttrium-90-labeled monoclonal antibody
	Abdominal pain, nausea, vomiting, diarrhea, peritonitis, bone marrow depression

Cervical Cancer Surgery followed by pelvic radiation therapy	Sexual dysfunction, diarrhea, fistula, small-bowel obstruction, ureteral stricture, cystitis, vaginal stricture, bladder perforation
Pelvic radiation therapy followed by surgery	Delayed wound healing, deep-vein thrombosis, adhesions, fistula formation, vaginal stricture
Intraoperative radiation therapy	Hemorrhage, infection, peripheral neuropathy, fistula formation, small bowel obstruction

Concomitant chemotherapy and pelvic radiation therapy
  Cisplatin
  5-Fluorouracil, mitomycin-C
	Hyperpigmentation, photosensitivity, vaginal stenosis, rectal ulcers, rectovaginal fistulas, small bowel obstruction, diarrhea, bone marrow depression, severe skin breakdown

5-Fluorouracil, cisplatin	Diarrhea, rectovaginal fistula, bone marrow depression, nephrotoxicity, rectal and vaginal mucositis
Mitomycin-C, cisplatin	Bone marrow depression, diarrhea, gastrointestinal bleeding, peripheral edema, bowel obstruction, photo-sensitivity to radiated field, vaginal stenosis, dry or moist desquamation

Neoadjuvent chemotherapy followed by radiation therapy and surgery
  Cisplatin and 5-fluorouracil
  Bleomycin, cisplatin, vincristine
  Bleomycin, vincristine, mitomycin-C,
    cisplatin
  Bleomycin, cisplatin, methotrexate
	Dry or moist desquamation, hyperpigmentation, diarrhea, fistula formation, bowel obstruction, photo-sensitivity, bone marrow depression, nausea, vomiting, pulmonary toxicity, vaginal stenosis, hemorrhagic cystitis

Biotherapy and radiation therapy with chemotherapy
  Cisplatin, 5-fluorouracil, interferon
  LC9018
	Malaise, headache, fever, skin reaction at injection site

Multimodal Treatment	Possible Enhanced Side Effects
Endometrial Cancer	
Surgery followed by adjuvant radiation therapy	
Intraperitoneal chromic phosphate	Diarrhea, fistula formation, bowel
Pelvic radiation therapy	obstruction, hemorrhagic cystitis,
Intravaginal radiation therapy	chronic enteritis, urethral stricture,
Intravaginal radiation therapy with pelvic	rectal ulcers. vaginal stenosis,
radiation therapy	sexual dysfunction
Surgery followed by radiation therapy followed by chemotherapy	Diarrhea, fistula formation, bowel obstruction, hemorrhagic cystitis,
Cyclophosphamide, doxorubicin, cisplatin	chronic enteritis, uretheral stricture, rectal ulcers, vaginal stenosis, sexual dysfunction
Hormonal agents: provera, depo-provera, megace	No enhanced side effects

reported an increased frequency of sexual activity after treatment (Bruner et al., 1993). Because of the high risk of side effects with these treatments, however, it is important for all patients, whether sexually active or not, to be instructed in the use of the vaginal dilator as outlined in the Patient Education Guidelines below.

Patient Education Guidelines for
Use of the Vaginal Dilator

♦ Start using the dilator 2 weeks after the last radiation-therapy treatment.

♦ Start with a small- or medium-size dilator and gradually increase the size. When the small size is easy to insert without discomfort, increase to the next largest size.

♦ Find a quiet, comfortable place to lie down undisturbed for 10 to 15 minutes. This may be in bed or in warm bath water.

♦ Apply a generous amount of a water-soluble lubricant to the rounded end of the dilator.

♦ Separate the labia and gently insert the dilator into the vagina as far as possible. Insert it to the point of pressure, never to the point of pain. Leave the dilator in place for 10 to 15 minutes. Turn the dilator in a circular motion or remove and reinsert it several times during this period.

♦ Use the dilator every day for 10 days, then every other day, gradually decreasing to 3 times a week. Those who are not sexually active need to continue on a maintenance schedule 3 times a week. Sexually active women may substitute the dilator for those times when intercourse does not occur.

Permission granted to reproduce these guidelines for educational purposes only.

Nursing Care of

The Patient Receiving Concomitant Cisplatin, 5-Fluorouracil, and Pelvic Radiation Therapy

Nursing Care	Rationale/Comments

◆ Assess hematological status
  ◆ Check CBC every week; check vital signs every week and as needed; monitor for signs and symptoms of infection or hemorrhage
  ◆ Collaborate with physician regarding blood transfusion as needed
  ◆ Teach patient and family about infection or hemorrhage precautions
	◆ Concomitant chemotherapy and radiation therapy puts patient at high risk of bone marrow depression; good perineal care will decrease risk of vaginal or rectal infection

◆ Assess GI and GU status
  ◆ Check mucous membranes, encourage mouth care every day
  ◆ Determine nutritional intake; dietary consultation as needed, weigh each week and notify physician if change in weight >10%
  ◆ Monitor for nausea and vomiting and collaborate with physician regarding prophylactic antiemetics
  ◆ Monitor for signs and symptoms of dehydration; encourage drinking 8–10 glasses of fluids/day unless contraindicated
  ◆ Assess for diarrhea; provide information on low-residue diet; collaborate with physician regarding antidiarrheal medication
  ◆ After completion of treatments, instruct on use of vaginal dilator
	◆ Chemotherapy and radiation therapy alter rapidly dividing tissue, including mucous membranes and the GI tract; patient is prone to weight loss, anorexia, nausea, vomiting, diarrhea, and dehydration. Measures to promote nutrition and fluid intake enhance tissue perfusion and healing of normal tissue. Pelvic irradiation increases risk of vaginal stenosis, and fibrosis; a dilator will maintain vaginal size for future pelvic exams, pap smears, and sexual activity

◆ Assess skin integrity
  ◆ Teach patients and families to check skin, especially skinfolds
  ◆ Provide written information on skin-care measures
  ◆ Inform patient of need to protect irradiated skin from sun
	◆ Skin is the first line of defense against infection; measures to maintain skin integrity will decrease risk of infection

◆ Assess renal status
  ◆ Check BUN/creatinine every week
  ◆ Monitor for changes in voiding
  ◆ Check urine for hematuria
	◆ Enhanced combined side effects are renal toxicity and hemorrhagic cystitis; monitoring BUN/creatinine, voiding, hematuria, and urine creatinine

Nursing Care	Rationale/Comments
◆ Assess renal status—*cont'd* ◆ Obtain 24-hour urine for creatinine clearance before cisplatin administration	clearance will help detect changes early, when preventive measures can be started

◆ Assess changes in self-image
  ◆ Determine patient's resources and social supports
  ◆ Encourage patien't to verbalize feelings
  ◆ Encourage strategies to enhance self-image (e.g., make-up, manicure, goal setting)
  ◆ Provide information on local and national resources and support groups
	◆ Diagnosis of gynecologic cancer, alopecia, side effects of chemotherapy, skin changes, and effects on sexual function, reproduction, and sexuality can have a major impact on self-image. Assessment of baseline self-image, available resources, social support, and future goals can help a patient make positive adjustment to these changes

◆ Assess and implement patient and family education
  ◆ Collaborate with other health care providers to ensure that patient education and care plan are consistent
  ◆ Provide schedule of treatment plan
  ◆ Anticipate side effects with strategies to prevent or alleviate them
  ◆ Teach symptoms to report
  ◆ Names and numbers to call for questions or to report symptoms
	◆ Knowledge of chemoradiotherapy schedule, anticipated side effects, and strategies to mitigate side effects can give patient and family a sense of control and prevent or minimize complications of treatment

❖ Summary

Multimodal therapy is increasingly being used in the treatment of gynecologic cancer to improve local control and to prevent distant relapse. Information gathered from multiple trials allows more individualization of treatment. The greatest benefit of these regimens is perhaps the improvement in disease-free survival rates; further trials will be needed to demonstrate any increase in overall survival rates. In addition, the benefits must be weighed against the enhanced combined side effects induced by these regimens. At present, perhaps the best hope for improved survival rates rests on better methods of early detection and prevention of these common female malignancies.

❖ References

Alberts D, Green S, Hannigan E, O'Toole R, Stock-Novack D, Anderson P, Surwit E, Malvyla V, Nahhas W, and Jolles C: Improved therapeutic index of carboplatin plus cyclophosphamide versus cisplatin plus cyclophosphamide: final report by the Southwest Oncology Group of a phase III randomized trial in stages III and IV ovarian cancer, J Clin Oncol 10:706–717, 1992.

Berman M and Berek J: Uterine corpus. In Haskell C, editor: Cancer treatment, ed 3, Philadelphia, 1990, WB Saunders Co, pp. 338–351.

Boente M, Berchuk A, and Bast R: Immunology of gynecologic cancers. In Hoskins W, Perez C, and Young R, editors: Principles and practice of gynecologic oncology, Philadelphia, 1992, JB Lippincott Co, pp. 117–135.

Bruner DW, Lanciano R, Keegan M, Corn B, Martin E, and Hanks G: Vaginal stenosis and sexual function following intracavitary radiation for the treatment of cervical and endometrial carcinoma, Int J Radiat Oncol Biol Phys 27:825–830, 1993.

Cannistra S: Cancer of the ovary, N Eng J Med 329:1550–1559, 1993.

Carney-Gersten P, Moore M, and Guiffre M: Intraperitoneal alpha interferon for ovarian cancer: a case report, Oncol Nurs Forum, 17:403–407, 1990.

Creasman W, Morrow CP, Bundy B, Homesley H, Graham J, and Heller P: Surgical pathologic spread patterns of endometrial cancer: a Gynecologic Oncology Group study, Cancer 60:2035–2041, 1987.

Crook J and Esche B: The uterine cervix. In Cox J, editor: Moss's radiation oncology rationale, technique, results, ed 7, St. Louis, 1994, Mosby, pp. 617–682.

Dauplat J, Legros M, Cindat P, Ferriere J, Ahmed S, and Plagne R: High-dose melphalan and autologous bone marrow support for treatment of ovarian carinoma with positive second-look operation, Gynecol Oncol 34:294–298, 1989.

de Leon CG, Kudelka A, Edwards C, Freedman R, Delclos L, and Kavanagh J: Combination therapy with 5-fluorouracil (5-FU), interferon alpha (IFN-α) and cisplatin (CDDP) for recurrent cervix cancer after radiation therapy, Pro Am Soc Clin Oncol 13:275, 1994 (abstract).

Delgado G, Goldson A, Ashayen E, Hill L, Petrilli E, and Hatch K: Intraoperative radiation in the treatment of advanced cervical cancer, Obstet Gynecol 63:246–252, 1984.

Dembo A: Abdominopelvic radiotherapy in ovarian cancer: a 10-year experience, Cancer 55:2285–2290, 1985.

Dembo A and Thomas G: The ovary. In Cox J, editor: Moss's radiation oncology rationale, technique, results, ed 7, St. Louis, 1994, Mosby, pp. 712–733.

Devine S, Vokes E, and Weichselbaum R: Chemotherapeutic and biologic radiation enhancement, Curr Opin Oncol 3:1090–1091, 1991.

DiSaia P and Creasman W: Clinical gynecologic oncology, ed 4, St. Louis, 1993, Mosby.

Dow KH: Principles of brachytherapy. In Dow KH and Hilderley L, editors: Nursing care in radiation oncology, Philadelphia, 1992, WB Saunders Co, pp. 16–29.

Eifel P, Ross J, Hendrickson M, Cox R, Kempson R, and Martinez A: Adenocarcinoma of the endometrium: analysis of 256 cases with disease limited to the uterine corpus: treatment comparisons, Cancer 52:1026–1031, 1983.

Einhorn N, Bygdeman M, and Sjoberg B: Combined radiation and surgical treatment for carcinoma of the uterine cervix, Cancer 4:720–723, 1980.

Epenetos A, Munro A, Stewart S, Ranpling R, Lambert H, McKenzie C, Soutter P, Rahmtulla A, Hooker G, Sivolapenko G, Snook D, Courtenay-Luck N, Dhokia B, Krausz T, Taylor-Papadimitriou J, Durbin H, and Bodmer W: Antibody-guided irradiation of advanced ovarian cancer with intraperitoneally administered radiolabelled monoclonal antibodies, J Clin Oncol 5:1890–1899, 1987.

Eriksson J and Walczak J: Ovarian cancer, Semin Oncol Nurs 6:214–227, 1990.

Fein D, Morgan L, Marcus R, Mendenhall W, Sombeck M, Freeman D, and Million R: Stage III ovarian carcinoma: an analysis of treatment results and complications following hyperfractionated abdominopelvic irradiation for salvage, Int J Radiat Oncol Biol Phys 29:169–176, 1994.

Friedlander M and Dembo A: Prognostic factors in ovarian cancer, Semin Oncol 18:205–212, 1991.

Fuks Z, Rizel S, and Biran S: Chemotherapeutic and surgical induction of pathological complete remission and whole abdominal irradiation for consolidation does not enhance the cure of stage III ovarian carcinoma, J Clin Oncol 6:509–516, 1988.

Gibbons S, Martinez A, Schray M, Podratz K, Stanhope R, Garton G, Weiner S, Brabbins D, and Malkasian G: Adjuvant whole abdominopelvic irradiation for high-risk endometrial carcinoma, Int J Radiat Oncol Biol Phys 21:1019–1025, 1991.

Grigsby P: Lack of proven efficacy of chemotherapy for patients with carcinoma of the uterine cervix, Semin Rad Oncol 4:30–33, 1994.

Gunderson L, Shipley W, Suit H, Epp E, Nardi G, Wood W, Cohen A, Nelson J, Battit G, Biggs P, Russell A, Rockett A, and Clark D: Intraoperative irradiation: a pilot study combining external-beam photons with "boost" dose intraoperative electrons, Cancer 49:2259–2266, 1982.

Hamilton T, Ozols R, and Longo D: Biologic therapy for the treatment of malignant common epithelial tumors of the ovary, Cancer 60:2054–2063, 1987.

Heath R, Rosenman J, Varia M, and Walton L: Peritoneal fluid cytology in endometrial cancer: its significance and the role of chromic phosphate (32P) therapy, Int J Radiat Oncol Biol Phys 15:815–822, 1988.

Hicks M, Piver S, Mas E, Hempling R, McAuley M, and Walsh D: Intraoperative orthovoltage radiation therapy in the treatment of recurrent gynecologic malignancies, Am J Clin Onc 16:497–500, 1993.

Hogan W, Littman P, Griner L, Miller C, and Mikuta J: Results of radiation therapy given after radical hysterectomy, Cancer 49:1278–1285, 1982.

Hoskins W, Perez C, Young R: Gynecologic tumors. In DeVita V, Hellman S, and Rosenberg S, editors: Cancer: principles and practice of oncology, ed 4, Philadelphia, 1993, JB Lippincott Co, pp. 1152–1225.

Jenkins B: Patients' reports of sexual changes after treatment for gynecological cancer, Oncol Nurs Forum 15:349–354, 1988.

John M and Flam M: Gynecologic system. In John M, Flam M, Legha S, and Phillips T, editors: Chemoradiation: an integrated approach to cancer treatment, Philadelphia, 1993, Lea & Febiger, pp. 374–383.

Kaye S, Lewis C, Paul J, Duncan I, Gordon H, Kitchener H, Cruickshank D, Atkinson R, Soukop M, Rankin E, Cassidy J, Davis J, Reed N, Crawford S, MacLean A, Swapp G, Sarkar T, Kennedy J, and Symonds R: Randomised study of two doses of cisplatin with cyclophosphamide in epithelial ovarian cancer, Lancet 340:329–333, 1992.

Kim R, Salter M, and Shingleton H: Adjuvant postoperative radiation therapy following radical hysterectomy in stage IB cancer of the cervix—analysis of treatment failure, Int J Radiat Oncol Biol Phys 14:445–449, 1988.

Kirsten F, Atkinson K, Coppleson J, Elliot P, Green D, Houghton R, Murray J, Russell P, Solomon H, Friedlander M, Swanson C, and Tattersall M: Combination chemotherapy followed by surgery or radiotherapy in patients with locally advanced cervical cancer, Br J Obstet Gynaecol 94:583–588, 1987.

Komaki R: The endometrium, the vagina, the vulva, and the female urethra. In Cox J, editor: Moss's radiation oncology rationale, technique, results, ed 7, St. Louis, 1994, Mosby, pp. 683–711.

Kong J, Peters L, Wharton JT, Ang KK, Delclos L, Gershenson D, Copeland L, Edwards C, Freedman R, Saul P, and Stringer C: Hyperfractionated split-course whole abdominal radiotherapy for ovarian carcinoma: tolerance and toxicity, Int J Radiat Oncol Biol Phys 14:737–743, 1988.

Kucera H, Vavara N, and Weghaupt K: Benefit of external irradiation in pathologic stage I endometrial carcinoma: a prospective clinical trial of 605 patients who received postoperative vaginal irradiation and additional pelvic irradiation in the presence of unfavorable prognostic factors, Gynecol Oncol 38:99–104, 1990.

Levin L, Simon R, and Hryniuk W: Importance of multiagent chemotherapy regimens in ovarian carcinoma: dose intensity analysis, J Nat Canc Inst 85:1732–1742, 1993.

MacDonald R, Thorogood J, and Mason M: A randomized trial of progestogens in the primary treatment of endometrial carcinoma, Br J Obstet Gynaecol 95:166–174, 1988.

Maitra A and Byfield J: Gynecologic cancer. In Lokich J and Byfield J: Combined modality cancer therapy: radiation and infusional chemotherapy. Chicago, 1991, Precept Press, Inc., pp. 209–214.

Malviya V, Han I, Deppe G, Malone J, Christensen C, Kim Y, and Ahmad K: High-dose-rate afterloading brachytherapy, external radiation therapy, and combination chemotherapy in poor-prognosis cancer of the cervix, Gynecol Oncol 42:233–238, 1991.

Maruyama Y, Bowen M, Vannagell J, Gallion H, DePriest P, and Wierzbicki J: A feasibility study of 252 Cf neutron brachytherapy, cisplatin, and 5-FU chemo-adjuvant and accelerated hyperfractionated radiotherapy for advanced cervical cancer, Int J Radiat Oncol Biol Phys 29:529–534, 1994.

McGuire W, Hoskins W, Brady M, Kucera P, Look K, Partridge E, and Davidson M: A phase III trial comparing cisplatin/cytoxan (PC) and cisplatin/taxol (PT) in advanced ovarian cancer, Proc Ann Meet Am Soc Clin Oncol 12, 1993 (abstract).

Million R, Rutledge F, and Fletcher G: Stage IV carcinoma of the cervix with bladder invasion, Am J Obstet Gynecol 113:239–246, 1972.

Mitchell M, Sandella J, and White L: Cervical cancer: the role of the human papillomavirus, Curr Iss in Ca Nurs Prac Updates 1:1–9, 1991.

Morrow CP, Bundy B, Homelsey H, Creasman W, Hornback N, Kurman R, and Thigpen JT: Doxorubicin as an adjunct following surgery and radiation therapy in patients with high-risk endometrial carcinoma, stage I and occult stage II: a Gynecologic Oncology Group study, Gynecol Oncol, 36:166–171, 1990.

Okawa T, Niibe H, Arai T, Sekiba K, Noda K, Takeuchi S, Hashimoto S, and Ogawa N: Effect of LC9018 combined with radiation therapy on carcinoma of the uterine cervix, Cancer 72:1949–1954, 1993.

O'Quinn A, Fletcher G, and Wharton JT: Guidelines for conservative hysterectomy after irradiation, Gynecol Oncol 9:68–79, 1980.

Ozols R: The current status of the treatment of ovarian cancer, Mediguide to Oncol 11(1):1–10, 1991.

Ozols R, Rubin S, Dembo A, and Robboy S: Epithelial ovarian cancers. In Hoskins W, Perez C, and Young R, editors: Principles and practice of gynecologic oncology, Philadelphia, 1992, JB Lippincott Co, pp. 731–781.

Pai L, Bookman M, Ozols R, Young R, Smith J, Longo D, Gould B, Frankel A, McClay E, Howell S, Reed E, Willingham M, Fitzgerald D, and Pastan I: Clinical evaluation of intraperitoneal *Pseudomonas* exotoxin immunoconjugate OVB3-PE in patients with ovarian cancer, J Clin Oncol 9:2095–2103, 1991.

Panici P, Scambia G, Baiocchi G, Greggi S, Ragusa G, Gallo A, Conte M, Battaglia F, Laurelli G, Rabitti C, Capelli A, and Mancuso S: Neoadjuvant chemotherapy and radical surgery in locally advanced cervical cancer, Cancer 67:372–379, 1991.

Park R, Gringsby P, Muss H, and Norris H: Corpus: epithelial tumors. In Hoskins W, Perez C, and Young R, editors: Principles and practice of gynecologic oncology, Philadelphia, 1992, JB Lippincott Co, pp. 663–693.

Perez C, Knapp R, DiSaia P, and Young R: Gynecologic tumors. In DeVita V, Hellman S, and Rosenberg S, editors: Cancer: principles and practice of oncology, ed 2, Philadelphia, 1985, JB Lippincott Co, pp. 1013–1081.

Perez C, Kurman R, Stehman F, and Thigpen J: Uterine cervix. In Hoskins W, Perez C, and Young R, editors: Principles and practice of gynecologic oncology, Philadelphia, 1992, JB Lippincott Co, pp. 591–662.

Peters W, Blasko J, Bagley C, Rudolph R, Smith M, and Rivkin S: Salvage therapy with whole-abdominal irradiation in patients with advanced carcinoma of the ovary previously treated by combination chemotherapy, Cancer 58:880–882, 1986.

Richards S and Hiratzka S: Vaginal dilation post pelvic irradiation: a patient education tool, Oncol Nurs Forum 13(4):89–91, 1986.

Richardson G, Scully R, Nikrui N, and Nelson J: Common epithelial cancer of the ovary: first of two parts. N Eng J Med 312:415–424, 1985.

Schray M, Martinez A, Howes A, Podratz K, Ballon S, Malkasian G, and Sikic B: Advanced epithelial ovarian cancer: salvage whole abdominal irradiation for patients with recurrent or persistent disease after combination chemotherapy, J Clin Oncol 6:1433–1439, 1988.

Shea I, Flaherty M, Elias A, Eder J, Antman K, Begg C, Schnipper L, Hei E, and Henner W: A phase I clinical and pharmacokinetic study of carboplatin and autologous bone marrow support, J Clin Oncol 7:651–661, 1989.

Shpall E, Clarke-Pearson D, Soper J, Berchuck A, Jones R, Bast R, Ross M, Lidor Y, Vanacek K, Taylor T, and Peters W: High-dose alkylating agent chemotherapy with autologous bone marrow support in patients with stage III/IV epithelial ovarian cancer, Gynecol Oncol 38:386–391, 1990.

Smalley R: Systemic treatment of squamous cell carcinoma of the cervix, Mediguide to Oncol 10:1–5, 1990.

Soper J, Creasman W, Clarke-Pearson D, Sullivan D, Vergadoro F, and Johnson W: Intraperitoneal chromic phosphate P32 suspension therapy of malignant peritoneal cytology in endometrial carcinoma, Am J Obstet Gynecol 153:191–196, 1985.

Souhami L, Gil R, Allan S, Canary P, Araujo C, Pinto L, and Silveira T: A randomized trial of chemotherapy followed by pelvic radiation therapy in stage IIIB carcinoma of the cervix, J Clin Oncol 9:970–977, 1991.

Souhami L, Seymour R, Roman T, Stanimir G, Trudeau M, Clark B, and Freeman C: Weekly cisplatin plus external-beam radiotherapy and high-dose-rate brachytherapy in patients with locally advanced carcinoma of the cervix, Int J Radiat Oncol Biol Phys 27:871–878, 1993.

Stehman F: Concurrent chemoradiation in carcinoma of the uterine cervix, Sem Oncol 19(suppl 11):88–91, 1992.

Stewart J, Hird V, Snook D, Dhokia B, Sivolapenko G, Hooker G, Papadimitriou JT, Rowlinson G, Sullivan M, Lambert H, Coulter C, Mason W, Soutter W, and Epenetos A: Intraperitoneal yttrium-90-labeled monoclonal antibody in ovarian cancer, J Clin Oncol 8:1941–1950, 1990.

Swenerton K, Jeffrey J, Stuart G, Roy M, Krepart G, Carmichael J, Drouin P, Stanimir R, O'Connell G, MacLean G, Kirk M, Canetta R, Koski B, Shelley W, Zee B, and Pater J: Cisplatin-cyclophosphamide versus carboplatin-cyclophosphamide in advanced ovarian cancer: a randomized phase III study of the National Cancer Institute of Canada clinical trials group, J Clin Oncol 10:718–726, 1992.

Thomas G, Dembo A, Fyles A, Gadalla T, Beale F, Bean H, Pringle J, Rawlings G, Bush R, and Black B: Concurrent chemoradiation in advanced cervical cancer, Gynecol Oncol 38:446–451, 1990.

Thompson L: Cancer of the cervix, Semin Oncol Nurs 6:190–197, 1990.

Walczak J and Klemm P: Gynecologic cancers. In Groenwald S, Frogge M, Goodman M, and Yarbro C, editors: Cancer nursing: principles and practice, ed 3, Boston, 1993, Jones & Bartlett, pp. 1065–1113.

Welander C: Use of interferon in the treatment of ovarian cancer as a single agent and in combination with cytotoxic drugs, Cancer 59:617–619, 1987.

Wingo P, Tong T, and Bolden S: Cancer statistics, 1995, CA Cancer J Clin 45:8–30, 1995.

Young R, Perez C, and Hoskins W: Cancer of the ovary. In DeVita V, Hellman S, and Rosenberg S, editors: Cancer: principles and practice of oncology, ed 4, Philadelphia, 1993, JB Lippincott Co, pp. 1226–1263.

Young R, Walton L, Ellenberg S, Homesley H, Wilbanks G, Decker D, Miller A, Park R, and Major F: Adjuvant therapy in stage I and stage II epithelial ovarian cancer: results of two prospective randomized trials, N Eng J Med 332:1021–1027, 1990.

Chapter 14

❖ *Head and*
Neck Cancers

Karen H. Baker
Jane E. Feldman

Head and neck cancers account for 5% of cancers diagnosed annually (Schleper, 1989) and approximately 140,000 deaths each year (Schottenfeld, 1992).

The upper aerodigestive tract is a complex system involved in the processes of oxygenation, nourishment, smell, taste, vision, hearing, and balance. In addition to physiologic considerations, patients with head and neck cancers face sociocultural concerns such as appearance.

The diagnosis is devastating for the patient and the family, and the outcome is often poor. This poor outcome may result from advanced disease at the time of diagnosis, older age, poor nutrition, associated medical problems, or additional new cancers within the upper aerodigestive tract. Many patients also do not seek medical attention until the tumor has spread to the lymph nodes or surrounding tissue and impairment and loss of function have progressed. Some areas of the head and neck allow enough space for a tumor to grow considerably in size before symptoms occur. In addition, symptoms such as sore throat, nasal congestion, ear pain, hoarseness, and coughing may mimic other more common head and neck problems, which may be treated without the diagnostician fully recognizing the true source of the problem. This is unfortunate because diagnosis and treatment of small lesions often have positive results and acceptable cure rates.

Tumors of the head and neck are multiple lesions generally associated with second primary cancers. The majority of these lesions occur at sites in the upper aerodigestive tract or the lungs where the cells have previously been exposed to similar environmental and behavioral risk factors. Nearly 10% of patients diagnosed with malignancies of the upper aerodigestive tract have a second, synchronous primary cancer at the time of diagnosis (Baker and Feldman, 1987).

❖ *Primary Sites*

There are many different primary sites in the head and neck—the lip and oral cavity, the pharynx (oropharynx, nasopharynx, hypopharynx), the larynx, the nasal cavity and nasal sinuses, the salivary glands, and the thyroid—each site having its own particular pattern of spread (Myers and LaSalle, 1991). Cancers of the head and neck are separate diseases based on distinct anatomic sites and lymphatic drainage.

Lip and Oral Cavity

The oral cavity extends from the vermillion border of the lips to the junction of the soft palate and the hard palate. The oropharynx is separated from the oral cavity by the tonsillar pillar, the soft palate, and the base of the tongue.

Early-stage lesions are often asymptomatic red lesions, called *erythroplakia,* or white lesions, called *leukoplakia.* All too often, the patient comes for treatment with an advanced lesion with extensive invasion of the skin, muscle, and the mandible or other adjacent structures.

Pharynx

The pharynx is divided into three areas: the oropharynx (below the soft palate and above the epiglottis), the nasopharynx (continuous with the nasal passages), and the hypopharynx (in the lower, laryngeal part of the pharynx). Each area may develop different characteristic symptoms.

Oropharynx

Many patients complain of a neck mass that "came up suddenly." The patient may have a history of vague symptoms such as sore throat, feeling of a lump in the throat, difficulty swallowing, or change in voice quality. Patients with advanced lesions may have a "hot potato" voice, ear pain, and malodorous breath that smells like necrotic tissue.

Nasopharynx

These patients usually complain of a painless neck mass and may also complain of nasal obstruction, bleeding, tinnitus, or otitis media caused by an obstructed eustachian tube.

Hypopharynx

The disease frequently progresses to advanced stages before diagnosis because of the "silent" nature of the hypopharynx. Patients may complain of enlarged neck nodes, unilateral sore throat, dysphagia, the sensation of something stuck in the throat that they can often point to, ear pain, bloody sputum, and weight loss. Up to 80% of patients have nodal metastasis at the time of diagnosis. The survival rate of patients with advanced disease is poor; the 5-year survival rate is only about 20% (Feldman and Baker, 1988).

Larynx

The larynx is composed of bone and cartilage joined by a complex of ligaments. The presenting symptoms are most often hoarseness, sore throat, ear pain, difficulty swallowing, and, in advanced cases, dyspnea and a significant weight loss.

Nasal Cavity and Paranasal Sinuses

Cancers of the nasal cavity and nasal sinuses are rare. Early-lesions may be superficial and ulcerative. Perineural spread is not uncommon. The patient may complain of numbness of the teeth or palate, the sensation of fullness, proptosis, visual changes, trismus, headache, nasal discharge, or bleeding.

Salivary Gland

The major salivary glands include the parotid, the submandibular, and the sublingual glands. The majority of salivary gland tumors occur in the parotid gland. Presenting symptoms will most often include a painless mass in front of or just below the jaw. There may be some discomfort associated with the mass, and patients with advanced disease may have weakness in the facial muscles or paralysis.

Thyroid

The thyroid gland is located between the sternocleidomastoid muscles adjacent to the trachea. Thyroid cancer comprises about 1% of all cancers. Patients are often diagnosed after an incidental finding of a painless thyroid mass. Only a small number of patients will have dysphagia, hoarseness, or airway obstruction; however, these are common findings in patients with more advanced disease (Baker and Feldman, 1993).

❖ Treatment

In treating cancers of the head and neck, there are three major goals. The first is to eradicate disease. The second, to minimize the loss of major functional categories —speech, involving the tongue and the larynx; respiration, involving the larnyx and the trachea; mastication-deglutition, involving the mandible, the teeth, the tongue, saliva, the palate, and the pharynx; and the special senses, including vision, hearing, taste, smell, and equilibrium. The third goal is to reach an acceptable cosmetic result (Baker and Feldman, 1987).

In general, early-stage lesions are treated equally well by surgery or by radiation. Often the treatment with the fewest side effects is chosen when the cure rates of two or more treatments are equal. For example, surgery is frequently chosen over radiation therapy in the treatment of tongue lesions to avoid radiation-induced xerostomia. For early-stage vocal cord lesions, radiation therapy is the standard of care because the voice is better preserved.

Oncologists often treat advanced disease with a combination approach that aims to improve local-regional control, to preserve organ function, and to reduce distant metastasis (Dimery and Hong, 1993). For many patients, the decision to use a second modality may be delayed until after the initial treatment has been administered and evaluated.

Quite often, surgery and radiation therapy are complementary—surgery for gross disease and radiation therapy for microscopic disease (Baker and Feldman, 1987). Although the immediate results of this treatment are often encouraging, survival is poor for patients with diagnosed advanced disease.

High-risk cancers necessitate radical treatments. Life-style issues and concerns contribute to the treatment decision. For example, the cost of each treatment, the location of the treatment facilities, family and work responsibilities, and the necessity of maintaining a rigorous schedule over several weeks versus one-time therapy may guide the patient to one particular option. Patients with medical problems severe enough to make anesthesia a considerable risk or with concomitant medical conditions are probably not candidates for surgery unless no other options are available. While high-grade tumors respond to radiation therapy, they also metastasize at an increased rate (Million and Cassisi, 1994a). The less differentiated tumors are infiltrative and have a higher incidence of lymph node involvement (Million and Cassisi, 1994a). (Grade and differentiation are discussed in Chapter 1.) Surgery and radiation therapy have equal rates of control (Million and Cassisi, 1994a). There is no difference between the two regarding the risk of a second malignancy developing or of neck disease and distant metastasis appearing later (more than 5 years) (Million and Cassisi, 1994a). One notable difference is that surgical complications occur shortly after the procedure, whereas some complications of radiation therapy can be delayed for an extended period (Million and Cassisi, 1994a).

Radiation Therapy

Radiation therapy may be curative or palliative. It is most often administered over several weeks in divided doses of approximately 2 Gy daily, 5 days each week, until a total of 60 to 70 Gy is reached. Hyperfractionation radiation, given in doses of approximately 1.8 Gy, twice or even more each day, spares healthy tissue in the treatment area and reduces the risk of tissue injury, often permitting higher total doses to be given (Cox et al., 1992).

Interstitial radiation therapy can be used alone or in combination with other modalities. A radioactive source (often iridium-192 or cesium-137) is implanted in narrow catheters directly into the tumor or very near the tumor bed (Figure 14-1). Early-stage oral tumors such as cancer of the lip, the floor of the mouth, and the anterior tongue respond to large doses delivered this way. Usually implants are temporary, but permanent seeds with low levels of radioactivity may be implanted into positive margins, nodes in the neck, or the base of the skull (Strohl, 1989).

To preserve the larynx and to maintain the patient's speech function, early-stage vocal cord cancer is often treated first with radiation rather than other therapies (Strohl, 1989). This is because surgery is more likely to save a patient who has undergone unsuccessful radiation therapy than radiation therapy is to salvage a surgical failure. Radiation therapy can also treat multiple lesions, predicted regional disease, and lymphatic drainage sites by encompassing them in the treatment field. Figure 14-2 indicates the typical radiation field for treatment of a cancer of the oral cavity.

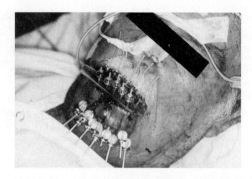

Fig. 14-1. Interstitial implant (brachytherapy) for squamous cell cancer of the lip.

Hyperthermia is a technique to enhance the effects of radiation therapy. Raising the temperature increases the circulatory rate and brings more oxygen to the area, increasing the radiosensitivity of the cells. Ultra-high-frequency tools such as microwave or ultrasound machines can heat tumors to a depth of 4 cm. When used with external-beam radiation therapy, hyperthermia has an additive effect (Busse and Bader, 1992; Strohl, 1989).

Surgery

The role of conventional surgery in the treatment of head and neck cancers is well described (Dimery and Hong, 1993; Million and Cassisi, 1994a, b, c, d). The cure rate is high for early-stage disease. Surgery is used if the cosmetic and functional results are acceptable, if the cancer has invaded bone or cartilage, or if the complications of radiation therapy are predicted to be severe.

Surgery often necessitates a resection with wide margins. The extent of resection may be based on numerous considerations such as the extent of disease, the likelihood of a cure, and the probability of rehabilitating the patient. Patients with diseased lymph nodes of the neck or suspected subclinical disease may require a neck dissection, as outlined in Table 14-1.

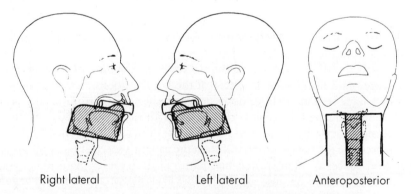

| Right lateral | Left lateral | Anteroposterior |

Fig. 14-2. Schematic representation of anatomic sites included in radiation fields used for extensive tumors in the lower aspect of the oral cavity. For small, well-differentiated tumors the field treating the low anterior part of the neck can be omitted in the absence of palpable disease. From Cooper JS: Carcinomas of the oral cavity and oropharynx. In Cox J, editor: Moss's radiation oncology: rationale, technique, results, ed 7, St. Louis, 1994, Mosby.

Table 14-1 Types of Neck Dissection

Type	Structures Involved	Nursing Interventions
Radical	◆ Sternocleidomastoid muscle (SCM) ◆ Internal jugular vein ◆ Deep cervical fat pad ◆ Contents of the submental and the submandibular triangles ◆ Spinal accessory nerve	Wound management; airway precautions; physical therapy when approved by physician; oral care; nutrition; pain management; swallowing therapy; flap and graft assessment; respiratory care. Head and facial edema may be problematic
Modified or functional	◆ Cervical lymph nodes N_0 with high risk ◆ Deep cervical fat pad ◆ Deep cervical lymphatics ◆ Attempt is made to save the SCM, the spinal accessory nerve, the internal jugular vein, or any combination	Close monitoring and assessment of airway, wounds, and swallowing. Surgery is less extensive, although similar care and precautions are required for modified or functional neck dissections
Supraomohyoid	◆ Removal of the contents of the submental and the submandibular triangles and the upper deep cervical fat pad ◆ Does not sacrifice the internal jugular vein	All of the above nursing interventions are appropriate, plus airway precautions are particularly critical because the patient is at risk for aspiration; tracheostomy may be present; swallowing and speech therapy
Posterior neck	◆ Removal of the contents of the posterior cervical triangle, the spinal accessory nerve, portions of the trapezius, and deep cervical musculature ◆ Usually associated with melanomas	All of the above nursing interventions are appropriate
Bilateral neck	Where bilateral or contralateral neck disease is a concern, surgery may be a combination of the following: ◆ Bilateral radical neck dissections with preservation of one jugular vein ◆ Radical neck dissection (side one) and functional neck dissection (side two) ◆ Bilateral functional neck dissections ◆ Supraomohyoid dissection (side two) and a functional, radical, or modified neck dissection (side one) ◆ Bilateral supraomohyoid dissections	Most extensive and disfiguring of the neck dissections, and nursing care is critical, especially for wound assessment and care; facial and head edema (possibly a major problem); eye care; oral care; respiratory and tracheostomy care; fluid and electrolyte balance and nutrition maintenance; self-esteem and self-image; aspiration precautions; speech and swallowing therapy; flap and graft care; pain management; and physical therapy

Adapted from Myers E and LaSalle D: Head and neck oncology: diagnoses, treatment, and rehabilitation, Boston, 1991. Little, Brown & Co.

The surgeon can use several different types of flaps and skin grafts to reconstruct extensive resections. Table 14-2 lists the sites of disease and corresponding surgical treatment procedures.

Neoadjuvant Radiation Therapy Followed by Surgery

Radiation therapy may be given before, during, or after surgery. The timing and the dosage of radiation remain open to debate; there is no uniform approach. The field of radiation includes the tumor and the draining lymph node regions (Brady and Davis, 1988).

The first dose of radiation given may be low, and then, after judging the response, the patient may receive a higher dose of radiation or have surgery. This is a common approach with cancers of the pyriform sinus and the larynx. Unresectable primary lesions are also treated in this manner. Inoperable diseased lymph nodes in the neck are included in the radiation field in an effort to make them resectable, but this often fails. In situations where the time required to heal after a major surgical procedure might delay the start of a postoperative course of radiation, preoperative radiation therapy is chosen. Other situations that necessitate preoperative radiation therapy include the presence of a synchronous (simultaneous) primary lesion or the invasion of the skin by the tumor (Hoffman, Crause, and Eschwege, 1992).

Surgery Followed by Radiation Therapy

Postoperative radiation is given when surgical margins have residual disease, multiple neck nodes are positive for disease, there is extracapsular invasion, tumor extends into the soft tissue of the neck, or transection of a tumor occurs during surgery (Brady and Davis, 1988; Hoffman, Crause, and Eschwege, 1992). Under optimal conditions, radiation therapy begins 4 to 6 weeks after surgery to allow for adequate wound healing.

Intraoperative Radiation Therapy

Intraoperative radiation therapy is the administration of a single dose of radiation directly to the open surgical area at the time of surgery. The initial success of this technique requires further study (Busse and Bader, 1992).

Neoadjuvant Radiation Followed by Surgery Followed by Adjuvant Radiation Therapy

Radiation administered before and after surgery is called "sandwich" therapy. Frequently one of the radiation courses is administered interstitially to deliver a high dose close to the tumor bed. This technique may be beneficial after surgery when it is expected that tissue will tolerate radiation poorly, but it is not widely used.

Adjuvant Chemotherapy

The role of chemotherapy in the management of cancers of the head and neck is not as clearly defined as the roles of radiation therapy and surgery. The principal

Table 14-2 **Surgical Options for Head and Neck Cancers**

Anatomic Site	Structures Involved and Surgical Approach	Expected Degree of Cosmetic or Functional Impairment	Nursing Interventions
Lip and oral cavity	Early lesion; intraoral excision vermilionectomy with a W- or U-shaped excision	No functional impairment; good cosmetic result	Observation; assistance; wound care; and oral care
	More advanced lesion; may include submandibular gland and duct; rim resection (mandible) if lesion is attached to the periosteum; may require reconstruction with graft or flap; composite resection (tongue, jaw, neck), hemimandibulectomy, and all or part of the tongue	Moderate to severe deformity; continuity of the mandible is preserved with rim resection; microvascular free flap for reconstruction causes mild to moderate deformity; swallowing and speech dysfunction result; aspiration may be a problem; composite resection for advanced lesions may result in severe functional and cosmetic impairment	Composite resection is extensive surgery; tracheostomy care; respiratory care; wound management; fistula management; speech and swallowing therapy; early ambulation; extensive patient education; oral care; self-image and self-esteem concerns; and odor control
Oropharynx	T_1 or T_2; wide local excision via transoral approach; healing by secondary intention or primary closure	None to minimal	Observation; assistance; and emotional support
	T_3 or T_4; mandibular split approach; skin graft, tongue or myocutaneous flap, or microvascular free flap	Moderate to severe; affects chewing, swallowing, speech, lip closure, and velepharyngeal competence; a prosthesis may be required	Tracheostomy care; respiratory care; speech and swallowing therapy; assistance with intraoral prosthesis; flap care; wound assessment and maintenance; and intraoral wound management
Thyroid	Partial or total thyroidectomy; advanced lesions may include surrounding structures; neck or mediastinal dissection	Minimal to severe depending on extent of resection, laryngeal nerve injury, and speech or voice impairment	Observe for airway compromise due to laryngeal edema, nerve paralysis, and hematoma; monitor Ca^{++} and Mg^{++} levels; thyroid hormone replacement; wound care; early ambulation; monitor for vocal cord paralysis

Data taken from Million RR and Cassisi NJ: Management of head and neck cancer: a multidisciplinary approach, ed 2, Philadelphia, 1994 a, b, c, and d, JB Lippincott Co, and from Myers E and LaSalle D: Head and neck oncology: diagnosis, treatment, and rehabilitation, Boston, 1991, Little Brown & Co.

Continued

Table 14-2 Surgical Options for Head and Neck Cancers—cont'd

Anatomic Site	Structures Involved and Surgical Approach	Expected Degree of Cosmetic or Functional Impairment	Nursing Interventions
Larynx, hypopharynx, and cervical esophagus	Laser excision of small tumors; vertical laryngectomy or hemilaryngectomy removes one half of the larynx	None to minimal; preserves the voice; tracheostomy may be required; impairment may be mild to moderate	Respiratory care; voice rest
	Horizontal or supraglottic laryngectomy removes the epiglottis and false cords	Preserves the voice; tracheostomy may be required; aspiration is likely; swallowing is difficult	Tracheostomy care and patient education; speech and swallowing therapy; oral care; aspiration may be problematic; aggressive respiratory care
	Total laryngectomy removes the complete larynx	Permanent tracheostomy; patient is an obligate neck breather; aphonia requires alternate speech method; impairment is moderate to severe	Laryngectomy or tracheostomy education; swallowing is resumed 1 week to 10 days after surgery; aspiration is not a problem unless fistula occurs; intensive speech therapy for alternative speech method; self-image and self-esteem concerns; refer patient to American Cancer Society for laryngectomy support group
	Laryngopharyngectomy removes the larynx and involved pharynx; reconstruction of the pharynx with flap or graft; a partial laryngopharyngectomy is done if there is no vocal cord paralysis	Permanent tracheostomy; obligate neck breather; aphonia requires alternate speech method; swallowing is difficult; moderate to severe impairment; temporary tracheostomy for partial laryngopharyngectomy	Care is same as for laryngectomy, but this surgery involves the pharynx also; observe for signs of fistula formation, especially at the stoma site; airway precautions; patient may require permanent gastrostomy; nutritional problems; complex nursing care; self-image problems; family education and involvement; patient education
	Esophagectomy with total laryngectomy with gastric pull-up	Stomach is pulled up into the neck; swallowing and nutritional problems; moderate to severe cosmetic and functional impairment	Same as above

Salivary gland	Superficial parotidectomy or deep lobe resection; local excision may be difficult because of perineural spread	Cosmetic impairment moderate to severe if the cranial nerve is involved; tumor-free margins may not be possible because of perineural tracking; functional impairment may be mild to severe depending on structures involved and extent of resection	Wound care; special needs if there is cranial nerve involvement (i.e., eye care, feeding needs, dry mouth care)
Nasal cavity and paranasal sinus	Most lesions are advanced at presentation; resection is determined by extent of lesion; en bloc resection of bone and soft tissue is desired (maxillectomy)	Cosmetic results can be very acceptable with prostheses or osseointegrated implants	Humidification; nasal irrigations; prosthesis management; speech and swallowing therapy; eating difficulties; eye care; self-image and self-esteem problems may be critical; flap and graft care; orbit care
	Craniofacial resection for advanced lesions; resection may include frontal sinus, ethmoid labyrinth, and the eye; may require reconstruction with vascularized flap; each operation is tailored to the extent of the disease	Mild to moderate cosmetic result	Same as above
	Radical surgery may include orbital exenteration	Moderate to severe deformity; prosthesis may be required	Same as above
Skull base	May involve multiple cranial nerves depending on site; may present with puzzling clinical picture; may involve resection of cranial nerves, vascular structures at the skull base, and the pituitary; most skull-base surgery involves retraction on the brain with associated central nervous system deficits	Mild to severe deformity and functional impairments depending on sites and extent of resection; possible cranial nerve deficits; CSF leak; decreased visual acuity or blindness; hormonal dysfunction; pituitary or hypothalamic dysfunction; speech impairment; visual or auditory hallucinations; seizures; dysphagia; behavior changes; ataxia; incoordination	There may be extensive cranial nerve deficits; occupation therapy assistance; refer patient to community organizations for assistance with sight and hearing losses; speech and swallowing therapy; family counseling and support

objective of adjuvant chemotherapy is to eradicate local microscopic and distant micrometastatic disease after the visible tumor has been resected (Hamasaki and Vokes, 1993; Norris and Cady, 1991).

Neoadjuvant Chemotherapy Followed by Surgery or Radiation Therapy

Neoadjuvant chemotherapy is given for advanced tumors to reduce or control tumor size with the intent of lessening the extent of surgery or radiation treatment needed and to eliminate micrometastatic disease (Adelstein et al., 1986; Harris and Smith, 1989; Morrison and Clark, 1992; Tannock, 1994). This approach may help preserve organs such as the larynx and even ultimately improve patient chances of survival (Marion, 1987; Taylor, 1993). Patients with advanced disease, poor chances of survival, or high risk of recurrence may be treated initially with chemotherapy. There is a trend toward giving chemotherapy before surgery or radiation therapy, although there is no clear benefit in terms of survival. The exact role and results of neoadjuvant chemotherapy continue to be investigated (Taylor et al., 1994; see the Research Highlight on page 243).

Concomitant Chemoradiotherapy

Concomitant chemoradiotherapy is given to enhance local control in resectable or unresectable disease, to improve tumor response, and ultimately to prolong survival by eradicating micrometastatic disease (Adelstein et al., 1986; Hamasaki and Vokes, 1993). Some of the antineoplastic agents such as 5-fluorouracil have a potentiating effect on radiation therapy and act as radiosensitizers (Verboke 1992; Jassem et al., 1992). The exact sequence of administration may vary: administering chemotherapy on specific days of radiation, alternating chemotherapy with radiation, or infusing chemotherapy over several days during radiation treatments.

   The literature abounds with combinations and sequences of chemotherapy, radiation therapy, and surgery. The concomitant approach, which benefits from the synergistic effect chemotherapeutic agents have on radiation therapy, is often favored (Dimery and Hong, 1993; Taylor, 1993). Patients with locally advanced disease and metastatic disease may benefit from chemotherapy. Even if the patient's chance of survival is not greatly affected, the need for less radical surgery is an advantage (Jassem et al., 1992).

Neoadjuvant Chemotherapy Followed by Concomitant Chemotherapy

Cisplatin and 5-fluorouracil have been administered as induction chemotherapy for patients with advanced disease for laryngeal preservation and then concomitantly with radiation therapy for patients with recurrent or metastatic disease for palliation (Hamasaki and Vokes, 1993).

Biotherapy

Biotherapy involves the use of agents derived from natural sources or agents that affect biological responses (Wujcik, 1993). Biological response modifiers (BRMs)

RESEARCH HIGHLIGHT

Taylor SG, Murthy AK, Vannetzel JM, Colin P, Dray DD, Caldarelli DD, Shott S, Vokes E, Showel JC, Hutchinson JC, Witt TR, Griem KL, Hartsell WF, Kies MS, Mittal B, Rebischung JL, Coupez DJ, Desphieux S, Bobin S, and LePajolec C: Randomized comparison of neoadjuvant cisplatin and fluorouracil infusion followed by radiation versus concomitant treatment in advanced head and neck cancer, J Clin Oncol 12:385–395, 1994.

Study A randomized trial between cisplatin given as 100 mg/m^2 over 15 minutes on day 1 plus 5-fluorouracil (5-FU) given as 1.0 g/m^2 by continuous infusion on days 1 to 5, repeated every 3 weeks for three cycles, followed by 70 Gy of radiation in 7 to 8 weeks versus cisplatin given as 60 mg/m^2 over 15 minutes on day 1 plus 5-FU given as 800 mg/m^2 by continuous infusion on days 1 to 5 plus 2 Gy of radiation on days 1 to 5, repeated every other week for seven cycles.

Sample The study included 215 patients with unresectable head and neck squamous cell cancers not previously treated with radiation or chemotherapy and a performance status of 0 to 2 who were stratified by extent of disease and performance status and then randomized for study.

Study aim To compare the efficacy and toxic side effects of two regimens of cisplatin plus 5-FU infusion and radiation given on a sequential schedule or a concomitant schedule to patients with unresectable head and neck cancers.

Findings The study analyzed a total of 214 patients. The complete response rates were similar for the two groups, but more patients in the concomitant treatment arm had partial responses and fewer patients in that arm had no change or progression of disease. Researchers observed similar rates of failure in the control of distant metastases for the concomitant-treatment arm and the sequential-treatment group (10% and 7%, respectively). However, there were divergent failure rates in treating regional disease (55% and 39%, respectively). The predominant toxic side effects included mucositis, leukopenia, thrombocytopenia, weight loss, vascular events such as stroke and arterial occlusion, elevated serum creatinine, and/or blood urea nitrogen. The two groups had an equal number of toxic side effects. The period of survival after treatment was similar for the two groups, although a significantly greater number of patients in the sequential arm died of their cancer.

Discussion Concomitant treatment offered improved disease control, especially regional disease, but the level of benefit depended on the experience of the treating institution. Translation of this benefit into improved survival rates is not yet evident because of a higher number of deaths from other causes in the concomitant arm.

---

augment the host's ability to respond to foreign bodies—in this case, cancer cells—and change the body's natural immune reaction to these cells (Parkinson and Schantz, 1992). One group of BRMs, the cytokines (interferons, interleukins, and colony-stimulating factors), are undergoing clinical and preclinical phase I and phase II trials for patients with advanced, recurrent, or metastatic cancers of the head and neck (Parkinson and Schantz, 1992). These substances are given alone, in combination with chemotherapy agents, or with other cytokines. The most common side effects of BRMs are flulike symptoms.

❖ Nursing Management

Combinations of treatment modalities lead to increased toxic side effects (see the Possible Side Effects from Multimodal Therapy in Head and Neck Cancers on page 245), the severity of which may require hospitalization for good management. The toxicities may necessitate either altered doses of chemotherapy or radiation therapy or delays in treatment. However, every effort should be made to give full doses and to keep treatment continuous to get the maximum benefit from each modality.

Problems faced by patients treated with multimodal therapy for head and neck cancer that may require nursing management include (1) delayed wound healing after surgery on a previously irradiated site; (2) alteration in nutrition and weight loss; (3) lower self-esteem because of hair loss and physical changes that cause difficulty with visible body functions such as eating, chewing, lip closure, or drooling; (4) education on ways to stop drinking alcohol and smoking cigarettes; (5) bone marrow depression; (6) nausea and vomiting; (7) alteration in coping abilities due to diagnosis, treatments, or disease progression; (8) airway maintenance; (9) oral care; (10) speech rehabilitation; (11) monitoring of swallowing ability and rehabilitation; (12) fistula control and management; (13) odor control from wounds or disease; and (14) precautions to avoid rupture of the carotid artery. Some of these problems are discussed in detail in Units III and IV; specific problems related to head and neck cancers are discussed below.

Airway

Most patients undergoing major resection involving the oral cavity, the tongue, the pharynx, or the larynx will return from the operating room with a tracheostomy tube in place to secure the airway. The tracheostomy may be permanent or temporary.

Laryngectomy is the removal of the larynx and placement of a permanent stoma. The patient will use a tracheostomy tube as a stent and to facilitate cleaning and suctioning after surgery. Patients may leave the tracheostomy tube out for short periods without fear of the stoma closing. Reinserting the tracheostomy tube is quite easy because the stoma is large and permanent. Nursing Care of the Airway is presented on page 248.

Patients who have had head and neck surgery without tracheostomy tubes need to have the airway carefully monitored as well. Edema of the tongue, the pharynx, or the larynx; aspiration of secretions or drainage; and postanesthesia respiratory complications such as pneumothorax, atelectasis, narcotic sedation, and depressed respiratory effort can cause airway emergencies.

Humidified oxygen administered by face mask, trach mask, or T-tube augments the oxygen reaching the patient's lungs and reduces the respiratory effort. It helps assure adequate oxygenation for flap and tissue perfusion, thins secretions, and moisturizes the mouth and the throat.

Oral Care

Oral complications of radiation therapy can be severe and debilitating, although meticulous oral care and preventive measures can greatly moderate the severity

Possible Side Effects from Multimodal Therapy in

Head and Neck Cancers

Multimodal Treatment	*Possible Enhanced Side Effects*
Radiation therapy followed by surgery	Delayed wound healing, fistula formation
Surgery followed by adjuvant radiation therapy	Fistula formation, hemorrhage, wound breakdown

Neoadjuvant chemotherapy followed by surgery
    Cisplatin, 5-fluorouracil
    Carboplatin, 5-fluorouracil
    Cisplatin, bleomycin, methotrexate
    Cisplatin, bleomycin, vincristine
    Paclitaxel, cisplatin
    Bleomycin, paclitaxel, cisplatin
    5-Fluorouracil, methotrexate
	No enhanced side effects

Neoadjuvant chemotherapy followed by radiation therapy
    Cisplatin, 5-fluorouracil
    Carboplatin, 5-fluorouracil
    5-Fluorouracil, methotrexate
	Photosensitivity

Cisplatin, bleomcyin, vincristine
    Cisplatin, paclitaxel
    Bleomycin, paclitaxel, cisplatin
    Cisplatin, bleomycin, methotrexate
	No enhanced side effects

Neoadjuvant chemotherapy followed by surgery followed by radiation therapy
    Cisplatin, 5-fluorouracil
    Carboplatin, 5-fluorouracil
    5-Fluorouracil, methotrexate
	Fistula formation, hemorrhage, wound breakdown, photosensitivity

Cisplatin, bleomycin, methotrexate
    Bleomycin, paclitaxel, cisplatin
    Cisplatin, bleomycin, vincristine
    Paclitaxel, cisplatin
	Fistula formation, hemorrhage, wound breakdown

Neoadjuvant chemotherapy followed by radiation therapy followed by surgery
    Cisplatin, 5-fluorouracil
    Carboplatin, 5-fluorouracil
    5-Fluorouracil, methotrexate
	Delayed wound healing, fistula formation, photosensitivity

Cisplatin, bleomycin, vincristine
    Cisplatin, bleomycin, methotrexate
    Paclitaxel, cisplatin
    Bleomycin, pacilitaxel, cisplatin
	Delayed wound healing, fistula formation

Data taken from Brady and Davis, 1988; Eifel and McClure, 1989; Harris and Smith, 1989; Mitchell, 1992; Taylor, 1991; Schenkier and Gelmon, 1994.

Continued

Multimodal Treatment	Possible Enhanced Side Effects
Conservative surgery followed by radiation therapy followed by adjuvant chemotherapy	
Cisplatin, 5-fluorouracil	Fistula formation, hemorrhage,
Carboplatin, 5-fluorouracil	wound breakdown, photosensitivity
5-Fluorouracil, methotrexate	
Cisplatin, bleomycin, methotrexate	Fistula formation, hemorrhage,
Cisplatin, bleomycin, vincristine	wound breakdown
Paclitaxel, cisplatin	Fistula formation, hemorrhage,
Bleomycin, paclitaxel, cisplatin	wound breakdown, radiation recall
Surgery followed by adjuvant chemotherapy	
Cisplatin, 5-fluorouracil	No enhanced side effects
Carboplatin, 5-fluorouracil	
5-Fluorouracil, methotrexate	
Cisplatin, bleomycin, methotrexate	
Cisplatin, bleomycin, vincristine	
Paclitaxel, cisplatin	
Bleomycin, paclitaxel, cisplatin	
Concomitant chemotherapy and radiation therapy	
Carboplatin, 5-fluorouracil	Severe mucositis, photosensitivity
Cisplatin, 5-fluorouracil	
5-Fluorouracil, methotrexate	Severe mucositis, photosensitivity, fibrosis, radionecrosis
Cisplatin, bleomycin, methotrexate	Severe mucositis, fibrosis, radionecrosis
Cisplatin, bleomycin, vincristine	Severe mucositis
Paclitaxel, cisplatin	Radiation recall
Bleomycin, paclitaxel, cisplatin	Severe mucositis, radiation recall
Neoadjuvant concomitant chemotherapy and radiation therapy followed by surgery	
Cisplatin, 5-fluorouracil	Mucositis, photosensitivity, fistula
Carboplatin, 5-fluorouracil	formation, delayed wound healing
5-Fluorouracil, methotrexate	Mucositis, photosensitivity, fibrosis, radionecrosis, delayed wound healing, fistula formation
Cisplatin, bleomycin, methotrexate	Mucositis, fibrosis, radionecrosis, delayed wound healing, fistula formation
Cisplatin, bleomycin, vincristine	Mucositis, delayed wound healing, fistula formation

Multimodal Treatment	Possible Enhanced Side Effects
Neoadjuvant concomitant chemotherapy and radiation therapy followed by surgery—*cont'd*	
Paclitaxel, cisplatin	Radiation recall, delayed wound healing, fistula formation
Bleomycin, paclitaxel, cisplatin	Mucositis, radiation recall, delayed wound healing, Fistula formation
Concomitant chemotherapy and biotherapy	
Cisplatin, 5-fluorouracil, interferon-α-2b	No enhanced side effects
Radiation therapy followed by adjuvant chemotherapy	
Cisplatin, 5-fluorouracil	Photosensitivity
Carboplatin, 5-fluorouracil	
5-Fluorouracil, methotrexate	
Cisplatin, bleomycin, methotrexate	No enhanced side effects
Cisplatin, bleomycin, vincristine	
Pacilitaxel, cisplatin	Radiation recall
Bleomycin, paclitaxel, cisplatin	

(Baker, 1987). (See the Patient Education Guidelines on page 249). The expected oral complications are the following:

♦ *Mucositis.* Mucositis usually occurs within 2 weeks of the start of treatment. In the early stages the mucosa is red and sore, becoming ulcerated and painful in the later stages. Local bacterial, fungal, or viral infections often occur and compound the problem. Mucositis usually resolves 2 to 6 weeks after the treatment ends.

♦ *Xerostomia.* Xerostomia occurs when the major salivary gland(s) are in the radiation field. Xerostomia may be permanent but frequently improves over time. It often takes up to a year to reach maximum improvement.

♦ *Dental disease.* The combination of decreased salivary pH, decreased salivary flow, and local infections increases the chances for dental caries, gingivitis, and other oral or dental problems.

♦ *Oral infections.* Yeast infections are a frequent problem, especially infections by *Candida albicans.* Bacterial infections also occur.

♦ *Osteoradionecrosis.* Osteoradionecrosis is bone death caused by high-dose radiation. Insufficient vascular supply is thought to cause the problem, but dental disease is also suspect.

♦ *Altered taste.* Taste changes may be permanent; however, some improvement can be expected 2 to 6 weeks after treatment ends. Taste changes can cause aversion to food and nutritional problems.

♦ *Trismus.* Trismus is difficulty opening the mouth and chewing; therapeutic exercises can minimize or prevent trismus.

Nursing Care of
The Airway

Nursing Care	Rationale/Comments
◆ Auscultate all lung fields carefully before and after suctioning or coughing	◆ Determine the effectiveness of intervention; listen to the right and left lungs, front and back, and to the tracheostomy tube
◆ Place stethoscope on neck alongside of trachea and listen to the air movements in the tube	◆ If the lumen is open, it will sound like wind passing through a tunnel; whistling or gurgling sounds may indicate an obstruction in the tube or upper airway
◆ For the first 24 to 48 hours after surgery, endotracheal suction may be necessary as often as every 2 hours	◆ Most patients with head and neck cancer have a long history of tobacco use and have copious secretions that require diligent respiratory surveillance
◆ Reduce suctioning frequency as soon as patient is able to mobilize own secretions	◆ Suctioning too frequently can traumatize the delicate tissues of the airway
◆ Oral suctioning may be necessary because secretions are often coughed up into the mouth during tracheal suctioning	◆ If the patient had oral surgery, the surgeon may restrict oral suctioning or leave orders for specific kinds of oral suctioning
◆ For a mucous plug, 2 to 3 ml saline squirted into the tracheostomy tube or stoma followed by coughing and/or suctioning will loosen and remove a mucous plug; repeat the procedure once or twice as needed	◆ Saline in the tracheostomy tube or the stoma lubricates the airway, stimulates coughing, and softens hard plugs; sometimes plugs can be propelled out of the tracheostomy with amazing force; always stand to the side of the patient
◆ After the patient has completely recovered from anesthesia and a strong cough reflex has returned, saline may be all that is required to clear the airway	◆ Stimulating a strong cough is more effective than suctioning to mobilize secretions

Speech Rehabilitation

After undergoing a total laryngectomy, patients will be unable to speak normally and must use an alternative method of communication. The three types of alaryngeal speech are intrinsic speech, prosthetic speech, and surgical-prosthetic speech (Goldstein and Merwin, 1994).

Intrinsic speech is usually esophageal. To produce esophageal speech, the patient brings air into the esophagus, traps the air, and then releases it with enough pressure to cause the top of the esophagus to vibrate. With intense speech therapy and practice, many patients learn to speak fluently this way. Esophageal speech training begins after surgical wounds have completely healed, usually 2 to 3 months

Patient Education Guidelines for

Oral Care During Radiation Therapy

♦ Follow this oral care plan throughout your radiation therapy and for 2 to 4 weeks after treatment.

♦ Look carefully at your mouth every day. Describe any changes to your dentist, doctor, or nurse.

♦ You may find that certain foods are difficult to chew or swallow and that acidic foods like orange juice, tomatoes, or pineapples are too strong. Soft, moist foods are the easiest to chew and swallow. Discuss any eating problems with your nurse or doctor.

♦ Brush with a soft toothbrush or a toothette and floss after meals and at bedtime. Use a plain fluoride gel for brushing. If you don't have natural teeth, swish and spit with a solution of salt water and hydrogen peroxide. Be sure to clean all the crevices where food particles can hide. You can make salt water by mixing 1 tsp of table salt in 1 quart of water.

♦ Swish and spit with an alkaline mouthwash after cleaning the mouth or as desired during the day. Swish and spit three to four mouthfuls each time. A simple and effective formula for alkaline mouth wash is 1 tsp of baking soda dissolved in 1 pint of salt water. Make a fresh mixture every morning to avoid bacterial growth in the solution.

♦ Swish and *swallow* with medicated mouth wash if ordered by your doctor. It is important to *swallow* medicated mouth wash if told to do so by your doctor because your doctor wants the medicine also to reach the back of your throat.

♦ Use an artificial saliva substitute as needed during the day and have water or other fluid available at all times. This helps to keep the mouth moist and comfortable.

♦ If you have teeth, your dentist will order a fluoride treatment, which is usually done at bedtime.

Permission granted to reproduce these guidelines for educational purposes only.

postoperatively. This type of a laryngeal speech may take a year or more to master. Some patients become frustrated with the slow progress or don't like the sound of esophageal speech and choose to use an artificial electronic larynx.

The electrolarynx is a battery-powered, hand-held device that produces vibrations. The vibrations become transformed into sound, which the tongue, the lips, and the cheeks shape into speech. Two commonly used types of electrolarynx are the Cooper-Rand and the Servox. The Cooper-Rand is an intraoral device consisting of an intraoral tube and a battery-powered tone generator. The sound is placed in the oral cavity through this intraoral tube. The Servox is a transcervical device. It has a battery-powered vibrating head that, when placed against the neck, transfers sound into the pharynx and the oral cavity. Patients are usually permitted to begin electrolaryngeal speech 10 days after surgery.

Surgical-prosthetic speech allows the patient to divert exhaled pulmonary air through a prosthesis that is implanted in a surgically placed tracheoesophageal puncture. The air passes from the trachea into the upper esophagus through a one-way valved prosthesis. The patient expels the air, causing the top of the esophagus to vibrate, much like the process for esophageal speech. The patient must have the manual dexterity and willingness to learn to remove, clean, and reinsert the prosthesis.

Speech and swallowing rehabilitation are closely related. They begin as soon as possible after surgical wounds have healed. The physician, speech pathologist, and nurse offer counseling and support as the patient begins the rehabilitative process.

Swallowing

Swallowing involves a coordinated series of actions. The swallow has been divided into three stages: oral, pharyngeal, and esophageal (Gay, Rendell, and Spiro, 1994). Surgery on head and neck cancers can affect any phase of swallowing. Surgery on the lip, the tongue, or the palate may affect the oral preparation or oral phase; surgery on the soft palate, the supraglottis, the nasopharynx, the pharyngeal wall, or the base of the tongue can affect the pharyngeal phase; surgery on the cervical esophagus may affect the esophageal phase. Box 14-1 lists some commonly encountered swallowing disorders. Swallowing therapy is initiated as early as the healing process permits.

Aspiration is the most dangerous problem resulting from impaired swallowing especially because the patient may be unaware that aspiration has occurred. Not every patient will cough and choke with aspiration. Some "silently" aspirate. These patients are at great risk for pneumonia and other pulmonary complications caused by food particles in the airway. Important nursing interventions include observation during feeding or meal time, reinforcement of swallowing techniques, auscultation of the lungs after meals, respiratory intervention such as suctioning, coughing, deep breathing, and documentation of suspected swallowing disorders.

Precautions to Avoid Carotid Artery Rupture

Carotid artery rupture is a potentially life-threatening event that occurs in 3% to 3.8% of extensive head and neck procedures (Everts, Cohen, and McMenomey, 1993). The patient with a neck wound and an exposed innominate or common

---

Box 14-1 Frequently Encountered Swallowing Disorders

- Inability to chew and form a bolus
- Inability to propel a bolus to the back of the oral cavity
- Inefficient chewing
- Premature swallow
- Failure of the epiglottis to close
- Regurgitation into the nasal cavity
- Incomplete lip closure
- Excessive dryness
- Unilateral food collection
- Food or liquid pooling in the vallecula

carotid artery is at risk for arterial rupture. Factors that may contribute to exposure of these major vessels are extensive radiation therapy, invasion by a tumor, tissue necrosis, wound breakdown, skin or flap necrosis, and infection or fistula formation with the resultant flow of saliva over the blood vessels (Everts, Cohen, and McMenomey, 1993; Schwarz and Yuska, 1989). The major nursing considerations are recognizing patients at risk for arterial rupture, counseling patients, teaching the staff, and preparing for the event. It is imperative that wounds be assessed with every dressing change and that any change in wound characteristics be documented and reported. Especially important to note are the color of the tissue, the amount and appearance of drainage, any change in wound appearance, the measurement of wound dimensions, odor, and the number of dressing changes required per shift.

Massive bleeding may not happen suddenly. There may be a "sentinel" bleed that heralds a pending hemorrhage. Any bleeding—even small amounts—raises a red flag and alerts the physician and the nurse that major bleeding may be imminent.

If a bleed should occur, the nursing actions are based on the ABCs: airway, breathing, and circulation. The first step is to secure the airway. If the patient is intubated, inflate the cuff of the tracheostomy tube or endotracheal tube to prevent aspiration and elevate the head of bed. Suction the tube and the oral cavity as needed. As the airway is being secured, call for assistance. After the airway is secured, the next step is to stop the bleeding. If the bleeding is external, apply firm pressure with a towel or gauze pads. If the bleeding is internal, the oral cavity and the oropharynx may be packed with fluff gauze or a vaginal pack (Schwarz and Yuska, 1989). Insert two large-bore intravenous access catheters and begin rapid infusion of IV fluid to maintain blood pressure. Patients who have had a sentinel bleed or who have a high likelihood of rupture should have venous access in place. Obtain blood for type and crossmatch or, if already ordered, prepare to infuse units per the physician's order. The patient should then be prepared for transfer to the operating room. This situation requires staff who are calm but decisive in their actions. A narcotic or antianxiety medication is frequently administered. After a bleeding event, observe the patient carefully for signs of new bleeding: unstable vital signs, changes in mental status, visual disturbances, or changes in level of consciousness.

Patients and family members will be very frightened, and they will need clear explanations. They should be counseled that a carotid artery may rupture, and decisions regarding treatment and resuscitation should be made beforehand because this event is often fatal.

Patients discharged to go home who are at risk for arterial rupture will require family counseling and assistance in case such an event occurs in the home. Discharge planning includes discussion with the home care nurse so that adequate home supplies are in place.

Fistula Control and Management

Salivary fistula management is a difficult but not uncommon problem following major head and neck surgery. When there is a break in the integrity of the suture line, the tissue in the oral cavity, or the oropharynx and saliva leaks into the adjacent tissue, a fistula can form. This saliva "bath" further breaks down the tissue and creates a passageway that eventually leads to an opening. This path often follows the surgical tract. Salivary fistula formation is discouraging for the patient because it often delays recovery and discharge. Early fistula formation may be seen as redness, swelling, or induration at a point along the cutaneous suture line. Salivary fistulas most often appear within the first week after surgery. Small fistulas often close with routine care, but larger fistulas may be persistent and not close for months or may require surgery for closure.

Nursing care of salivary fistulas involves keeping the skin clean and dry, collecting or diverting the saliva flow, and controlling odor. Light packing with sterile medicated gauze strips may be helpful. Caution is needed when packing a fistula because pressure may further erode the surrounding tissue. Managing a large salivary fistula is a nursing challenge, and often the enterostomal therapist is consulted for creative ideas on skin care, salivary flow diversion and collection, and odor control. If the salivary fistula is draining near the tracheostoma or laryngestoma, great care is required to protect the airway. Carotid artery precautions are necessary if the fistula is near the artery.

Other nursing considerations for the head and neck cancer patient are pain control; flap, graft, and wound management; facial lymphedema; pulmonary complications; chylous fistula formation; and nutritional management.

❖ Summary

Care of the patient with cancer of the head and neck is complex and challenging. Nurses can assist these patients at several critical points in the recovery and rehabilitation process by providing specialized nursing care, timely and relevant teaching, and counseling interventions. Teaching patients about treatments, side effects, and self-care activities is pivotal to patient recovery and rehabilitation. After treatments are complete, many patients with head and neck cancer return to work and resume their roles in the home, the workplace, and the community.

❖ References

Adelstein DJ, Sharan VM, Damm C, Earle AS, Shah AC, Haria CD, Trey JE, Carter SG, and Hines JD: Chemoradiation therapy as initial management in patients with squamous cell carcinoma of the head and neck, Canc Treat Rep 70:761–767, 1986.

Baker KH: Oral care for head and neck cancer patients undergoing radiation therapy, Navy Med Nov–Dec:7–9, 1987.

Baker KH and Feldman JE: Cancers of the head and neck, Canc Nurs 10:293–299, 1987.

Baker KH and Feldman JE: Thyroid cancer: a review, Oncol Nurs Forum 20:95–104, 1993.

Brady LW and Davis WL: Treatment of head and neck cancer by radiation therapy, Semin Oncol 15:29–38, 1988.

Busse PM and Bader SB: Radiation therapy for head and neck cancer. In Snow GB and Clark JR, editors: Multimodal therapy for head and neck cancer, New York, 1992, Thieme Medical Publishers, Inc.

Cooper JS: Carcinomas of the oral cavity and oropharynx. In Cox JD, editor: Moss's radiation oncology: rationale, techniques, results, St. Louis, 1994, Mosby, pp. 169–213.

Cox JD, Pajak TF, Marcial VA, Coia L, Mohiuddin M, Fu KF, Selim HM, Byhardt RW, Rubin P, Ortiz HG, and Martin L: Interruptions adversely affect local control and survival with hyperfractionated radiation therapy of carcinomas of the upper respiratory and digestive tracts, Cancer 69:2744–2748, 1992.

Dimery IW and Hong WK: Overview of combined modality therapies for head and neck cancer, J Nat Canc Inst 85(2):95–107, 1993.

Eifel PJ and McClure S: Severe chemotherapy-induced recall of radiation mucositis in a patient with non-Hodgkin's lymphoma of Waldeyer's ring, Int J Radiat Oncol Biol Phys 17:907–908, 1989 (letter).

Everts EC, Cohen JI, and McMenomey SO: Surgical complications. In Cummings CW, Fredrickson JM, Harker LA, Krause CJ, and Schuller DE, editors: Otolaryngology head and neck surgery, ed 2, St. Louis, 1993, Mosby, pp. 1673–1690.

Feldman JE and Baker KH: The psychodynamics of prolonged treatment in a patient with cancer of the hypopharynx, Cancer Nurs 11:362–367, 1988.

Gay T, Rendell J, and Spiro J: Oral and laryngeal muscle coordination during swallowing, Laryngoscope 104:341–349, 1994.

Goldstein L and Merwin G: Speech and rehabilitation after total laryngectomy. In Million RR and Cassisi NJ: Management of head and neck cancer: a multidisciplinary approach, ed 2, Philadelphia, 1994, JB Lippincott Co, pp. 449–504.

Hamasaki VK and Vokes EE: Chemotherapy and combined modality therapy in head and neck cancer, Cur Opin Oncol 5:508–517, 1993.

Harris LL and Smith S: Chemotherapy in head and neck cancer, Semin Oncol Nurs 5:174–181, 1989.

Hoffman HT, Crause CJ, and Eschwege F: Combined surgery and radiotherapy. In Snow GB and Clark JR, editors: Multimodal therapy for head and neck cancer, New York, 1992, Thieme Medical Publishers, Inc, pp. 76–94.

Jassem J, Dewitt L, Keus R, and Bartelink H: Concomitant chemotherapy and radiotherapy. In Snow GB and Clark JR, editors: Multimodal therapy for head and neck cancer, New York, 1992, Thieme Medical Publishers, Inc, pp. 126–146.

Marion J: Chemotherapy and immunotherapy of head and neck tumors. In Thawley SE and Panjie WR, editors: Comprehensive management of head and neck tumors, Philadelphia, 1987, WB Saunders Co, pp. 1885–1896.

Million RR and Cassisi NJ: General principles for treatment of cancers of the head and neck: the primary site. In Million RR and Cassisi NJ: Management of head and neck cancer: a multidisciplinary approach, ed 2, Philadelphia, 1994a, JB Lippincott Co, pp. 61–74.

Million RR and Cassisi NJ: General principles for treatment of cancers of the head and neck: nasopharynx. In Million RR and Cassisi NJ: Management of head and neck cancer: a multidisciplinary approach, ed 2, Philadelphia, 1994b, JB Lippincott Co, pp. 599–626.

Million RR and Cassisi NJ: General principles for treatment of cancers of the head and neck: nasal cavity, ethmoid and sphenoid sinuses. In Million RR and Cassisi NJ: Management of head and neck cancer: a multidisciplinary approach, ed 2, Philadelphia, 1994c, JB Lippincott Co, pp. 573–598.

Million RR and Cassisi NJ: General principles for treatment of cancers of the head and neck: pharynx. In Million RR and Cassisi NJ: Management of head and neck cancer: a multidisciplinary approach, ed 2, Philadelphia, 1994d, JB Lippincott Co, pp. 505–532.

Mitchell EP: Gastrointestinal toxicity of chemotherapeutic agents, Semin Oncol 19:566–579, 1992.

Morrison BW and Clark JR: Induction chemotherapy. In Snow GB and Clark JR, editors: Multimodal therapy for head and neck cancer, New York, 1992, Thieme Medical Publishers, Inc, pp. 95–112.

Myers E and LaSalle D: Head and neck oncology: diagnosis, treatment, and rehabilitation, Boston, 1991, Little, Brown & Co.

Norris CM Jr and Cady B: Head, neck, and thyroid cancer. In Holleb AI, Fink DJ, and Murphy GP, editors: Textbook of clinical oncology, Atlanta, 1991, American Cancer Society, pp. 306–328.

Parkinson DR and Schantz SP: Immunobiological therapy for head and neck cancer. In Snow GB and Clark JR, editors: Multimodal therapy for head and neck cancer. New York, 1992, Thieme Medical Publishers, Inc, pp. 147–159.

Schenkier T and Gelmon K: Paclitaxel and radiation-recall dermatitis, J Clin Oncol 12:439, 1994 (letter).

Schleper J: Prevention, detection, and diagnosis of the head and neck cancers, Semin Oncol Nurs 5:139–149, 1989.

Schottenfeld D: In Newell GR and Hong WK, editors: The biology and prevention of aerodigestive tract cancers, New York, 1992, Plenum Press, pp. 1–20.

Schwarz SS and Yuska CM: Common patient care issues following surgery for head and neck cancer, Semin Oncol Nurs 5:191–194, 1989.

Strohl RA: Radiation therapy for head and neck cancers, Semin Oncol Nurs 5:166–173, 1989.

Tannock IF: General principles of chemotherapy. In Million RR and Cassisi NJ: Management of head and neck cancer: a multidisciplinary approach, ed 2, Philadelphia, 1994, JB Lippincott Co, pp. 143–156.

Taylor SG: Head and neck cancer. In Pinedo HM, Longo DI, and Chabner BA, editors: Cancer chemotherapy and biological response modifiers annual 14, Toronto, 1993, Elsevier Science Publishers BV, pp. 427–441.

Taylor SG: Head and neck cancer. In Lokich JJ and Byfield JE: Combined modality cancer therapy: radiation and infusional chemotherapy. Chicago, 1991, Precept Press, Inc, pp. 75–98.

Taylor SG, Murthy AK, Vannetzel JM, Colin P, Dray M, Caldarelli DD, Schott S, Vokes E, Showel JL, Hutchinson JC, Witt TR, Griem KL, Hartsell WF, Kies MS, Mittal B, Rebischung JL, Coupez DJ, Desphieux JL, Bobin S, and LePajolec C: Randomized comparison of neoadjuvant cisplatin and fluorouracil infusion followed by radiation versus concomitant treatment in advanced head and neck cancer, J Clin Oncol 12:385–395, 1994.

Verboken JB: Adjuvant chemotherapy for advanced squamous cell carcinoma of the head and neck. In Snow GB and Clark JR, editors: Multimodal therapy for head and neck cancer. New York, 1992, Thieme Medical Publishers, Inc, pp. 112–126.

Wujcik D: An odyssey into biologic therapy, Oncol Nurs Forum 20:879–887, 1993.

Chapter **15**

❖ *Hematopoietic and Immunologic Cancers*

Kimberly A. Rumsey

Cancers of the hematopoietic and immune systems are diseases in which there is a proliferation of malignant cells that derive originally from the bone marrow, the thymus, and lymphatic tissue (Carson and Callaghan, 1991). The two most common types of hematopoietic and immunologic malignancies are leukemia and lymphoma, in that order.

❖ *Leukemia*

Leukemia refers to a group of hematologic malignancies that affect the bone marrow and lymphoid tissue, resulting in proliferation of dysfunctional cells. Leukemia accounts for approximately 8% of cancers in the United States. During 1995 an estimated 25,700 new cases of leukemia were diagnosed and 20,400 leukemia-related deaths occurred (Wingo, Tong, and Bolden, 1995).

The bone marrow is the site where *hematopoiesis,* the differentiation and maturation of the blood cells, occurs within the body. Typically hematopoiesis is a highly regulated process. Leukemia occurs when regulatory control of the differentiation and maturation of a specific type of cell is lost, which results in the arrested development of that cell. An arrest that occurs early in the process of differentiation and maturation results in acute leukemia; chronic leukemia involves more mature cells. As these leukemic cells proliferate and accumulate in the bone marrow, the resultant lack of space and nutrients limits the production of healthy cell lines.

255

The leukemic cells essentially replace the bone marrow, and they eventually spill into the peripheral blood. There are four subgroups of leukemia: acute lymphocytic leukemia, acute myelogenous leukemia, chronic lymphocytic leukemia, and chronic myelogenous leukemia. Table 15-1 lists the most common clinical manifestations associated with the different types of leukemia.

Acute Lymphoblastic Leukemia

Acute lymphoblastic leukemia (ALL) involves the uncontrolled proliferation of immature lymphocytes. ALL is the most common childhood leukemia but accounts for only 15% to 20% of adulthood leukemias (Maguire-Eisen, 1990; Mitus and Rosenthal, 1991).

Treatment

The medical management of ALL focuses on removing all leukemic cells from the body. Treatment can be divided into two stages. The first stage, remission-induction therapy, involves the use of chemotherapeutic agents to eradicate all detectable leukemic cells, to induce a complete remission, and to restore bone marrow function. *Complete remission* is defined as the state when bone marrow aspirate contains less than 5% lymphoblasts and extramedullary disease has been eliminated. Postremission therapy, including consolidation and maintenance treatments, is administered to eliminate all remaining, undetectable leukemic cells (Devine and Larson, 1994).

Remission-induction therapy using an anthracycline (usually daunorubicin), vincristine, asparaginase, and prednisone results in complete remission 70% to 75% of the time (Hoeltzer and Gale, 1987). Although treatment usually begins in the hospital, after complete remission has been achieved, the patient can be treated on an outpatient basis.

Central nervous system (CNS) prophylaxis is included in the treatment regimen because leukemic cells have the ability to infiltrate the CNS and because the chemotherapeutic agents used in the treatment of ALL do not cross the blood-brain barrier. Methotrexate administered directly into the cerebrospinal fluid (CSF) through the intrathecal or intraventricular route is the CNS prophylactic treatment of choice (Henderson, 1983). Radiation can be administered to the cranium in fractionated doses for a total of 24 Gy (Henderson, 1983; Mitus and Rosenthal, 1991).

Because the long-term survival rate for ALL patients is low, therapy is administered after remission to eradicate undetectable leukemic cells. Patients may require maintenance chemotherapy for 2 to 3 years. Generally the same drugs used in remission-induction therapy apply to postremission treatment, with the addition of methotrexate and 6-mercaptopurine (Lachant and Skeel, 1991).

If the patient should experience a relapse after postremission therapy is complete, treatment based on high-dose cytarabine with the addition of idarubicin or mitoxantrone produces approximately a 65% second-remission rate (Hiddemann et al., 1987; Nooter et al., 1990). Patients who experience an early relapse but have good prognostic factors may be eligible for bone marrow transplantation (Mortimer et al., 1989; Vogelsang, 1989) (see Chapter 6, Bone Marrow Transplantation).

Table 15-1   Clinical Manifestations of Leukemia

	Anorexia	Bleeding	Bruising	Bone or Joint Pain	Exercise Intolerance	Fatigue	Fever	Headache	Hepatic Enlargement	Infection	Lymphadenopathy	Pallor	Shortness of Breath	Splenic Enlargement	Sweats	Weight Loss	Comments
Acute lymphocytic leukemia	—	D	D	D	—	D	D	D	—	D	D	D	—	—	—	—	May be nonsymptomatic at diagnosis
Acute myelogenous leukemia	—	D	—	D	—	D	—	—	D	D	D	D	D	—	D	—	Infections are unresponsive to antibiotics; patients may have coagulation abnormalities
Chronic lymphocytic leukemia	—	L	—	—	D	D/L	—	—	—	—	D	—	—	D	L	L	May be nonsymptomatic at diagnosis
Chronic myelogenous leukemia	D	L	—	D	D	D/L	D/L	—	D/L	—	L	D	—	D/L	L	D/L	>85% have the Philadelphia chromosome; manifestations of blast stage resemble those of acute leukemia

D = May be present at diagnosis
L = May indicate late stage of disease

Acute Myelogenous Leukemia

Acute myelogenous leukemia (AML), sometimes referred to as acute nonlymphocytic leukemia (ANLL), involves the uncontrolled proliferation of myeloid, monocyte, erythroid, or megakaryocyte cells. AML is the most common type of adult
leukemia in the United States (Mitus and Rosenthal, 1991).

Treatment

The management of AML focuses on eliminating leukemic cells. Figure 15-1 presents a synopsis of treatment options. Induction therapy and postremission therapy
also apply to the treatment of AML. Remission-induction therapy using cytarabine
and an anthracycline will produce complete remission in 50% to 75% of patients;
however, the duration of remission is only 4 to 8 months (Champlin, 1988). Postremission therapy can increase the duration of the remission to 10 to 15 months
(Wolff et al., 1987).

Consolidation therapy, given immediately after remission-induction therapy,
involves the administration of one to two additional courses of remission-induction
drugs or high-dose therapy (Wolff et al., 1987). The use of drugs other than those
used to induce remission may help decrease the chance of the leukemia becoming
resistant to the chemotherapy (Gale and Foon, 1987). Overall, the rate of second
remission is low (20%), and the long-term survival rate is less than 5% (Mitus and
Rosenthal, 1991). Bone marrow transplantation is another postremission option and
is recommended for patients who are less than 50 years of age, in their first remission,
and have a human leukocyte antigen (HLA) matched donor. It is also an option for
high-risk patients with poor prognostic factors (Gale, Armitage, and Butturini, 1989).

Chronic Lymphocytic Leukemia

Chronic lymphocytic leukemia (CLL) is characterized by the proliferation and accumulation of mature lymphocytes that are immunologically dysfunctional. CLL is
the most common leukemia in the United States, and it accounts for approximately
30% of all leukemia cases (Collins, 1990; Mitus and Rosenthal, 1991). Despite
advances in the treatment of CLL, the median survival period remains 4 to 6 years
(Morrison, 1994).

Treatment

One of the most difficult decisions regarding the treatment of CLL is when to initiate therapy. Disease-related symptoms (weight loss, fatigue, sweats, and fever),
progressive cytopenias (decrease in all blood cell lines) requiring transfusion, and
repeated infections that require antibiotics are three indications for therapy
(Cheson, 1990). Patients whose disease is in an early stage should be observed for
several months to see how the disease progresses (Rai et al., 1984; Silbar and Stahl,
1990). Single-agent chemotherapy with or without corticosteroids is indicated as
the disease begins to progress. Chlorambucil and cyclophosphamide are the
common therapeutic agents used. These agents are well tolerated, and each produces a response rate of 60% and complete remission in approximately 10% to 20%
of patients (Gale and Foon, 1987). Combination chemotherapy with either CVP

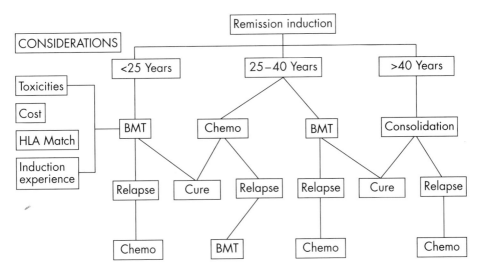

Fig. 15-1. Acute myelogenous leukemia treatment sequence. From Wujcik D: Options for postremission therapy in acute leukemia, Semin Oncol Nurs 6(1):25–30, 1990.

(cyclophosphamide, vincristine, and prednisone) or CHOP (cyclophosphamide, doxorubicin, vincristine [Oncovin], and prednisone) is used in more advanced stages of CLL (Gale and Foon, 1987). Fludarabine, a relatively new chemotherapeutic agent, may also be used to treat patients with advanced CLL, especially those who did not benefit from standard chemotherapy (Keating et al., 1989).

Other therapies used in the treatment of CLL include splenectomy, radiation therapy, and leukapheresis. Splenectomy is a palliative therapy used in patients with hemolytic anemia, thrombocytopenia, pancytopenia, or splenomegaly to decrease the pain. Splenectomy also reduces the white blood cell count and improves the red blood cell and platelet counts. Local radiation therapy, given in fractionated doses, works to control symptoms associated with lymphadenopathy and hypersplenism. Leukapheresis, a process that removes leukocytes from the blood, is used to immediately decrease the number of circulating lymphocytes; however, once leukapheresis has ended, the number of lymphocytes increases.

Chronic Myelogenous Leukemia

Chronic myelogenous leukemia (CML) involves the myeloid stem cell and is characterized by increased production of granulocytes, especially the neutrophils. The hallmark of CML is the presence of the Philadelphia chromosome (Ph), which can serve as a diagnostic marker. CML accounts for about 20% to 30% of adulthood leukemias in the United States (Carson and Callaghan, 1991; Mitus and Rosenthal, 1991).

Treatment

Treatment for CML is generally palliative. Currently allogeneic bone marrow transplantation offers the only chance of cure; however, the best time to perform the transplant remains controversial. The best results are achieved if the transplant is done early in the chronic stage and in patients who have not received busulfan therapy (Delage, Ritz, and Anderson, 1990; Snyder and McGlave, 1990).

Single-agent oral chemotherapy with busulfan or hydroxyurea is the most common therapy for CML. Used in the chronic stage, these agents control the growth of malignant cells and the symptoms associated with the disease. They do not eradicate the disease, however, and patients continue to have the Philadelphia chromosome. In spite of treatment, CML will progress to the terminal stage, at which point the disease is generally unresponsive to treatment (Collins, 1990). Combination chemotherapy involving a variety of agents has also been attempted, but it produces significant toxic side effects without improving the rate of survival from CML.

Alpha interferon (IFN-α) controls myeloid proliferation and reduces the number of Ph-positive cells. IFN-α has demonstrated a complete hematologic response rate of 70% (Talpaz et al., 1987). Researchers have also investigated combination chemotherapy using IFN-α and other agents that seem effective against CML. IFN-α with hydroxyurea produces rapid control of the disease and with longer duration than other regimens (Kantarjian et al., 1993).

❖ *Malignant Lymphomas*

The malignant lymphomas, Hodgkin's disease (HD) and non-Hodgkin's lymphoma (NHL), originate in the lymphatic system. This group of cancers represents the seventh most common malignancy in the United States. Lymphomas are one of the most studied malignancies, and one of the most curable. Although they share a few minor similarities, HD and NHL are considerably different.

Hodgkin's Disease

Hodgkin's disease accounts for less than 1% of all cancers in the United States (McFadden, 1993). Statisticians estimate that in 1995 7800 new cases of HD were diagnosed and 1450 HD-related deaths occurred (Wingo, Tong, and Bolden, 1995). Peak incidence occurs in the second decade of life and after age 45. HD is one of the most curable of all malignancies and one of the few for which conventional treatment is accepted.

Because patients with HD have a generally favorable prognosis—even patients with advanced disease—it is imperative to choose the treatment regimen carefully. Correct staging, the presence of prognostic indicators, and knowledge of the toxic effects related to various treatments are important considerations when choosing therapy. Aggressive therapy is usually appropriate for treating patients with poor prognostic factors such as being older than 60; having bulky mediastinal disease, cancer at a late stage, B symptoms (fever, night sweats, weight loss), lymphocyte depletion histology, or many Reed-Sternberg cells, and being male.

Treatment

The current treatment recommendations for HD are fairly standard and generally accepted. The goal of treatment is to cure the patient while avoiding treatment-associated complications. After a patient has achieved remission, the physician may recommend that the patient undergo bone marrow harvest and storage in case the malignancy recurs (Vose, Bierman, and Armitage, 1990).

Oncologists use radiation therapy curatively in most patients with early-stage disease and negative laparotomy (Cornbleet et al., 1985; McFadden, 1993; Moore and Cabanillas, 1993). Radiation therapy is generally administered to the involved nodal areas, including the mantle, the para-aortic-splenic pedicle, and pelvic regions (Figure 15-2) in fractionated doses for a total dose of 40 to 44 Gy. Studies show that extending the treatment fields to include adjacent, disease-free nodes helps obtain the desired cure rates (Eyre and Farver, 1991).

The standard and most commonly used chemotherapy regimens for treatment of HD include MOPP (mechlorethamine, vincristine [Oncovin], procarbazine, and prednisone) and ABVD (doxorubicin [Adriamycin], bleomycin, vinblastine, and dacarbazine). Each regimen can be administered separately in 28-day cycles, or alter-

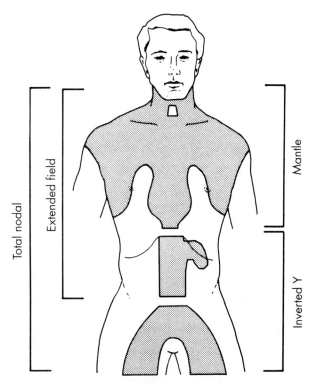

Fig. 15-2. Standard radiation fields for Hodgkin's disease. Mantle—from mandible to diaphragm; lungs, heart, spinal cord, and humeral heads are shielded. Inverted Y—from diaphragm to ischial tuberosities, including the spleen if not removed; spinal cord, kidneys, bladder, rectum, and gonads are shielded. Extended field—involves mantle zone and uppermost inverted-Y zone; does not include the pelvic, inguinal, or femoral nodes. Total nodal —mantle zone and complete inverted-Y zone. From McFadden ME: Malignant lymphomas. In Groenwald SL, Goodman M, Frogge MH, and Yarbro CH, editors: Cancer nursing: principles and practice, ed 3, Boston, 1993, Jones & Bartlett Publishers.

nating the regimen from cycle to cycle. When used separately, MOPP and ABVD produce expected remission rates of 80% to 85% in previously untreated patients, and 60% to 70% of those patients can expect long-term survival (McFadden, 1993). Combination therapy produces the same response rates but is thought to be superior because it avoids drug cross-resistance and prevents overlapping toxic effects to organs (Bonnadonna, Valagussa, and Santoro, 1986; Goldie, Coldman, and Guaduskus, 1982).

Patients with bulky disease and those with poor prognostic factors receive a combination of chemotherapy and radiation therapy (Henkelman, Hagemester, and Fuller, 1988). Combined-modality therapy can reduce the total dose of radiation necessary for disease eradication. This is especially important in children and adolescents, because it allows the administration of additional doses of chemotherapy and/or radiation therapy should the disease recur. Approximately 20% of patients will have residual or recurrent disease after the initial treatment. High-dose chemotherapy with bone marrow transplantation is another option for patients who experience recurrent disease (Vose, Bierman, and Armitage, 1990).

Non-Hodgkin's Lymphoma

Non-Hodgkin's lymphoma (NHL) refers to a heterogenous group of malignancies caused by the uncontrolled proliferation of abnormal lymphocytes. NHL resembles HD but does not have the characteristic Reed-Sternberg cell. It is estimated that 50,900 new cases of NHL were diagnosed in 1995 and that 22,700 NHL-related deaths occurred (Wingo, Tong, and Bolden, 1995).

Treatment

The histologic type, the extent of the disease, and the patient's performance status are the most important factors considered when determining treatment for NHL (Longo et al., 1993). The histologic type indicates the natural history of the lymphoma, and the treatment is based on the aggressiveness of the disease. For example, the natural history of a high-grade lymphoma may be only a few weeks' duration, and it will therefore be treated very aggressively. Because the majority of patients with NHL have disseminated disease at the time of diagnosis, the extent of disease, or staging, is a minor consideration. Because of the highly toxic therapies used for NHL, performance status is very important in determining appropriate treatment.

Controversy surrounds the thought that treatment of low-grade, or indolent, NHL alters the natural history of the disease (Young et al., 1988). Indolent lymphomas are sensitive to various chemotherapy regimens, which have a rate of complete remission of 60% to 70%, but the remissions only last a short time. Most patients experience several remissions and subsequent relapse and eventually die of their disease (Young, 1987). The most common chemotherapeutic agents used to treat low-grade lymphomas are cyclophosphamide and prednisone. Radiation (40 Gy) administered to the tumor and adjacent nodes is reported to provide a disease-free duration of 10 years in early-stage NHL (Paryani et al., 1983), and total body irradiation can result in complete remission in many patients with indolent NHL, although the remission is short-lived (McFadden, 1993). Fludarabine has produced second remissions in some patients with previously treated low-grade NHL (Hochster et al., 1992).

The treatment of choice for the more aggressive NHLs (intermediate and high-grade) is combination chemotherapy. For localized aggressive NHL, radiation administered to the site of disease has had some success; however, the risk of relapse in unirradiated sites is high. This risk can be decreased by combining radiation therapy with chemotherapy (McFadden, 1993). Regimens such as CHOP and BACOP (bleomycin, doxorubicin [Adriamycin], cyclophosphamide, vincristine [Oncovin], and prednisone) produce long-term remission in 35% to 45% of patients. Other combinations using methotrexate with leucovorin or cytosine arabinoside as a prophylactic CNS treatment have also been developed and have been reported to improve the long-term survival rate (Longo et al., 1993). More recently, researchers report new high-dose chemotherapy regimens developed in an attempt to improve patients' chances of long-term survival (Sweetman, Mead, and Whitehouse, 1991; Vitolo et al., 1992; Zuckerman, LoBuglio, and Reeves, 1990). Studies combining biotherapy and chemotherapy have also shown promise (see the Research Highlight below).

For patients with recurrent or unresponsive aggressive NHL, the chance of remission is minimal, and cure is rare. These patients have decreased bone marrow reserve as a result of previous therapy and therefore cannot tolerate additional treatment (McFadden, 1993). High-dose chemotherapy followed by bone marrow transplantation produces durable second remissions in some patients (Bitran et al.,

---

RESEARCH HIGHLIGHT

Solal-Celigny P, Lepage E, Brousse N, Reyes F, Haioun C, Leporrier M, Peuchmaur M, Bosly A, Parlier Y, Brice P, Coiffier B, and Gisselbrecht C: Recombinant interferon alfa-2b combined with a regimen containing doxorubicin in patients with advanced follicular lymphoma, N Eng J Med 329:1608–1614, 1993.

Study Patients received chemotherapy alone or chemotherapy with interferon alfa-2b. The chemotherapy regimen consisted of cyclophosphamide given as 600 mg/m^2, doxorubicin given as 25 mg/m^2, teniposide (VM-26) given as 60 mg/m^2, and prednisone given as 40 mg/m^2 (CHVP) monthly for six cycles and then every 2 months for 1 year. Interferon was administered at a dose of 5 million units 3 times weekly for 18 months.

Sample The study included 242 patients with advanced low-grade follicular non-Hodgkin's lymphoma.

Study aim To evaluate the benefit of concomitant administration of interferon alfa-2b with a doxorubicin-based regimen in patients with follicular non-Hodgkin's lymphoma.

Findings The patients who received CHVP with interferon alfa-2b experienced a higher response rate (85% vs 69%), a longer period of event-free survival (34 months vs 19 months), and higher rate of survival at 3 years (86% vs 69%).

Discussion Patients who received CHVP with interferon had a 12% incidence of grade 3 neutropenia compared with a 2% incidence in patients who received CHVP alone. Cardiac toxicity caused the cessation of doxorubicin treatment in one patient. Treatment with interferon was stopped in 13 patients (11%) because of adverse reactions to the interferon, the most common of which was fatigue (7 patients).

Possible Side Effects from Multimodal Therapy in

Hematopoietic and Immunologic Cancers

Multimodal Treatment	*Possible Enhanced Side Effects*
Leukemia	
Chemotherapy with prophylactic cranial radiation therapy	
Daunorubicin, vincristine, asparaginase, prednisone	Cerebella, neurotoxicity, alopecia
Chemobiotherapy	
Hydroxyurea with interferon	Fatigue
High-dose chemotherapy with total body radiation therapy followed by bone marrow transplantation	
Cyclophosphamide, etoposide, busulfan	Nausea, vomiting, mucositis, bone
Carboplatin	marrow depression, diarrhea,
Cisplatin	esophagitis, organ toxicity,
Ifosfamide	photosensitivity
Cytosine	
Non-Hodgkin's Lymphoma	
Chemotherapy followed by radiation therapy followed by chemotherapy	
Cyclophosphamide, vincristine, prednisone	Nausea, vomiting, mucositis, diar-
Cyclophosphamide, vincristine, procarbazine, prednisone	rhea, organ toxicity (depends on site irradiated), bone marrow toxicity,
Bleomycin, doxorubicin, cyclophosphamide, vincristine, prednisone	increased risk of acute nonlym- phocytic leukemia
Cyclophosphamide, doxorubicin, vincristine	
Cyclophosphamide, vincristine, methotrexate, cytarabine	
Methotrexate, bleomycin, doxorubicin, vincristine, cyclophosphamide, dexamethasone	
Concomitant chemobiotherapy	
Cyclophosphamide, doxorubicin, teniposide, prednisone, interferon alfa-2	Increased white blood cell count, fatigue
Hodgkin's Disease	
Chemotherapy and mantle radiation therapy	
Mechlorethamine, vincristine, procarbazine, prednisone	Breast cancer, acute leukemia, thyroid disease, photosensitivity, dysphagia, nausea, vomiting, bone marrow depression, pulmonary toxicity

Data taken from Billingham et al., 1977; Biti et al., 1994; Fraser and Tucker, 1989; Hancock, Cox, and McDougall, 1991; Hancock, Tucker, and Hoppe, 1993; Rubin, Constine, and Nelson, 1992; Showel, Hoover, and Deutsch, 1993; Solal-Celigny et al., 1993; and Yahalom et al., 1992.

Multimodal Treatment	Possible Enhanced Side Effects
Doxorubicin, bleomycin, vinblastine, dacarbazine	Radiation recall esophagitis, radiation recall dermatitis, mucositis, bone marrow depression, cardiac and pulmonary toxicity
Chemotherapy and inverted-y radiation therapy Mechlorethamine, vincristine, procarbazine, prednisone Doxorubicin, bleomycin, vinblastine, dacarbazine	Nausea, vomiting, diarrhea, bone marrow depression, photosensitivity

1990; Freedman, Takvorian, and Anderson, 1990; Gribben et al., 1989; Troussard et al., 1990).

❖ *Nursing Management*

Nurses need to have astute assessment skills when caring for patients with hematopoietic and immunologic malignancies because these patients may experience various side effects related to the disease and/or its treatment. Possible Side Effects from Multimodal Therapy are presented on page 264. As already discussed, these malignancies commonly affect the CNS, and nurses and family members are often the first to detect this complication. It is therefore imperative that family members learn the signs and symptoms of CNS involvement. Nurses should assess patient mobility, sensory difficulties, cognition, and self-care abilities during each interaction with the patient. Subtle changes may indicate spinal cord compression or metastasis to the CNS. Other problems associated with the disease include myelosuppression, disseminated intravascular coagulation (DIC) (see the Nursing Care table on page 266), which is a bleeding disorder characterized by uncontrolled bleeding and clot formation, and superior vena cava syndrome (see Chapter 9, Lung Cancer). These complications can be life threatening and require immediate action from the health care team.

Radiation therapy and chemotherapy can cause major side effects that significantly affect the patient's quality of life. Complications associated with radiation therapy depend on the site of treatment. For example, if the mantle is irradiated, the patient may experience loss of taste, dry mouth, redness of skin, hair loss in that region, dysphagia, nausea, and vomiting. Complications associated with chemotherapy depend on the specific agents used. The most common complication related to the treatment regimen is severe, prolonged myelosuppression, which requires blood transfusions (see Patient Education Guidelines on page 267). The severity and duration of myelosuppression can delay the treatment plan and/or require a decrease of the dosage, which may adversely affect the outcome of the treatment. One of the most disturbing treatment-related issues regarding these malignancies are the delayed effects of treatment that produce lifelong problems such as infertility, pericarditis,

Nursing Care of

The Patient with Disseminated Intravascular Coagulation (DIC)

Nursing Care	Rationale/Comments
◆ Assess for evidence of bleeding and/or thrombosis: ◆ Skin and mucous membranes— petechiae, ecchymosis, purpura, pallor, frank blood or oozing from venipuncture and wound sites (bone marrow biopsy site, etc.) ◆ Pulmonary—crackling, wheezing, or stridor when lungs are auscultated; dyspnea, tachypnea, cyanosis, hemoptysis, or chest pain ◆ Cardiovascular—tachycardia, hypotension, diminished peripheral pulses, palpitations, or angina ◆ Renal—peripheral edema, oliguria, hematuria ◆ Gastrointestinal—abdominal distention, decreased bowel sounds, positive guaiac stool test ◆ Neurologic—headache, blurred vision, vertigo, changes in mental status	◆ Early detection and prompt intervention provide the best prognosis
◆ Monitor laboratory values for abnormalities that may indicate bleeding, including complete blood count, platelet count, prothrombin time, partial thromboplastin time, thrombin time, fibrinogen level, fibrin-split products	◆ Early detection and prompt intervention provide the best prognosis; use the lab values to determine patient's response to treatment
◆ Institute safety measures: assist with ambulation; keep side rails elevated at all times	◆ Increased potential for injury related to clot forming in the microcirculation, low platelet levels, consumption of clotting factors, and clot dissolution
◆ Monitor fluid volume and prevent deficits ◆ Measure intake and output ◆ Administer fluids, blood, and blood products	◆ Detects dehydration and hemodynamic instability
◆ Provide patient and family education	◆ The more the patient and family understand, the less anxious and more cooperative they will be

Patient Education Guidelines for

Blood Component Transfusions

◆ Chemotherapy used to treat cancer destroys normal cells at the same time as they destroy cancer cells. Some of the cells most severely affected by this include cells in your blood (red blood cells, white blood cells, and platelets).

◆ Your nurse and your physician will periodically monitor the number of these cells by doing a complete blood count (CBC) with a differential and platelet count.

◆ If the counts get too low or if you begin to have symptoms of low blood counts, a blood transfusion may be required.

◆ The types of components commonly transfused include the following:
  ◆ Red blood cells
  ◆ Platelets
  ◆ Plasma
  ◆ Cryoprecipitate

◆ We will draw blood from you periodically to ensure that the donor's blood type matches yours. We also will double-check to ensure that you receive the correct blood. The blood bank screens all donors and blood for diseases such as hepatitis and HIV, so the chance of your receiving infected blood is minimal.

◆ Your nurse or physician will discuss how your family and friends can donate blood directly to you or replace blood taken from the blood bank.

◆ You may receive medications prior to the transfusion to decrease the incidence or severity of side effects.

◆ The most common side effects of transfusions are fever and chills. Your nurse will monitor you frequently throughout the transfusion. Notify the nurse if you begin to feel any of these symptoms.

Permission granted to reproduce these guidelines for educational purposes only.

---

cardiomyopathy, pneumonitis, and secondary malignancies. It is important for patients and family members to be aware of the long-term effects of the malignancy and the resources available to them for support and assistance.

❖ Summary

Although very complex, caring for patients with hematopoietic and immunologic malignancies can also be challenging and satisfying. Nurses can have a major impact on the quality of life of patients and families. Relationships are formed that may last for years.

❖ References

Billingham MF, Bristow MR, Glatstein E, Mason JW, Masek MA, and Daniels JR: Adriamycin cardiotoxicity: endomyocardial biopsy evidence of enhancement by irradiation, Am J Surg Path 1:17–23, 1977.

Biti G, Cellai E, Magrini SM, Papi MG, Ponticelli P, and Boddi V: Second solid tumors and leukemia after treatment for Hodgkin's disease: an analysis of 1121 patients from a single institution, Int J Radiat Oncol Biol Phys 29:25–31, 1994.

Bitran JD, Williams SF, Moormeier J, and Mick J: High-dose combination chemotherapy with thiotepa and autologous hematopoietic stem cell reinfusion in the treatment of patients with relapsed refractory lymphoma, Semin Oncol 17:39–42, 1990.

Bonnadonna G, Valagussa P, and Santoro A: Alternating non-cross resistance combination chemotherapy or MOPP in stage IV Hodgkin's disease, Ann Int Med 104:739–746, 1986.

Carson C and Callaghan ME: Hematopoietic and immunologic cancers. In Baird SB, McCorkle R, and Grant M, editors: Cancer nursing: a comprehensive textbook, Philadelphia, 1991, WB Saunders Co, pp. 536–566.

Champlin R: Acute myelogenous leukemia: biology and treatment, Mediguide to Oncol 8:1–9, 1988.

Cheson BD: The acute leukemias. In Wittes RE, editor: Manual of oncology therapeutics, Philadelphia, 1990, JB Lippincott Co, pp. 251–260.

Collins PM: Diagnosis and treatment of chronic leukemia, Semin Oncol Nurs 6:31–43, 1990.

Cornbleet MA, Vitolo U, Ultman JE, Golomb HM, Oleske D, Griem ML, Ferguson DJ, and Miller JB: Pathologic stages of IA and IIA Hodgkin's disease: results of treatment with radiotherapy alone (1968–1980), J Clin Oncol 3:758–768, 1985.

Delage R, Ritz J, and Anderson KC: The evolving role of bone marrow transplantation in the treatment of chronic myelogenous leukemia, Hematol Clin N Am 4:369–388, 1990.

Devine SM and Larson RA: Acute leukemia in adults: recent developments in diagnosis and treatment, CA-Cancer J Clin 44:326–352, 1994.

Eyre HJ and Farver ML: Hodgkin's disease and non-Hodgkin's lymphoma. In Holleb AI, Fink DJ, and Murphy GP, editors: Textbook of clinical oncology, Atlanta, 1991, American Cancer Society, pp. 377–396.

Fraser MC and Tucker MA: Second malignancies following cancer therapy, Semin Oncol Nurs 5:43–55, 1989.

Freedman AS, Takvorian T, and Anderson KC: Autologous bone marrow transplant in B-cell non-Hodgkin's lymphoma: very low treatment-related mortality in 100 patients in sensitive relapse, J Clin Oncol 8:784–791, 1990.

Gale RP, Armitage JO, and Butturini A: Is there a role of autotransplants in acute leukemia?, Bone Marrow Transplant 4:217–219, 1989.

Gale RP and Foon KA: Therapy of acute myelogenous leukemia, Semin Hematol 24:40–54, 1987.

Goldie JH, Coldman AJ, and Guaduskus GA: Rationale for use of alternating non-cross resistant chemotherapy, Canc Treat Rep 66:439–449, 1982.

Gribben JG, Linch DC, Singer CR, McMillan AK, Jarrett M, and Goldstone AH: Successful treatment of refractory Hodgkin's disease by high-dose combination chemotherapy and autologous bone marrow transplant, Blood 73:340–344, 1989.

Hancock SL, Cox RS, and McDougall IR: Thyroid disease after treatment of Hodgkin's disease, N Eng J Med 325:599–605, 1991.

Hancock SL, Tucker MA, and Hoppe RT: Breast cancer after treatment of Hodgkin's disease, J Natl Cancer Inst 85:25–31, 1993.

Henderson ES: Acute lymphocytic leukemia. In Williams WJ, Beutler E, Erslev AJ, and Lichtman MA, editors: Hematology, New York, 1983, McGraw-Hill, pp. 970–978.

Henkelman GC, Hagemester FB, and Fuller LM: Two cycles of MOPP and radiotherapy for stage IIIA and IIIB Hodgkin's disease, J Clin Oncol 6:1293–1302, 1988.

Hiddemann W, Kretzman H, Straif K, Wolf-Dieter L, Mertelsma R, Planaker M, Donhuijsen-Ant R, Lengfelder E, Arlin Z, and Buchner T: High-dose cytosine arabinoside in combination with mito-xantrone for the treatment of refractory acute myeloid and lymphoblastic leukemia, Semin Oncol 14:73–77, 1987.

Hochster HS, Kim K, Green MD, Mann RB, Neiman RS, Oken MM, Cassileth PA, Stott P, Ritch P, and O'Connell MJ: Activity of fludarabine in previously treated non-Hodgkin's low-grade lymphoma: results of an Eastern Cooperative Group study, J Clin Oncol 10:28–32, 1992.

Hoeltzer D and Gale RP: Acute lymphoblastic leukemia in adults: recent progress, future directions, Semin Hematol 24:27–39, 1987.

Kantarjian HM, Diesseroth A, Kurzrock R, Estrov Z, and Talpaz M: Chronic myelogenous leukemia: a concise update, Blood 82:691–703, 1993.

Keating MJ, Kantarjian H, Talpaz M, Radman J, Koller C, Barlogie B, Velasquez W, Plumkett H, Friedrich EJ and McCredie KB: A new agent with major activity against chronic lymphocytic leukemia, Blood 74:19–25, 1989.

Lachant NA and Skeel RT: Acute leukemias. In Skeel RT, editor: Handbook of cancer chemotherapy, Boston, 1991, Little, Brown & Co, pp. 284–311.

Longo DL, DeVita VT, Jaffe ES, Mach P, and Urba WJ: Lymphocytic lymphomas. In Devita VT, Hellman S, and Rosenberg SA: Cancer: principles and practice of oncology, ed 3, Philadelphia, 1993, JB Lippincott Co, pp. 1859–1927.

Maguire-Eisen M: Diagnosis and treatment of adult acute leukemia, Semin Oncol Nurs 6:17–24, 1990.

McFadden ME: Malignant lymphomas. In Groenwald SL, Goodman M, Frogge MH, and Yarbro CH, editors: Cancer nursing: principles and practice, ed 3, Boston, 1993, Jones & Bartlett Publishers, pp. 1200–1228.

Mitus AJ, and Rosenthal DS: Adult leukemias. In Holleb AI, Fink DJ, and Murphy GP, editors: Textbook of clinical oncology, Atlanta, 1991, American Cancer Society, pp. 410–432.

Moore DF and Cabanillas F: What constitutes a "cure" in lymphoma?, Leuk Lymph 11(3–4):161–163, 1993.

Morrison VA: Chronic leukemias, CA-Cancer J Clin 44:353–377, 1994.

Mortimer J, Blinder MA, Schulman S, Applebaum FR, Buckner CD, Clift RA, Sanders JE, Storb R, and Thomas ED: Relapse of acute leukemia after marrow transplantation: natural history and results of subsequent therapy, J Clin Oncol 7:50–57, 1989.

Nooter K, Sonneveld P, Oostrum R, Herweijer H, Hagenbeek T, and Valerio D: Overexpression of the *mdrl* gene in blast cells from patients with acute myelocytic leukemia is associated with decreased anthracycline accumulation that can be restored by cyclosporine, Int J Cancer 45:262–268, 1990.

Paryani SB, Hoppe RT, Cox RS, Colby TV, Rosenberg SA, and Kaplan HS: Analysis of non-Hodgkin's lymphomas with nodular and favorable histologies, stage I and II, Cancer 52:2300–2307, 1983.

Rai KR, Sawintsky A, Jagathambal K, Gartenhaus W, and Phillips E: Chronic lymphocytic leukemia, Med Clin Am 68:697–711, 1984.

Rubin P, Constine LS, and Nelson DF: Late effects of cancer treatment: radiation and drug toxicity. In Perez CA and Brady LW, editors: Principles and practice of radiation oncology, ed 2, Philadelphia, 1992, JB Lippincott Co, pp. 124–161.

Showel J, Hoover SV, and Deutsch S: Radiation-recall, Int J Radiat Oncol Biol Phys 24:929, 1993 (letter).

Silbar R and Stahl R: Chronic lymphocytic leukemia and related diseases. In Williams WJ, Beutler E, Erslev AJ, and Lichtman MA, editors: Hematology, New York, 1990, McGraw-Hill, pp. 1005–1024.

Snyder DS and McGlave PB: Treatment of chronic myelogenous leukemia with bone marrow transplantation, Hematol Clin N Am 4:535–557, 1990.

Solal-Celigny P, Lepage E, Brousse N, Reyes F, Haioun C, Leporrier M, Peuchmaur M, Bosly A, Parlier Y, Brice P, Coiffier B, and Gisselbrecht C: Recombinant interferon alfa-2b combined with a regimen containing doxorubicin in patients with advanced follicular lymphoma, N Eng J Med 329:1608–1614, 1993.

Sweetman JW, Mead GM, and Whitehouse JMA: Intensive weekly combination chemotherapy for patients with intermediate-grade and high-grade non-Hodgkin's lymphoma, J Clin Oncol 9:2202–2209, 1991.

Talpaz M, Kantarjian HM, McCredie KB, Keating MJ, Truliio J, and Gutterman J: Clinical investigation of human alpha interferon in chronic myelogenous leukemia, Blood 69:1280–1288, 1987.

Troussard X, Leblond V, Kuentz M, Milpied M, Jauet JP, Cordonnier C, Leporrier M, and Vernant JP: Allogeneic bone marrow transplantation in adults with Burkitts's lymphoma or acute lymphoblastic leukemia in first remission, J Clin Oncol 8:809–812, 1990.

Vitolo U, Bertini M, Brusomolino E, Cavaller GB, Comotti B, Gallo E, Ghio R, Levis A, Luxi G, Menegheini V, Novero D, Orsucci L, Rota-Scalabrini D, Tarella C, Todeschini G, Viero P, Barbui T, Bernasconi C, Perona G, Pileri A, and Resegotti L: MACOP-B treatment in diffuse large-cell lymphoma: identification of prognostic groups in an Italian multicenter study, J Clin Oncol 10:219–227, 1992.

Vogelsang GB: Bone marrow transplantation, Mediguide to Oncol 9:1–6, 1989.

Vose JM, Bierman PJ, and Armitage JO: Hodgkin's disease: the role of bone marrow transplantation, Semin Oncol 17:749–757, 1990.

Wingo PA, Tong T, and Bolden S: Cancer statistics, 1995, CA-Cancer J Clin 45:8–30, 1995.

Wolff SN, Herzig RH, Phillips CL, Lazarus HM, Greer JP, Stein RS, Ray WA, and Herzig GP: High-dose cytosine arabinoside and daunorubicin as consolidation therapy for acute nonlymphocytic leukemia in first remission: an update, Semin Oncol 14:12–17, 1987.

Yahalom J, Petrek JA, Biddinger PW, Kessler S, Dershaw DD, McCormick B, Osborne MP, Kinne DA, and Rosen PP: Breast cancer in patients irradiated for Hodgkin's disease: a clinical and pathologic analysis of 45 events in 37 patients, J Clin Oncol 10:1674–1681, 1992.

Young RC: Combination chemotherapy in advanced non-Hodgkin's lymphoma, Adv Oncol 3(2):20–26, 1987.

Young RC, Longo DL, Glatstein E, Ihde DC, Jaffe ES, and DeVita VT: The treatment of indolent lymphomas; watchful waiting vs aggressive combined modality, Semin Hematol 24(suppl 2):11–16, 1988.

Zuckerman KS, LoBuglio AF, and Reeves JA: Chemotherapy of intermediate- and high-grade non-Hodgkin's lymphomas with a high-dose doxorubicin-containing regimen, J Clin Oncol 8:248–259, 1990.

Chapter 16

❖ *Malignant Melanoma*

Alice J. Longman

The past several decades have seen a dramatic increase in the incidence of malignant melanoma. The incidence is rising faster than any other cancer, with an overall increase of about 4% each year (American Cancer Society, 1995; Friedman et al., 1991). In 1995, statisticians expect to see more than 34,000 diagnoses of malignant melanoma (Wingo, Tong, and Bolden, 1995). Caucasians are 10 times more likely than African Americans to develop malignant melanoma. The 5-year survival rate is 84%, although, when detected and treated early, malignant melanoma is highly curable. An estimated 7200 persons will die from malignant melanoma in 1995 (Wingo, Tong, and Bolden, 1995).

Ninety percent of melanomas arise in the skin, and the rest develop in the eye and the mucous membranes of the mouth and the anus (Longman, 1991). The prognosis is good if the lesion is localized and thin. Two phases of growth, radial and vertical, occur in malignant melanoma (Lawler, 1991). Malignant melanoma grows in a horizontal fashion in the epidermis during the *radial phase*. As the tumor continues to grow, the atypical cells descend into the underlying tissues, activity known as the *vertical phase*. In the vertical phase, neoplastic cells have an increased potential for metastasis.

The characteristic features of early malignant melanoma can best be remembered by thinking of ABCD: *A* for asymmetry, *B* for border irregularity, *C* for color variegation, and *D* for diameter (Friedman et al., 1991) (Box 16-1). The prognosis depends on the depth of invasion, the anatomic site, the presence or absence of ulceration, and the thickness and growth pattern of the tumor. Therefore, nurses should be especially mindful of and teach the early warning signs of malignant melanoma (Friedman et al., 1991). Look for the following changes in moles:

Color, especially in relation to the spread of color
Size, especially sudden enlargement
Shape, in relation to the margins
Elevation, especially sudden elevation

Surface, especially scaliness or crusting
Surrounding skin, especially redness
Sensation, including itching and tenderness
Consistency, including softening

❖ *Treatment*

The mainstay of treatment for malignant melanoma is surgery. However, microscopic disease can remain, causing recurrence of the disease (Miller et al., 1995).

Surgery

The diagnosis of malignant melanoma is usually made by an excisional biopsy, which entails removal of the lesion as well as 2 to 3 mm of normal tissue surrounding the lesion. The exception may be very large lesions, in which case an incisional biopsy (only a piece of the lesion is removed) may be the treatment of choice. Wide local excision includes the full thickness of skin and subcutaneous fat. Opinions differ regarding management of the defect after excision of a melanoma. Direct closure is possible and recommended if the margin is 2 millimeters or less (Holmstrom, 1992). For some defects, a free graft or a skin flap may be necessary. Many surgeons advocate nodal dissection for later stages of the disease, although its necessity is controversial in stage I (Holmstrom, 1992).

Surgery is also used for palliation of disease and symptomatic involvement. Surgical removal of a solitary lesion is recommended if the lesion is accessible.

Chemotherapy

The usefulness of adjuvant chemotherapy (as an addition to surgery) remains questionable in the treatment of malignant melanoma. For the treatment of disseminated melanoma the agent with the most consistent activity is dacarbazine. The nitrosoureas (carmustine, lomustine, semustine, and chlorozotocin) have also been used in metastatic disease. Other single agents that oncologists have used with varying success include the vinca alkaloids, melphalan, cisplatin, and procarbazine (Lawler, 1991). Clinical trials combining the hormonal agents tamoxifen (McClay and McClay, 1994) or megestrol acetate (Nathanson, Meelu, and Losada, 1994) with other chemotherapeutic agents remain inconclusive.

Box 16-1 Clinical Features of Early Malignant Melanoma

Asymmetry of Shape: One half of the lesion does not match the other half.

Border Irregularity: Lack of distinct edge in border.

Color Variegation: Pigmentation is not uniform.

Diameter Change: Greater than 6 mm.

Radiation Therapy

Many oncologists regard metastatic or recurrent melanoma as radiation-resistant. However, although melanoma may be a radiation-resistant tumor, not all tumor cells are resistant. For local recurrence of gross residual disease, large individual dose fractions sometimes prove effective. Under investigation is the combination of hyperthermia and radiation. For elderly patients with lesions in areas unsuitable for surgery, radiation therapy may be the treatment of choice. Patients often benefit from radiation therapy for palliation of symptoms. For relief of neurologic symptoms, radiation in conjunction with steroids may offer relief (Loescher and Booth, 1990).

Surgery Followed by Adjuvant Biotherapy

Experimental adjuvant studies are being conducted that use the patient's own tumor after surgical excision and radiation therapy to kill melanoma cells. The melanoma cells, prepared as a vaccine, are injected back into the patient to stimulate the body's antigen-antibody response to fight the melanoma (Miller et al., 1995). Interferon alpha is also used investigationally as an adjuvant treatment (Barth and Morton, 1995).

Chemobiotherapy

Interleukin-2 (IL-2) followed by high-dose cisplatin (Demchak et al., 1991) or dacarbazine and cisplatin (Flaherty et al., 1993) improves the response rate in metastatic disease when compared with any of these agents used alone. Falkson, Falkson, and Falkson (1991) compared treatment with dacarbazine alone to treatment with dacarbazine plus interferon alpha-2b and found an increased survival rate in the group that received the combination drugs (see Research Highlight on page 274). By giving concomitant chemotherapy (carmustine, cisplatin, and dacarbazine), hormonal therapy (tamoxifen), and biotherapy (IL-2 and interferon alpha-2a), Richards and colleagues (1992) were again able to increase the rate of response to treatment.

❖ Uveal Melanoma

The iris, the ciliary body, and choroid portions of the eye may be sites of uveal melanoma. Some of the predisposing factors include ocular melanocytosis, ocular nevi, and neurofibromatosis. An important risk factor may be intermittent, intense exposure to ultraviolet radiation (Loescher and Booth, 1990; Longman, 1992).

Tumors that affect the iris and ciliary body respond well to local resection. Choroidal melanoma may require enucleation (removal of the eye), although this is controversial because many researchers think it leads to tumor cell dissemination and metastases. The most common nonenucleation therapy is radiation therapy.

❖ Nursing Management

Strategies for the reduction of the incidence of malignant melanoma involve professional education, increasing public awareness, prevention, and early detection.

```
┌─ RESEARCH HIGHLIGHT ──────────────────────────────────────
```

Falkson CI, Falkson G, and Falkson HC: Improved results with the addition of interferon alfa-b to dacarbazine in the treatment of patients with metastatic malignant melanoma, J Clin Oncol 9:1403–1408, 1991.

Study Patients were randomized to receive dacarbazine given as 200 mg/m² continuous infusion for 5 days on a 28-day schedule or interferon alfa-2 given as 15 mU/m² intravenously 5 days a week for 3 weeks and then 10 mU/m² subcutaneously 3 times a week as well as the same dacarbazine treatment described above, which started 28 days after the interferon was initiated.

Sample The study included 64 patients with confirmed metastatic malignant melanoma. The median age was 64, and 43 patients were male. All had good performance status (ECOG 0 to 1); none had concurrent malignancy, cardiac disease, or brain metastasis.

Study aim To see whether or not the addition of interferon alfa-2b to dacarbazine improved response to treatment.

Findings The study documented an objective response by 20% of the patients on dacarbazine alone and 53% of the patients on both dacarbazine and interferon alfa-2b. Of the patients on dacarbazine alone, 2 had a complete response (no evidence of disease), whereas 10 patients on dacarbazine and interferon alfa-2b had a complete response.

Discussion The interferon alfa-2b greatly improved response to treatment, although side effects were more severe in the group receiving both agents. Both groups experienced about the same nausea and vomiting, but the group receiving combined therapy had greater bone marrow depression, more flulike symptoms, and neurologic toxicity ranging from mild headache to confusion. This study used a small sample size and needs to be repeated with more patients, but it demonstrates that there is a role for interferon alfa-2b with dacarbazine for patients with metastatic melanoma. Implications for nurses include treatment of increased side effects.

Malignant melanoma, if detected and treated early, is a highly curable disease. Caucasians who have developed one malignant melanoma have a 5% risk of developing a new melanoma (Seidman et al., 1985) and need to be closely monitored.

Screening

Educating health professionals and the public about the hazards of excessive exposure to ultraviolet radiation is of the utmost importance. There are five factors to consider in the exposure of the skin to ultraviolet radiation. These include the time of day when exposure occurs, the geographical area where exposure occurs, the altitude or weather conditions, the time of year, and the length of exposure (Loescher, 1993; Longman, 1992)(Box 16-2).

To avoid dangerous exposure, the National Cancer Institute, the American Cancer Society, the Skin Cancer Foundation, and the American Academy of Dermatology recommend minimizing excessive sun exposure between the hours of

Box 16-2 Arizona Sun Awareness Project

Southern Arizona receives one of the highest intensities of ultraviolet radiation in the United States. People living in southern Arizona are at risk for developing malignant melanoma because of the intensity of sunlight, the latitude (32 degrees north), and the altitude (2410 feet) and because Arizona has clear skies for more than 190 days of the year.

The National Oceanic and Atmospheric Administration, which is studying ozone concentration, has confirmed the high intensity of ultraviolet radiation in southern Arizona with the use of a Robertson-Berger sunburn meter. The meter detects solar ultraviolet radiation with a wavelength shorter than 333 nanometers (UV-B), the response varying with decreasing wavelengths. The data produced by the meter have been termed the *sunburn unit* (SBU). The SBU is equal to a minimal erythema dose or the amount of UV-B radiation that will produce redness within 24 hours after exposure.

The Robertson-Berger sunburn meter at the Arizona Health Sciences Center prints the sun-intensity data on paper tape every 30 minutes. The sun-intensity index is reported to the local newspapers and television stations for inclusion in their weather reports. A sample report follows:

Minutes in Sun Today to Redden Skin

Time	Minutes
9 A.M.	40
10 A.M.	21
11 A.M.	17
Noon	16
1 P.M.	14
2 P.M.	22
3 P.M.	23
4 P.M.	32

From Arizona Sun Awareness Project, University of Arizona Cancer Center.

10:00 A.M. and 3:00 P.M., when ultraviolet rays are the most intense; staying aware that surfaces such as sand, snow, or water can reflect more than half of the ultraviolet radiation that bombards the skin, and avoiding tanning parlors because the UV-A radiation emitted by tanning booths damages the deep layers of the skin.

Dermatologists advocate the use of sunscreens during sun exposure for all persons over 12 years of age (Bargoil and Erdman, 1993). For children under 12 years of age, sunscreens formulated for adults should not be used because children are more sensitive to the chemicals in adult formulas. For infants under 6 months of age, physicians do not recommend the use of sunscreens, and parents therefore should keep them out of direct sunlight. Recommendations for using sunscreens include a sun-protection factor (SPF) of 15 or more, applying it at least 15 minutes before every exposure to the sun, and reapplying it at least every 2 hours thereafter. Waterproof sunscreens are available for use when swimming or by those who perspire heavily (Bargoil and Erdman, 1993; Berwick et al., 1991; Lawler and Schreiber, 1989; Loescher and Booth, 1990; Longman, 1992). Other protective behaviors include wearing cover-up clothing such as a long-sleeved shirt and long pants of a loose fabric, a wide-brimmed hat, and sunglasses.

Health professionals and the general public should know about skin pigmentation and the erythema caused by the sun (Table 16-1). The harmful effects of sun exposure begin in childhood, and the effects may appear by the time a person reaches young adulthood. People with fair skin, blue or green eyes, blond or red hair, and freckles have a higher risk of sun damage.

Early Detection

Early detection of malignant melanoma should occur as part of an individual's routine health care. Those persons with atypical moles, familial atypical moles, and melanoma syndrome are at high risk for the development of malignant melanoma. Those at high risk should have skin examinations every 3 to 6 months, along with baseline and follow-up photographs of atypical moles (Loescher, 1993). They should also learn skin self-examination techniques (see Patient Education Guidelines on page 277).

Friedman et al. (1991) described the technique of epiluminescence using the dermatascope (dermoscopy) to examine pigmented lesions. The technique uses mineral oil placed on the surface of the lesion. The mineral oil allows the examiner to see through the stratum corneum of the skin. They caution that more work has to be done to establish the positive predictive value of this skin assessment technique.

Skin assessment and examination are key to early detection of malignant melanoma. The examination requires good lighting, and a magnifying glass may be used if necessary. A thorough examination must include the following steps:

- Inspection and palpation of all accessible skin surfaces
- Assessment of preexisting lesions on the skin such as nevi
- Inspection of the scalp and entire hairline
- Inspection of the face, the lips, and the neck
- Inspection and palpation of all surfaces of the upper extremities
- Inspection and palpation of the skin of the back, the buttocks, and the back of the legs

Table 16-1   Skin Types and Skin Reactions

Skin Type	Skin Reactions
1	Burns easily and severely; tans little or not at all
2	Burns easily and severely; tans minimally or lightly
3	Burns moderately; tans approximately average
4	Burns minimally; tans easily
5	Burns rarely; tans easily and substantially
6	Never burns; tans profusely

Patient Education Guidelines for

Skin Cancer Screening and Examination

♦ Skin cancer screening can be part of routine preventive health care. It can occur in the home, in the workplace, and in the community.

♦ Skin cancer awareness has increased as the incidence of malignant melanoma in the world has risen.

♦ To screen for skin cancer, health professionals conduct a total body examination.

♦ For the examination, individuals should undress to their underwear.

♦ Ask if the individual has noted suspicious lesions or if there are changes in any existing nevi.

♦ The ABCDs can identify potential malignant lesions and are easy to teach.

♦ The assessment of each region of the body is essential. A complete examination begins with the scalp and proceeds downward.

♦ Urge individuals to do skin self-examination. The procedure is essentially the same as that done by health professionals.

♦ For individuals at high risk, monthly skin self-examination is recommended.

♦ Guidelines for high-risk individuals include routine skin self-examination, examination by a dermatologist twice a year, and screening of other family members.

Permission granted to reproduce these guidelines for educational purposes only.

The skin should also be assessed for changes in existing moles such as size, shape, color, and history of itching or burning in existing moles (Longman, 1992).

The nursing management of patients with malignant melanoma depends on the treatment modality. A diagnosis of malignant melanoma naturally raises concerns in the patient and the family, and both patient and family should be included in nursing care planning (Lawler, 1991; Loescher and Booth, 1990; Longman, 1992).

Short-term Treatment Strategies

After excision of the lesion, the patient receives instruction regarding the prevention of infection and trauma at the excision site. Those patients having split-thickness skin grafts should have the donor and recipient sites protected and monitored for infection and hemorrhage (Lawler, 1991) (see Nursing Care of the Skin Graft Site on page 278). For those with lymph node dissection, instruction is given about protection of the involved extremity from infection and trauma. In some patients, lymphedema may occur, but elevating the extremity can minimize risk of its occurrence.

Nursing interventions include management of side effects related to multimodal therapy (see Possible Side Effects on page 279). Nurses need to use an open approach with patients in discussing management of any treatment problems.

Nursing Care of

The Skin Graft Site

Nursing Care	Rationale/Comments
◆ Inspect the site daily and assess for edema, hematoma, infection, or fluid collection under the graft	◆ Indicates a problem or potential problem with healing
◆ Assess the viability of the graft (color, temperature)	◆ Grafts do not have their own blood supply; normally it takes about 2 weeks for a new blood supply to develop

◆ Apply the dressing as ordered
  ◆ Single layer of fine-mesh gauze directly over the graft
  ◆ Several thicknesses of padding
  ◆ Cover with a pressure bandage placed firmly
	◆ Fine-mesh gauze allows visual monitoring without disruption of the site when the dressing is changed; unless instructed to do so, do not remove fine-mesh gauze when changing dressings, because this will disturb the graft and may interfere with the development of a new blood supply for the graft; padding of the dressing provides protection from graft movement (graft may not be sutured but just placed at site) and from patient scratching when asleep; the pressure dressing also helps prevent graft movement and fluid buildup underneath the graft

◆ If possible, the graft site should be elevated, and the patient should be instructed not to lie on the graft site	◆ This allows better circulation and enhances blood supply; warm compresses may be prescribed for the same reason; there is no sense of feeling at the graft site for several months, so care must be taken not to burn the patient
◆ Encourage the patient to avoid coffee, tea, chocolate, and other sources of caffeine; encourage patient to stop or decrease smoking	◆ Caffeine and nicotine cause venous constriction and may inhibit the graft from developing its own blood supply
◆ After the dressing is no longer needed, cocoa butter or lanolin is used two to three times a day to lubricate the site	◆ Moisturizers or creams remove crustiness and keep the graft soft and pliable
◆ Long-term care includes avoiding direct sunlight and sources of heat unless closely monitored	◆ The graft is sensitive to the sun and will burn easily; until sensation to the site returns (up to 6 months after surgery), the site is at risk for burns

Possible Side Effects from Multimodal Therapy in **Melanoma**

Multimodal Treatment	Possible Enhanced Side Effects

Surgery followed by adjuvant biotherapy
   Interleukin-2
   Tumor necrosis factor
   Monoclonal antibodies
	No enhanced side effects

Autologous vaccine	Transient (12 hours) urticaria at injection site
Concomitant chemotherapy and biotherapy Interleukin-2 and high-dose cisplatin	Increased risk of nephrotoxicity, fatigue
Dacarbazine and interferon alfa-2b	Increased bone marrow depression, increased incidence and severity of flulike syndrome, fatigue, diarrhea, increased risk of infection, increased neurotoxicity
Carmustine, cisplatin, dacarbazine, tamoxifen, interleukin-2, interferon alpha-2b	Fatigue, nausea and vomiting, vitiligio-like depigmentation (milky white skin patches), idiopathic thrombocytopenia

Data taken from Demchak et al., 1991; Falkson, Falkson, and Falkson, 1991; Miller et al., 1995; Richards et al., 1992.

Long-term Treatment Strategies

Patients with malignant melanoma should be evaluated at regular intervals for local recurrence or metastatic disease. Follow-up is based on the recurrence rate for melanomas of different thickness. Evaluations should take place every 3 to 6 months for 2 years, then every 6 months for up to 5 years, and yearly thereafter (Lawler, 1991; Loescher and Booth, 1990; Longman, 1992). The importance of evaluation at regular intervals must be stressed to the patient, who must also make changes in life-style to reduce skin exposure to UV rays and further development of any lesions. For nurses, patients, and families, educational materials are available from such institutions as the American Cancer Society (e.g., *Prevention and Early Detection of Malignant Melanoma*), the National Cancer Institute (e.g., *What You Need to Know About Melanoma*), the Skin Cancer Foundation (e.g., *The Melanoma Letter*), and the American Academy of Dermatology (e.g., *Melanoma Skin Cancer*).

❖ Summary

Nurses are in a unique position to be advocates for those at risk of and for those being treated for malignant melanoma. The best-known treatments to date are prevention, early detection, and prompt treatment.

❖ *References*

American Cancer Society: American Cancer Society facts and figures—1995. Atlanta, 1995, American Cancer Society.

Bargoil SC and Erdman LK: Safe tan: an oxymoron, Cancer Nurs 16:139–144, 1993.

Barth A and Morton DL: The role of adjuvant therapy in malignant melanoma, Cancer 75:726–734, 1995.

Berwick M, Bolognia JL, Heer C, and Fine JA: The role of the nurse in skin cancer prevention, screening, and early detection, Semin Oncol Nurs 7:64–71, 1991.

Demchak PA, Mier JV, Robert NJ, O'Brien K, Gould JA, and Atkins MB: Interleukin-2 and high-dose cisplatin in patients with metastatic melanoma: a pilot study, J Clin Oncol 9:1821–1830, 1991.

Falkson CI, Falkson G, and Falkson HC: Improved results with the addition of interferon alfa-2b to dacarbazine in the treatment of patients with malignant melanoma, J Clin Oncol 9:1403–1408, 1991.

Flaherty LE, Robinson W, Redman BG, Gonzalez R, Martino S, Kraut M, Valdivieso M, and Rudolph AR: A phase II study of dacarbazine and cisplatin in combination with outpatient-administered interleukin-2 in metastatic malignant melanoma, Cancer 71:3520–3525, 1993.

Friedman RJ, Rigel DS, Silverman MK, Kopf AW, and Vossaert KA: Malignant melanoma in the 1990s: the continued importance of early detection and the role of physician examination and self-examination of the skin, CA-Cancer J Clinic 41:201–226, 1991.

Holmstrom H: Surgical management of primary melanoma, Semin Surg Oncol 8:336–369, 1992.

Kelly PP: Skin cancer and melanoma awareness campaign, Oncol Nurs Forum 18:927–931, 1991.

Lawler PE and Schreiber S: Cutaneous malignant melanoma: nursing's role in prevention and early detection, Oncol Nurs Forum 16:345–352, 1989.

Lawler PE: Cutaneous malignant melanoma, Semin Oncol Nurs 7:26–35, 1991.

Loescher LJ: Skin cancer prevention and detection update, Semin Oncol Nurs 9:184–187, 1993.

Loescher LJ and Booth A: Skin cancer. In Groenwald SL, Frogge MH, Goodman M, and Yarbro CH, editors: Cancer nursing: principles and practice, ed 2, Boston, 1990, Jones & Bartlett Publishers, pp. 999–1014.

Longman AJ: Skin cancers. In Baird S, McCorkle R, and Grant M, editors: Cancer nursing: a comprehensive textbook, Philadelphia, 1991, WB Saunders Co, pp. 637–646.

Longman A: Skin cancer. In Clark J and McGee R, editors: Core curriculum for oncology nursing, ed 2, Philadelphia, 1992, WB Saunders Co, pp. 488–498.

McClay EF and McClay ME: Tamoxifen: is it useful in the treatment of patients with metastatic melanoma?, J Clin Oncol 12:617–626, 1994.

Miller K, Abeles G, Oratz R, Zeleniuch-Jacquotte A, Cui J, Roses DF, Harris MN, and Bystryn J: Improved survival of patients with melanoma with an antibody response to immunization to a polyvalent melanoma vaccine, Cancer 75:495–502, 1995.

Nathanson L, Meelu MA, and Losada R: Chemohormone therapy of metastatic melanoma with megestrol acetate plus dacarbazine, carmustine, and cisplatin, Cancer 73:98–102, 1994.

Richards JM, Mehta M, Rammings K, and Skosey P: Sequential chemoimmunotherapy in the treatment of metastatic melanoma, J Clin Oncol 10:1338–1343, 1992.

Seidman H, Mushinski MH, Gelb SK, and Silverberg E: Probabilities of eventually developing cancer or dying—United States, 1985, CA Cancer J Clin 35:36–56, 1985.

Wingo PA, Tong T, and Bolden S: Cancer statistics, 1995, CA Cancer J Clin 45:8–30, 1995.

Chapter 17

❖ *Sarcomas*

Jeannine M. Brant

Sarcomas are malignancies derived from connective tissues in the body. They may occur anywhere in the body but most frequently develop in the extremities, usually the legs. Sarcomas are a rare form of cancer and comprise 1% of all malignancies. The American Cancer Society projects that there will be 6000 new cases of sarcoma diagnosed in 1995 and approximately 3600 deaths from the disease (Wingo, Tong, and Bolden, 1995).

Historically sarcomas had an extremely poor prognosis. The standard treatment was amputation or radical resection. Recently, multimodal therapy has dramatically decreased the incidence of local recurrence, metastatic spread, and radical surgery. Limb-sparing surgery combined with radiation therapy and chemotherapy has greatly improved the quality of life for patients.

Sarcomas are divided into soft tissue sarcomas (STS) and musculoskeletal sarcomas (MS). Distinctions between the different types are outlined in Table 17-1. Some of the most common sarcomas—rhabdomyosarcoma, osteosarcoma, and Ewing's sarcoma—occur primarily in children and young adults and will be discussed more thoroughly in Chapter 19, Pediatric-specific Cancers.

❖ *Treatment*

Although STS and MS are both categorized as sarcomas, they have unique characteristics and respond differently to chemotherapy and radiation therapy. Each tumor must be evaluated by histologic type, location, stage, and age of the patient in order to plan an appropriate treatment regimen (Malawer, Link, and Donaldson, 1993; Yang et al., 1993).

Musculoskeletal Sarcomas

Before the advent of multimodal therapy, the prognosis for MS was grave. Local control was obtained by radical surgery and amputation; however, many patients relapsed and died from metastatic disease. Oncologists used adjuvant and neoadjuvant therapy for MS to try to control the highly prevalent microscopic spread of the

Table 17-1 Characteristics of Sarcomas

Type of Sarcoma	Host Factors	Patient Assessment	Common Locations	Metastatic Pattern
Musculoskeletal Sarcomas				
Chondrosarcoma	Affects ages 30–60; most common in people over 55 years old, and more common in males than females	Dull, aching pain at the tumor site; pain may not always be present	Pelvic bones, long bones, scapula, ribs	Slow-growing, locally invasive; metastatic sites: lungs, heart
Ewing's sarcoma	80% of patients are less than 30 years old; predominant in caucasians	Pain at the tumor site with increasing persistence and severity	Long bones, pelvis	Metastasizes early; metastatic sites: lungs, lymph nodes, skull
Osteosarcoma	Affects ages 10–25; more common in males than females	Pain and a palpable mass at the tumor site; pain usually increases at night; advanced presenting symptoms: anemia, weight loss, increased serum alkaline phosphatase level	Femur, tibia, humerus	Metastasizes quickly to the lungs
Soft Tissue Sarcomas				
Angiosarcoma	Affects the elderly; more males affected than females	Multifocal, enlarging purple lesions usually found on the scalp	Head and neck	Usually high-grade, metastasizes early
Fibrosarcoma	Affects all age groups	May appear as scars; hard fibrous lesions may be felt on deep and superficial palpation	Abdominal wall, extremities	Local recurrence common; metastasizes to the lungs at variable rates
Leiomyosarcoma	Median age is 60 years old	Pain at tumor location; GI or GU bleeding; cutaneous lesions may be painless	Viscera: uterus, GI tract, retroperitoneum	Metastatic in more than 50% of patients to peritoneum, liver, lungs
Liposarcoma	Mean age is 50s; affects more males than females	Firm and nodular tumor on palpation, usually painless; multicentric origins	Thigh, popliteal space, inguinal/gluteal regions, retroperitoneum	Metastasizes to lymph nodes and lungs; metastatic spread is highly variable
Malignant fibrous histiocytoma	Affects people more than 40 years old	Fever, neutrophilia, eosinophilia	Lower extremities, trunk, retroperitoneum	May metastasize to distant sites, less often to lymph nodes
Rhabdomyo-sarcoma	Most common in children	Grapelike lesions, exophthalmos, proptosis	Head and neck, genitouri-nary tract, trunk, extremities	High rate of local recurrence and early metastases to many organs
Synovial sarcoma	Most common in second through fourth decades of life	Painful, hard masses usually near joints and tendons	Extremities, abdominal wall	High rate of local recurrence, metastasizes to lymph nodes

disease. The most common site for disease spread is the lungs (Malawer, Link, and Donaldson, 1993).

Surgery Followed by Adjuvant Chemotherapy

The goal of adjuvant therapy of MS is to eradicate microscopic disease after surgical resection of the local tumor. Unfortunately, many musculoskeletal sarcomas are relatively drug resistant. Tumors respond in various ways, depending on the histologic tumor type and the specific chemotherapeutic agents used. Tumors treated with methotrexate have shown a response rate of 0% to 80%. The rate of response to doxorubicin is approximately 26%, to cisplatin 33%, and to ifosfamide 33%. Other single agents that demonstrate some ability to elicit tumor response include cyclophosphamide, melphalan, mitomycin-C, dacarbazine, and dactinomycin. Responses can be partial or complete. The 5-year survival rate for many intensive, adjuvant, combination chemotherapy regimens is about 60% (Malawer, Link, and Donaldson, 1993).

Neoadjuvant Chemotherapy Followed by Surgery

Neoadjuvant chemotherapy has become the most favored treatment for MS. It is administered to eradicate potential microscopic disease shortly after diagnosis and before the local sarcoma is surgically resected. This form of treatment eliminates the possibility of having to delay chemotherapy to allow surgical wounds to heal. Neoadjuvant chemotherapy may also facilitate limb-sparing surgery by shrinking the tumor before the operation and allowing for a more conservative resection. It allows the physician to evaluate the tumor's responsiveness to particular chemotherapeutic agents and to tailor the adjuvant chemotherapy according to the tumor's sensitivity. In addition, neoadjuvant chemotherapy allows for the formation of a customized endoprosthesis (internal prosthesis for limb-sparing surgery), which may take up to 3 months (Bacci et al., 1993; Malawer, Link, and Donaldson, 1993; Piasecki, 1993; Ruggieri et al., 1993) (see the Research Highlight on page 284).

Soft Tissue Sarcomas

The goal of multimodal treatment for STS is to completely excise all tumors and to preserve limb and body function without affecting long-term survival (Brennan et al., 1991).

Surgery

After diagnosis, the tumor is evaluated for immediate resectability. Resectability depends on the vascularity of the tumor and tumor adherence to adjacent structures. Resection is likely to be performed initially if it will spare limbs and if the tumor can be removed safely with wide margins. The surgeon performs an en bloc resection by removing all previous biopsy tracks along the tumor and also removing generous margins that include associated muscles, tendons, and fascial tissue. Margins should include normal tissue surrounding the tumor in all directions: 2 cm of normal tissue for low-grade tumors and more than 4 cm for high-grade tumors (Blum et al. 1993). Surgery with wide surgical margins may be the only treatment for small, low-grade tumors (Tran et al., 1992).

RESEARCH HIGHLIGHT

Ruggieri P, DeCristofaro R, Picci P, Bacci G, Biagini R, Casadei R, Ferraro A, Ferruzi A, Fabbri N, Cazzola A, and Campanacci M: Complications and surgical indications in 144 cases of nonmetastatic osteosarcoma of the extremities treated with neoadjuvant chemotherapy, Clin Orthop and Related Res 295:226–238, 1993.

Study Patients received two cycles of neoadjuvant chemotherapy consisting of doxorubicin, methotrexate, and cisplatin followed by radical or limb-sparing surgical resection. Good responders (more than 90% necrosis) received an additional two cycles of doxorubicin, ifosfamide, methotrexate, cisplatin, and etoposide, and poor responders (less than 90% necrosis) received three additional cycles of the same.

Sample The study included 144 patients with high-grade, extracompartmental, nonmetastic osteosarcoma.

Study aim To determine joint, orthopedic, and functional complications associated with neoadjuvant chemotherapy, surgery, and adjuvant chemotherapy.

Findings The continuous disease-free survival (DFS) rate was 79% in good responders and 72% in poor responders. Of patients who had limb-sparing surgery, 65% experienced one or more complications, including nerve palsies, graft fractures, and polyethylene bearings wearing out in reconstructive devices. There were no complications in amputee patients. Function was measured at more than 50% in 77% of patients who had limb-sparing surgery and more than 50% in 64% of amputee patients.

Discussion Patients who underwent limb-sparing surgeries experienced significant complications, although the reconstructive procedure influenced the complications more than the actual surgery. Neoadjuvant chemotherapy also influenced the incidence and severity of the complications. The therapeutic ratio must be weighed carefully so that benefits will outweigh the risks for each individual patient.

Table 17-2 discusses the advantages and disadvantages of the three most common methods of reconstruction. The reconstruction may include a metal artificial replacement, bone allografts (bone transplanted from another individual), or bone autografts (bone transplanted from one area of the patient to another) (Piasecki, 1993; Piasecki, 1992).

Surgery Followed by Adjuvant Radiation Therapy
Adjuvant radiation therapy is frequently used in the treatment of high-grade tumors because they have a significant degree of local recurrence. It is also used if the surgical margins are too small or contain some residual tumor. Adjuvant radiation therapy can significantly decrease local recurrence in STS and is becoming a standard treatment (Morton, Antman, and Tepper, 1993; Ricci et al., 1992; Tran et al., 1992). The various histological types of STS have variable responses to radiation. Liposarcomas are the most radiosensitive, whereas leiomyosarcomas and fibrosarcomas are the least responsive. Angiosarcomas have a wide variation of radiosensitivity (Ricci et al., 1992). Although adjuvant radiation therapy has decreased local recurrence in many cases, the overall survival rate in many STSs depends to a large degree on the adequacy of the surgical resection; that is, if the surgeon has obtained

Table 17-2   Methods of Reconstruction Following Limb-Sparing Surgery

Surgical Procedure	*Advantages*	*Disadvantages*
Arthrodesis (fusion)	Tolerates running, jumping; revision surgery less likely	Results in stiff joint; complications: infection, nonunion of the implant to the bone
Arthroplasty (artificial metal and/or allograft joint)	Allows joint mobility	Joint will not tolerate high-impact activity; complications: infections, implant fracture, loosening of implant, nonunion of the implant to the bone
Intercalary allograft (allograft secured to host bone by screws and metal plates)	Can be sized in surgery; provides joint mobility and stability	Degenerative arthritis can occur over time; must limit weight-bearing activity until allograft is healed to the host bone (6–12 months); adjuvant chemotherapy may be delayed until allograft has healed; complications: infection, nonunion of the implant to the bone, allograft fracture

wide, clear, disease-free margins. This is especially true if the tumor is not radiosensitive (Testolin et al., 1992; Wanebo et al., 1992).

Surgery with Neoadjuvant Radiation Therapy
Neoadjuvant radiation therapy can render some locally unresectable tumors resectable for limb-sparing procedures. Before the use of neoadjuvant radiation therapy, amputation and radical resection were frequently the only options. The radiologist can also use smaller radiation fields in neoadjuvant therapy compared to those used in adjuvant radiation therapy because the field does not need to encompass surgical margins (Cartwright, 1983). Neoadjuvant radiation therapy is especially valuable in determining the radioresponsiveness of the specific tumor before surgical intervention (Ricci et al., 1992). The preoperative treatment course generally begins with 50 Gy given as 2 Gy daily 5 days per week for 5 weeks. A rest period and tumor-evaluation period then occur after neoadjuvant radiation therapy. Surgical resection with wide surgical margins is then done, if possible, followed by a 15-Gy boost of radiation therapy (Springfield, 1993). A decision tree for the treatment of STS appears in Figure 17-1. This standard therapy algorithm does not consider current clinical trials or "last-resort" chemotherapy administration.

Surgery with Adjuvant Chemotherapy
The role of adjuvant chemotherapy in adult STS is unknown at this time and is limited to advanced disease, high-grade disease, and clinical trials. The combination of doxorubicin (80 mg/m^2) and ifosfamide (3750 mg/m^2) yields a 34% overall response. The combination of doxorubicin (40 mg/m^2), mitomycin-C (8 mg/m^2), and cisplatin (60 mg/m^2) produces a similar response rate of 31%. Other combination regimens with doxorubicin or an alternative anthracycline such as epirubicin

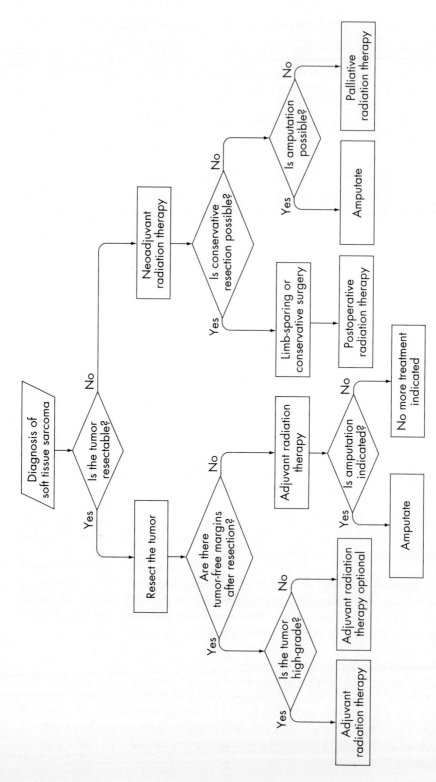

Fig. 17-1.   Multimodal therapy for soft tissue sarcomas.

have produced similar results (Blum et al., 1993; Edmonson et al., 1993; Harstrick et al., 1993).

Surgery with Neoadjuvant Chemotherapy and Radiation Therapy
Regional neoadjuvant intraarterial chemotherapy has been used in STS of the extremities to deliver the chemotherapy directly to the tumor. The patient receives this chemotherapy in combination with reduced doses of radiation therapy followed by limb-sparing surgery. The 3-year disease-free survival rate has reached 59%, but it is uncertain whether this multimodal approach is superior to other treatments (Issels et al., 1993; Soulen et al., 1992).

❖ *Nursing Management*

The nurse's role begins with the initial diagnosis of the sarcoma and extends through the rehabilitative period. Patients with MS and STS must confront potential changes in body image, body function, and emotional state in relation to the cancer, diagnosis, surgery, and body alteration. The nurse has a role to play in the multidisciplinary team in regard to discussing treatment options with patients facing amputation or limb-sparing procedures.

Amputation

When amputation is planned, the patient will likely have fears regarding postoperative pain, disability, and disfigurement. The nursing plan includes assisting the patient and significant others in coping with the loss. Patients are encouraged to express their fears and concerns regarding amputation and related dysfunction. The nurse and the prosthetist can provide valuable information regarding the prosthesis, functional expectations, and the rehabilitation plan.

Postoperative care includes wound management. The stump is elevated for the first 24 hours following surgery to prevent dependent edema. The stump is wrapped with elastic bandages to help decrease the swelling so that the stump shrinks back to its original size. Within 3 to 6 weeks, the individual may be fitted for a temporary prosthesis. A permanent prosthesis is fitted approximately 3 months after surgery. The delayed prosthesis fitting allows for wound inspection following surgery and for elastic wraps and stump shrinkers to prepare the stump for the prosthesis. The prosthetist may also apply a prosthesis directly after surgery. The advantage of the immediate fitting is that it decreases stump edema because of the pressure of the fitting on the stump. Patients are also likely to ambulate earlier and to adjust more quickly emotionally because of the immediate limb replacement (Piasecki, 1992).

The nursing plan also includes the management of potential phantom pain. Phantom pain involves painful sensations at the site of the missing limb. The individual may feel severe cramping, throbbing, and burning in former anatomical locations of the amputated limb (Piasecki, 1993). Phantom pain occurs in approximately 50% to 75% of patients following the first week of surgery, but it may persist for months to years. The pathophysiology is not clearly understood, but the pain most likely results from the interruption of nerve pathways (Jensen

Nursing Care of

The Person with Phantom Pain

Nursing Care	Rationale/Comments

◆ Encourage positive coping techniques
  ◆ Rest and relaxation
  ◆ Diversion and distraction
  ◆ Hypnosis
	◆ Informing patients of the potential for phantom stump pain is important to eliminate feelings of mental anguish; behavioral and relaxation therapy may decrease chronic phantom pain and facilitate coping

◆ Use thermal and mechanical stimuli to decrease pain
  ◆ Heat
  ◆ Cold
  ◆ Wrap stump with elastic wraps
  ◆ Percuss and massage the stump
  ◆ Apply the prosthesis
  ◆ Acupuncture
	◆ A variety of mechanical and thermal interventions have been tried to alleviate stump pain; all are easy, inexpensive techniques with varied results that can be tried in the hospital or the home setting

◆ Elevate the stump	◆ Decreases stump edema and lessens pain

◆ Assess and medicate for pain as needed
  ◆ Narcotic analgesics
  ◆ Nonnarcotics
  ◆ Muscle relaxants
  ◆ Antidepressants
  ◆ Anticonvulsants
  ◆ Beta blockers
  ◆ Local anesthetics
	◆ Narcotic and nonnarcotic analgesics are most commonly used for phantom pain; antidepressants may be indicated for peripheral neuropathy and anticonvulsants for "shooting" neuropathic pain; beta blockers have been used with mixed responses; local anesthetics may be used to determine which patients may benefit from a nerve block

◆ Assist with and monitor effectiveness of nerve blocks when indicated	◆ Used to block pain at the nerve; long-term relief is infrequent, but some patients may benefit from repeated blocks
◆ Apply and monitor response to TENS (transcutaneous electric nerve stimulation) unit when indicated	◆ Approximately 50% of patients may respond to TENS, but success is generally short-term

and Rasmussen, 1989; Loeser, 1990; Piasecki, 1993). Some of the nursing and medical interventions used to treat phantom pain are listed in the Nursing Care table above).

Long-term care of the stump includes individual daily assessment for pressure sores, redness, pain, or any other abnormalities. The individual must also learn to care for the prosthetic device. Patient Education Guidelines for Stump and Prosthesis Care are presented on page 289.

Patient Education Guidelines for

Stump and Prosthesis Care

◆ Wash the stump daily with a mild soap and water.

◆ Avoid using skin care products and alcohol on the stump.

◆ Inspect the stump daily for the following:
  ◆ Redness
  ◆ Pressure sores
  ◆ Abrasions

◆ Report any changes to your nurse or physician.

◆ Change the stump sock daily. Make sure the sock fits properly (no folds or wrinkles).

◆ Put on the prosthesis before getting out of bed in the morning and keep it on until bedtime.

◆ Thoroughly clean the prosthesis socket daily with soap and water.

◆ Never adjust the prosthesis on your own. Visit the prosthetist every 1 or 2 months during the first year after the operation.

Permission granted to reproduce these guidelines for educational purposes only.

Limb-sparing Surgery

Limb-sparing surgery takes approximately 6 hours because of the complexity of the vascular network, the tendons, and the nerves. This increases the potential for post-operative infection, hemorrhage, deep-vein thrombosis, nerve injury, and pulmonary complications. Patients must be taught about coughing and deep breathing after surgery to prevent pulmonary complications. Prophylactic postoperative anticoagulation, sequential compressive devices, and antiembolic stockings are frequently used to prevent hypercoagulation. Prophylactic antibiotics are used to prevent infection (Piasecki, 1993).

Postoperative pain is often severe and is initially managed with epidural or intravenous opioids. Oral opioids are prescribed as pain decreases, and patients frequently take opioids throughout the initial rehabilitation period, which may last up to a couple of months (Piasecki, 1993).

Patients may also experience side effects from neoadjuvant and adjuvant radiation therapy and chemotherapy. These side effects may occur in the middle of recovery from surgery. Possible Side Effects from Multimodal Therapy in Sarcoma are presented on page 290.

❖ Summary

Bone and soft tissue sarcomas are rare, but they have the potential to impose great suffering on individuals. The advent of multimodal therapy has greatly improved the overall survival rate and the quality of life of patients with MS and STS. Multi-

Possible Side Effects from Multimodal Therapy in

Sarcoma

Multimodal Treatment	Possible Enhanced Side Effects
Musculosketetal Sarcoma	
Surgery followed by adjuvant chemotherapy	
Cisplatin, doxorubicin	No enhanced side effects
Methotrexate, bleomycin, cyclophosphamide, dactinomycin, doxorubicin	
Etoposide, cyclophosphamide, cisplatin, doxorubicin	
Doxorubicin, ifosfamide, dacarbazine	
Neoadjuvant chemotherapy followed by surgery	
Cisplatin, doxorubicin	No enhanced side effects
Methotrexate, bleomycin, cyclophosphamide, dactinomycin, doxorubicin	
Etoposide, cyclophosphamide, cisplatin, doxorubicin	
Doxorubicin, ifosfamide, dacarbazine	
Soft-Tissue Sarcoma	
Surgery followed by adjuvant radiation therapy— external beam	Lymphedema
Surgery followed by adjuvant radiation therapy— brachytherapy	Delayed wound healing, soft tissue necrosis
Surgery followed by adjuvant radiation therapy and chemotherapy	
Etoposide, ifosfamide	No enhanced side effects
Doxorubicin, ifosfamide	Increased skin reaction, chronic infection at surgical site
Vindesine, doxorubicin, cyclophosphamide	
Doxorubicin, dacarbazine	
Cyclophosphamide, vincristine, doxorubicin, dacarbazine	
Doxorubicin, ifosfamide, dacarbazine	
Neoadjuvant radiation therapy followed by surgery	Lymphedema, delayed wound healing

Data taken from Arbeit, Hilaris, and Brennen, 1987; Karakousis and Perez, 1994; Shiu et al., 1991; Stinson et al., 1991.

modal therapy has also created new challenges in patient care because of limb-sparing surgery and the rehabilitation associated with this procedure. Nurses have a unique role in educating patients about the disease process, treatment options, and rehabilitation and in helping patients cope with the alteration in body image and life-style.

❖ References

Arbeit JM, Hilaris BS, and Brennen MF: Wound complications in the multimodality treatments of extremity and superficial truncal sarcomas, J Clin Oncol 5:480–488, 1987.

Bacci G, Picci P, Ferrari S, Ruggieri P, Casadei R, Tienghi A, del Prever AB, Gherlinzoni F, Mercuri M, and Monti C: Primary chemotherapy and delayed surgery for nonmetastatic osteosarcoma of the extremity, Cancer 72:3227–3238, 1993.

Blum RH, Edmonson J, Ryan L, and Pelletier L: Efficacy of ifosfamide in combination with doxorubicin for the treatment of metastatic soft tissue sarcoma, Cancer Chemother Pharma 31(suppl 2):S238–S240, 1993.

Brennan MF, Casper ES, Harrison LB, Shiu MA, Gaynor J, and Hajdu SI: The role of multimodality therapy in soft tissue sarcomas, Ann Surg 214:328–338, 1991.

Cartwright S: Adult soft tissue sarcomas: an overview, Radiography 49(582):131–150, 1983.

Edmonson JH, Ryan LM, Blum RH, Brooks JSJ, Shiraki M, Frytak S, and Parkinson DR: Randomized comparison of doxorubicin alone versus ifosfamide plus doxorubicin or mitomycin, doxorubicin, and cisplatin against advanced soft tissue sarcomas, J Clin Oncol 11:1269–1275, 1993.

Harstrick A, Bokemeyer C, Schmoll HJ, Kohne-Wompner CH, Knipp H, Schoffski P, Anagnou J, Wipperman B, Neumann S, and Poliwoda H: A pilot study of rapidly alternating therapy epirubicin/dacarbazine and ifosfamide as first-line therapy for metastatic soft tissue sarcoma in adults, Cancer Chemother Pharma 31(suppl 2): S217–S221, 1993.

Issels RD, Bosse D, Abdel-Rahman S, Starck M, Panzer M, Jauch KW, Stiegler H, Berger H, Sauer H, Peter K, and Wilmanns W: Preoperative systemic etoposide/doxorubicin chemotherapy combined with regional hyperthermia in high-risk sarcoma: a pilot study, Cancer Chemother Pharma 31(suppl 2):S233–S237, 1993.

Jensen TS and Rasmussen P: Phantom pain and related phenomena after amputation. In Wall PD and Melzack R, editors: Textbook of pain, ed 2, New York, 1989, Churchill Livingstone, pp. 508–543.

Karakousis CP and Perez RP: Soft tissue sarcomas in adults, CA Cancer J Clin 44:200–210, 1994.

Loeser JD: Pain after amputation: phantom limb and stump pain. In Bonica JJ, Loeser JD, Chapman CR, and Fordyce WE, editors: The management of pain, ed 2, Philadelphia, 1990, Lea & Febiger, pp. 244–256.

Malawer MM, Link MP, and Donaldson SS: Sarcomas of the bone. In DeVita VT, Hellman S, and Rosenberg SA, editors: Cancer: principles and practice of oncology, ed 4, Philadelphia, 1993, JB Lippincott Co, pp. 1509–1562.

Morton DL, Antman KH, and Tepper J: Soft tissue sarcoma. In Holland JF, Frei E III, Bast RC Jr, Kuff DW, Morton DL, and Weichselbaum RR, editors: Cancer medicine, ed 3, Philadelphia, 1993, Lea & Febiger, pp. 1858–1887.

Piasecki P: Bone and soft tissue sarcoma. In Groenwald SL, Frogge MH, Goodman M, and Yarbro CH, editors: Cancer nursing: principles and practice, ed 3, Boston, 1993, Jones & Bartlett Publishers, pp. 877–902.

Piasecki P: Update in orthopaedic oncology, Orthop Nurs 11:36–43, 1992.

Ricci SB, Milani F, Gramaglia A, Ricci PB, and Borsa G: On extravisceral soft tissue sarcomas: effectiveness of radiation treatment and problems of radiotherapy and radiosurgical treatment, Panminerva Medica 34:69–76, 1992.

Ruggieri P, DeCristofaro R, Picci P, Bacci G, Biagini R, Casadei R, Ferraro A, Ferruzzi A, Fabbri N, Cazzola A, and Campanacci M: Complications and surgical indications in 144 cases of nonmetastatic osteosarcoma of the extremities treated with neoadjuvant chemotherapy, Clin Ortho Related Res 295:226–238, 1993.

Shiu MH, Hilaris BS, Harrison LB, and Brennen MF: Brachytherapy and function-saving resections of soft tissue sarcoma arising in the limb, Int J Radiat Oncol Biol Phys 21:1485–1492, 1991.

Soulen MC, Weissmann JR, Sullivan KL, Lackman RD, Shapiro MJ, Bonn J, Weiss AJ, and Gardiner GA: Intraarterial chemotherapy with limb-sparing resection of large STS of the extremities, J Vascular Interventional Radiology 3:659–663, 1992.

Springfield D: Liposarcoma, Clin Ortho Related Res 289:50–57, 1993.

Stinson SF, DeLaney TF, Greenberg J, Yang JC, Lampert MH, Hicks JE, Venzon D, White DE, Rosenberg SA, and Glatstein EJ: Acute and long-term effects on limb function of combined modality limb-sparing therapy for extremity soft tissue sarcoma, Int J Radiat Oncol Biol Phys 21:1493–1499, 1991.

Testolin A, Possa F, Fior SD, Bolzicco GP, Panizzoni GA, and Gasparini G: Surgical and adjuvant radiation therapy of resectable retroperitoneal soft tissue sarcomas in adults, Tumori 78:388–391, 1992.

Tran LM, Mark R, Meier R, Calcaterra TC, and Parker RG: Sarcomas of the head and neck: prognostic factors and treatment strategies, Cancer 70:169–177, 1992.

Wanebo HJ, Koness J, MacFarlane JK, Eilber FR, Byers RM, Elias EG, and Spiro RH: Head and neck sarcoma: report of the head and neck sarcoma registry, Head and Neck 14:1–7, 1992.

Wingo PA, Tong T, and Bolden S: Cancer statistics, 1995, CA Cancer J Clin 45:8–30, 1995.

Yang JC, Rosenberg SA, Glatstein EJ, and Antman KH: Sarcomas of soft tissues. In DeVita VT, Hellman S, and Rosenberg SA, editors: Cancer: principles and practice of oncology, ed 4, Philadelphia, 1993, JB Lippincott Co, pp. 1436–1488.

Chapter *18*

❖ *Primary Brain Tumors*

Jeannine M. Brant

The American Cancer Society estimates that there will be 17,200 tumors of the brain and central nervous system diagnosed in 1995 and 13,300 deaths. Brain tumors are the second leading cause of death from cancer in children under 15, the third leading cause of death from cancer in men ages 15 to 24, and the fourth leading cause of death from cancer in women ages 15 to 24 (Wingo, Tong, and Bolden, 1995). Despite clinical advances, brain tumors characteristically have a high degree of morbidity and mortality.

❖ *Treatment*

Multimodal therapy is widely used in the treatment of brain tumors, and yet for some histologic types the prognosis remains poor. The isolated physiologic location of the brain makes treatment difficult. A lining of endothelial cells called the blood-brain barrier separates the brain from the spinal fluid. The lipid membranes of the endothelial cells regulate the diffusion of molecules and drugs across the membrane. Fat-soluble drugs cross the blood-brain barrier, whereas water-soluble drugs do not. Investigational therapies focus on ways to disrupt the blood-brain barrier so that the treatment can penetrate the tumor, potentiate chemotherapy and radiation therapy, and sensitize the brain tumor cells, resulting in greater cell kill (Wegmann, 1993). These new treatments, in combination with standard treatment modalities, are providing longer periods of survival for many patients.

Primary brain tumors are named for the origin of the neuroglial cell or other nervous system cell from which they are derived. Table 18-1 outlines characteristics of the more common brain tumors.

Surgery

Surgery is most often the initial treatment of choice for primary brain tumors. The neurosurgeon evaluates the tumor for potential resectability, taking into considera-

Table 18-1   Characteristics of Primary Brain Tumors

Type of Tumor	Cellular Characteristics	Common Locations	Host Factors and Presentation
Glioblastoma multiform	Multiple foci of origin; highly malignant, infiltrative, hemorrhagic and cystic regions; areas of necrosis; frequent mitosis	Cerebral hemispheres, frontal lobe	More common in men; increased incidence in fifth and sixth decades
Astrocytoma	Regular and uniform cells; slight increase in cellularity; usually no clear border between tumor and surrounding normal tissue	May occur in any area of the brain	Mean age at presentation is 35; seizures most common presenting symptom
Ependymoma	Small, round, uniform nuclei; differentiation highly variable from low-grade to anaplastic	Cerebral hemispheres, ventricles	Peak incidence age 5 and age 34; may present with ICP and hydrocephalus
Medulloblastoma	Highly proliferative; metastasizes quickly to the spinal axis	Cerebellum	Peak incidence in first decade of life; second peak occurs from ages 20 to 30
Meningioma	Generally slow-growing; some variants are more malignant	Cerebral hemispheres, cerebellum, pituitary region, optic nerve	More common in women, usually present in third to sixth decades
Oligodendroglioma	Multinucleated giant cells; abundant necrotic zones; proliferation of blood vessels; calcification within tumor and in adjacent tissue; vary in grade of malignancy; small, round, uniform nuclei	Frontal, parietal, and temporal lobes	Occur most often in young and middle-aged adults; seizures common

ICP = Intracranial pressure

tion the location, size, histologic type, and encapsulation of the tumor, the patient's overall condition, and the patient's neurologic status. The goal of surgery is to remove as much of the tumor as possible while preserving neurologic function. Surgeons generally totally excise tumors that are encapsulated and located in areas of the brain that will not cause deficits. Gliomas are generally infiltrative and cannot be totally resected, but they can be debulked as aggressively as possible (Wegmann, 1993). The aggressiveness of the resection relates directly to the overall survival of the patient (Chandler et al., 1993; Simpson et al., 1993; Willis, 1991).

Surgery with Adjuvant Chemotherapy

Oncologists commonly give adjuvant chemotherapy following surgery. Oligodendroglioma is very chemosensitive, whereas gliomas and many other tumors are relatively drug resistant. The lack of responsiveness is related to the anatomic separation by the blood-brain barrier and the variable blood flow within the tumor bed. This prevents chemotherapy from completely penetrating the tumor. Nitrosoureas, including carmustine and lomustine, are often the chemotherapeutic agents of choice. They penetrate the blood-brain barrier and reach the tumor (Fine and Antman, 1992; Wegmann, 1993).

A variety of other agents may be used to kill more cells or to allow greater penetration by the chemotherapy (Levin, Gutin, and Leibel, 1993; Prados and Wilson, 1993). Investigators have shown that the drug angiotensin II increases tumor blood flow, suggesting the possibility of an enhanced chemotherapy response (Tomura et al., 1993). Spiromustine (a combination of mechlorethamine and phenytoin) is used in clinical trials to transport chemotherapeutic agents to the tumor (Resio and DeVroom, 1986). Further clinical trials are needed to determine the effectiveness and toxicity of these regimens.

Chemotherapy given through the carotid arteries directly delivers a greater dose of drug to the tumor bed. Intracarotid chemotherapy is usually given after surgery and before radiation therapy (Calvo et al., 1989; Recht et al., 1990). Oncologists have also given high doses of chemotherapy in a single course in an attempt to prevent drug resistance by the tumor and to deliver large doses of chemotherapy to all areas of the brain and overcome the brain's variable blood flow. Although complete and partial responses have been reported, the median survival rate is not significantly improved. Patients can experience major central nervous system and other organ toxicities, as well as septicemia and death (Fine and Altman, 1992). Autologous bone marrow transplant provides another chemotherapy alternative.

Surgery with Adjuvant Radiation Therapy

External-Beam Radiation Therapy

Patients frequently receive radiation therapy after surgery to eliminate residual tumor cells. The treatment varies according to the tumor location and histologic type and the condition of the patient. Medulloblastomas are very radiosensitive, whereas most others are not. Brain tumor cells are generally hypoxic, and this limits the radiosensitivity. Radiation dosages vary from 40 to 80 Gy delivered over 4 to 8 weeks, although doses greater than 60 Gy are associated with brain necrosis (Larson et al., 1990). Radiation is traditionally administered as one treatment per day 5 days per week. More recently, clinicians have used hyperfractionated radiation therapy (lower doses of radiation therapy given more than once a day) to increase the number of cells killed and to decrease side effects from the radiation (Prados et al., 1993; Prados and Wilson, 1993). Initially the radiation therapy may increase neurologic side effects due to swelling and radiation necrosis, thus increasing the intracranial pressure (ICP) (Prados and Wilson, 1993; Wegmann, 1993; Willis, 1991).

Investigation continues into agents that might sensitize tumors or enhance the radiation therapy. Lonidamine has been used as a radiosensitizer and has shown that it can enhance radiation therapy and chemotherapy (Guglielimi et al., 1991). Bromodeoxyuridine (BUdR) has been given in clinical trials as an intracarotid radiosensitizer in malignant gliomas (Hegarty et al., 1990).

Brachytherapy

Brachytherapy involves implantation of radioactive sources into the tumor bed in the brain by an open craniotomy or through a stereotactic technique. Radiation sources include iodine-125, iridium-192, californium-252, cesium-177, and radium-226 (Willis, 1991). Brachytherapy allows the radiation to penetrate directly to the tumor bed, minimizing destruction of the normal surrounding tissue. It is most often used as a boost in conjunction with external-beam therapy or chemotherapy (Prados et al., 1992; Scharfen et al., 1992; Sneed et al., 1992).

Radiosurgery

Radiosurgery is a type of radiation therapy used to treat small intracranial lesions and spare the surrounding tissue. A stereotactic frame targets the tumor very precisely. The frame is aligned with the tumor using MRI, CT, and angiography. Radiation is then delivered three-dimensionally to the tumor site. Radiosurgery differs from external-beam radiation therapy in several ways: small volumes are treated, single fractions are commonly used, alignment requires additional time and care, and radiation-therapy beams spare surrounding tissue as they intersect at the central tumor location. Radiosurgery is a useful treatment modality for malignant gliomas (Larson et al., 1990; Loeffler et al., 1992).

Hyperthermia

Hyperthermia is an investigational adjunct treatment used to enhance both radiation therapy and chemotherapy. The brain tumor is heated to 42.5°C through such techniques as whole body heating, isolated perfusion of the tumor (requiring the placement of cannula in the tumor bed), ultrasound, radiofrequency, or microwaves. Schedules vary according to specific clinical trials (Guthkelch et al., 1991; Page, Ricca, and Dohan, 1990).

Biotherapy

Various experimental studies focus on combined modality treatment involving surgery, radiation therapy, and biotherapy. The biotherapy regimens include the use of interferon, monoclonal antibodies, tumor-infiltrating lymphocytes (TIL), and lymphokine-activated killer (LAK) cells. Further research is needed to determine the role of biotherapy for treating brain tumors (Bioardi et al., 1991; Hayes, 1992; Jereb et al., 1989) (see the Research Highlight below).

❖ Nursing Management

Postoperative Care

After a craniotomy, the patient will be in the intensive care unit under close observation. The nurse should be aware of potential complications of the operation, which include intracranial bleeding, cerebral edema, and water intoxication. A thorough neurologic assessment can detect changes in the patient's level of consciousness, intracranial pressure, or motor function. The patient is monitored carefully for seizures, which can occur because of postoperative edema. Prophylactic anticonvulsants are frequently administered and may be continued throughout the course of the disease. Cerebral edema is treated with corticosteroids, osmotic diuretic therapy, fluid restriction, hyperventilation, hypothermia, and anesthetics. An increase in temperature indicates infection. Infections most frequently involve the cranial wound or the cerebral spinal fluid (Wegmann, 1993) (see Nursing Care of the Patient After a Craniotomy on page 298).

RESEARCH HIGHLIGHT

Mortimer JE, Crowley J, Eyre H, Weiden P, Eltringham J, and Stuckey WJ: A phase II randomized study comparing sequential and combined intraarterial cisplatin and radiation therapy in primary brain tumors, Cancer 69:1220–1223, 1992.

Study Patients in arm I received 150 mg cisplatin intraarterial (IA) every 21 days in 2 doses followed by 55.8 Gy of radiation therapy. Patients in arm II received the same treatment as those in arm I but received it concomitantly.

Sample The study included 27 patients age 15 and older who had a confirmed diagnosis of malignant glioma.

Study aim To help determine the role of IA cisplatin in potentiating radiation therapy for malignant gliomas using sequential and concomitant administration regimens.

Findings Twenty-seven percent of patients in each arm experienced an objective tumor response. Thromboembolic complications with the IA chemotherapy were 14%. The median survival period for patients was 9.6 months in arm I and 10.8 months in arm II.

Discussion Significant complications included difficulty cannulating the artery and thromboembolism. Toxicity may outweigh therapeutic benefit for many patients. The role of IA cisplatin remains unknown, and further investigation is needed.

Nursing Care of

The Patient After a Craniotomy

Nursing Care	*Rationale/Comments*

◆ Monitor vital signs every hour for 24 hours or until stable
  ◆ Temperature
  ◆ Blood pressure
  ◆ Heart rate
  ◆ Respirations
	◆ Patient may develop a local incision infection post-operatively or an infection in the cerebrospinal fluid (meningitis) as a result of the surgery; other changes in vital signs such as increased heart rate and blood pressure may indicate an increase in intracranial pressure (ICP)

◆ Assess patient's level of consciousness	◆ Patient arousal and level of consciousness are indicators of a patient's status postoperatively; a decreased level of consciousness may indicate an increase in ICP

◆ Monitor patient's neurologic signs and symptoms
  ◆ Reflexes
  ◆ Pupil response
  ◆ Strength
  ◆ Movement
	◆ Hemiparesis, weakness, and pupil changes may indicate an increase in ICP and cerebral edema; these signs may also reveal neurologic deficits resulting from the surgery

◆ Monitor intracranial pressure (ICP) and manage prophylactically
  ◆ Corticosteroids
  ◆ Osmotic diuretic therapy
  ◆ Elevate head of bed
  ◆ Fluid restriction
	◆ Corticosteroids decrease cerebral edema caused by the surgery, whereas osmotic diuretics pull fluid from the brain area to eliminate swelling and pressure; these medications are used prophylactically to maintain a normal ICP; elevating the head of the bed promotes venous drainage from the head, which decreases edema and ICP

◆ Discourage activities that increase ICP
  ◆ Valsalva maneuver
  ◆ Coughing and sneezing
  ◆ Anxiety and overstimulation
	◆ Any type of straining activity increases ICP and should be avoided

◆ Monitor and medicate for seizure activity	◆ Seizures may result from the tumor or from cranial disturbance during surgery and are usually treated effectively with anticonvulsant therapy

◆ Assess for signs and symptoms of hemorrhage
  ◆ Increased ICP
  ◆ Swelling and edema over the incision
	◆ Patients may develop intracranial bleeding or a subdural hematoma postoperatively

◆ Provide support to the patient and family during recovery phase
  ◆ Education about recovery
  ◆ Emotional support
	◆ Information regarding the patient's neurologic status, ICP monitoring, and progress may alleviate the family's fears and anxieties about the surgery; physical and mental deficits may also become apparent postoperatively, and the family will require additional support

Chemotherapy

Patients who receive intracarotid chemotherapy may experience an exacerbation of neurologic symptoms as well as side effects of the specific drugs given. The increased neurologic symptoms occur when the chemotherapy is effective and the tumor cells die but the brain does not rid itself of the dead cells in an efficient manner. If the patient has had an Ommaya reservoir implanted as a means of giving chemotherapy, the nurse will also need to address care of the reservoir (Jereb et al., 1989). Possible Side Effects from Multimodal Therapy are listed below.

Brachytherapy

Intracranial interstitial radiation therapy (brachytherapy) involves placing radioactive sources in the cranial tissue and using a radiation level high enough possibly to warrant a lead head shield. The shield is formed over the head, and the patient wears it from the operating room to the nursing unit and keeps it on until the radiation level returns to a safe level. The patient is placed in a private room and visitation is minimized. The nurse is responsible for educating the patient and family about the lead head shield, radiation precautions, and the need for isolation (Willis, Rittenmeyer, and Hitchon, 1986).

Possible Side Effects from Multimodal Therapy in Brain Tumors

Multimodal Therapy	Possible Enhanced Side Effects

Surgery with adjuvant chemotherapy
   Hydroxyurea, 5-fluorouracil
   Cyclophosphamide, vincristine
   Carmustine
   Lomustine
	Neurotoxicity

Surgery followed by adjuvant cranial radiation therapy	Alopecia, neurotoxicity, loss of cognitive function, intracranial edema

Surgery followed by cranial radiation therapy and biotherapy
   Interferon
   Monoclonal antibodies
   Tumor necrosis factor
	Alopecia, neurotoxicity, intracranial edema, fatigue

Surgery followed by cranial radiation therapy with chemotherapy
   Hydroxyurea, lomustine, procarbazine, vincristine
   Carmustine
   Procarbazine, lomustine, vincristine
	Alopecia, neurotoxicity, loss of cognitive function, intracranial edema

Data taken from Kramer and Moore, 1989; Rozenthal and Kinsella, 1991.

Patient Education Guidelines for

Changes in Physical and Mental Status

♦ *Gait Changes* You may experience changes in your gait or unsteadiness when walking. Sit on the edge of the bed before standing. Use assistive devices (walker, cane) to help with walking. You may benefit from physical therapy and rehabilitation.

♦ *Physical Deficits* You may experience hemiparesis or one-sided weakness. Use assistive devices for eating and writing. You may likely benefit from occupational therapy; that is, if your dominant hand is paralyzed or weak, you may need to train the nondominant hand to help with eating, dressing, and bathing.

Purchase clothing with velcro fasteners, large buttons, or snaps. Use slip-on or velcro-close shoes.

Rearrange your house so that items are easy to reach.

♦ *Memory Loss* You may experience short-term or long-term memory loss. To deal with this, put items in the same place each time. Maintain a daily routine whenever possible. Use notes and reminders—for example, grocery lists, where the car is parked, and things to do.

♦ *Personality Changes* You may experience personality changes. Try to maintain as much of your normal life-style as possible.

Permission granted to reproduce these guidelines for educational purposes only.

Hyperthermia

The nurse is often responsible for monitoring the administration of hyperthermia. Hyperthermia may be delivered in several ways, although the most common method involves implanting heat sources. Initially, the patient goes to the operating room to have an intracranial catheter inserted. After having the scalp shaved, the patient undergoes general anesthesia. The catheter is placed using stereotactic techniques, and the procedure lasts approximately 2 to 3 hours. The patient returns to the intensive care unit, and the catheter is connected to a heat source. The target temperature is 105 to 107.6°F. The nurse must stay alert to postoperative craniotomy complications as described earlier. Neurologic symptoms may worsen temporarily because of surgical destruction of some normal tissue and because of tumor infiltration and edema. During the procedure, the patient may complain of a headache that is relieved by analgesics. The patient experiences no heat sensation (Edwards, Stupperich, and Welsh, 1991).

Psychosocial Issues

Patients with brain tumors are likely to experience fear and anxiety related to the diagnosis and the potential manifestations of the disease. They often express concern with changes in mentation and function. The oncology team needs to address patients and families candidly in regard to the benefits and risks of the treatment modalities, including potential alterations in physical function, mentation, and the general side effects caused by treatment. Radiation necrosis, a complication of high-dose cranial radiation therapy that causes irreversible and progressive destruction of brain tissue, should be addressed. Body-image changes associated with hair loss from treatment are also significant and cause distress. All treatments must be carefully discussed with the patient and family, especially in instances where the prognosis is poor. Patient Education Guidelines for Changes in Physical and Mental Status are presented on page 300.

❖ Summary

Multimodal therapy for the treatment of brain tumors is used extensively, and new experimental therapies are on the horizon. It is important for the health care team to assess carefully potential treatment modalities for each individual patient. The therapeutic ratio of benefits and risks is best discussed in conjunction with the patient and significant others.

❖ References

Bioardi A, Silvani A, Milanesi I, Munari L, Broggi G, and Botturi M: Local immunotherapy (β-IFN) and systemic chemotherapy in primary glial tumors, Ital J Neurol Sci 12:163–169, 1991.

Calvo FA, Dy C, Henriques I, Hidalgo V, Bilbao I, and Santos M: Postoperative radical radiotherapy with concurrent weekly intraarterial cisplatinum for treatment of malignant glioma: a pilot study, Radiother Oncol 14:83–88, 1989.

Chandler KL, Prados MD, Malec M, and Wilson CB: Long-term survival in patients with glioblastoma multiforme, Neurosurgery 32:716–720, 1993.

Edwards DK, Stupperich TK, Welsh DM: Hyperthermia treatment for malignant brain tumors; nursing management during therapy, J Neurosc Nurs 23:34–38, 1991.

Fine HA and Antman KH: High-dose chemotherapy with autologous bone marrow transplantation in the treatment of high-grade astrocytomas in adults: therapeutic rationale and clinical experience, Bone Marrow Transplant 10:315–321, 1992.

Guglielmi A, Bruzzone E, Gentile SL, Barra S, Mori A, Bacigalupa A, Rosso R, Vitale V, Giaretti W, Fronsina G, Arena G, Rossi O, Abbondandolo A, and Sobrero A: Radiation treatment plus CCNU plus the radiosensitizer lonidamine in malignant gliomas operated, Anticancer Res 11:1779–1782, 1991.

Guthkelch AN, Carter LP, Cassady JR, Hynynen KH, Iacono RP, Johnson PC, Obbens EAMT, Roemer RB, Seeger JF, Shimm DS, and Stea B: Treatment of malignant brain tumors with focused ultrasound hyperthermia and radiation: results of a phase I trial, J Neuro-Oncol 10:271–284, 1991.

Hayes RL: The cellular immunotherapy of primary brain tumors, Rev Neurol 148(6–7):454–466, 1992.

Hegarty TJ, Thornton AF, Diaz RF, Chandler WF, Ensminger WD, Junck L, Page MA, Gebarski SS, Hood TW, Stetson PL, Tankanow RM, McKeever PE, Lichter AS, Greenberg HS: Intra-arterial bromodeoxyuridine radiosensitization of malignant gliomas, Int J Radiat Oncol Biol Phys 19:421–428, 1990.

Jereb B, Petric J, Lamovec J, Skrbec M, and Soss E: Intratumor application of human leukocyte interferon-alpha in patients with malignant brain tumors. Am J Clin Onc 12(1): 1–7, 1989.

Kramer J and Moore IM: Late effects of cancer therapy on the central nervous system, Semin Oncol Nurs 5:22–28, 1989.

Larson DA, Gutin PH, Leibel SA, Phillips TL, Sneed PK, and Wara WM: Stereotaxic irradiation of brain tumors, Cancer 65:792–799, 1990.

Levin VA, Gutin PH, and Leibel S: Neoplasms of the central nervous system. In DeVita VT Jr, Hellman S, and Rosenberg SA editors: Cancer: principles and practice of oncology, ed 4, Philadelphia, 1993, JB Lippincott Co, pp. 1679–1737.

Loeffler JS, Alexander E III, Shea WM, Wen PY, Fine HA, Kooy HM, and Black P: Radiosurgery as part of the initial management of patients with malignant gliomas, J Clin Oncol 10:1379–1385, 1992.

Mortimer JE, Crowley J, Eyre H, Weiden P, Eltringham J, and Stuckey WJ: A phase II randomized study comparing sequential and combined intraarterial cisplatin and radiation therapy in primary brain tumors, Cancer 69:1220–1223, 1992.

Page RC, Ricca GF, and Dohan FC: Hyperthermia for the treatment of brain tumors. In Bischer HI, editor: Consensus on hyperthermia for the 1990s, New York, 1990, Plenum Press, pp. 145–153.

Prados MD, Gutin PH, Phillips TL, Wara WM, Sneed PK, Larson DA, Lamb SA, Ham B, Malec MK, and Wilson CB: Interstitial brachytherapy for newly diagnosed patients with malignant gliomas: The UCSF experience, Int J Radiat Oncol Biol Phys 24:593–597, 1992.

Prados MD, Wara WM, Edwards SB, and Cogen PH: Hyperfractionated craniospinal radiation therapy for primitive neuroectodermal tumors: early results of a pilot study, Int J Radiat Oncol Biol Phys 28:431–438, 1993.

Prados MD and Wilson CB: Neoplasms of the central nervous system. In Holland JF, Frei E III, Bast RC Jr, Kuff DW, Morton DL, and Weichselbaum RR, editors: Cancer medicine, ed 3, Philadelphia, 1993, Lea & Febiger, pp. 1080–1119.

Recht L, Fram RJ, Strauss G, Fitzgerald TJ, Liepman M, Lew R, Kadish S, Sherman D, Wilson J, Greenberger J, Egan P, and Silver D: Preirradiation chemotherapy of supratentorial malignant primary brain tumors with intracarotid cis-Platinum (CDDP) and i.v. BCNU, Am J Clin Oncol 13:125–131, 1990.

Resio MJ and DeVroom HL: Spiromustine and intracarotid artery cisplatin in the treatment of glioblastoma multiforme, J Neurosci Nurs 18:13–22, 1986.

Rozenthal JM and Kinsella TJ: Brain tumor. In Lokich JJ and Byfield JE: Combined modality cancer therapy: radiation and infusional chemotherapy, Chicago, 1991, Precept Press, pp. 215–239.

Scharfen CO, Sneed PK, Wara WM, Larson DA, Phillips TL, Prados MD, Weaver KA, Malec M, Acord P, Lamborn KR, Lamb SA, Ham B, and Gutin PH: High activity iodine-125 interstitial implant for gliomas, Int J Radiat Oncol Biol Phys 24:583–591, 1992.

Simpson JR, Horton J, Scott C, Curran WJ, Rubin P, Fischback J, Isaacson S, Rotman M, Asbell SO, Nelson JS, Weinstein AS, and Nelson DF: Influence of location and extent of surgical resection on survival of patients with glioblastoma multiforme: results of three consecutive Radiation Therapy Oncology Group (RTOG) clinical trials, Int J Radiat Oncol Biol Phys 26:239–244, 1993.

Sneed PK, Gutin PH, Prados MD, Phillips TL, Weaver KA, Wara WM, and Larson DA: Brachytherapy of brain tumors, Stereotact Funct Neurosurg 59:157–165, 1992.

Tomura N, Kato T, Kanno I, Shishido F, Inugami A, Uemura K, Higano S, Fujita H, Mineura K, and Kowada M: Increased blood flow in human brain tumor after administration of angiotensin II: demonstration by PET, Computer Med Imag Graph 17:443–449, 1993.

Wegmann, JA: Central nervous system cancers. In Groenwald SL, Frogge MH, Goodman M, and Yarbro CH, editors: Cancer nursing: principles and practice, ed 3, Boston, 1993, Jones & Bartlett Publishers, pp. 959–983.

Willis D: Intracranial astrocytoma: pathology, diagnosis, and clinical presentation, J Neurosci Nurs 23:7–14, 1991.

Willis D, Rittenmeyer H, and Hitchon P: Intracranial interstitial radiation, J Neurosci Nurs 18:153–156, 1986.

Wingo PA, Tong T, and Bolden S: Cancer statistics, 1995, CA- Cancer J Clin 45:8–30, 1995.

Chapter *19*

❖ *Pediatric-specific Cancers*

Marcia E. Rostad

Nearly 7500 children under the age of 15 contract cancer in the United States annually (Bleyer, 1990). Statisticians predict that the prevalence of childhood cancer survivors among young adults will increase from the current 1 in 1000 persons to 1 in 900 persons by the year 2000. Successful treatment of childhood cancer can be partially attributed to the multimodal approach used to treat certain malignancies. These childhood malignancies include neuroblastoma, Wilms' tumor, rhabdomyosarcoma, and bone tumors such as osteosarcoma and Ewing's sarcoma.

❖ *Neuroblastoma*

Neuroblastoma is a malignant tumor that arises from neural crest cells, which are responsible for the formation of the central nervous system (Brodeur and Castleberry, 1993). This common pediatric tumor accounts for 10% of all childhood malignancies. Spontaneous regression and induced maturation to benign ganglioneuroma have been observed in infants. Some researchers speculate that neuroblasts may normally exist in fetuses and very young infants and that these neuroblasts eventually differentiate into normal cells (Brodeur and Castleberry, 1993).

Treatment

The presenting symptoms of a child with neuroblastoma typically include a primary tumor along the sympathetic nervous system, which encompasses the cervical, thoracic, adrenal, and pelvic areas (Brodeur and Castleberry, 1993). Initially, parents and pediatricians may attribute signs and symptoms to normal pediatric problems. As a result, by the time it is detected, the disease may be widely disseminated.

After diagnostic evaluation, the surgeon generally attempts a resection. Complete resection of the primary tumor improves long-term survival (Haase et al.,

1991). In some cases only a biopsy or partial resection with lymph node samples is possible because of involvement of vital structures (e.g., the abdominal aorta, the liver, the kidney[s], and the spinal cord). The amount of residual tumor serves as the baseline measure from which to evaluate the effectiveness of adjuvant therapy.

Pediatric Oncology Group (POG) stage A patients are treated with surgical resection alone and closely monitored for disease recurrence. Stage A patients receive additional therapy if disease recurs (Brodeur and Castleberry, 1993). (See Chapter 1 for a discussion on staging.)

Surgery Followed by Adjuvant Chemotherapy, with or without Radiation Therapy, Followed by Surgery

Multimodal therapy is standard procedure with POG stage B patients older than 1 year (Brodeur and Castleberry, 1993). Postoperative cyclophosphamide and doxorubicin given every 21 days for 5 courses has increased the 4-year survival rate from 42% to 93% (Bowman et al., 1991). If the chemotherapy has less of an effect than desired, radiation therapy may be used (Brodeur and Castleberry, 1993). The late effects associated with radiation therapy may be more manageable than those associated with the continuation of cytotoxic agents, especially the cardiotoxic effects of doxorubicin on the young developing heart. After chemotherapy or combined chemotherapy and radiation therapy, the patient undergoes complete resection again to remove remaining disease and to evaluate the effectiveness of the therapy.

A cure is less likely in children older than 1 year even when therapy is aggressive. For infants (less than 1 year of age) with stage C or D neuroblastoma, postsurgical courses of cyclophosphamide and doxorubicin are administered, followed by several courses of cisplatin and teniposide if only a partial remission occurs (Bowman et al., 1991). Radiation therapy is usually not indicated. Postchemotherapy surgery usually removes any remaining tumor and aids in the evaluation of the therapy's effectiveness.

Neoadjuvant Chemotherapy Followed by Surgery with or without Radiation Therapy

In children older than 1 year of age who exhibit symptoms of POG stage C or D neuroblastoma, the surgeon will attempt a resection, but the timing of this surgery is made on an individual basis (Shamberger et al., 1991). The child receives neoadjuvant chemotherapy to decrease the size of the tumor; the surgeon may then perform a resection without risk to the integrity of nearby vital organs and vascular structures. The tumor also takes on a more manageable appearance after chemotherapy. The chemotherapy plan includes a carefully orchestrated regimen of multiple agents such as vincristine, cyclophosphamide, cisplatin, doxorubicin, and teniposide (Brodeur and Castleberry, 1993). After chemotherapy, the tumor becomes more encapsulated, making it easier to remove surgically from surrounding structures and less likely to induce high blood loss (Shamberger et al., 1991).

The purpose of radiation therapy is to eliminate residual tumor, shrink unresectable tumors, control disseminated disease, and manage symptoms in end-stage disease. External-beam radiation to the tumor site and surrounding area may total 15 to 30 Gy, with fractionated doses of 1.5 to 4 Gy, depending on the child's age, tumor volume, and the tumor's location. The radiation oncologist may also elect to give intraoperative radiation therapy during the postchemotherapy surgical resection (Brodeur and Castleberry, 1993).

Children with aggressive or advanced-stage neuroblastoma may benefit from chemotherapy given as intensive myeloablative consolidation therapy followed by autologous bone marrow transplantation (ABMT) (Matthay et al., 1993). Pre-ABMT protocols include various combinations of chemotherapy agents such as cisplatin, teniposide, etoposide, and melphalan with total body irradiation. This is followed by the infusion of autologous bone marrow that has been purged of detectable tumor cells. The initial response to this therapy has been favorable, with an average overall progression-free survival rate of 44% at 3 years (Matthay et al., 1993). Sites of relapse correlate with sites of original disease, including bone, bone marrow, and primary tumor site if not completely resected.

❖ Wilms' Tumor

Wilms' tumor is a malignant tumor of the kidney and the most common abdominal tumor in children (Exelby, 1991). It arises from embryonic renal cells, occurs largely in infants and preschool children, and is occasionally associated with congenital genitourinary abnormalities. Refinement of effective treatment regimens have resulted in a 5-year survival rate of approximately 90% (Exelby, 1991).

Treatment

Currently children with Wilms' tumor can be treated following the National Wilms' Tumor Study Four (NWTS-4) protocols (Green et al., 1993; Green et al., 1991). The main objective of the NWTS-4 protocols is to improve overall survival using the least amount of treatment possible.

Favorable Histology: Surgery Followed by Adjuvant Chemotherapy
In nearly all cases, the involved kidney is removed (National Wilms' Tumor Study Committee [NWTSC], 1991). A simple nephrectomy has replaced the radical nephrectomy usually done in the past with equally good results (NWTSC, 1991). During the operative procedure, regional lymph node sampling ensures accurate staging. The surgeon attempts to excise all tumor with the kidney, but this is not always possible. In contrast to neuroblastoma, the surgeon is not aggressive if removing the entire mass proves difficult. Intraoperative spillage of the tumor adversely affects the outcome, increasing the rate of relapse nearly twofold (NWTSC, 1991). In cases when part of the tumor is left behind, postoperative abdominal radiation therapy and chemotherapy yield good control rates (NWTSC, 1991).

Chemotherapy for Wilms' tumor consists of dactinomycin and vincristine administered according to a variable schedule over 3 to 6 months for children with a stage I tumor and favorable histology and over 6 to 15 months for children with a stage II tumor and favorable histology. Radiation therapy is usually not indicated in early-stage Wilms' tumor (Kim, Nesbit, and Levitt, 1992; Thomas et al., 1991).

Favorable Histology: Surgery Followed by Adjuvant Chemotherapy with Radiation Therapy
Children with a stage III tumor and favorable histology get treated with dactino-mycin, vincristine, and doxorubicin over 6 to 15 months and children with a stage IV tumor get treated at more frequent intervals, using maximum-tolerated doses for 15 months (Green et al., 1991).

Children with stage III and IV Wilms' tumors also receive radiation therapy. Radiation therapy is administered concomitantly with chemotherapy beginning as soon as the child becomes stable after surgery. Because a delay in starting radiation therapy after surgery has been associated with higher relapse rates, it is recommended that therapy begin no later than 9 days after surgery (Green et al., 1993).

The current NWTS treatment protocol recommends the use of six daily fractionated radiation treatments of 1.8 Gy directed to the kidney area, including the flank, and crossing over the midline to include the bilateral para-aortic nodes (Kim, Nesbit, and Levitt, 1992) (Figure 19-1). This dose should be reduced to 1.5 Gy daily when a large volume, such as the whole abdomen, is irradiated.

Metastases to the liver and the lungs are also treated with radiation therapy (Kim, Nesbit, and Levitt, 1992). If pulmonary metastases occur, both lungs receive radiation regardless of the extent and location of nodules. Daily fractionated doses of 1.5 Gy for a total dose of 12 Gy are usually administered.

The role of radiation therapy for a bilateral Wilms' tumor is less clear than for a unilateral tumor. In some cases radiation is reserved for only those children who have persistent or progressive disease after chemotherapy (Kim, Nesbit, and Levitt, 1992). Intraoperative radiation therapy has been implemented as a means to irradiate more precisely the actual part of the kidney involved with tumor (Halberg et al., 1991). However, the use of radiation therapy in smaller total doses to spare the kidney from damaging effects has proven ineffective (Kirkbride and Plowman, 1992).

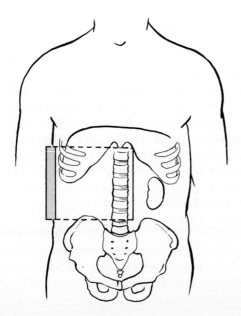

Fig. 19-1. Tumor-bed irradiation for Wilms' tumor when the tumor is on the right side. The fields extend across the midline to include the entire width of the vertebral bodies. The shaded area indicates the necessity of shielding the tangential abdominal wall. From Kim TH, Nesbit ME, and Levitt SH: Wilm's tumor. In Levitt SH, Khan FM, and Potish RA, editors: Levitt and Tapley's technological basis of radiation therapy: practical clinical applications, ed 2, Philadelphia, 1992, Lea & Febiger.

The fourth National Wilms' Tumor Study has attempted to define better several aspects of future treatment for this childhood malignancy (Green et al., 1991). This study is evaluating the economic impact of two different treatment strategies, one of which requires fewer visits to the clinic because the dosages are intensified as the frequency of administration decreases. Other questions explored by the study include the role of chemotherapy in stage I patients, the possibility of avoiding pulmonary radiation in stage IV patients, the role of prenephrectomy (neoadjuvant) chemotherapy, the elimination of doxorubicin from treatment to avoid cardiotoxicity, and the long-term late effects of treatment.

Unfavorable Histology: Surgery Followed by Adjuvant Chemotherapy
Followed by Adjuvant Radiation Therapy
Children with Wilms' tumor, and unfavorable histology, regardless of stage, receive chemotherapy using stage IV favorable histology regimens. Postoperative radiation concomitant with chemotherapy is recommended for all patients with anaplastic Wilms' tumor at stages II, III, and IV (Kim, Nesbit, and Levitt, 1992). Radiation therapy starts immediately after the child has stabilized from surgery. For children older than 41 months, the same fields and dosages used for tumors of favorable histology apply. Children younger than 41 months receive age-adjusted dosages to avoid detrimental late effects of therapy.

Bilateral Tumors: Neoadjuvant Chemotherapy with Adjuvant Radiation Therapy
The role of surgery in treating a bilateral Wilms' tumor is not as clear as in treating a unilateral Wilms' tumor. A general rule has been to excise the kidney that has the largest lesion and to perform a partial nephrectomy of the less affected kidney (NWTSC, 1991; Rao and Fleming, 1994). This leaves the remaining kidney with as much renal parenchyma as possible to avoid renal failure. However, tumors that resist treatment or progress while being treated can threaten the viability of the remaining kidney. A recent study randomized children with bilateral disease to initial surgical resection followed by chemotherapy or to biopsy followed by chemotherapy and then surgical resection (Shaul et al., 1992). The findings of this study showed no difference in survival between patients who had initial surgery or those who had initial chemotherapy. Even though children who received chemotherapy before surgery did not avoid the eventual need for unilateral total nephrectomy, postponing surgery provided time to evaluate which kidney to remove (the one less responsive to therapy or the one with less functional capability). The use of neoadjuvant chemotherapy in cases of a bilateral Wilms' tumor may soon become standard practice.

There are rare cases where bilateral nephrectomies are determined to be the best choice. When this occurs, the child receives renal dialysis until a kidney transplant can be considered 12 to 18 months later (Rao and Fleming, 1994).

❖ *Rhabdomyosarcoma*

Sarcomas result when mesenchymal cells fail to develop normally into fibrous tissue, muscle, cartilage, and bone. Rhabdomyosarcoma (RMS) is a malignant tumor that arises from mesenchymal tissue and is the most common soft tissue sarcoma in persons under 21 years of age (Raney et al., 1993). Nearly 50% of all cases are diagnosed in children under 5 years of age (Wexler and Helman, 1994).

Treatment

All Clinical Groups: Surgery

During the first clinical trials conducted to treat rhabdomyosarcoma, a surgicopathologic staging system (the Clinical Grouping System) was initiated (Wexler and Helman, 1994). This system, based on the resectability of the lesion, is beginning to lose favor to the more modern TNM (tumor, node, metatastases) method of staging. However, until that transition is complete, the categorization of tumor factors into clinical groups still occurs today.

The role of surgery in the management of RMS depends on the site of presentation and the extent of tumor involvement. Surgical intervention may be limited solely to the biopsy of the lesion, or it may be extensive (Rao and Fleming, 1994). More limited procedures have replaced the radical surgery used in the past for some RMS of the head and neck. The addition of radiation therapy and chemotherapy can produce results surpassing the overall results initially obtained by surgery and can also preserve normal anatomic structures.

The surgical approach to RMS tumors of the extremities is generally more aggressive than to tumors of the head and neck (Rao and Fleming, 1994). Although amputation is discouraged, wide local excision is often employed initially or following multimodal therapy. The surgeon resects a 2-cm margin of normal tissue around the tumor to help ensure the removal of microinvading malignant cells. If the surgeon excises a smaller margin of normal tissue, postoperative radiation therapy is instituted (Rao and Fleming, 1994).

Rhabdomyosarcoma of the testes is usually surgically managed with an orchiectomy and retroperitoneal node dissection (Rao and Fleming, 1994). Surgery follows chemotherapy for RMS of the bladder or the bladder and the prostate, but not in all cases. Radiation therapy alone may be all that is necessary for RMS of the bladder if the tumor responds well to chemotherapy. Surgical procedures may include a partial cystectomy or a prostatectomy. The extent of tissue and nodal excision depends greatly on local involvement of the tumor and whether the tumor has distant metastases. All patients receive postoperative radiation therapy.

A simple hysterectomy and partial vaginectomy is indicated for RMS of the uterus or cervix (Rao and Fleming, 1994). A partial vaginectomy may be all that is necessary if there is only local occurrence of the tumor. Chemotherapy and radiation therapy follow surgery.

Clinical Group I: Surgery Followed by Adjuvant Chemotherapy

Children with localized disease are treated with vincristine and dactinomycin [actinomycin D] (VA) without radiation therapy. This treatment plan, refined over two decades, has become the "gold standard" for cure of patients with nonalveolar Clinical Group I (completely resectable) tumors. Current randomized clinical trials treat children with different triple-drug combinations without regard to histology in an effort to improve overall outcomes. These combinations include VAC (vincristine, dactinomycin [actinomycin D], cyclophosphamide), VAI (vincristine, dactinomycin [actinomycin D], ifosfamide), and VIE (vincristine, ifosfamide, etoposide) (Wexler and Helman, 1994).

Clinical Groups II toIV: Surgery Followed by Concomitant Chemoradiotherapy

Treatment for Clinical Group II patients (locally extensive, nonmetastatic tumors) generally lasts 1 year. For children in Clinical Group II with nonalveolar tumors, treatment with VA and radiation therapy appears adequate (Wexler and Helman, 1994). Exceptions include children whose tumors originate from other than the paratesticular region or the head and neck. These cases are more difficult to treat and require the addition of doxorubicin.

Children who have unfavorable histology and disease sites at the time of diagnosis may be treated for as long as 2 years with three-agent combination therapy, which includes VAdriaC (vincristine, doxorubicin [Adriamycin], cyclophosphamide); VAC plus cisplatin; or VadriaC-VAC plus cisplatin and etoposide.

Management strategies for patients with distant metastatic disease are disappointing (Wexler and Helman, 1994). Intensive regimens of combination agents are given aggressively over a minimum of 2 years, but most patients develop recurrent metastatic disease 18 to 24 months after diagnosis. Only 20% of these children will be curable. Newer chemotherapy treatment protocols in combination with other treatment modalities are needed to improve the outlook for children with advanced RMS.

Radiation therapy plays an important role in local eradication of residual tumor as well as in other sites of bulky tumor spread. Without radiation therapy, local recurrence rates soar to as high as 75% (Raney et al., 1993). Radiation therapy is indicated in all cases of pediatric RMS with the exception of localized, completely resected Clinical Group Stage I patients. Children with Clinical Group II incompletely resected tumors generally receive a total dose of 40 Gy of conventional fractionated radiation therapy administered concomitantly with chemotherapy. Radiation therapy begins approximately 2 months after the initiation of chemotherapy (Wexler and Helman, 1994). The site to be irradiated includes the extent of the tumor prior to initial treatment plus a margin of 2 to 5 cm. Most children with residual disease (Clinical Group III) receive conventional fractionated radiation therapy to a total dose of 40 to 50 Gy or a total dose of nearly 60 Gy administered as 1.1 Gy hyperfractionated therapy twice daily. Regionally positive lymph nodes are treated with full radiation doses as well. Areas of distant metastasis (Clinical Group IV) may also be irradiated. However, radiation to these areas may not affect the overall outcome because many children with advanced RMS will not survive their disease. Other radiation-therapy techniques include intraoperative radiation therapy and radiation implants.

Rhabdomyosarcoma continues to present treatment challenges. Although the overall survival rate of patients with early-stage disease has exceeded 80%, the 3-year survival rate of those with advanced disease is not even half of that (Wexler and Helman, 1994). Dose-intensive therapies with aggressive supportive therapies, precision brachytherapy, and newer surgical techniques may help improve this dismal outcome (Raney et al., 1993).

❖ *Osteosarcoma*

Osteosarcoma is a primary malignant bone tumor that commonly occurs in children. It derives from primitive bone-forming cells and appears more frequently in adolescents and young adults than in young children (Link and Eilber, 1993).

Treatment

Neoadjuvant Chemotherapy Followed by Surgery Followed by Adjuvant Chemotherapy
Osteosarcoma tends to spread locally and through the bloodstream to the lungs if not treated with systemic therapy. Most of the children have local disease at the time of diagnosis, but the disease will almost certainly spread to distant sites if systemic therapy is not applied.

Chemotherapy for the treatment of bone tumors improves the overall rate of survival (Meyers et al., 1992). Systemic therapy is administered before or after surgery (Horowitz et al., 1993; Link and Eilber, 1993). Newer treatment protocols call for the administration of chemotherapy preoperatively to contain and shrink the tumor as well as postoperatively to destroy tumor cells that may remain after tumor resection and to treat any micrometastasis that may have occurred.

Multiagent regimens are used for the treatment of osteosarcoma (Link and Eilber, 1993). Combination protocols include high-dose methotrexate with leucovorin rescue plus vincristine with or without doxorubicin; bleomycin, cyclophosphamide, and dactinomycin; doxorubicin plus cisplatin alternating with etoposide and cyclophosphamide (Cassano, et al., 1991; Link and Eilber, 1993). The duration of neoadjuvant and adjuvant therapy depends on a multitude of variables, including the presentation characteristics and response of the tumor to therapy. Preoperative therapy usually lasts from 3 to 6 months, but it may last longer; postoperative therapy may last as long as 1 year (Bacci et al., 1993) (See the Research Highlight on page 311).

Intraarterial chemotherapy has been administered to children with osteosarcoma preoperatively. A short 2-hour infusion of cisplatin is given every 14 days for 3 courses, which results in varying degrees of tumor necrosis at the time of resection (Quintana et al., 1991). Children have also received intraarterial cisplatin in combination with systemic agents such as doxorubicin to treat local as well as distant disease (Yasko and Lane, 1991).

Following initial chemotherapy, surgery may be performed if the tumor is located in an accessible area such as a rib or in an extremity. The type and extent of surgery depends on the location of the tumor, its size, and whether it has spread. If the tumor is small and accessible, local excision is usually performed.

The decision to amputate or to attempt the salvage of an affected extremity involves several considerations (Link and Eilber, 1993), including the responsiveness of the tumor to neoadjuvant chemotherapy. If the tumor has diminished in size, limb salvage can be considered. However, if disease has progressed during chemotherapy, an amputation should be performed and the chemotherapy regimen altered. Amputation may be the best choice in certain situations even when limb salvage is possible. In the young and growing child, amputation may be favored

---

Bacci G, Picci P, Ferrari S, Ruggieri P, Casadei R, Tienghi A, del Prever AB, Gherlinzoni F, Mercuri M, and Monti C: Primary chemotherapy and delayed surgery for nonmetastatic osteosarcoma of the extremities, Cancer 72:3227–3238, 1993.

Study Patients received two cycles of neoadjuvant high-dose methotrexate followed by cisplatin given intraarterially and doxorubicin. Postoperatively the good responders (those having more than 90% tumor necrosis) received three more cycles of these drugs. Poor responders received these same agents plus ifosfamide and etoposide.

Sample The study included 164 patients with localized osteosarcoma of the extremity.

Study aim To increase the number of good responders by using more aggressive chemotherapy and to improve the prognosis of poor responders by using different salvage chemotherapy.

Findings There were 109 children (66% of all patients) free of disease at an average follow-up time of 54 months. The 5-year, actuarial, continuously-disease-free survival rate was 63%, 52 children experienced metastases, and 3 had local recurrence.

Discussion It is possible to cure more than 60% of children with localized osteosarcoma of an extremity with aggressive neoadjuvant chemotherapy. The use of aggressive chemotherapy may help avoid amputation. Ifosfamide and etoposide may be effective in children who do not respond to preoperative chemotherapy.

---

because of potential discrepancies in the size of limbs as a result of radiation therapy. In addition, the salvaged limb may have less function than the limited function imposed by an artificial limb (Aboudalfia and Malawer, 1992).

The location of the tumor chiefly determines the extent of the amputation. Tumors of the distal tibia necessitate a below-the-knee amputation, whereas an above-the-knee amputation or knee disarticulation is appropriate for tibial and fibular lesions. Distal femoral lesions require a high, above-the-knee amputation. A hip disarticulation or hemipelvectomy is performed for proximal femur tumors. Amputation procedures require the excision of 8 to 10 cm of normal tissue beyond the border of the original tumor (Eilber, 1994).

Limb salvage involves more complicated procedures than amputations, but it can be considered if the size of the primary tumor has diminished markedly after chemotherapy or radiation therapy. Any portion of the bone invaded by the tumor is excised along with a margin of 5 to 8 cm of normal tissue. The bony defect is then replaced with a metallic endoprosthesis and joint replacement or, less commonly, with cadaver allografts or a combination of cadaver allografts and endoprosthesis (Aboudalfia and Malawer, 1992; Link and Eilber, 1993). The operation must leave adequate skin and muscle to cover the resection site to allow the wound to heal and to aid in the restoration of motor power.

Limb salvage has numerous other contraindications. These include major neurovascular involvement of the tumor or loss of substantial neurovasculature at the time of tumor resection, pathologic fractures, infection of the biopsy site, extensive muscle involvement, and immature skeletal age, which will result in a difference of 6 to 8 cm or more in leg length (Aboudalfia and Malawer, 1992).

Radiation therapy does not work effectively against osteosarcoma because the disease is highly radioresistant. Radiation therapy for prophylaxis or treatment of osteosarcoma pulmonary metastases is currently being investigated (Link and Eilber, 1993).

Studies have reported long-term survival rates as high as 80% in children with osteosarcoma who exhibit low-risk factors (Link and Eilber, 1993) such as localized disease, favorable tumor histology, small tumor size, tumor location away from the main axis of the body, complete surgical resection of the tumor, short duration of symptoms, and patient age (older than 10). Children with high-risk factors or those who relapse have a long-term survival rate as low as 13%. Newer therapies that incorporate biologic response modifiers and cutting-edge technologies may hold the key to overcoming treatment failures (Link and Eilber, 1993).

❖ Ewing's Sarcoma

Ewing's sarcoma is an undifferentiated bone tumor (Horowitz et al., 1993). It occurs most frequently in the second decade of life. Ewing's sarcoma may also occur in soft tissues. Ewing's sarcoma occurs as often in an extremity as on the body's central axis. Common sites for tumor occurrence include the distal and proximal sites of the extremities, the pelvis, and the chest wall.

Treatment

Neoadjuvant Chemotherapy Followed by Radiation Therapy

The treatment of Ewing's sarcoma with chemotherapy usually involves a combination of agents. Successful regimens include vincristine, dactinomycin, doxorubicin, and cyclophosphamide (Yasko and Lane, 1991) or ifosfamide plus etoposide (Meyer et al., 1992).

Current data supports the use of chemotherapy before radiation therapy to treat distant metastases and to reduce the size of the primary tumor (Horowitz et al., 1993). The reduction in tumor size allows the use of a smaller radiation field, thereby sparing nearly normal tissues from the damaging effects of radiation. Radiation doses of 45 to 50 Gy at 1.8 to 2 Gy daily fractions have become the routine approach in irradiating Ewing's sarcoma tumors and surrounding tissues. It is not uncommon for an additional boost of radiation to be delivered to the tumor alone. Newer radiation techniques include hyperfractionated radiation and intraoperative radiation therapies. In hyperfractionated radiation, doses are delivered 6 hours apart, twice daily. The theory is that smaller radiation fractions delivered more frequently allow enough time for the damaged normal cells to repair themselves but do not allow the damaged tumor cells, which require more time to repair themselves, time to recover. Intraoperative radiation therapy may be more damaging to large tumors that fail to regress satisfactorily with chemotherapy and external radiation. Local doses as high as 20 Gy have been administered in the operating room during surgical resection.

Neoadjuvant Chemotherapy Followed by Radiation Therapy with or without Surgery
Following chemotherapy and radiation therapy, surgery may not be possible. Inoperable examples include Ewing's sarcoma located on the pelvis or in the proximal end of an extremity. An extensive presentation of the tumor, such as involvement of the entire shaft of the femur, also makes amputation unlikely. Metastatic spread of the tumor to other organ systems also rules against amputation.

If the child is an appropriate candidate for surgery, a decision is made to amputate or to perform a limb-salvage procedure. The same surgical considerations regarding osteosarcoma apply to the child with Ewing's sarcoma.

The prognosis for children with Ewing's sarcoma is difficult to predict (Horowitz et al., 1993). Children with local disease and children who are diagnosed at a young age do better than other children and can probably expect a long-term survival rate of 50% to 70%.

❖ Nursing Management

Children who receive multimodal cancer therapy are susceptible to the same treatment-related complications as adults. However, because of the child's young age, immature organ systems, and continuous physical and mental growth and development these complications have additional and greater consequences. The physical consequences of cancer treatment include organ system dysfunction, a delay or permanent retardation in physical growth, and loss of a limb or organ. Psychosocial consequences of cancer treatment include learning disabilities, difficulty in adapting to wellness, and potentially disabling fears of disease recurrence. Possible Side Effects from Multimodal Therapy are listed on page 314.

Special Considerations

Before administering chemotherapy to a child, the oncologist must consider how the agent will be delivered and how the acute side effects can best be managed. Immediate attention should be given to inserting a permanent vascular access device. A tunneled catheter, an implanted port, or a short-term nontunneled device can be used in children (Keegan-Wells and Steward, 1992; Marcoux et al., 1990). The type of device selected will depend on several factors: the length of therapy, the agents used, the potential need for supportive therapies, the child's age, the child's stage of development, the availability and responsibility of a caregiver, and the child's choice of device. If the course of cancer therapy is expected to last more than 1 year, if the chemotherapeutic agents will be administered as long infusions, and if there is a potential for frequent infusion of blood components, antimicrobial agents, and total parenteral nutrition, a tunneled catheter may work best. If the child is older or has the ability to overcome the fear of needle sticks, an implanted port may be appropriate. The status of the primary caregiver will greatly affect which device to insert. An implanted port may be best if there is concern regarding the caregiver's ability to comply with the daily care a tunneled catheter requires. Short-term, nontunneled catheters are useful if the therapy is brief and the child has

Possible Side Effects from Multimodal Therapy in
Pediatric Cancers

Multimodal Treatment	Possible Enhanced Side Effects*
Neuroblastoma	
Surgery followed by adjuvant chemotherapy followed by surgery	
Cyclophosphamide, doxorubicin Cisplatin, teniposide	No enhanced side effects
Surgery followed by adjuvant chemotherapy followed by adjuvant radiation therapy followed by surgery	
Cyclophosphamide, doxorubicin	Adhesions, fistula formation, poor wound healing, cardiotoxicity (if radiation to the chest), nephrotoxicity (if radiation to the pelvis), small bowel obstruction (if radiation to the pelvis), increased bone marrow depression, secondary cancers
Neoadjuvant chemotherapy followed by surgery followed by radiation therapy	
Vincristine, cyclophosphamide, cisplatin, doxorubicin, teniposide	Adhesions, fistula formation, increased bone marrow depression, cardiotoxicity (if radiation to the chest), nephrotoxicity (if radiation to the pelvis), small bowel obstruction (if radiation to the pelvis), secondary cancers
Wilms' Tumor	
Nephrectomy followed by chemotherapy	
Dactinomycin, vincristine	Renal dysfunction
Nephrectomy followed by chemotherapy followed by pelvic radiation	
Dactinomycin, vincristine, doxorubicin	Renal dysfunction, increased bone marrow depression
Nephrectomy followed by concomitant chemoradiotherapy (radiation to the pelvis)	
Dactinomycin, vincristine, doxorubicin	Renal dysfunction, increased bone marrow depression, fistula formation
Neoadjuvant chemotherapy followed by nephrectomy	
Dactinomycin, vincristine, doxorubicin	No enhanced side effects

*Depends on the site of treatment; only some common sites are listed here.

Arbeit, Hilaris, and Brennen, 1987; DeLaat and Lampkin, 1992; Fraser and Tucker, 1989; Hobbie et al., 1993; Moore and Ruccione, 1993; Rubin, Constine, and Nelson, 1992.

Multimodal Treatment	Possible Enhanced Side Effects*
Rhabdomyosarcoma	
Surgery followed by adjuvant chemotherapy	
Vincristine, dactinomycin	No enhanced side effects
Vincristine, dactinomycin, cyclophosphamide	
Vincristine, dactinomycin, ifosfamide	
Vincristine, ifosfamide, etoposide	
Surgery followed by adjuvant radiation therapy	No enhanced side effects
Surgery followed by adjuvant concomitant chemoradiotherapy	
Vincristine, dactinomycin, cyclophosphamide	Facial asymmetry (if treatment site is head), impaired fertility (if treatment site is testes), cardiotoxicity (if treatment site is chest), ototoxicity (if treatment site is head), increased bone marrow depression (if treatment site is pelvic area), secondary cancers
Vincristine, doxorubicin, cyclophosphamide, cisplatin	
Vincristine, dactinomycin, cyclophosphamide, cisplatin, etoposide	
Osteosarcoma	
Neoadjuvant chemotherapy followed by surgery followed by adjuvant chemotherapy	
Methotrexate, vincristine	No enhanced side effects
Methotrexate, vincristine, doxorubicin	
Bleomycin, cyclophosphamide, dactinomycin	
Doxorubicin, cisplatin, etoposide, cyclophosphamide	
Ewing's Sarcoma	
Neoadjuvant chemotherapy followed by radiation therapy	
Vincristine, dactinomycin, doxorubicin, cyclophosphamide	No enhanced side effects (if only extremity involved; otherwise side effects are site-specific)
Ifosfamide, etoposide	
Neoadjuvant chemotherapy followed by radiation therapy followed by surgery	
Vincristine, dactinomycin, doxorubicin, cyclophosphamide	Deformity or shortening of affected limb, delayed wound healing (other side effects are site-specific)
Ifosfamide, etoposide	

adequate vasculature. Nursing Care of the Child Preparing to Undergo a Procedure is presented on page 316.

Dehydration secondary to the nausea and vomiting associated with chemotherapy and, in some cases, radiation therapy, is a significant problem in children. It can

Nursing Care of

The Child Preparing to Undergo a Procedure

Nursing Care	Rationale/Comments

◆ Assess the situation in intervention preparation
  ◆ The child's developmental and chronological age
  ◆ The potential hazards of the procedure
  ◆ Mechanisms that can balance the hazards and the child's ability to cope with the stress of the procedure
	◆ The child's outward behavior may not be an accurate reflection of his or her anxiety; a better understanding can be obtained by recognizing those fears and issues relevant to a child's developmental and chronological age; technical and emotional aspects associated with a particular procedure will also help identify issues that most concern the child (e.g., pain, separation, unfamiliar surroundings, strangers); how the child and family deal with threatening situations will alert the nurse to coping strengths and weaknesses and what interventions may be useful

◆ Plan for effective interventions ◆ Provide ongoing emotional support of the child and parents	◆ Ongoing emotional support before and after a procedure will provide the child with a sense of reassurance and acknowledge his or her fears and concerns; emotional support of parents will help them support, reassure, and console the child
	Infant Provide constant verbal and physical efforts to soothe and comfort the infant; maintain parents' presence to assist with consoling but not with restraining
	Toddler Let the child know it is all right to cry; inform the child what will please you, because toddlers are eager to please; maintain parents' presence if the child experiences separation anxiety
	Preschooler Offer ample opportunities for questions and provide simple, consistent answers, let the child know ways in which he or she may cooperate
	School-age child Identify misconceptions that can propagate unrealistic fears, a private setting may encourage the child to be more open and forthcoming about feelings
	Adolescent Provide opportunities for active involvement in planning and conducting the procedure; consider having another adolescent with similar experiences help in the preparation; be sensitive about adolescents' need for privacy

From Manion J: Preparing children for hospitalization, procedures, or surgery. In Craft MJ and Denehy JA, editors: Nursing interventions for infants and children, Philadelphia, 1990, WB Saunders Co.

Nursing Care	*Rationale/Comments*
◆ Facilitate emotional expression, personal interaction, and play	◆ To help develop a relationship of trust, a single individual should be responsible for most of the preparation; individuals who will be involved with the procedure should also participate
	Structured and unstructured play provide a mechanism to impart information through an activity a child can readily identify with; play with miniature models, puppets, and toy medical instruments can help the child verbalize fears, concerns, and anger, and signal his or her level of comprehension, coping, and acceptance
	Infant Play after the procedure can restore a sense of normalcy and signal completion of the event
	Toddlers Provide opportunities to handle equipment, if appropriate; keep sessions short because of children's limited attention spans
	Preschooler Use actual equipment and allow child to act out the procedure on dolls or stuffed animals; puppet play is ideal for identifying a child's feelings
	School-age child Provide specific information about the procedure and discuss the body parts involved
	Adolescent Provide rationale for the procedure and discuss the body parts involved
◆ Provide procedural and sensory information	◆ Children are not only concerned about the procedure to be done to their bodies; they are equally concerned about how the procedure will feel afterwards; children are most concerned about pain, mutilation of body parts, and loss of privacy
	When describing procedures, use words that children can easily understand; avoid technical terms such as injection, anesthesia, incision, and MRI; a short description of these terms will be better understood (needle, medicine to help you go to sleep, small opening, pictures of inside of you); avoid words that are threatening such as shot, cut open, and dye; some terms will require an explanation because they can be confusing for the child: OR table, ICU, bed pan, and draw your blood, for example

Continued

Nursing Care	Rationale/Comments
◆ Recognize variables affecting preparation strategies	◆ Variables can make preparation ineffective if they are not considered when developing a plan for preparing the child for a procedure
◆ Optimal timing of the preparation	◆ Toddlers' and preschoolers' conceptions of time center around activities of daily living; the child should be informed of the time of procedures as they correlate to daily activities (lunch time, nap time); these children should receive preparation shortly before the event occurs to avoid developing exaggerated fears; school-age children and adolescents have good concepts of time and should begin to receive preparation as soon as the procedure is scheduled
◆ Involvement of the family	◆ An assessment of the family as a unit will identify members who will be most accessible and available to assist in procedure preparation; involvement of at least one parent is important because the child depends on a parent for comfort, security, protection from harm, and reassurance
◆ Physiologic status	◆ The urgency of the situation or the child's illness can make preparation short or impossible; in these situations, a postprocedural debriefing when the child is stable is beneficial; postprocedural debriefing can help the child understand why the procedure was conducted, resolve feelings of fear or anger, and establish a level of trust with health care providers
◆ Psychological status	◆ An assessment of individual coping styles will help to identify which interventions to implement; active, coping children have a heightened awareness of situations and might experience increased stress; children who are avoidant copers (copes by avoiding an issue) do best with information that is supportive and reassuring in nature rather than detailed; children who show both of these styles do best with general information limited to the procedure

rapidly lead to electrolyte imbalance and weight loss. For the infant or toddler, nausea or vomiting may significantly reduce nutritional intake. Numerous antiemetic agents and various combinations of antiemetic agents may be given as long as measures are taken to administer correct pediatric doses and to minimize side effects. Extrapyramidal reactions (muscle jitteriness and facial grimaces) frequently occur in children who have received certain antiemetic agents, primarily the phenothiazines and metoclopramide. To minimize this side effect, diphenhydramine can be administered concomitantly. Behavioral interventions are effective for children who experience persistent nausea.

If the child experiences oral or esophageal mucositis, intravenous administration becomes the only reliable route for giving analgesics. Children need to be medicated with an appropriate analgesic. The oral and intravenous routes (if child has a vascular access device) are preferred over injections and suppositories because of children's fears of needle sticks and rectal penetration. The child with cancer may also experience pain directly caused by the tumor, as an outcome of surgery, or as a side effect of chemotherapy or radiation therapy. Parent Education Guidelines for Sedation in the Child Receiving Radiation Therapy appear below (From Bucholtz JD: Issues concerning the sedation of children for radiation therapy, Oncol Nurs Forum 19:649–655, 1992).

Parent Education Guidelines for

Sedation in the Child Receiving Radiation Therapy

♦ *The Need for Sedation*   Your child will need to lie still during each radiation treatment. To help your child do this, it will be necessary to give your child special medicines to put him or her to sleep for a short period of time. Two different types of medications used are: sedatives and general anesthesia.

♦ *Sedatives*   Sedatives are medicines that can make a child feel sleepy or that make him or her actually fall asleep. These medications can be given orally, rectally, or by injection into the muscle or vein.

The medication your child will receive is called _____

Possible side effects include _____

_____

♦ *Monitoring Your Child*   Your child's vital signs (pulse, respirations, temperature, and blood pressure) will be measured before each treatment. The nurse will stay with your child until he or she is asleep. Once your child is asleep and ready for treatments to begin, the nurse will leave the room and watch your child from a television monitor. Afterwards the child will be watched closely in the radiation department until fully awake. Your child's vital signs will be measured during this time. After your child is safely awake, you may all go home.

♦ *General Anesthesia*   The radiation therapy team has recommended that your child receive general anesthesia for sedation. This decision was based on different factors that your child's doctor will discuss with you. Some of these factors include how complicated the treatments will be, how long each treatment will last, and your child's reaction to sedatives in the past. General anesthesia will be given by an anesthesiologist (a doctor who specializes in putting patients to sleep). Your child cannot eat or drink for 6 hours before being anesthetized. Your child will have an IV and be put to sleep with an IV medication.

Permission granted to reproduce these guidelines for educational purposes only.

Continued

Your child's pulse, respirations, and blood pressure will be constantly monitored throughout the treatment by special equipment. After the treatment is completed, your child will go to the postanesthesia care unit (PACU). The nurses in the PACU will closely monitor your child's recovery. Parents are usually permitted to be with their child at this time, but always check with the PACU nurses. Certain circumstances may come up that may not always make this possible. After your child safely wakes up, the PACU nurses will let you take him or her home.

♦ *Discharge Care*   Your child may temporarily feel confused, frightened, or irritable after waking up. It is important to comfort your child and help him or her understand that the treatment is over and that it is time to go home. Some children may return to normal play activities once home, while others may feel tired and have little energy. It is generally all right for the child to resume the activity he or she chooses (i.e., play or rest). The child may eat after treatment, but start with liquids first. You may feed your child when he or she is able to drink without feeling sick. Please call the radiation department at the following number if there is something about your child that concerns you or if your child has any of the following complications:

Vomiting
Difficult to waken
Fever of more than 100°F
Extreme crying or fussiness

Phone number: _____

Psychosocial Issues

The psychosocial sequelae of pediatric cancer therapy depend a great deal on the individual child. It cannot be assumed that all children will suffer lifelong psychosocial consequences directly related to therapy. However, as the children mature, how they adjust to wellness and adulthood should be closely monitored for any problems possibly associated with therapy. Because cancer therapy for children has changed so dramatically in recent years, studies conducted 10 to 20 years ago that documented moderate to severe psychological impairment may not apply today. Children who receive high doses of cranial radiation and intrathecal methotrexate experience cognitive dysfunction and learning disorders. This late effect is demonstrated by poor social and emotional skills as well as problems performing in school, especially in handwriting, reading, and math. These children may need special education to help deal with these discrepancies (Hymovich and Roehnert, 1989).

With more children surviving cancer, attention has refocused on the long-term effects of treatment such as cardiomyopathy and second cancers. These long-term effects are the result of organ toxicity incurred during therapy. Some of these effects can be adequately treated or compensated for, whereas others may result in permanent disabilities. Long-term effects of treatment are discussed in Unit III.

❖ Summary

Progress against pediatric cancers continues with the implementation of multi-modal therapy. Current successes can be contributed, in part, to a multidisciplinary approach to care and to the development of supportive therapies such as antimicrobial agents, growth factors, and blood-component therapy. The consequences of intensive therapies, however, are only now being fully understood. As more children survive their cancers, the late effects of therapy will become evident. Only time will tell what the future holds for these children as they enter adulthood.

❖ References

Aboudalfia AJ and Malawer MM: Limb-sparing surgery for osteosarcoma, Cont Oncol 2(9):20–32, 1992.

Arbeit JM, Hilaris BS, and Brennan MF: Wound complications in the multimodality treatment of extremity and superficial truncal sarcomas, J Clin Oncol 5:480–488,1987.

Bacci G, Picci P, Ferrari S, Ruggieri P, Casadei R, Tienghi A, del Prever AB, Gherlinzoni F, Mercuri M, and Monti C: Primary chemotherapy and delayed surgery for nonmetastatic osteosarcoma of the extremities, Cancer 72:3227–3238, 1993.

Bleyer WA: The impact of childhood cancer on the United States and the world, CA-Cancer J Clin 40:355–367, 1990.

Bowman LC, Hancock ML, Santana VM, Hayes FA, Kun L, Parham DM, Furman WL, Rao BN, Green AA, and Crist WM: Impact of intensified therapy on clinical outcome in infants and children with neuroblastoma: the St. Jude Children's Research Hospital experience, 1962 to 1988, J Clin Oncol 9:1599–1608, 1991.

Brodeur GM and Castleberry RP: Neuroblastoma. In Pizzo PA and Poplack DG, editors: Principles and practice of pediatric oncology, ed 2, Philadelphia, 1993, JB Lippincott Co, pp. 739–767.

Cassano WF, Graham-Pole J, and Dickson N: Etoposide, cyclophosphamide, cisplatin, and doxorubicin as neoadjuvant chemotherapy for osteosarcoma, Cancer 68:1899–1902, 1991.

DeLaat CA and Lampkin BC: Long-term survivors of childhood cancer: evaluation and identification of sequelae of treatment, CA-Cancer J Clin 42:263–282, 1992.

Eilber FR: Malignant tumors of bone. In McKenna RJ and Murphy GP, editors: Cancer surgery, Philadelphia, 1994, JB Lippincott Co, pp. 657–662.

Exelby PR: Wilms' tumor 1991: clinical evaluation and treatment, Urol Clin No Am 18:589–597, 1991.

Fraser MC and Tucker MA: Second malignancies following cancer, Semin Oncol Nurs 5:43–55, 1989.

Green DM, D'Angio GJ, Beckwith JB, Breslow NE, Finklestein JZ, Kelalis P, and Thomas PRM: Wilms' tumor (nephroblastoma, renal embryoma). In Pizzo PA and Poplack DG, editors: Principles and practice of pediatric oncology, ed 2, Philadelphia, 1993, JB Lippincott Co, pp. 713–737.

Green DM, Finklestein JZ, Breslow NF, and Beckwith JB: Remaining problems in the treatment of patients with Wilms' tumor, Pedia Clin No Am 38:475–488, 1991.

Haase G, O'Leary MC, Ramsay NKC, Romansky SG, Stram DO, Seeger RC, and Hammond GD: Aggressive surgery combined with intensive chemotherapy improves survival in poor-risk neuroblastoma, J Pedia Surg 26:1119–1124, 1991.

Halberg FE, Harrison MR, Salvatierra O, Longaker MT, Wara WM, and Phillips TL: Intraoperative radiation therapy for Wilms' tumor in situ or ex vivo, Cancer 67:2839–2843, 1991.

Hobbie W, Ruccione KS, Moore I, Truesdell S: Late effects in long-term survivors. In Foley GV, Fochtman D, and Mooney KH, editors: Nursing care of the child with cancer, ed 2, Philadelphia, 1993, WB Saunders Co, pp. 482–486.

Horowitz ME, DeLaney TF, Malawer MM, and Tsokos MG: Ewing's sarcoma family of tumors: Ewing's sarcoma of bone and soft tissue and the peripheral primitive neuroectodermal tumors. In Pizzo PA and Poplack DG, editors: Principles and practice of pediatric oncology, ed 2, Philadelphia, 1993, JB Lippincott Co, pp. 795–821.

Hymovich DP and Roehnert JE: Psychosocial consequences of childhood cancer, Semin Oncol Nurs 5:56–62, 1989.

Keegan-Wells D and Steward JL: The use of venous access devices in pediatric oncology nursing practice, J Pedia Oncol Nurs 9(4):159–169, 1992.

Kim TH, Nesbit ME, and Levitt SH: Wilms' tumor. In Levitt SH, Khan FM, and Potish RA, editors: Levitt and Tapley's technological basis of radiation therapy: practical clinical applications, ed 2, Philadelphia, 1992, Lea & Febiger, pp. 377–381.

Kirkbride P, and Plowman PN: Radiotherapy to the surviving kidney after unilateral nephrectomy in bilateral Wilms' tumor, Brit J Radiol 65(774):510–516, 1992.

Link MP and Eilber F: Osteosarcoma. In Pizzo PA and Poplack DG, editors: Principles and practice of pediatric oncology, ed 2, Philadelphia, 1993, JB Lippincott Co, pp. 841–866.

Marcoux C, Fisher S, and Wong D: Central venous access devices in children, Pedia Nurs 16(2): 123–133, 1990.

Matthay KK, Atkinson JB, Stram DO, Selch M, Reynolds CP, and Seeger RC: Patterns of relapse after autologous purged bone marrow transplantation for neuroblastoma: a Children's Cancer Group pilot study, J Clin Oncol 11:2226–2233, 1993.

Meyer WH, Kun L, Marina N, Roberson P, Parham D, Rao B, Fletcher B, and Pratt CB: Ifosfamide plus etoposide in newly diagnosed Ewing's sarcoma of bone, J Clin Oncol 10:1737–1742, 1992.

Meyers PA, Heller G, Healey J, Huvos A, Lane J, Marcove R, Applewhite A, Vlamis V, and Rosen G: Chemotherapy for nonmetastatic osteogenic sarcoma: the Memorial Sloan-Kettering experience, J Clin Oncol 10:5–15, 1992.

Moore IM and Ruccione KS: Late effects of cancer treatment. In Groenwald SL, Goodman M, Frogge MH, and Yarbro CH, editors: Cancer nursing: principles and practice, ed 3, Boston, 1993, Jones & Bartlett Publishers, pp. 840–858.

National Wilms' Tumor Study Committee: Wilms' tumor: status report, 1990, J Clin Oncol 9:877–887, 1991.

Quintana J, Beresi V, DelPozo H, Latorre JJ, Henriquez A, Chamas N, Diaz V, Geldres V, Sepulveda L, Macho L, and Dolz G: Intra-arterial cisplatin given prior to surgery in osteosarcoma: grade of necrosis and size of tumor as major prognostic factors, Amer J Pedia Hemat Oncol 13:269–273, 1991.

Raney RB, Hays DM, Tefft M, and Triche TJ: Rhabdomyosarcoma and the undifferentiated sarcomas. In Pizzo PA and Poplack DG, editors: Principles and practice of pediatric oncology, ed 2, Philadelphia, 1993, JB Lippincott Co, pp. 769–794.

Rao BN and Fleming ID: Surgery for pediatric cancer. In McKenna RJ and Murphy GP, editors: Cancer surgery, Philadelphia, 1994, JB Lippincott Co, pp. 577–600.

Rubin R, Constine LS, and Nelson DF: Late effects of cancer treatment: radiation and drug toxicity. In Perez CA and Brady LW, editors: Principles and practice of radiation oncology, ed 2, Philadelphia, 1992, JB Lippincott Co, pp. 124–161.

Shamberger RC, Allarde-Segundo A, Kozakewich HPW, and Grier HE: Surgical management of stage III and IV neuroblastoma resection before or after chemotherapy? J Pedia Surg 26:1113–1118, 1991.

Shaul DB, Srikanth MM, Ortega JA, and Mahour GH: Treatment for bilateral Wilms' tumor: comparison of initial biopsy and chemotherapy to initial surgical resection in the preservation of renal mass and function, J Pedia Surg 27:1009–1015, 1992.

Thomas PRM, Tefft M, Compaan PJ, Norkool P, Breslow NE, and D'Angio GJ: Results of two radiation therapy randomizations in the Third National Wilms' Tumor Study, Cancer 68:1703–1717, 1991.

Wexler LH and Helman LJ: Pediatric soft tissue sarcomas, Cancer J Clin 44:211–247, 1994.

Yasko AW and Lane JM: Chemotherapy for bone and soft-tissue sarcomas of the extremities, J Bone Joint Surg 73-A(8):1263–1271, 1991.

UNIT III

SIDE EFFECTS

Chapter 20

❖ *Gastrointestinal Side Effects*

Rebecca Hawkins

Cancer treatments can affect the gastrointestinal (GI) tract in various ways. These include nausea, vomiting, mucositis, constipation, diarrhea, and decreased appetite. Most of these side effects, if not managed aggressively, can have deleterious outcomes, such as increased debilitation, dehydration, dysphagia, malnutrition, and decreased treatment tolerance. Some patients may abandon or delay treatment, leading to inadequate cancer care.

❖ *Nausea and Vomiting*

Nausea and vomiting are well known by both health care providers and the general public. Less understood are the advances that have been made in controlling these side effects. Nausea and vomiting are thought to be mediated by the vomiting center (VC) located in the lateral reticular formation of the medulla oblongata in the brain (Figure 20-1). Input from the GI tract, the pharynx, and various sympathetic nerves can stimulate the vomiting center via the vagal visceral afferent fibers (Hogan, 1990; Rhodes, 1990).

The central nervous system provides input to the VC by both physiologic and psychologic mechanisms. An example of a physiologic mechanism is direct stimulation to the midbrain from increased intracranial pressure. Psychogenic factors can lead to nausea and vomiting by stimulating the cortex and the limbic system through emotional and sensory stimuli (Hogan, 1990; Rhodes, 1990).

The chemoreceptor trigger zone (CTZ) plays a major role in nausea and vomiting. The CTZ is a separate area of the brain located in the floor of the fourth ventricle, outside the blood-brain barrier. The CTZ acts like a sensing mechanism that detects noxious substances such as chemotherapeutic agents or their metabolites and sends an afferent signal to the VC, resulting in nausea and vomiting (Shannon-Bodnar, 1990). The exact mechanism of the cause of nausea and vomiting is still unknown, and current studies continue to explore this phenomenon.

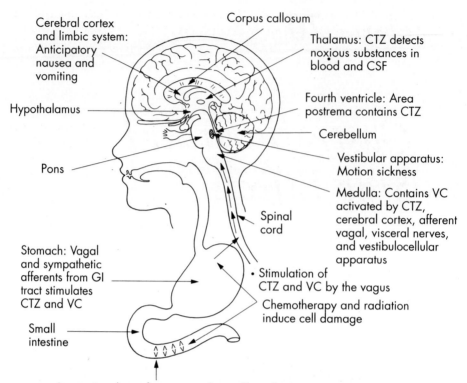

Serotonin release from enterochromaffin cells: Serotonin activates
5-HT₃ receptors on visceral and vagal afferents, sending messages
to CTZ and VC, site of action of 5-HT₃ antagonist

Fig. 20-1. Various pathways that can lead to nausea and vomiting from cancer treatments.
VC = vomiting center; CTZ = chemoreceptor trigger zone; CSF = cerebral spinal fluid. From
Camp-Sorrell D: Chemotherapy: toxicity management. In Groenwald SL, Goodman M, Frogge
MH, and Yarbro CH, editors: Cancer nursing principles and practice, ed 3, Boston, 1993, Jones
& Bartlett Publishers.

Effects from Surgery

Postoperative nausea and vomiting have been attributed to both anesthetic-related
and patient-related factors. Greater frequency of nausea and vomiting has been
noted in pediatric patients, female patients, obese patients, anxious patients,
patients with delayed gastric emptying, and patients with a history of motion sick-
ness (Watcha and White, 1992). Certain types of anesthetic drugs (nitrous oxide,
etomidate, ketamine, propofol, and inhaled agents), deeper levels of anesthesia,
anesthesia via mask, gastric distention, and suctioning during surgery are also associated with a higher incidence of nausea and vomiting (Watcha and White, 1992).

Manipulation of the bowel during surgery may result in paralytic ileus or complete bowel obstruction, causing nausea and vomiting, abdominal pain, cramping,
or bloating (Burke and Levenback, 1994; Iwamoto, 1992). Postoperative factors

related to nausea and vomiting include pain, dizziness, change of position, ambulation, time of first oral intake, and use of opioid analgesics (Watcha and White, 1992).

Effects from Chemotherapy

The incidence of chemotherapy-induced nausea and vomiting varies according to the chemotherapeutic agent, the dose, and the emetic potential (Table 20-1). Other factors such as schedule, route of administration, administration rate, anxiety, previous adverse experiences to chemotherapy, concomitant treatments, and individual patient factors influence the incidence of nausea and vomiting (Graves, 1992).

Effects from Radiation Therapy

Radiation therapy to the brain, the esophagus, and the abdomen causes nausea and vomiting. However, nausea and vomiting may also result from emotional responses such as stress, depression, or anxiety (Strohl, 1989). Nausea and vomiting can occur within 2 hours of therapy, or not until several days after beginning treatment (Hogan, 1990; Strohl, 1989).

Effects from Biotherapy

The exact cause of nausea and vomiting from biological response modifiers is uncertain. The incidence is also unknown; however, in one National Biotherapy Study Group trial in which interleukin-2 (IL-2) was used, the frequency was 80% (Sharp, 1993). Although the frequency will vary, nausea and vomiting completely dissipate after completion of the therapy (Iwamoto, 1992). The biological agents that most commonly produce nausea and vomiting are interleukin-2 (IL-2), tumor necrosis factor (TNF), and lymphokine-activated killer (LAK) cells (Iwamoto, 1992).

Effects from Multimodal Therapy

The combination of interferon and cisplatin causes more nausea and vomiting than expected from each agent (Sznol and Longo, 1993). The increased toxicity occurs even when cisplatin is given on varying schedules of every 3 to 4 weeks, days 1 and 8 of a 28-day cycle, or weekly. The interferon is given three times a week. Concomitant thoracic radiation therapy and cisplatin are associated with severe nausea and vomiting, as is surgery of the GI tract followed by concomitant chemotherapy and radiation therapy to the GI tract. High-dose chemotherapy and total body irradiation followed by bone marrow transplantation is also associated with severe nausea and vomiting.

Nursing Management of Nausea and Vomiting

Assessment is an ongoing process. The patient's previous history, expectations, and emotional status and the type and emetogenicity of the cancer treatment should be assessed before planning interventions to control side effects. Box 20-1 provides

Table 20-1 Emetogenic Potential of Chemotherapeutic Agents

Incidence	Agent	Onset (hours after administration)	Duration (in hours)
Very high (>90%)	Cisplatin	1–6	24–48+
	Dacarbazine	1–3	1–12
	Mechlorethamine	2–5	8–24
	Melphalan (HD)	3–6	6–12
	Streptozocin	1–6	12–24
	Cytarabine (HD)	2–4	12–24
High (60%–90%)	Carmustine	2–4	4–24
	Cyclophosphamide	4–12	12–24
	Procarbazine	24–27	Variable
	Etoposide (HD)	4–6	24+
	Semustine	1–5	12–24
	Lomustine	4–6	12–24
	Dactinomycin	2–5	24
	Plicamycin	1–6	12–24
Moderate (30%–60%)	Doxorubicin	4–6	6+
	Mitoxantrone	4–6	6+
	5-Fluorouracil	3–6	24+
	Mitomycin-C	1–4	48–72
	Carboplatin	4–6	12–24
	Daunorubicin	2–6	24
	Asparaginase	1–4	2–12
	Hexamethylmelamine	1–4	—
Low (10%–30%)	Bleomycin	3–6	—
	Cytarabine	6–12	3–12
	Etoposide	3–8	—
	Melphalan	6–12	—
	6-Mercaptopurine	4–8	—
	Methotrexate	4–12	3–12
	Vinblastine	4–8	—
	Hydroxyurea	—	—
	Teniposide	—	—
	Navelbine	4–8	—
Very low (<10%)	Vincristine	4–8	—
	Chlorambucil	48–72	—
	Busulfan	—	—
	Thioguanine	—	—
	Hormones	—	—
	Steroids	—	—

HD = High dose
Reprinted with permission from Camp-Sorrell D: Chemotherapy: toxicity management. In Groenwald SL, Frogge MH, Goodman M, and Yarbro CH, editors: Cancer nursing: principles and practice, ed 3, Boston, 1993, Jones & Bartlett Publishers.

Box 20-1 Nursing Assessment Guidelines for Nausea and Vomiting

Initial and Pretreatment Assessment

- Prior history of nausea and vomiting
  - Pregnancy
  - Previous cancer treatment and side effects
  - "Nervous stomach"
- Patient's or family's understanding or beliefs regarding proposed cancer therapy or therapies and side effects
- Current or previous cancer treatment
- Level of patient's or family's emotional status*
- Patient's current nutritional status and oral intake
  - Height
  - Baseline weight
  - Diet history, including personal eating patterns and sociocultural preferences
- Current side effects from cancer*
  - Weight
  - Pain
  - Nausea and vomiting
  - Anorexia
  - Altered taste
  - Sore mouth
  - Fatigue
  - Alterations in bowel or bladder function
- Baseline laboratory data
  - CBC and differential*
  - Platelet count*
  - Electrolytes*
  - Total protein
  - Total iron-binding capacity
  - Serum iron
  - Albumin
- Age (older patients have lower risk of nausea and vomiting)
- Current history of alcohol or drug abuse (have lower risk of nausea and vomiting)
- Current use or willingness to try nonpharmacologic treatments for nausea and vomiting
  - Hypnosis
  - Imagery
  - Distraction
  - Relaxation
- Emetic potential of cancer treatment
- Effectiveness of antiemetic regimen; compliance and side effects*

*Complete prior to each treatment.

guidelines for an assessment related to nausea and vomiting. It should be used before each treatment.

The management of nausea and vomiting requires continuous assessment and evaluation of current interventions used to control symptoms. Individual responses to treatments vary; therefore a flexible approach is important. Individuals can respond to treatment-related nausea and vomiting by developing anticipatory nausea and vomiting (ANV). ANV occurs when nausea and/or vomiting are induced before administration of cancer treatment. Cues such as a sight, sound, or smell are paired with the sensation to vomit, evoking the symptom. Pharmacologic and nonpharmacologic interventions can be employed to minimize nausea and vomiting.

Pharmacologic Interventions
Antiemetic drugs are the most frequently used intervention for the management of nausea and vomiting. Antiemetic drugs can be combined to achieve greater efficacy. In addition, newer antiemetics, such as the serotonin antagonists, have dramatically improved the management of nausea and vomiting. A clear understanding of antiemetic classifications will assist the health care provider in achieving greater control of nausea and vomiting. Table 20-2 provides a summary of antiemetic drugs by classification.

Nonpharmacologic Interventions
Behavioral techniques such as relaxation, guided imagery, distraction, and hypnosis are useful in the management of nausea and vomiting, including anticipatory nausea and vomiting (Morrow and Hickok, 1993; Wickham, 1989).

Progressive muscle relaxation allows the patient to achieve a state of relaxation in anticipation of, or in response to, a variety of situations that may produce tension or anxiety. The technique involves learning to relax by actively tensing and then relaxing specific muscle groups in a progressive manner. It can often be combined with guided imagery (Morrow and Hickok, 1993).

Guided imagery is visualization of pleasant, soothing images or scenes while in a relaxed state. These images decrease tension and anxiety and provide a distraction from unpleasant experiences. An audio- or videotape can help stimulate visualization (Morrow and Hickok, 1993).

Aerobic exercise has shown to provide relief from cancer-therapy-induced nausea and vomiting (Winningham and MacVicar, 1988). The mechanism of action is uncertain, but nausea and vomiting have a strong psychologic component, and exercise can improve mood (Winningham and MacVicar, 1988).

Behavioral interventions need to be practiced until they become "second nature." It is not appropriate to teach behavioral interventions when the patient is nauseous or vomiting. Other nursing interventions for nausea and vomiting are listed in the Nursing Management box on page 334.

Patient Education
Providing the patient and family with information on how to manage nausea and vomiting allows them to participate in care and gives them a greater feeling of control. Guidelines for patient education (see page 335) help ensure that patients and families are well-prepared to assist in the management of nausea and vomiting.

Table 20-2 Antiemetic Therapy

Classification	Drugs	Availability/ Dose	Schedule	Duration/ Half-Life	Comments
Benzodiazepines					
Mechanism of Action: CNS depressant; interferes with afferent nerves from cerebral cortex; sedative	Lorazepam	Tablet: 1–3 mg po or sublingual IV: 0.5–2.5 mg	Every 3–4 hours	4–8 hours/ half-life 10–15 hours	Reduces anticipatory nausea and vomiting; may aggravate CNS effects of ifosfamide; use with caution in patients with hepatic and renal dysfunction
Common Side Effects: Sedation, amnesia, confusion	Diazepam	Tablet: 2–4 mg IV: 2–10 mg	Every 4–6 hours	4–8 hours/ half-life 30–40 hours	
Butyrophenones					
Mechanism of Action: Dopamine antagonist in the CTZ, esophagus, and stomach	Droperidol	IM: 2.5–10 mg IV: 0.5–2.5 mg	Every 3–4 hours	2–4 hours/ half-life 10 hours	Diphenhydramine 25–50 mg po or IV will prevent EPS; EPS is more common in young patients; may have additive effects; use caution in patients with cardiac disorders
Common Side Effects: Sedation, hypotension, tachycardia, EPS	Haloperidol	Tablet: 3–5 mg IM: 1–2 mg IV: 1–3 mg	Every 4 hours	2–6 hours/ half-life 12–18 hours	
Cannabinoids					
Mechanism of Action: Suppression of pathways to VC is speculated	Nabilone	Tablet: 2 mg	Every 3 hours	4–6 hours	Classified as a schedule II drug; may be difficult to obtain in outpatient setting; elderly patients generally do not tolerate side effects; generally used for second-line antiemetic therapy
Common Side Effects: Sedation, dizziness, dysphoria, dry mouth, disorientation, impaired concentration, orthostatic hypotension, tachycardia	Dronabinol	Tablet: 5–10 mg	Every 4 hours	4–6 hours	
Steroids					
Mechanism of Action: Antiprostaglandin synthesis activity?	Dexamethasone	Tablet: 10–40 mg IV: 4–20 mg	Every 3 hours	Half-life 2–3 hours	Rapid infusion causes perineal itching and burning
	Solu Medrol	IV: 125–250 mg	Every 3 hours		

Continued

Table 20-2 Antiemetic Therapy—cont'd

Classification	Drugs	Availability/Dose	Schedule	Duration/Half-Life	Comments
Steroids—cont'd					
Common Side Effects: Insomnia, euphoria, anxiety, hypertension, edema					
Antihistamines					
Mechanism of Action: Histamine H1 receptor antagonist	Diphenhydramine	Tablet: 25–50 mg IM/IV: 12.5–50 mg	Every 3–4 hours	Half-life 5–8 hours	Prevents acute dystonic reactions; use cautiously in patients with hepatic dysfunction
Common Side Effects: Sedation, hypotension					
Serotonin Inhibitor					
Mechanism of Action: Serotonin receptor; (5-HT3) antagonist	Ondansetron	IV: .15 mg/kg 30 min. before chemotherapy and then x 3 or as a single 32 mg dose Tablet: 8 mg x 4	Every 4 hours	Half-life 3–4 hours	Transient elevations of LFTs may occur with cisplatin and ondansetron; single-dose of ondansetron or granisetron is sufficient for a 24-hour period; BMY has caused moderate to severe hypotension; ECG changes have been observed with BMY use; neither ondansetron nor granisetron recommended for delayed or anticipatory nausea and vomiting
Common Side Effects: Hypotension, headache, constipation, minimal sedation	Granisetron	IV: 10 μg/kg Tablet: 1 mg	Every 8 hours Every 12 hours	Half-life 8–10 hours	
	Batanopride (BMY-25801; investigational)	IV: 1.2–8 mg/kg	2–3 hours x 3 doses		
Phenothiazine					
Mechanism of Action: Blocks dopamine receptor in the CTZ; inhibits VC by blocking autonomic afferent impulses via vagus nerve	Prochlorperazine	Tablet: 5–25 mg Sustained release: 10–30 mg po IM/IV: 5–20 mg Rectal: 25 mg	Every 4–6 hours Every 10–12 hours Every 3–4 hours Every 4–6 hours	3–4 hours 10–12 hours 3–4 hours 3–4 hours	Administer IV dose over 15–30 minutes; EPS more common in persons <30 years of age; side effects can be cumulative in the elderly; do not exceed 5 mg min

Phenothiazine—cont'd

Common Side Effects: Sedation, orthostatic hypotension, EPS, dizziness, drowsiness

Drug	Dose	Schedule	Onset	Comments
Promethazine	Tablet: 12.5–25 mg IM/IV: 10–25 mg Rectal: 25 mg	Every 4–6 hours	3–4 hours	with IV dose; dystonia can occur with chlorpromazine, especially with IM; chlorpromazine generally second-line antiemetic therapy; diphenhydramine can prevent EPS and dystonia; sustained-release form can prevent delayed nausea
Triethylperazine	Tablet: 10 mg IM: 10 mg Rectal: 10 mg	Every 4–6 hours	3–4 hours	
Chlorpromazine	Tablet: 25–50 mg IM/IV: 25–50 mg Rectal: 25–100 mg	Every 4–6 hours	3–4 hours	and vomiting; for intractable nausea and vomiting, perphenazine can be administered as continuous IV infusion with a 5 mg loading dose and then at 1 mg per hour
Perphenazine	Tablet: 4 mg IM/IV: 5 mg	Every 4–6 hours	3–4 hours	

Substituted Benzamide

Mechanism of Action: Dopamine antagonist; accelerates gastric emptying and small bowel transit; CTZ

Drug	Dose	Schedule	Onset	Comments
Metoclopramide	Tablet: 5–10 mg IV: 1–3 mg/kg	Every 6 hours Every 2–3 hours for 3–5 doses	2–3 hours/ Half-life 4–6 hours	EPS more common in young patients; administer over 15 minutes to prevent intense anxiety; use cautiously in patients with renal dysfunction

Common Side Effects: Sedation, diarrhea, anxiety, EPS, fatigue, headache

VC = Vomiting Center; CTZ = Chemoreceptor Trigger Zone; EPS = Extrapyramidal Symptoms
Revised from Camp-Sorrell D: Chemotherapy: Toxicity management. In Groenwald SL, Frogge MH, Goodman M, and Yarbro CH, editors: Cancer nursing: principles and practice, ed 3, Boston, 1993, Jones & Bartlett Publishers.

Nursing Management of
Nausea and Vomiting

◆ Maintain comfort
  ◆ Provide odor-free environment
  ◆ Give adequate analgesia
  ◆ Reposition the patient
  ◆ Provide a comfortable bed or chair for chemotherapy administration
  ◆ Minimize stimuli such as sights, sounds, or smells
◆ Provide an antiemetic
  ◆ Assess compliance and effectiveness of antiemetic from previous treatment
  ◆ Adjust antiemetic if needed
  ◆ Administer antiemetic as ordered 30 minutes before chemotherapy
◆ Provide antiemetic measures in chemotherapy administration
  ◆ Offer a cold washcloth for the patient's forehead if nauseated
  ◆ Slow infusions of highly emetic agents, if necessary, or increase their dilution (Perry, 1993)
◆ Maintain nutrition
  ◆ Offer suggestions for high-calorie and nutritional foods
  ◆ Encourage eating favorite foods in small frequent meals, but avoid favorite foods during highly emetic periods
  ◆ Offer and encourage nutritional supplements if needed
  ◆ Suggest eating cold or room-temperature foods when nauseated
  ◆ Refer to dietitian if necessary
◆ Encourage patient participation
  ◆ Educate patient and family regarding nausea and vomiting and its management
  ◆ Encourage the use of diaries to note usage of medications, side effects, and episodes of nausea and vomiting

Using antiemetics correctly will reduce or prevent episodes of nausea and vomiting. It is important to stress to the patient and family that if an intervention is not effective, diet and drug modifications will be continued until symptoms are controlled.

❖ *Mucositis*

Mucositis is inflammation and ulceration of the mucosa. Mucositis can occur anywhere there is mucosal lining (e.g., the oral cavity, the esophagus, the upper and lower gastrointestinal tracts, the rectum, and the vagina) (Beck, 1992). Mucositis of the oral cavity (stomatitis) and the esophagus (esophagitis) will be discussed in this section.

The oral and esophageal mucosa is comprised of nonkeratinized squamous epithelial cells, salivary glands, and ectopic sebaceous glands. The epithelium regenerates every 10 to 14 days. This continuous and rapid proliferation of the epithelial stem cells makes the mucosa extremely susceptible to the cytotoxic effects of chemotherapy, radiation therapy, and biotherapy (Beck, 1992; Graham, 1993).

Managing stomatitis and esophagitis is an important nursing function, because the patient's inability to communicate, eat, or drink may lead to weight loss,

Patient Education Guidelines for

Nausea and Vomiting

Some cancer treatments can cause nausea and vomiting.

◆ Discuss the use of your antiemetic (antinausea medication) with your health care provider. Understand when and how to use the medicine and its potential side effects. Take the antiemetic as prescribed, whether needed or not, for 48 hours after chemotherapy.

◆ The following dietary management steps help prevent or minimize nausea and vomiting:
   ◆ Carbonated beverages help curb nausea
   ◆ Eat cold food instead of hot food
   ◆ Eat small, frequent meals
   ◆ Avoid smelling foods directly because the smell may cause nausea
   ◆ Eat crackers or hard candy when nausea occurs
   ◆ Avoid greasy foods, which take longer to digest

◆ Ask someone else to cook if the smell makes you nauseated.

◆ Use strategies such as distraction, relaxation, music, and guided imagery.

◆ Immediately report uncontrolled vomiting or more than three episodes of vomiting to your physician or nurse.

Permission granted to reproduce these guidelines for educational purposes only.

malnutrition, and decreased quality of life. Early stomatitis is described as a burning sensation, although no abnormalities of the mucosa may be visible. As stomatitis progresses, there may be increased sensitivity to heat, cold, or spicy or salty foods. Advanced stomatitis is manifested by erosions or ulcers of the mucosa and moderate to severe pain.

Esophagitis is inflammation of the esophageal lining. It is caused by chemotherapy and radiation damage to the mucosa. Patients often have dysgeusia, with extreme cases leading to dehydration, malnutrition, and pain that may require intravenous narcotics such as morphine or dilaudid to control it.

Effects from Surgery

Surgery can affect the mucosa directly and indirectly. The direct effects from surgery are seen in head and neck cancers, where surgery itself causes alterations in the integrity of the oral mucosa and the possible loss of salivary tissue (Beck, 1992). Indirectly, cancer surgery may result in drying of the mucosa because of fluid and nutritional deficits, the side effects of medications, or alterations in respiratory patterns. This drying of the mucosa decreases the mucosal integrity, increasing the risk for mucositis.

Effects from Chemotherapy

Chemotherapeutic agents known to cause mucositis have a direct and an indirect effect on the mucosa. The direct effect is the cessation of epithelial replication. This results in thinning of the epithelium, leading to ulceration about 2 to 3 weeks after the administration of chemotherapy. The indirect effect is the result of myelosuppression, when infection or bleeding of the oral mucosa may occur (Wujcik, 1992).

Chemotherapeutic agents associated with mucositis are 5-fluorouracil, dactinomycin, doxorubicin, bleomycin, daunorubicin, and vinblastine. The drug dose and administration rate affect the degree of mucositis (Wujcik, 1992). In patients who receive high doses of chemotherapy, as many as 40% will have an earlier onset of mucositis. It can occur with greater severity and with greater incidence of infection (Mitchell, 1992; Wujcik, 1992).

Effects from Radiation Therapy

Patients given radiation therapy to the head and neck, lung, and upper spinal cord can expect to get mucositis. The extent depends on the site and on the cumulative dose, depth, penetration, and the number and frequency of the radiation treatments. Generally mucositis is noted at doses of 20 Gy or more and begins 1 to 2 weeks after treatment has started. It may persist for several weeks following cessation of therapy (Beck, 1992; Dudjak, 1987).

Initially the mucosa takes on a white appearance, which is due to a decrease in mitotic activity by the epithelial cells. As these cells are lost, they are not sufficiently replaced by the epithelial stem cells, which results in thinning and increasing inflammation. When treatment doses reach the range of 25 Gy, erythema develops. A fibrinous exudate may appear, noted as a white or tan glistening membrane. The membrane is easily removed, even with slight trauma, and an ulcer will develop (Dudjak, 1987).

Effects from Biotherapy

Biological response modifiers most associated with mucositis are interleukin-2 (IL-2) and lymphokine-activated killer (LAK) cells. The exact mechanism is still unknown, although it may be the result of direct damage from the IL-2 or IL-2-induced secretions of other lymphokines such as gamma interferon (Beck, 1992). Mucositis has been estimated to develop in 13% to 46% of patients receiving 1000 units of IL-2 three times a day.

Effects from Multimodal Therapy

Current cancer treatment includes an aggressive multimodal approach, which increases the incidence, intensity, and duration of mucositis. These side effects can be seen much earlier than with single-modality therapy.

Prior radiation therapy increases the likelihood of epithelial damage to the GI mucosa when chemotherapy is administered (Mitchell, 1992). Damaged GI epithelium creates an environment at high risk for GI moniliasis (candidiasis) (Mitchell, 1992), presenting as a diffuse exudate in the oral mucosa and as ulcerations and diffuse erosions in the esophagus and the stomach. Patients at greatest risk are those on any combination of chemotherapy, radiation therapy, corticosteroids, and antimicrobials (Mitchell, 1992).

Radiation therapy to the oral cavity, neck, lung, or mediastinum given concurrently with some chemotherapy agents increases the incidence and severity of mucositis. Severe mucositis can also result from high-dose chemotherapy and total body irradiation followed by bone marrow transplantation. These side effects are due to intense, combined, simultaneous damage by both therapies.

Mucosal radiation recall (a reactivation of a mucosal reaction noted at a previously irradiated site) occurs when dactinomycin or doxorubicin is given months or even years after radiation has been administered (Mitchell, 1992).

5-Fluorouracil combined with interferon increases the incidence and severity of mucositis (Sznol and Longo, 1993).

Nursing Management of Mucositis

Oral assessment should be integrated into the routine physical examination of every cancer patient. The frequency of the assessment depends on the potential for mucositis development. High-risk patients need to have a routine systematic oral assessment performed at least once, and up to four times a day, utilizing a standardized assessment guide (Graham, 1993). Patients at high risk for mucositis include (1) those with hematological cancers and head and neck cancers, (2) patients less than 20 years of age, (3) those with limitations in performing their own care, (4) those with poor oral hygiene, (5) those who use alcohol and tobacco, and (6) those who use oxygen therapy (Beck, 1992; Sonis and Clark, 1991).

Oral assessment should be performed systematically to obtain complete and accurate data. The examination requires a good source of lighting, the use of gloves, a tongue blade, and a dental mirror. The exam should begin with a careful examination of the lips, the tongue, and the oral mucosa. The tongue blade is useful for depressing the tongue, and the mirror allows a look at the dorsal surface of the tongue, the uvula, and the oropharynx. Particular attention should be given to the color, moisture, texture, and integrity of the oral mucosa. The teeth should be checked for color, shine, debris, and dental disease. The amount and quality of saliva should be evaluated. Ask the patient about any changes in taste, voice, ability to swallow, and comfort (Beck, 1992).

Using a standardized oral-assessment guide expedites documentation of the oral cavity. There are several oral assessment guides available. One example is the Beck Oral Cavity Assessment form shown in Table 20-3.

Nursing management and patient education focus on cleanliness, moisturizing, maintaining mucosal integrity, and promoting comfort (Beck, 1992). Although the most effective solution or oral protocol has not been determined, several combinations of baking soda, hydrogen peroxide, and saline have been effective. Good oral hygiene and maintaining oral mucosal integrity help to decrease infection.

Complications from mucositis can be minimized with a good diet, oral hygiene, and prophylactic medications. A well-balanced diet is recommended. The patient should avoid foods containing sugars because they can be a source for bacteria. Avoiding oral irritants such as tobacco will reduce the pain from mucositis. Routine oral hygiene, including brushing, flossing, and rinsing the teeth, must be initiated. Early detection of mucositis allows early intervention and treatment.

Table 20-3   The Oral Cavity Assessment Form
Directions: 1. Determine rating for each category. 2. Add up ratings. 3. Institute care based on ratings total score.

Category	Rating	1	2	3	4
Lips	1 2 3 4	Smooth, soft, pink, moist, and intact	Slightly dry, wrinkled, reddened areas	Dry, rough, swollen, inflammatory line of demarcation	Very dry, inflamed, cracked, blistered, ulcerated, and bleeding
Tongue	1 2 3 4	Smooth, firm, pink, moist, and intact	Papillae prominent particularly at base, dry, pink with reddened areas	Raised, red papillae all over tongue giving peppered appearance: (very dry and swollen), coating at base	Very dry, thick, grooved and coated; tip very red and demarcated, sides blistered
Oral mucosa	1 2 3 4	Smooth, pink, moist, and intact	Pale, slightly dry, reddened areas or white pustules	Red, dry, inflamed, edematous, ulcerated	Very red, shiny, edematous with blisters and/or ulcerations
Teeth or dentures	1 2 3 4	Shiny, no debris, well fitting	Slightly dull with slight debris, slightly loose	Dull with debris on half of visible enamel; loose with areas of irritation	Very dull, covered with debris, unable to wear due to irritation
Saliva	1 2 3 4	Thin, watery, sufficient saliva quantity	Saliva amount increased	Saliva scant, mouth dry	Saliva thick, ropy, viscid, or mucid

Total score: Mild dysfunction: 6–10, Moderate dysfunction: 11–15, Severe dysfunction: 16–20.

From Beck SL and Yasko JM: Guidelines for oral care, Newbury Park, California, 1984, Sage Publications.

Patient Education Guidelines for

Potential Mucositis

◆ Brush your teeth gently with a soft toothbrush or toothettes four times a day.
◆ Rinse your mouth three to four times a day with oral rinse as prescribed by your physician or nurse.
◆ Examine your mouth daily for redness, bleeding, or white patches.
◆ Check with your physician or nurse before having dental work done.
◆ Call your physician or nurse if the following symptoms occur:
  ◆ White patches in mouth
  ◆ Sores in mouth
  ◆ Bleeding from the gums
  ◆ Temperature above 100°F
◆ Avoid the following to help lessen mouth pain if sores develop:
  ◆ Highly acidic foods (orange juice, tomato juice)
  ◆ Spicy foods
  ◆ Alcoholic beverages
  ◆ Commercial mouthwashes containing alcohol
  ◆ Smoking
  ◆ Poorly fitting dentures
◆ Eat a well-balanced diet and avoid foods with a high sugar content.

Permission granted to reproduce these guidelines for educational purposes only.

Prophylactic use of antifungal and antiviral agents for patients at risk for severe neutropenia may decrease the incidence of infection or its severity. Acyclovir has been given orally to prevent herpes simplex, especially in patients undergoing bone marrow transplantation (Camp-Sorrell, 1991; Wujcik, 1992).

Before initiation of therapy, a complete dental examination is recommended, because good dentition helps to reduce the risk of infection. Extraction and repair of diseased teeth minimize oral treatment complications (Jansma et al., 1992).

Mucositis is a side effect that requires patient involvement. The more information and understanding the patient and family have regarding mucositis, the greater the chance of minimizing complications. (See the Patient Education Guidelines above.)

❖ Constipation and Diarrhea

Constipation is defined as the infrequent passing of hard and dry stool, usually accompanied by discomfort. Constipation may result in pain, poor nutrition, or bowel obstruction, and, if not properly managed, it can lead to improper use of laxatives (Gootenberg and Pizzo, 1991; Levy, 1991). Diarrhea is defined as an increase in stool volume and liquidity, usually occurring three to four times per day. Diarrhea can lead to systemic problems such as lethargy, weakness, dehydration, and electrolyte loss (Levy, 1991). Without immediate management, cancer treatments may have to be discontinued until the diarrhea is resolved. Both may adversely affect the quality of life of the patient with cancer.

Factors that can potentially alter bowel function include medication with opioids or antiemetics, decreased nutrition, decreased fluid intake, immobility, and cancer therapy. The absorption of water into the colon regulates bowel function, expressed as either constipation, diarrhea, or "normal" bowel function. The intestines absorb the nutrients and fluids taken in by the patient. The small intestines absorb most of the nutrients, whereas the colon absorbs only water and electrolytes (Canty, 1994; Levy, 1991). Alteration in fluid intake or alteration of the GI mucosa will influence the consistency of the stool.

Effects from Surgery

Constipation following abdominal or pelvic surgery results from ileus (decreased bowel motility). The exact mechanism for the decrease in bowel motility is unknown, but it appears to be related to opening the peritoneal cavity and is aggravated by extensive manipulation of the bowel during lengthy surgical procedures. For most people, the ileus is minimal and will resolve spontaneously (Clarke-Pearson et al., 1993). Constipation may be exacerbated by patient immobility and opioid pain medication. Small bowel obstruction from adhesions can occur.

Following abdominal surgery, diarrhea can occur as a common consequence of the bowels' return to their normal function (Clarke-Pearson et al., 1993). However, prolonged or multiple episodes of diarrhea may represent more serious problems such as partial bowel obstruction, colitis, or bacterial or parasitic infections (Clarke-Pearson et al., 1993). Patients undergoing resection of the small bowel or the loss of the ileocecal valve will have shortened transit time, resulting in chronic diarrhea and accompanying electrolyte loss (Burke and Levenback, 1994).

Effects from Chemotherapy

Vincristine and vinblastine are the chemotherapeutic agents most frequently associated with constipation. This results from nerve stimulation along the GI tract, which decreases peristalsis and causes paralytic ileus (Camp-Sorrell, 1991).

Diarrhea can be caused by 5-fluorouracil, cisplatin (Cascinu et al., 1994; Petrelli et al., 1993), methotrexate, dactinomycin, doxorubicin, and daunorubicin (Levy, 1991). These drugs cause mucositis. Because the bowel lining is so irritated, it cannot absorb fluid, thereby causing diarrhea.

Effects from Radiation Therapy

When radiation is delivered to the abdomen, pelvis, or the lower thoracic and lumbar spine, the incidence of diarrhea can reach 80%. Diarrhea generally develops after the bowel has received 18 to 22 Gy, which usually occurs about the second week of radiation therapy (Danielsson et al., 1991; Henriksson, Franzen, and Littbrano, 1991). Radiation-induced diarrhea can be chronic, persisting 5 to 15 years after the completion of radiation therapy (Levy, 1991). The cause is directly attributed to the damage done to the epithelial cells during radiation therapy, which causes edema of the intestinal wall. The short cell cycle of these cells makes them highly sensitive to radiation (Henriksson, Franzen, and Littbrano, 1991).

Effects from Biotherapy

Diarrhea is also a side effect of treatment with biological response modifiers, especially IL-2, which has an incidence as high as 84% (Callendo, Joyce, and Altmiller, 1993; Iwamoto, 1992). The mechanism of action is unknown (Callendo, Joyce, and Altmiller, 1993).

Effects from Multimodal Therapy

GI-tract surgery followed by concomitant chemotherapy and radiation therapy—with or without biotherapy—increases the incidence of severe chronic diarrhea. Neoadjuvant radiation therapy followed by rectal surgery results in diarrhea. This phenomenon is increased when 5-fluorouracil is given concomitantly.

Dactinomycin, bleomycin, doxorubicin, and 5-fluorouracil enhance radiation therapy, especially if given concurrently, but result in a higher incidence of diarrhea (von der Masse, 1994). Concurrent chemotherapy and radiation therapy increase the incidence of severe enteritis in children (Mitchell, 1992). In animal studies, cytarabine protects the intestines from damage if given 12 hours before radiation therapy (von der Masse, 1994). No documentation was found on cytarabine's protective effect in human clinical trials.

Interferon, when given with 5-fluorouracil and leucovorin, increases the incidence and severity of diarrhea (Sznol and Longo, 1993), as does levamisole when given with 5-fluorouracil.

Nursing Management of Constipation and Diarrhea

Assessment of bowel function is necessary to identify diarrhea or constipation and to manage the patient experiencing either side effect. A careful history of the patient's bowel habits before treatment will provide a baseline to determine the degree of alteration. Individual elimination patterns differ greatly, ranging from one to three bowel movements per day to one bowel movement every three days (Canty, 1994). The change in the patient's elimination pattern from the baseline is more important than the actual number of daily bowel movements.

Current and previous use of medications, including laxatives, should be assessed. Many drugs are known to cause constipation or diarrhea. Dietary factors that can cause diarrhea include caffeine and alcohol, whereas chocolate and cheeses can cause constipation. Other considerations include metabolic abnormalities such as hypercalcemia, which will cause constipation, and hypocalcemia, which will cause diarrhea. Box 20-2 provides guidelines for accurately assessing bowel function.

Nursing management of constipation and diarrhea begins with the anticipation of situations that lead to alterations in bowel function. Prevention is best, but if this proves impossible, providing specific interventions to alleviate complications is

---

Box 20-2 Nursing Assessment Guidelines for Bowel Function

- Cancer history
  - Type of cancer
  - Potential for disease invasion of bowels
  - Presentation with bowel obstruction
- Elimination patterns
  - Baseline (before cancer)
  - Current pattern of elimination
  - Character, frequency, and time of day of elimination
- Medication use
  - History of laxative use or abuse
  - Current medication history
  - Current and past cancer treatment (location of surgery and/or radiation therapy and types of chemotherapeutic agents)
- Diet history
  - Dietary fiber intake (6–10 g of dietary fiber/day is recommended)
  - Fluid intake (eight 8-oz glasses of fluid/day is recommended)
- Exercise and activity
  - Daily exercise helps to increase peristalsis
- Potential metabolic sources
  - Risk of hypercalcemia
  - Risk of hypocalcemia

---

necessary. Usually, dietary interventions alone do not succeed in reversing constipation. Pharmacologic interventions that can be coupled with nonpharmacologic approaches such as increasing the patient's activity and intake of fluid and fiber are usually required.

Laxatives or stool softeners usually relieve constipation. Laxatives stimulate defecation by (1) osmotic properties that cause fluid absorption into the bowel, which softens the stool, (2) acting directly on the mucosa and decreasing the absorption of water, and (3) increasing intestinal motility, which decreases absorption of salt and water because of decreased transient time (Canty, 1994).

Other pharmacologic therapies include the use of suppositories and enemas. Suppositories usually induce elimination within 30 minutes by stimulating the rectal mucosa to increase contractility (Canty, 1994). Enemas with sodium phosphate add bulk. Mineral oil enemas lubricate the stool, and saline enemas cause fluid retention in the intestinal lumen, allowing the stool to move easier. Soapsud enemas cause irritation to the mucosa and stimulate defecation (Canty, 1994). The most important goal is to retain and augment normal bowel motility and to develop a bowel regimen and regular function. Many times constipation can be prevented by using a stool softener in combination with a bulking agent.

The management of diarrhea usually requires pharmacologic intervention. Before pharmacologic treatment begins, the cause of diarrhea such as infection (viral, parasitic, or bacterial), intestinal obstruction, laxative abuse, and tumor recurrence should be ruled out. Prompt management of diarrhea is essential to prevent dehydration, electrolyte imbalance (sodium and potassium), and skin breakdown in the perianal area.

The treatment of choice for diarrhea caused by cancer therapy is Imodium (loperamide), a long-acting opioid agonist derived from butyramide. Diphenoxylate combined with atropine is another antidiarrheal agent. Codeine has a powerful constipating effect but is usually not used as first-line therapy because of its systemic side effects. Sandostatin is a useful antidiarrheal agent for high-volume diarrhea that is not responsive to other agents (Levy, 1991). Psyllium, a bulking agent, is also used for watery diarrhea to create a gel, thereby thickening and slowing the diarrhea.

Alterations in bowel function require careful patient education to minimize the effects of constipation and diarrhea. Explaining the cause of constipation and diarrhea may help the patient to cope more effectively. The Patient Education Guidelines listed below will guide the nurse in providing this education.

Patient Education Guidelines for

Constipation and Diarrhea

Diarrhea
- ◆ Eat foods high in fiber.
- ◆ Notify your nurse or physician if you have more than three watery stools per day.
- ◆ Eat foods high in sodium and potassium if you are experiencing diarrhea.
- ◆ Drink at least eight 8-oz glasses of fluid a day to prevent dehydration.
- ◆ Avoid the following:
  - ◆ Milk products
  - ◆ Raw fruits and vegetables
  - ◆ Beans and peas
  - ◆ Spicy or fatty foods
  - ◆ Caffeine
  - ◆ Alcohol and tobacco
- ◆ Take antidiarrheal medication as ordered.
- ◆ Be sure your rectal area is clean and dry after each episode of diarrhea.
- ◆ Nutmeg added to foods may decrease diarrhea.
- ◆ A&D ointment may be used to soothe the rectal area.

Constipation
- ◆ Report to your nurse or physician when stools are hard to pass, or if you do not have a bowel movement for 2 days.
- ◆ Drink at least eight 8-oz glasses of fluid/day. Hot liquids are best.
- ◆ Try to exercise daily.
- ◆ Use medications for your bowel as instructed by your physician or nurse.
- ◆ Eat foods high in fiber.

Permission granted to reproduce these guidelines for educational purposes only.

❖ *Anorexia and Cachexia*

Anorexia, the lack of desire to eat, affects 15% to 40% of patients at the time of cancer diagnosis and 80% of patients with advanced disease (Nelson, Walsh, and Sheehan, 1994). The exact etiology is unclear but it relates to five factors: abnormal increased synthesis of serotonin, which stimulates a feeling of satiety; alteration in taste and smell acuity, possibly related to a decrease in serum zinc levels; cancer treatments; food aversions; and an inability to digest nutrients (Robuk and Fleetwood, 1992).

Cachexia is characterized by loss of body weight, adipose tissue, visceral protein, and skeletal muscle (Robuck and Fleetwood, 1992); early satiety, weakness; asthenia; anemia; and abnormalities in protein, lipid, and carbohydrate metabolism (Langstein and Norton, 1991). Cachexia is attributed to anorexia, metabolic changes that increase energy needs, and the loss of nutrients (Robuck and Fleetwood, 1992).

The mechanism of action for anorexia differs from that for cachexia, although the two are related. In anorexia, cancer cells appear to have priority over normal cells for getting nutrients. As the tumor grows, body mass decreases and patients lose weight, despite eating a normal diet. In cachexia, a hypermetabolic state exists that is thought to be related to the tumor and to less efficient production of glucose (Robuck and Fleetwood, 1992).

Effects from Surgery

Several types of cancer surgery may result in alterations in nutrition. Surgeries of the head and neck can lead to mechanical defects causing obstructions, disturbances in motor and sensory function, fistula formation, aspiration, and anorexia. Other surgeries involving the GI tract can lead to malabsorption of nutrients, dumping syndromes, loss of digestive enzymes, fistulas, obstructions, and severe metabolic complications. In addition, the stress response to surgery leads to a hypermetabolic state, resulting in elevated levels of protein synthesis and energy expenditure. Often the cachectic patient with cancer requires nutritional repletion before surgery (Robuck and Fleetwood, 1992).

Effects from Chemotherapy

Chemotherapeutic agents can affect the nutritional status of a patient with cancer. Chemotherapy interferes with the replication of rapidly multiplying cells, including the mucosal cells of the GI tract. Side effects of stomatitis, diarrhea, nausea, vomiting, and mucosal ulcers impede normal digestion and absorption of nutrients, leading to anorexia and weight loss, resulting in malnutrition (Robuck and Fleetwood, 1992).

Effects from Radiation Therapy

Depending on the location and the dose of radiation, side effects may contribute to anorexia and cachexia. When the abdominal organs receive radiation, nausea, vomiting, diarrhea, and intestinal malabsorption occur. When radiation is given to the chest, mediastinum, or lungs, side effects of dysgeusia and esophagitis can develop (Robuck and Fleetwood, 1992; Skipper, Szeluga, and Groenwald, 1993). Stomatitis can occur after radiation therapy in the oral cavity.

Effects from Biotherapy

The relation of biotherapy to anorexia-cachexia syndrome is not fully understood. Studies have documented that biotherapy causes diarrhea, nausea, vomiting, taste alterations, and mucositis (Viele and Moran, 1993). What is clear is that cytokines such as tumor necrosis factor, interferons, and interleukins appear to play a role in cancer cachexia and, when given as therapy, may eventually have the potential for reversing or adding to the anorexia-cachexia syndrome (Langstein and Norton, 1991).

Effects from Multimodal Therapy

Nutritional alterations are compounded in patients receiving multimodal therapy who are considered at high risk for the development of anorexia or cachexia. Patients who receive both chemotherapy and radiation therapy to the GI tract—with or without surgery—have a high incidence of weight loss due to malabsorption. The combination of radiation therapy and surgery can lead to increased incidence of intestinal obstruction, adhesions, or fistula formation, all of which can affect nutrition.

Nursing Management of Anorexia and Cachexia

Careful assessment of anorexia and cachexia can guide the nurse in planning beneficial interventions. Box 20-3 provides guidelines to be utilized for this assessment.

The treatments for the malnourished patient that involve specialized nutritional interventions such as total enteral nutrition (TEN) or total parenteral nutrition (TPN) remain controversial. TPN has been shown to benefit malnourished patients with GI cancers undergoing surgery. However, no improvement in tolerance or response was noted in patients undergoing chemotherapy (Eng-Hen and Lowery, 1991; Nelson, Walsh, and Sheehan, 1994). In fact, some studies conclude that TPN may stimulate tumor growth, and patients were found to have a lower rate of survival. These studies, however, are felt to be flawed because of small sample sizes and because patients in the control group had a lesser extent of disease (Nelson, Walsh, and Sheehan, 1994). TPN has also been correlated with pneumothorax and infection, although these complications may be overemphasized in relation to benefits (Nelson, Walsh, and Sheehan, 1994). Beneficial effects of TPN include a decreased rate of sepsis and better wound healing (Eng-Hen and Lowery, 1991).

Other controversial interventions include the drug cyproheptadine, an antihistamine with antiserotonergic properties. Doses of cyproheptadine at 8 mg three times per day were shown in one study to increase appetite but in another study were found to have only mild appetite stimulation with no significant weight gain (Nelson, Walsh, and Sheehan, 1994; Loprinzi, Goldberg, and Burnham, 1992). Hydrazine sulfate, an experimental cytotoxic antineoplastic agent, which is not commercially available in the United States, has been studied for its antineoplastic effects

---

Box 20-3 Nursing Assessment Guidelines for Anorexia-Cachexia

Nutritional History

◆ Note the patient's current height, weight, and history of weight loss
◆ Take a diet history of current food and fluid intake: note the type, amount, and frequency of intake; usually a 3-day history is more accurate and a written diary is more accurate than memory
◆ Assess how patient's mood or relationships with others affects nutritional intake
◆ Determine ability to prepare and obtain food of nutritional value
◆ Assess available help with food preparation (family, friends, Meals-on-Wheels)

Assessment for Severe Weight Loss and Malnutrition

◆ Assess degree of weight loss against chart of standard height and weight for age
◆ Patients at 5th percentile or below are considered severely underweight
◆ A weight loss of 10 percentiles on a standard weight-and-height chart is a reasonable standard for severe weight loss
◆ Anthropometric measurements (triceps skin-fold measurements) indicate moderate malnutrition at the 5th to 10th percentile and severe malnutrition at less than the 5th percentile
◆ Low serum albumin levels
   Mild = 3.0 gm/100 ml
   Moderate = 2.5–3.0 gm/100 ml
   Severe = <2.5 gm/100 ml
◆ Decreased transferrin (decline along with albumin is an early indicator of malnutrition)
◆ Electrolyte imbalance such as decreased nitrogen and decreased calcium

Symptoms Affecting Anorexia and Cachexia

◆ Taste and smell alterations
◆ Stomatitis and xerostomia
◆ Alterations in bowel function (constipation, diarrhea, and fistulas)
◆ Nausea and vomiting
◆ Alterations in mechanical functioning (inability to chew, swallow, or digest)
◆ Pain

---

and its ability to ameliorate the effects of cancer-associated anorexia and cachexia, After 30 years of study, investigators felt that hydrazine sulfate did not have a significant antitumor effect. Since that time, studies have focused on its role in combating anorexia and cachexia, but to date they remain inconclusive (Loprinizi, Goldberg, and Burnham, 1992; Nelson, Walsh, and Sheehan, 1994).

Anabolic steroids and corticosteroids have been suggested as appetite stimulants. However, side effects such as osteoporosis, immunosuppression, psychosis, and gastrointestinal bleeding have raised concerns and have decreased enthusiasm for extensive investigation (Loprinzi, Goldberg, and Burnham, 1992; Nelson, Walsh, and Sheehan, 1994).

Patient Education Guidelines for

Anorexia and Cachexia

◆ Eat six small meals a day.
◆ Eat high-protein, high-calorie foods. Use protein supplements if necessary.
◆ Drink a glass of wine or beer before meals, if your physician approves.
◆ Increase the amount of seasoning in foods to help increase the taste.
◆ Provide foods in a pleasant atmosphere to improve the appetite.
◆ Weigh yourself weekly and call your physician or nurse if you have lost more than 3 pounds in a week.
◆ Take medication to improve the appetite if ordered.
◆ Have others prepare the food if cooking bothers you.
◆ Add 1 tablespoon of nonfat powdered milk to foods to increase the protein.
◆ Use high-fat products such as whole milk and butter.

Permission granted to reproduce these guidelines for educational purposes only.

The most recognized and utilized drug for anorexia and cachexia is megestrol acetate, a progestational hormone. Several studies have demonstrated that megestrol acetate increases the appetite of patients suffering from cancer-induced anorexia and cachexia and of those with HIV disease. Three randomized double-blind clinical trials have reported significant weight gain in individuals taking megestrol acetate. The optimal dose has been established at 1600 mg per day. One main consideration in using megestrol acetate is cost, although compared to other treatments such as enteral or parenteral nutrition, it is the most economical.

As with all symptom management, patient education is paramount. The patient and family should be taught simple, specific techniques to improve the appetite in hopes of decreasing cachexia. Lack of appetite and weight loss are very distressing to family members. Patients need high-calorie and high-protein supplements or foods to maintain nutritional requirements. It may improve the appetite to consume alcohol or to avoid overextending the stomach by eating small meals frequently. The Patient Education Guidelines on this page will guide the nurse in providing this education.

❖ Summary

The gastrointestinal side effects experienced by patients are some of the most distressing and potentially debilitating they will face. However, most of these side effects can be managed with a variety of interventions. Patients receiving multimodal therapy have a greater incidence of these side effects. Patients need to be reminded that symptom control will be tailored and changed according to their individual responses and needs. Emphasis on the dramatic improvements that have been made must be stressed to support and alleviate the fears of patients and families. The management of those who receive multimodal treatment is challenging and requires great sophistication in assessment, management, and interventions.

❖ *References*

Beck SL: Prevention and management of oral complications in the cancer patient, Curr Iss Cancer Nurs Prac 1(6): 1–12, 1992.

Beck SL and Yasko JM: Guidelines for oral care, Newbury Park, California, 1984, Sage Publications.

Burke TW and Levenback C: Gastrointestinal tract. In Orr JW and Shingleton HM, editors: Complications in gynecological surgery: prevention, recognition, and management, Philadelphia, 1994, JB Lippincott Co, pp. 103–130.

Callendo G, Joyce D, and Altmiller M: Nursing guidelines and discharge planning for patients receiving recombinant interleukin-2, Semin Oncol Nurs 9(3)(suppl 1):25–31, 1993.

Camp-Sorrell D: Chemotherapy: toxicity management. In Groenwald SL, Frogge MH, Goodman M, and Yarbro CH, editors: Cancer nursing: principles and practice, ed 3, Boston, 1993, Jones & Bartlett Publishers, pp. 331–365.

Camp-Sorrell D: Controlling adverse effects of chemotherapy, Nursing 21(4):34–32, 1991.

Canty SL: Constipation as a side effect of opioids, Oncol Nurs Forum 21:739–745, 1994.

Cascinu S, Feldeli A, Feldeli SL, and Catalano G: Control of chemotherapy-induced diarrhea with octreotide, Oncology 51:70–73, 1994.

Clarke-Pearson DL, Olt GJ, Rodriguez G, and Boente M: Preoperative and postoperative care. In Gershensen DM, Dechenney AL, and Curry SL, editors: Operative gynecology, Philadelphia, 1993, WB Saunders Co, pp. 29–83.

Danielsson A, Nyhlin H, Persson H, Stendahl U, Stenling R, and Suhr O: Chronic diarrhea after radiotherapy for gynecological cancer: occurrence and aetiology, Gut, 32:1180–1187, 1991.

Dudjak LA: Mouth care for mucositis due to radiation therapy, Cancer Nurs 10:131–140, 1987.

Eng-Hen N and Lowery SF: Nutritional support and cancer cachexia, Hematol Oncol Clin No Am 5:161–184, 1991.

Gootenberg JE and Pizzo PA: Optimal management of acute toxicities of therapy, Pedia Clin No Am 38:269–297, 1991.

Graves T: Emesis as a complication of cancer chemotherapy: pathophysiology, importance, and treatment, Pharmacotherapy 12:337–345, 1992.

Graham KM: Reducing the incidence of stomatitis using a quality assessment and improvement approach, Cancer Nurs 16:117–122, 1993.

Henriksson R, Franzen L, and Littbrano B: Prevention of irradiation-induced bowel discomfort by sucrafate: a double-blind, placebo-controlled study when treating localized pelvic cancer, Am J Med 91(suppl 2a):2a-151s–2a-157s, 1991.

Hogan CM: Advances in the management of nausea and vomiting, Adv Oncol Nurs 25:475–497, 1990.

Iwamoto RR: The impact of nutrition on the quality of life of persons with cancer, Quality of Life: A Nursing Challenge 1:15–21, 1992.

Jansma J, Vissink A, Spijkervet FK, Roodenburg JLN, Panders AK, Vermey A, Szabo BG, and Johanne's-Gravenmade E: Protocol for the prevention and treatment of oral sequelae resulting from head and neck radiation, Cancer 70:2171–2180, 1992.

Langstein HN and Norton JA: Mechanisms of cancer cachexia, Hematol Oncol Clin No Am 5:103–123, 1991.

Levy MH: Constipation and diarrhea in cancer patients, Cancer Bull 43:412–422, 1991.

Loprinzi RM, Goldberg RM, and Burnham NL: Cancer-associated anorexia and cachexia, Drugs 43:499–506, 1992.

Mitchell EP: Gastrointestinal toxicity of chemotherapy agents, Semin Oncol 19:566–579, 1992.

Morrow GR and Hickok JT: Behavioral treatment of chemotherapy-induced nausea and vomiting, Oncol 7:83–94, 1993.

Nelson KA, Walsh D, and Sheehan FA: The cancer anorexia-cachexia syndrome, J Clin Oncol 12:213–225, 1994.

Petrelli NJ, Rodriguez-Bigas M, Rustum Y, Herra L, and Creaven P: Bowel rest, intravenous hydration, and continuous high-dose infusion of octreotide acetate for the treatment of chemotherapy-induced diarrhea in patients with colorectal carcinoma, Cancer 72:1543–1546, 1993.

Rhodes VA: Nausea, vomiting, and retching, Nurs Clin No Am 25:885–900, 1990.

Robuck JT and Fleetwood JB: Nutritional support of the patient with cancer, Focus Crit Care 19:129–138, 1992.

Sharp E: Case management: hospitalized IL-2 patients, Semin Oncol Nurs 9(suppl 1):14–19, 1993.

Shannon-Bodnar R: The physiology of nausea and vomiting, Oncol Patient Care 1:1–12, 1990.

Skipper A, Szeluga DJ, and Groenwald SL: Nutritional disturbances. In Groenwald SL, Frogge MH, Goodman M, and Yarbro CH, editors: Cancer nursing: principles and practice, Boston, 1993, Jones & Bartlett Publishers, pp. 620–643.

Sonis S and Clark J: Prevention and management of oral mucositis induced by antineoplastic therapy, Oncology 5:11–12, 1991.

Strohl RA: Radiation therapy and resulting emesis, Oncology Nursing Perspectives: Management of Treatment-Induced Side Effects 6:11–15, 1989.

Sznol M and Longo DL: Chemotherapy drug interactions with biological agents, Semin Oncol 20:80–92, 1993.

Viele CS and Moran TA: Nursing management of the nonhospitalized patient receiving recombinant interleukin-2, Semin Oncol Nurs 9(suppl 1):20–24, 1993.

von der Masse H: Complications of combined radiotherapy and chemotherapy, Semin Rad Oncol 4:81–94, 1994.

Watcha MF and White PF: Postoperative nausea and vomiting, Anesth 77:162–184, 1992.

Wickham R: Managing chemotherapy-related nausea and vomiting: the state of the art, Oncol Nurs Forum, 16:563–574, 1989.

Winningham ML and MacVicar MG: The effect of aerobic exercise on patient report of nausea, Oncol Nurs Forum 15:447–450, 1988.

Wujcik D: Current research in side effects of high-dose chemotherapy, Semin Oncol Nurs 8:102–112, 1992.

Chapter *21*

❖ *Cutaneous Reactions*

Maureen E. O'Rourke

When using multimodal therapy, it is important to maintain the integrity of the integumentary system as the first line of defense against infection. To understand fully the side effects of multimodal therapy and the damage they can cause, a discussion of the cutaneous effects of each individual modality follows.

❖ *Effects from Radiation Therapy*

Radiation-induced cutaneous toxicities result from disruption of the reproductive activity of the cells in the basal and suprabasal layers (Pennings et al., 1970; Rubin and Casarett, 1968). Cellular oxygenation and an increased proportion of cells in the G_2 and M phases of the cell cycle enhance radiosensitivity (Sitton, 1992a). In addition, the extent of tissue damage is affected by the total radiation dose and the volume and location of tissue irradiated, the fractionation schedule, and the type of energy source utilized (O'Rourke, 1987). Host-specific factors, including light skin complexion, anatomic variations such as obesity and increased skin folds, concomitant use of photosensitizing medications, concurrent illnesses, and compromised nutritional status, can also modify cutaneous reactions (Parker and Juillard, 1988).

The effects of ionizing radiation on the skin can be classified as early and late (or delayed) reactions. Although some variability has been noted in the literature, early effects are generally categorized as occurring during or within 6 months of treatment. Delayed effects are those occurring more than 6 months after treatment (Fajardo, 1982). Table 21-1 outlines several distinct phases of skin response. The standard treatment is 1.8 to 2 Gy per day.

Transient Early Erythema

Transient early erythema occurs within a few hours of radiation exposure, increases in intensity with cumulative doses of 2 to 8 Gy, and subsides in 24 to 48 hours.

Table 21-1   Cutaneous Responses to Radiation Therapy

Phase	Time to Occurrence After Radiation Therapy	Duration	Pathophysiology	Frequency
Transient early erythema	Hours	24–48 hours	Local inflammatory response; increased capillary permeability	Common
Main erythematous reaction	3–6 weeks	Variable	Dry or moist desquamation from loss of epidermal basal cells	Common
Late-phase erythema	8–16 weeks	Variable	Dermal ischemia and necrosis from loss of endothelium	Uncommon
Late skin damage	14–52 weeks and beyond	Can last years	Unclear; dermal atrophy, subcutaneous induration, telangiectasias	Common

The early erythematous reaction is inflammatory in nature, resulting from activation of proteolytic enzymes and increased capillary permeability (Hopewell, 1990). Additional early effects include increased pigmentation related to activation of the melanocytes and the subsequent transfer of melanin to the keratinocytes (Dutreix, 1986).

Hopewell (1990) noted two other special cases of early skin responses: acute ulceration and acute dermal necrosis. Acute ulceration, seen within the first 14 days of treatment, is associated with an early loss of the epidermis and dermal tissues caused by cell death during the interphase of the cell cycle. Acute dermal necrosis is associated with low-energy β radiation, occurs within the first 10 days of treatment, and is characterized by death of keratinocytes located in the upper viable layers of the epidermis.

Main Erythematous Reaction

The main erythematous reaction appears 3 to 6 weeks after initial radiation exposure and is related to loss of epidermal basal cells, which causes a dry or a moist desquamation (Hopewell, 1990). Dry desquamation is characterized by flaking dry skin and pruritis, with a threshold dose of 10 Gy. Moist desquamation generally develops after 15 Gy, when the basal layer is unable to recover, resulting in exposure of the dermis with a fibrous exudate and painful ulceration. Repair is generally complete within 2 weeks after radiation therapy ends (Dutreix, 1986). The repopulation of the basal cell layer after radiation damage takes place as the clonogenic cells from within the radiated area itself proliferate. If an area of skin completely loses its clonogenic epithelial cells, the desquamation must heal totally as a result of division and migration of viable cells from the edges of the radiated area. Especially when a large area receives high doses of radiation, sterilizing all clonogenic cells in that area, cell migration is largely ineffective in repopulating the area. In such situations, secondary ulceration and infection may develop (Hopewell, 1990).

Late-phase Erythema

Late-phase erythema is associated with dermal ischemia and possible necrosis and is seen 8 to 16 weeks after radiation therapy. This reaction is associated with edema after threshold doses of approximately 15.4 Gy, and is characterized by a dusky or mauve appearance to the skin. Histological findings include a reduction in capillary density, diminished dermal blood flow, and a loss of endothelial cells (Hopewell, 1990). Factors influencing the progression of this reaction, or its recovery, are poorly understood.

Late Skin Damage

Late skin damage is characterized by dermal atrophy and thinning of the dermal tissue as well as subcutaneous induration and fibrosis. The mechanisms for these injuries are uncertain. The first phase of this reaction appears between 14 and 20 weeks after radiation treatment, and a later phase occurs after 52 weeks. Skin breakdown and necrosis may occur years after radiation and may be precipitated by even slight trauma to the skin. After an episode of moist desquamation, skin atrophy begins at 3 months and progresses but stabilizes by the fourth year. Such reactions involve the epidermis, the dermis, and subcutaneous tissues. The mechanisms involved in late skin damage and the recovery process are poorly understood (Dutreix, 1986).

Telangiectasia is a spidery blemish in the skin, caused by atypical dilation of superficial dermal capillaries, a common late reaction in human skin. Rarely seen earlier than 52 weeks after the completion of radiation therapy, they may increase in severity and quantity for up to 10 years after radiation, with progression related to dose and fraction size (Turesson and Notter, 1986).

Although few investigations have looked into the effects of radiation on the glandular structures of the skin, with the exception of the hair follicles, none of the skin appendages appear to play a major role in the response of the skin to radiation (Hopewell, 1990). Some dysfunction of the eccrine and the sebaceous glands may occur, with eccrine gland activity returning more readily than sebaceous gland activity. Diminished sebaceous gland activity contributes to the overall dryness and fragility of atrophic skin (Shimm and Cassady, 1994).

Radiosensitivity of the hair varies according to its growth rate, with rapidly growing scalp hair being the most radiosensitive, followed in decreasing order by the male beard, eyebrows, axilla hair, pubic hair, and fine body hair. Damage to the germinal epithelium of the hair follicle occurs after a threshold dose of 4 to 5 Gy. Epilation (hair loss) is delayed because the hair adheres to the follicle (Shimm and Cassady, 1994). Low radiation doses (25 to 30 Gy) generally cause a temporary decrease in the growth rate without epilation, whereas higher doses may cause temporary alopecia within the treatment field. After epilation, researchers have noted alterations in the growth rate, texture, and color of hair. Regrowth usually begins within 2 months after treatment (Sitton, 1992a); however, high-dose radiation (45 Gy or more) may result in permanent hair loss (Hilderly, 1993).

Hyperthermia is thought to have no role in the curative treatment of tumors in humans, but numerous studies have demonstrated its synergistic effect in combination with ionizing radiation (Horsman and Overgaard, 1992). The cytotoxic mechanism of heat appears to be multifaceted: damage to cell and nuclear membranes, damage to lysosomes that causes a release of digestive enzymes, and ultimately cell death (Brandt and Harney, 1989). Nutrient-deficient, hypoxic cells with low pH are more sensitive to hyperthermia, as are typically radioresistant cells in S phase (Hall and Cox, 1994).

Hyperthermia enhances radiation-induced skin reactions. Howard and colleagues (1987) noted an increased incidence of severe skin reactions in patients with superficial tumors treated with hyperthermia and radiation over those treated with radiation alone. Skin reactions range from local discomfort and transient erythema to edema and blisters.

A final factor is the occurrence of secondary skin cancers as a consequence of radiation exposure. The mean latency period for the induction of skin cancer is estimated at 24.5 years (Dutreix, 1986). A lifetime skin dose of 20 Gy (substantially lower than doses used to treat malignancies) is thought to impart a high risk of skin cancer (Charles, 1986), although calculations of risk are highly variable and complicated by the inability to quantify the interactive effect of ionizing radiation and ultraviolet radiation (Fry, 1990).

❖ Effects from Chemotherapy

As with radiation-induced cutaneous toxicity, the rapidly proliferating cells of the epidermis and mucosal surfaces, as well as the cells of the hair and nails, are vulnerable to cytotoxic agents. The cutaneous side effects of chemotherapy are the result of direct toxicity, but they may also be a harbinger of systemic toxicity (DeSpain, 1992). Whereas some chemotherapeutic agents rarely cause skin problems, specific agents cause distinctive cutaneous toxicities. In some cases these unique toxicities have been documented as solitary episodes and have not been subsequently observed. Skin manifestations are best interpreted in light of the patient's total clinical picture, including concomitant medication use, blood products, and antecedent skin conditions (DeSpain, 1992). The major patterns of chemotherapy-induced cutaneous toxicity include alopecia, hyperpigmentation, nail disorders, photosensitivity, extravasation injury, and hypersensitivity reactions.

Alopecia

Although not life-threatening, alopecia is one of the most psychologically damaging side effects of chemotherapy. Mitotically active hair follicles are susceptible to the damaging effects of chemotherapy. The degree of alopecia varies but relates directly to the pharmacokinetics and plasma half-life of the drugs used (Keller and Blausey, 1988). Hair loss usually begins during the second week after a single treatment of chemotherapy and becomes most noticeable within 1 to 2 months. Hair growth resumes 1 to 2 months after the therapy ends. Chemotherapeutic agents causing severe alopecia include cyclophosphamide, ifosfamide, 5-fluorouracil, dactinomycin, daunorubicin, doxorubicin, bleomycin, vindesine (DeSpain, 1992), and paclitaxel (Dorr and Von Hoff, 1994). Moderate alopecia has been associated with mechlorethamine, thiotepa, methotrexate, vinblastine, vincristine, etoposide, carmustine, and hydroxyurea (DeSpain, 1992). Mitomycin-C, mitoxantrone, and melphalan have also been associated with alopecia. In addition, a variety of commonly prescribed nononcological drugs may induce alopecia, as well as such conditions as malnutrition, stress, iron deficiency, anemia, and lupus erythematosus (Keller and Blausey, 1988).

Hyperpigmentation

Numerous chemotherapeutic agents are associated with hyperpigmentation, commonly the alkylating agents and antitumor antibiotics. This condition is mainly a cosmetic concern and is rarely associated with systemic toxicity. Pigmentation changes occur in diffuse and localized patterns and may involve the skin, the teeth, the hair, the nails, and mucous membranes. The pathogenesis of such changes is poorly understood, although studies have focused on deviations in melanin stimulation and distribution within the dermis. Postinflammatory changes have also been implicated. In most cases, hyperpigmentation subsides over time and may completely resolve. In rare cases, skin changes are permanent (DeSpain, 1992).

Busulfan-induced hyperpigmentation represents a unique presentation that some have linked to underlying pulmonary fibrosis (Bronner and Hood, 1983). Its presentation mimics Addison's disease, with hyperpigmentation extending over the trunk, the neck, the abdomen, and volar creases, accompanied by weight loss, hypotension, nausea, vomiting, and anorexia, but not alopecia. Mucous membrane involvement is rare, however, and levels of melanocyte-stimulating hormone and adrenal cortical hormone remain normal. The syndrome resolves fully after discontinuation of busulfan (DeSpain, 1992).

Hyperpigmentation related to drug-induced photosensitivity (an adverse skin reaction triggered by exposure to normally harmless doses of sunlight) has been reported with cyclophosphamide, dactinomycin, methotrexate, and 5-fluorouracil. Serpiginous (winding, creeping) hyperpigmentation overlying veins in the absence of phlebitis or sclerosis has been reported with 5-fluorouracil. The suggested mechanism is endothelial fragility, which allows leakage of the offending drug into surrounding soft tissue (Hrushesky, 1976).

Hyperpigmentation of the veins used for administering chemotherapy is also common. Up to one third of patients report localized hyperpigmented linear streaks appearing approximately 1 month after the administration of bleomycin. The streaks and areas of hyperpigmentation reportedly appear over pressure points following a trauma such as friction or scratching. The pathophysiology remains unknown but is thought to be related to vasodilation and increased tissue concentration of bleomycin, and is generally not permanent (deBast et al., 1971).

Hyperpigmentation of the oral mucosa and the tongue, especially in blacks, has been reported after treatment with doxorubicin, busulfan, cyclophosphamide, and 5-fluorouracil (Dunagin, 1982). Clinicians also report that cisplatin causes a gingival line of hyperpigmentation resembling a "lead line" (Ettinger and Freeman, 1979).

Topical application of mechlorethamine has also been associated with hyperpigmentation. Although the mechanism of action is unknown, Vonderheid (1984) suggests a direct melanogenic effect or a postinflammatory effect. Topical application of thiotepa has been associated with leukoderma and depigmentation, including the documented loss of melanocytes (Harben, Cooper, and Rodman, 1979), whereas systemic administration of this same agent produces erythematous eruptions followed by hyperpigmentation (Herzig et al., 1988).

Nail Disorders

Nail changes due to chemotherapy include pigmentation changes secondary to melanin deposits in the nail plate and a variety of effects related to toxicity of the mitotically active nail matrix. Transverse white bands or nail depressions (Beau's lines) involving all 10 fingernails have been reported. The lines result from the reduction or temporary cessation of mitotic activity in the nail, which continues as the nail grows. Onycholysis, the partial separation of the nail plate from the bed, has been noted after treatment with bleomycin, doxorubicin, and 5-fluorouracil. Brittle and dystrophic nails have been reported with 5-fluorouracil and hydroxyurea (DeSpain, 1992).

Photosensitivity

Dacarbazine, methotrexate, 5-fluorouracil, procarbazine, and vinblastine may cause photosensitive reactions (Medical Letter, 1986). Symptoms include exaggerated sunburn type of reactions, often accompanied by stinging and urticaria. The reaction is thought to occur via a phototoxic mechanism involving UVB light (DeSpain, 1992). Patients receiving photodynamic therapy that involves intravenous administration of a photosensitizing agent followed by laser treatment of superficial tumors in the bladder, the pleura, the head and neck, the bronchus, the chest wall, or the peritoneal cavity (Dachowski and Delaney, 1992) may experience severe erythematous phototoxic reactions. They subsequently are highly sensitive to direct and indirect sunlight and sometimes to artificial lighting. This may persist up to 1 month after treatment (DeSpain, 1992).

Hypersensitivity

Although hypersensitive reactions to chemotherapy happen infrequently, they are sometimes associated with systemic hypersensitivity and do not appear to be dose related. Type I immediate-hypersensitivity reactions are manifested by urticaria and angioedema and may be associated with anaphylaxis. The chemotherapeutic agent asparaginase most often produces such reactions, although other agents such as cisplatin, busulfan, chlorambucil, cyclophosphamide, doxorubicin, etoposide, melphalan, methotrexate, mitotane, paclitaxel, and procarbazine have also been implicated. Clinicians have also described type III serum-sickness reactions with urticaria following treatment with asparaginase and procarbazine (DeSpain, 1992). Chemotherapeutic agents have caused erythema multiforme, characterized by erythematous wheals on the extremities and on mucous membranes. However, most reports involved patients at risk for infection or those taking multiple medications; thus the etiology is indeterminate (DeSpain, 1992).

Exanthematous drug rashes characterized by macular papular eruptions have been associated with a variety of chemotherapeutic agents. The pathogenesis of these remains unclear but is thought to involve multiple immune-mediated pathways. An example is topical application of mechlorethamine, which is associated with contact dermatitis.

Wood and Ellerhorst-Ryan (1984) reported delayed skin reactions in eight patients 2 weeks to 6 months after receiving intravenous mitomycin-C. The reactions included fibrosis, erythema along the venous walls, skin crusting, ulceration, and deep tissue necrosis. The authors postulated that these reactions could represent an allergic response or a synergism between mitomycin-C and other antineoplastic agents concurrently administered to the patient.

High-dose cytarabine therapy is associated with cutaneous toxicity in 3% to 72% of patients. It begins with erythema of the hands and feet and progresses to painful swelling, bullae formation, and desquamation. The pathogenesis is unclear, although it is thought to be multifactorial (Richards and Wujcik, 1992). Other agents have been associated with acral erythema, including cyclophosphamide, doxorubicin, 6-mercaptopurine, 5-fluorouracil, methotrexate, hydroxyurea, and mitotane. The syndrome is sometimes referred to as palmar-plantar erythema, hand-foot syndrome, or erythrodysesthesia syndrome (DeSpain, 1992).

Miscellaneous Integumentary Conditions

Degenerative changes in the sweat glands associated with neutrophilic infiltration have been reported with numerous chemotherapeutic agents. It has been suggested that cytotoxic drugs are secreted or concentrated in the eccrine glands in the absence of inflammation, causing this local toxicity. Dactinomycin has been associated with a distinctive folliculitis. An acute erythematous rash involving the face and neck has been observed in patients receiving plicamycin one day prior to severe hematologic, renal, hepatic, and electrolyte abnormalities and has been suggested as an indication for the discontinuation of therapy (DeSpain, 1992).

Curran, Luce, and Page (1990) presented an analysis of 539 cases of venous flare reaction associated with the administration of doxorubicin. None were associated with anaphylaxis, and the manifestations of the flare reactions included urticaria, pain and stinging, erythema at the injection site and along the vein, and edema—all manifestations of an inflammatory response. Although the overall incidence of flare reactions is not well documented, this study reported 17.5%.

Hormonal agents are relatively uncommon causes of cutaneous toxicity. The systemic use of corticosteroids is associated with acne, characterized by multiple erythematous pustules that appear as early as 2 weeks after the initiation of therapy. Long-term use is associated with skin fragility, easy bruising, telangiectasias, striae, atrophy, poor wound healing, infections, and hirsutism. Chronic use of androgens may cause hirsutism, acne, and temporal balding (DeSpain, 1992).

❖ Effects from Biotherapy

Biotherapy is an evolving area of research, and documentation regarding side effects and their management continues to grow. Investigators report several patterns of cutaneous reactions. Interferon has been associated with a pruritic eruption extending over the trunk and extremities that responds to antihistamines. One third of patients experience mild alopecia (DeSpain, 1992); however, excessive growth of the eyelashes has also been observed (Foon and Dougher, 1984). High doses (10 million units/m^2 and above) have been reported to cause cyanosis of the nail beds and oral mucosa (Grunberg et al., 1987). Rashes have also been reported following administration of granulocyte-macrophage colony-stimulating factor (Steger et al., 1992). Erythematous reactions following administration of interleukin-2 (IL-2) are well documented and thought to be cutaneous manifestations of a more widespread capillary-leak syndrome in which edematous fluid leaks between endothelial cells of the capillary walls (Gaspari et al., 1987). Other documented cutaneous complications include superficial punctate cutaneous erosions (minute spots or depressions) of the trunk, erosions occurring in surgical scars, and diffuse hair thinning within 12 weeks of IL-2 therapy (Gaspari et al., 1987).

❖ Effects from Multimodal Therapy

The majority of cases of enhanced skin effects occur when chemotherapy and radiation therapy are administered concurrently (Phillips and Fu, 1976); however, previous radiation of tissue may enhance drug reactions (Figure 21-1). This phenomenon was first observed in patients following treatment of Wilm's tumor with radiation and dactinomycin (D'Angio, Farber, and Maddock, 1959). Doxorubicin and a variety of other antineoplastic agents have subsequently demonstrated similar effects (Donaldson, Glick, and Wilbur, 1974). More recently a radiation recall reaction was reported associated with the administration of vinblastine in a patient treated for AIDS-related Kaposi's sarcoma (Nemechek and Corder, 1992), and in two patients with breast cancer treated with paclitaxel (Shenkier and Gelmon, 1994). Phillips (1980) describes this "recall phenomenon" as a skin reaction occurring within the radiation portal when chemotherapy is administered following radiation therapy, which may be more severe than the original skin reaction to radiation. He proposes that this may not represent actual recall of radiation damage, but rather the addition of chemotherapeutic cell kill to damage already caused to the stem cell population in the basal layer.

The potential for enhanced skin effects exists whenever the multimodal approach is utilized, regardless of the timing (i.e., chemotherapy administered before, during, or after radiation therapy) (O'Rourke, 1987). For example, reactions to the sun are enhanced in the irradiated field if the patient has also received a chemotherapy agent that causes photosensitivity.

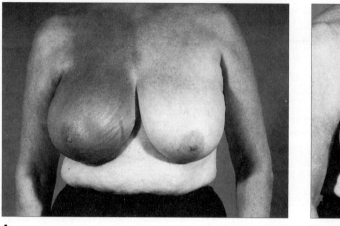
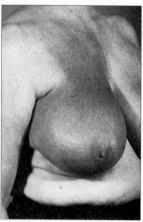

A   **B**

Fig. 21-1.   A and **B,** Erythematous skin reaction of the right breast in a 51-year-old patient who was treated with 46 Gy to the entire right breast in 25 fractions followed by a 19-Gy boost to the primary tumor via an iridium-192 three-plane implant. She then was scheduled to receive six cycles of CMF (cyclophosphamide, methotrexate, and 5-fluorouracil) chemotherapy. This reaction developed on day 8 of the third cycle of chemotherapy. Note the lines of demarcation defining the radiation portal.

Treatment plans involving both surgery and radiation therapy are increasingly common. Controversy continues in regard to the optimal timing of such regimens, although postoperative treatments are generally delayed until adequate tissue repair has taken place. Potential complications of surgery include delayed wound healing and infection, adhesion formation, fibrosis, abscess formation, dehiscence, and evisceration. Fistula formation may be exaggerated when radiation is administered preoperatively or when surgery must be performed on previously irradiated tissue (Scofield, Liebman, and Popkin, 1991). Intraoperative radiation therapy is now being employed with selective tumors as a method of applying radiation directly to the tumor and of bypassing penetration through the skin and the potential related cutaneous toxicities.

❖ *Nursing Management*

Assessment should be ongoing throughout the course of therapy, and the foci should be based on an understanding of the potential cutaneous toxicities of multimodal therapies. Adjuvant treatment can contribute to an increased risk of cutaneous reactions. Nurses must consider the temporal relationship between the therapies administered and the onset of skin eruptions when attempting to identify the offending agent.

Systematic assessment of the integumentary system, including the skin, the nails, and the hair, must take place before the initiation of any therapy to determine the patient's baseline status. Because most patients receive therapy in crowded outpatient settings, the nurse should take extra care to maintain patient privacy during skin assessments. Skin inspection focuses on color, moisture, texture, and temperature, with special attention given to any areas of prior radiation and surgical scars (McNally and Strohl, 1991). The nurse queries the patient about concomitant medications such as photosensitizing agents, including over-the-counter agents that may influence skin reactions.

Ongoing assessment includes not only the radiation portal but also the radiation exit site (Iwamoto, 1994). Evaluation of the patient's current skin-care and hair-care regimen is an important consideration. If the patient is receiving radiation therapy to the head or chemotherapy, which will cause alopecia, hair dryers and harsh chemicals may damage already fragile hair. Ointments, creams, lotions, and deodorants may unintentionally enhance skin reactions by creating a bolus effect in the treatment areas when the patient receives radiation therapy.

Many commercially available deodorants contain metallic substances that interact with the photons emitted from radioactive sources and cause radiation scatter, which increases skin reactions. Particular attention is paid to areas at high risk for cutaneous reactions to radiation such as skinfolds in the axilla, under the breasts, behind the ears, and in the perineum, the groin, and gluteal folds. Facial skin is especially vulnerable due to the thinness of the epidermal layer. Patients receiving radiation to the perineal area may experience severe skin reactions related to moisture and friction, or they may develop diarrhea caused by concurrent use of radiation and 5-fluorouracil. Stoma appliances and skin barriers can act as a bolus material and enhance skin reactions (Iwamoto, 1994).

In cases of dry or moist desquamation, the area of the lesion should be measured. Clinical photographs taken for comparison over time can enhance the documentation. Drainage should be inspected for color, consistency, and amount, and cultures should be obtained. Nutritional assessment should consider the increased metabolic demands for wound healing, including caloric needs, and vitamins A, B complex, and C intake to promote capillary stability, wound contraction, and epithelialization (O'Rourke, 1987). Dietary consultation may be indicated.

Elderly clients may be at risk for increased cutaneous complications. The physiologic changes that accompany the aging process include decreased distribution of subcutaneous fat on the extremities; general thinning of the dermis and epidermis; diminished elasticity and turgor of the dermis; atrophy; dryness; and partial disappearance of capillaries, with a loss of dilating capacity in the remaining vessels (Timiras, 1972). These changes predispose the elderly to radiation-induced skin damage. In addition, the normal physiologic changes of aging that affect drug absorption, distribution, metabolism, and elimination (Timiras, 1972) may potentiate cutaneous effects of chemotherapy (O'Rourke, 1987).

Patient education before treatment is essential to minimize potential side effects. Patients and family members should be instructed on skin care and given recommendations to avoid lotions, powders, and other products that may enhance radiation effects and irritate sensitive tissue. Wearing loose cotton clothing washed in a mild detergent helps prevent skin irritation. Shaving in the area of the treatment portal should be avoided. Patients must protect themselves from sun exposure during treatment and thereafter by applying sunscreen that has a sun-protection factor (SPF) of 40 and by wearing protective clothing. Sun Precautions, Inc. (Seattle, Washington) markets the only FDA-approved sun-protective clothing (Solumbra), which maintains an SPF of 30+, even when wet. Teaching should include the expected acute skin effects of exposure to radiation therapy (tanning, erythema, dryness) and also the potential delayed effects (dermal ischemia, telangectasia). The importance of follow-up appointments for continued assessment should be emphasized. Patient Education Guidelines for Skin Care During Concurrent Chemoradiotherapy appear below.

Erythematous Reactions and Dry Desquamation

Although treatment recommendations vary greatly in the literature, conservative approaches are emphasized in practice. Early recommendations advised against washing the irradiated area (Strohl, 1988). More recently, gentle washing with warm water and mild soap using the hands rather than a washcloth to minimize friction is recommended (Sitton, 1992b). Frosch and Kligman (1979) gauged the irritant qualities of 18 common soaps and only rated Dove soap as mild. Iwamoto

---

Patient Education Guidelines for

Skin Care During Concurrent Chemoradiotherapy

◆ The site to be irradiated will be outlined. This is the area that needs special care. If the outline starts to fade, the radiation therapist will darken it. After completion of all your radiation treatments, these marks will fade in 7 to 14 days.

◆ Wash this area by letting the shower water drip indirectly over the area (if for instance your chest is the site of treatment, stand with your back to the shower and let the water hit your shoulders and trickle down your chest) or by wringing a wet washcloth over the area. Do not rub the area with the washcloth.

◆ It should not be necessary to use soap in the treatment area, but, if needed, use *only* Dove soap.

◆ Wear only cotton clothing over the treatment area. Wash clothes that come in contact with the treatment area with baby detergent, such as Ivory Snow.

◆ Avoid exposing the site to extremes of temperature. This includes heating pads, hot shower water, and ice packs.

◆ Avoid tight-fitting clothing such as elastic belts and girdles over the treatment area.

◆ Avoid the sun during treatment and after treatment. Use a sunscreen with an SPF of 40 or higher.

◆ Check the skin daily for increased redness, openings of the skin, and infection or drainage. Report these to your nurse or physician. Don't try any skin-care remedies without consulting your nurse or physician.

Permission granted to reproduce these guidelines for educational purposes only.

(1994) suggests using only unperfumed, nondeodorant soaps. Topical application of hydrocortisone creams or ointments, Aquaphor, hydrous lanolin, or A&D ointment have been suggested (Sitton, 1992b). Sitton (1992b) advised applying hydrocortisone to moist, noninfected skin after bathing. Although topical steroids may decrease pruritus, prolonged use can lead to thinning of the skin and delayed wound healing. Preparations containing alcohol, phenol, or menthol should be avoided because of their irritant properties, as should hydrophobic preparations such as petroleum jelly, which may trap bacteria and are difficult to remove from the skin.

The use of cornstarch to soothe irritated skin is controversial. Sitton (1992b) advises against it, noting its propensity for promoting fungal growth. Strohl (1988) recommends its use when the skin is dry and itchy. If used, it should be used sparingly to avoid clumping. The use of nonperfumed, hydrophilic moisturizing lotions that contain no metal compounds had also been recommended (Iwamoto, 1994). If flecks of metal are on the skin, they affect the radiation beam during treatment.

Moist Desquamation

Treatment recommendations are conservative. They include gentle cleansing with a half-strength solution of hydrogen peroxide or a Domeboro solution applied as soaks or wet dressings, followed by saline rinses. Hydrogen peroxide is useful for cleansing and for removing purulent debris; however, if used at full strength it can damage granulation tissue. Systemic analgesics may be needed to manage pain.

Gauze dressings and tape should be avoided. Hydrocolloid dressings such as Duoderm and Tegasorb, which come in a variety of shapes, have been utilized for the management of moist desquamation wounds (Margolin et al., 1990; Sitton, 1992b). The advantages of such dressings include enhanced patient comfort, avoidance of skin maceration from the accumulation of fluid under film dressings, and ease of application (dressings contour easily to awkward skin surfaces such as inframammary folds). Margolin and colleagues (1990) documented the use of occlusive hydrocolloid dressings in 20 patients experiencing moist desquamation secondary to radiation treatment. No wound infections occurred and the mean healing time was 12 days. The major difficulty was melted gel, which patients found particularly bothersome in the hot weather.

Moisture-vapor-permeable (MVP) dressings (e.g., Tegaderm and Opsite) have also been studied. In a randomized trial, patients using MVP dressings had an average healing time of 19 days compared to 24 days for the hydrous lanolin group; however, the differences were not statistically significant (Shell, Stauntz, and Grimm, 1986). The advantage of MVP dressings is their ability to provide an occlusive, moist environment to promote healing and patient comfort. Radiation may be administered through MVP dressings without creating a bolus effect, presently a disadvantage of hydrocolloid dressings (Sitton, 1992b). MVP dressings are difficult to maintain in areas such as skinfolds and the axilla, which are prone to moist desquamation reactions. Further nursing research is needed to compare MVP dressings and hydrocolloid dressings in terms of variables such as wound healing, infection, and patient comfort. Nursing Management of the Patient with Moist Desquamation is presented on page 362.

Nursing Management of

The Patient with Moist Desquamation

◆ Avoid dry gauze dressings and tape.

◆ Use gentle washing.

◆ The area can be treated with half-strength hydrogen peroxide or Domoboro solution soaks applied for 15 to 30 minutes 3 or 4 times a day. For perianal areas, the patient can use a sitz bath of tepid water and Burow's solution.

◆ Continuous wet dressings will keep the area moist, promote healing, and increase patient comfort by decreasing itchiness.

◆ If the patient is currently receiving radiation therapy, a moisture-vapor-permeable (MVP) dressing can be applied every 3 to 4 days. Change it as needed when drainage builds up under the dressing.

◆ If radiation therapy is completed, or if the patient is on a treatment break, a hydrocolloid dressing can be applied every 3 to 5 days. Change the dressing more frequently if gel seepage occurs.

◆ Monitor for infection.

◆ Provide pain medication as needed.

Hypersensitivity

A comprehensive allergy history should be documented in the patient's record before the administration of any chemotherapeutic agents. Baseline vital signs provide a measure for comparison in the event that a patient develops an allergic or hypersensitive reaction. Skin testing should be performed before the administration of drugs such as bleomycin, which have shown a propensity to cause hypersensitivity responses. In the event of a localized hypersensitive response, do not remove the intravenous line. Administer diphenhydramine and/or hydrocortisone per the physician's orders. Monitor vital signs every 15 minutes for 1 hour. If the patient is sensitized, avoid using the agent again unless it is critical to the overall treatment plan. In this case, premedication with antihistamines or corticosteroids may be necessary (Oncology Nursing Society [ONS], 1992).

Flare reactions may occur during the administration of doxorubicin or daunorubicin. Immediately stop administering the drug, but do not discontinue the intravenous line. These reactions must be differentiated from extravasation. If extravasation is not suspected, flush the vein with saline. Continue flushing and observe for resolution of the flare reaction (ONS, 1992). Reassure the patient that this reaction is transient and usually resolves within 30 minutes (Curran, Luce, and Page, 1990). If resolution does not occur, administer 25 mg to 50 mg of hydrocortisone and/or 25 mg to 50 mg of diphenhydramine intravenously, as a physician orders. Flush the line again with saline. Once the flare resolves, resume the infusion at a slower rate. Before administering the drug in the future, consider premedication with antihistamines and/or glucocorticoids. Administering doxorubicin or daunorubicin at a slower rate with greater fluid volume may prevent future occurrences (ONS, 1992).

Alopecia

Hair preservation interventions are limited. Numerous researchers have investigated the use of scalp hypothermia with varying results. Parker (1987) demonstrated its efficacy in a small sample of patients with breast cancer who received cyclophosphamide, methotrexate, and fluorouracil therapy. Giaccone and colleagues (1988) also showed the benefit of hypothermia in a randomized, controlled study of patients receiving doxorubicin; however, decreased scalp perfusion during hypothermia may provide a sanctuary for tumor cell proliferation and may result in a decreased cell kill. Hypothermia is thus not recommended for patients with leukemia or lymphoma, sarcomas, breast malignancies, lung, renal, or gastric tumors (Keller and Blausey, 1988). In January 1990, the FDA rescinded clearance for the manufacturers of scalp-cooling devices to market these products for prevention of chemotherapy-induced alopecia. To date no manufacturers have provided the FDA with evidence of their safety and efficacy or received FDA approval.

Drugs such as Minoxidil have failed to demonstrate their effectiveness in preventing alopecia (Denes and Seely, 1994; Granai et al., 1991). Current research efforts include evaluation of potential hair-protective agents such as Imuvert (a biological response modifier) (Hussein et al., 1990) and 1,25-dihydroxyvitamin D_3 (Jiminez and Ynis, 1992). Interventions focus predominantly on minimizing the psychosocial trauma associated with hair loss and altered body image. Patient preparation is essential, and a number of measures have been suggested to minimize or camouflage the loss. A professional haircut may diminish the effect of thinning hair. Hair stylists should avoid using harsh chemicals, curling irons, and dryers set at high temperatures. Braiding the hair or tying it in a pony tail may break more fragile hairs than leaving it loose. For patients with long hair, a short cut may make the hair-loss process seem less dramatic. Wearing wigs, turbans, and stylish hats may enhance a positive self-image (Keller and Blausey, 1988).

Patients should be informed that hair loss is temporary and that hair will regrow after the treatment has stopped. Hair generally returns in 2 to 6 months. Potential changes in color and texture should be discussed. Patients may receive conflicting information about available hair-preservation techniques, and the advantages and disadvantages of these should be discussed openly. The nurse should encourage patients to share their concerns and inform them about local support groups as well as the American Cancer Society and National Cosmetology Association's Look-Good–Feel-Better program.

Delayed Wound Healing

Surgery performed on previously radiated skin should be followed by meticulous care to the site. Healing will be slow, and infection or abscess formation can occur. Documentation of the size (including depth), drainage, and appearance of the wound at least twice a week will allow caregivers to evaluate healing. Photographic documentation, taken from the same angle each time, provides accurate comparisons to assess progress and to determine if the wound care is effective.

❖ Summary

Multimodal therapy is now the mainstay of cancer treatment. Although it has led to dramatic improvements in patient survival, the enhanced effects on normal tissues cannot be overlooked. Patients often receive their care from multiple specialists, but nurses are in a pivotal position to consider the overlapping effects of the multimodal therapy. There is a growing body of nursing research regarding the management of cutaneous toxicities; however, much work remains to be done before the interventions can be scientifically substantiated.

❖ References

Brandt BB and Harney J: An overview of interstitial brachytherapy and hyperthermia, Oncol Nurs Forum 16:833–841, 1989.

Bronner AK and Hood AF: Cutaneous complications of chemotherapeutic agents, J Am Acad Derm 9:645–663, 1983.

Charles MW: Introduction and update on localised irradiation accidents: recent developments in the dosimetry of superficial tissues, Brit J Radiol 19(suppl):1–7, 1986.

Curran CF, Luce JK, and Page JA: Doxorubicin-associated flare reactions, Oncol Nurs Forum 17:387–389, 1990.

Dachowski LJ and Delaney TF: Photodynamic therapy: the NCI experience and its nursing implications, Oncol Nurs Forum 19:63–67, 1992.

D'Angio GJ, Farber S, and Maddock CL: Potentiation of x-ray effects by actinomycin D, Radiol 73:175–177, 1959.

deBast AE, Morianne N, Wanet J, Ledoux M, Achten G, and Kenis Y: Bleomycin in mycosis fungoides and reticulum cell lymphoma, Arch Derm 104:508–512, 1971.

Denes AE and Seely K: Failure of topical Minoxidil to accelerate hair growth following chemotherapy, Proc Am Soc Clin Oncol 13:446, 1994 (abstract).

DeSpain JD: Dermatologic toxicity. In Perry MC, editor: The chemotherapy sourcebook. Baltimore, 1992, Williams & Wilkins, pp. 531–547.

Donaldson SS, Glick JM, and Wilbur JR: Adriamycin activating a recall phenomenon after radiation therapy, Ann Int Med 83:407–408, 1974.

Dorr RT and Von Hoff DD: Cancer chemotherapy handbook, ed 2, Norwalk, Connecticut, 1994, Appleton & Lange.

Dunagin WG: Clinical toxicity of chemotherapeutic agents: dermatologic toxicity, Semin Oncol 9:14–22, 1982.

Dutreix J: Radiotherapy studies in skin: clinical and experimental, Brit J Radiol 9(suppl):22–28, 1986.

Ettinger LJ and Freeman AI: The gingival platinum line. A new finding following cisdichlorodiamine platinum (II) treatment, Cancer 44:1882–1884, 1979.

Fajardo L: Skin. In Fajardo L, editor: Pathology of radiation injury, New York, 1982, Masson Publishing Co, pp. 186–199.

Foon KA and Dougher G: Increased growth of eyelashes in a patient given leukocyte A interferon, N Eng J Med 311:1259, 1984.

Frosch P and Kligman A: The soap chamber: a new method for assessment of the irritancy of soaps, J Am Acad Derm 1:35–41, 1979.

Fry RJ: Radiation protection guidelines for the skin, Int J Radiat Biol 57:829–839, 1990.

Gaspari A, Lotze MT, Rosenberg SA, Stern JB, and Katz SI: Dermatologic changes associated with interleukin-2 administration, JAMA 25:1624–1629, 1987.

Giaccone G, DiGiulio F, Morandini MP, and Calciati A: Scalp hypothermia in the prevention of doxorubicin-induced hair loss, Cancer Nurs 11:170–173, 1988.

Granai CO, Frederickson H, Gajewski W, Goodman A, Goldstein A, and Baden H: The use of Minoxidil to attempt to prevent alopecia during chemotherapy for gynecologic malignancies, Eur J Gyn Oncol 12:129–132, 1991.

Grunberg SM, Kempf RA, Venturi CL, and Mitchell MS: Phase I study of recombinant β-interferon given by four hour infusion, Cancer Res 47:1174–1178, 1987.

Hall EJ and Cox JD: Physical and biologic basis of radiation therapy. In Cox JD, editor: Moss's radiation oncology, ed 7, St. Louis, 1994, Mosby, pp. 3–66.

Harben DJ, Cooper RH, and Rodman OC: Thiotepa-induced leukoderma, Arch Derm 115:973–974, 1979.

Herzig R, Fay J, Herzig G, MaMaistre CF, Wolff S, Egorin M, Frei-Lahr D, Brown R, Standjord S, Coccia P, Giannone L, Norris D, Weick J, Rothman S, Bolwell B, and Lowder J: Phase I–II studies with high-dose thiotepa and autologous marrow transplantation in patients with refractory malignancies, Proc Am Soc Clin Oncol 7:74, 1988 (abstract).

Hilderly L: Radiotherapy. In Groenwald SL, Frogge MH, Goodman M, and Yarbro CH, editors: Cancer nursing: principles and practice, ed 3, Boston, 1993, Jones & Bartlett Publishers, pp. 235–269.

Hopewell JW: The skin: its structure and response to ionizing radiation, Int J Radiat Biol, 57:751–773, 1990.

Horsman MR and Overgaard J: Simultaneous and sequential treatment with radiation and hyperthermia: a comparative assessment. In Handl-Zeller L, editor: Interstitial hyperthermia, New York, 1992, Springer-Verlag Wien, pp. 11–33.

Howard GCW, Sathiaseelan V, Freedman L, and Bleehen NM: Hyperthermia and radiation in the treatment of superficial malignancy: an analysis of treatment parameters, response, and toxicity, Int J Hyperthermia 3:1–8, 1987.

Hrushesky WJ: Serpentine supravenous fluorouracil hyperpigmentation, JAMA 236:138, 1976.

Hussein AM, Jimenez JJ, McCall CA, and Yunis AA: Protection from chemotherapy-induced alopecia in a rat model, Science 249:1564–1566, 1990.

Iwamoto R: Radiation therapy. In Otto S, editor: Oncology nursing, ed 2, St. Louis, 1994, Mosby, pp. 467–492.

Jiminez JJ and Ynis AA: Protection from chemotherapy-induced alopecia by 1,25-dihydroxyvitamin D_3, Cancer Res 52:5123–5125, 1992.

Keller JF and Blausey LA: Nursing issues and management in chemotherapy-induced alopecia, Oncol Nurs Forum 15:603–607, 1988.

Margolin SG, Breneman JC, Denman DL, LaChapelle P, Weckback L, and Aron BS: Management of radiation-induced moist skin desquamation using hydrocolloid dressing, Cancer Nurs 13:71–80, 1990.

McNally J and Strohl R: Skin integrity, impairment of: related to radiation therapy. In McNally J, Somerville E, Miaskowski C, and Rostad M, editors: Guidelines for oncology nursing practice, ed 2, Philadelphia, 1991, WB Saunders Co, pp. 236–240.

Medical Letter, Inc: Drugs that can cause photosensitivity, Medical Letter 28(713):49–52, 1986.

Nemechek PM and Corder MC: Radiation recall associated with vinblastine in a patient treated for Kaposi's sarcoma related to acquired immune deficiency syndrome, Cancer 70:1605–1606, 1992.

Oncology Nursing Society: Cancer chemotherapy guidelines. Recommendations for the management of vesicant extravasation, hypersensitivity, and anaphylaxis, Pittsburgh, 1992, Oncology Nursing Society.

O'Rourke ME: Enhanced cutaneous effects in combined modality therapy, Oncol Nurs Forum, 14(6):31–35, 1987.

Parker R: The effectiveness of scalp hypothermia in preventing cyclophosphamide-induced alopecia, Oncol Nurs Forum 14(6):49–53, 1987.

Parker RG and Juillard GJF: Skin: the basic model for relating dose, time, and fractionation, Front Radiat Ther Oncol 22:53–61, 1988.

Pennings NS, Fulton JE, Weinstin GD, and Frost P: Location of proliferating cells in human epidermis, Arch Derm 101:323–327, 1970.

Phillips TL: Tissue toxicity of radiation-drug interactions. In Sokol GH and Maickel RP, editors: Radiation-drug interactions in the treatment of cancer, New York, 1980, John Wiley and Sons, pp. 175–200.

Phillips TL and Fu KK: Quantification of combined radiation therapy and chemotherapy effects on critical normal tissues, Cancer, 37:1186–1200, 1976.

Richards C and Wujcik D: Cutaneous toxicity associated with high-dose cytosine arabinoside, Oncol Nurs Forum 19:1191–1195, 1992.

Rubin P and Cassarett GW: Clinical radiation pathology, Philadelphia, 1968, WB Saunders Co.

Scofield RP, Liebman MC, and Popkin JD: Multimodal therapy. In Baird SB, McCorkle R, and Grant M, editors: Cancer nursing: a comprehensive textbook, Philadelphia, 1991, WB Saunders Co, pp. 344–354.

Shell J, Stauntz F, and Grimm J: Comparison of moisture vapor permeable (MVP) dressings to conventional dressings for management of radiation skin reactions, Oncol Nurs Forum 13(1):11–16, 1986.

Shenkier T and Gelmon K: Paclitaxel and radiation-recall dermatitis, J Clin Oncol 12:439, 1994 (letter).

Shimm DS and Cassady RJ: The skin. In Cox JD, editor: Moss's radiation oncology: rationale, techniques, results, ed 7, St. Louis, 1994, Mosby, pp. 99–118.

Sitton E: Early and late radiation-induced skin alterations. Part 1: mechanisms of skin changes, Oncol Nurs Forum 19:801–807, 1992a.

Sitton E: Early and late radiation-induced skin alterations. Part II: nursing care of irradiated skin, Oncol Nurs Forum 19:907–912, 1992b.

Steger GG, Locker G, Rainer H, Mader RM, Seider AE, Gnant MFX, Aberer W, and Jakesz R: Cutaneous reactions to GM-CSF in inflammatory breast cancer, N Eng J Med 327:286, 1992.

Strohl RA: The nursing role in radiation oncology: symptom management of acute and chronic reactions, Oncol Nurs Forum 15:430–434, 1988.

Timiras PS: Decline in homeostatic regulation. In Timiras PS, editor: Developmental physiology and aging, New York, 1972, MacMillan Co, pp. 542–563.

Turesson I and Notter G: The predictive value of skin telangiectasia for late radiation effects in different normal tissues, Int J Radiat Oncol Biol Phys 12:603–609, 1986.

Vonderheid EC: Topical mechlorethamine chemotherapy, Int J Derm 23:180–186, 1984.

Wood HA and Ellerhorst-Ryan JM: Delayed adverse skin reactions associated with mitomycin-C administration, Oncol Nurs Forum 11(4):14–18, 1984.

Chapter 22

❖ *Hematologic Toxicities*

Dawn Camp-Sorrell

Hematopoiesis is a continuous process that begins with pluripotent stem cells in the bone marrow and progresses to the development of mature, functional, circulating blood cells. The hematopoietic process is complex (Figure 22-1). Pluripotential stem cells are "uncommitted"; that is, they can differentiate into one of several types of committed stem cells that in turn mature into one particular type of blood cell (DiJulio, 1991; Erslev and Weiss, 1983).

Hematopoiesis is regulated by hematopoietic growth factors called colony-stimulating factors (CSFs) or colony-stimulating units (CSUs). These highly specific, hormonelike glycoproteins are endogenous substances that stimulate progenitor and precursor cells of all major blood cell lines to differentiate and mature. Progenitor cells are early ancestors of mature blood cells. Precursor cells belong to a specific lineage and develop immediately into mature blood cells. Specific hormonal signals can stimulate production of stem cells to maintain homeostasis (Haeuber, 1991). Under conditions of stress such as infection, hemorrhage, or bone marrow depletion, stem cell production can increase markedly (Wujcik, 1993a).

Stem cells committed to the myeloblast line mature into granulocytes (white blood cells) that further differentiate into neutrophils, basophils, or eosinophils (see Figure 22-1). Other types of white blood cells include monocytes and lymphocytes (Table 22-1).

Neutrophils are commonly referred to as the first line of defense in response to bacterial infection because they neutralize and localize bacteria. Immature neutrophils are known as *bands*. Basophils contain large amounts of heparin and histamine, and they accumulate at sites of inflammation. Heparin is involved in the mechanism of clot prevention in the microcirculation, and the histamine enhances the allergic response to antigens. Eosinophils play a role in inflammatory and allergic reactions and in combatting parasitic infections. Granulocytes have a life span of 2 to 3 days in the tissue and 6 to 8 hours in the bloodstream.

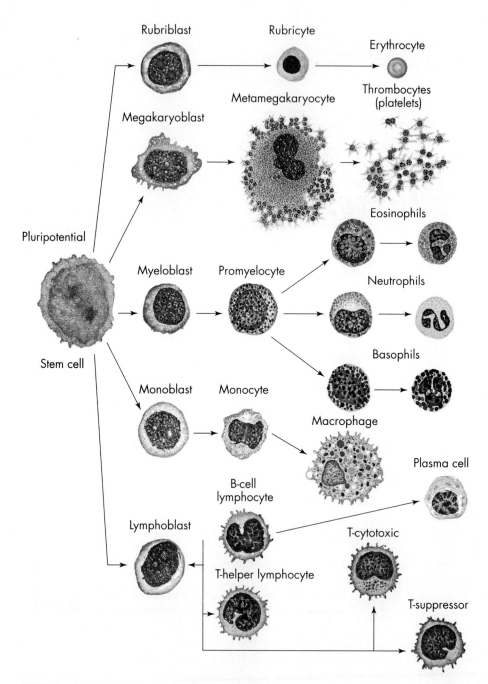

Fig. 22-1. Components of blood derived from a single stem cell. From Belcher AE: Cancer nursing, St. Louis, 1992, Mosby, 1992.

Table 22-1   Normal Laboratory Values for Complete Blood Count

Blood Component	Normal Value
Hemoglobin	Men: 14–16.5 g/dl Women: 12–16 g/dl
Hematocrit	Men: 42%–51% Women: 37%–47%
Platelets	145,000–364,000 per mm^3
White Blood Count	5,000–10,000 per mm^3

Differential of WBC*

Lymphocytes	15%–52% of WBC
Neutrophils (segs) (polys)	35%–73%
Bands	0%–11%
Monocytes	2%–14%
Eosinophils	0%–5%
Basophils	0%–2%

*Differential always adds up to 100% under normal conditions.

Stem cells committed to the monoblast line mature into monocytes. The function of monocytes is to remove damaged cells and the debris of dead cells from circulation, to interact with lymphoid cells during certain phases of immunologic reactions, and to act as a defense against certain microorganisms such as toxoplasma (DiJulio, 1991; Rostad, 1991; Wujcik, 1993a). Monocytes can live for months to years unless destroyed while defending the body against microorganisms (Alkire and Collingwood, 1990).

Stem cells committed to the lymphoblast line mature into lymphocytes. Lymphocytes, which further differentiate into T- or B-lymphocytes, enable the immune system to distinguish self from nonself or foreign antigens. T-lymphocytes are responsible for cell-mediated immunity, which has a dominant effect in delayed hypersensitivity reactions, graft-versus-host disease, and antitumor immunity. B-lymphocytes, which differentiate into plasma cells or memory cells, are responsible for humoral-mediated immunity. Plasma cells secrete specific immunoglobulins that target antigens for destruction. Memory cells are stored until needed for bacteria and allergic reactions. Intact cellular and humoral immunity both provide protection against viral, fungal, and parasitic infections (DiJulio, 1991; Rostad, 1991; Wujcik, 1993a). Mature lymphocytes have a life span of 100 to 300 days.

The primary role of erythrocytes is threefold: to transport hemoglobin that carries oxygen from the lungs to the peripheral tissues, to transport carbon dioxide to the lungs, and to maintain the blood's pH. Mature red blood cells (RBCs) normally live about 120 days in circulation.

Platelets prevent clotting by maintaining the vein's integrity to prevent bleeding. They adhere to injured tissue and to each other to form a clot. Platelets circulate for

7 to 10 days. By adulthood, production of red blood cells, white blood cells, and platelets occurs mainly in the flat bones such as the sternum, the ribs, the skull, and the proximal ends of long bones (DiJulio, 1991).

❖ Hematologic Toxicity

Myelosuppression is a reduction in bone marrow function that results in a reduced release of red blood cells (anemia), white blood cells (leukocytopenia), and platelets (thrombocytopenia) into the peripheral circulation. Myelosuppression is also known as bone marrow depression or bone marrow suppression.

Effects from Surgery

The administration of anesthesia and the trauma and stress of surgery can be immunosuppressive. Immunosuppression has been found to occur from 1 to 3 days after surgery (Riboli et al., 1984). Patients with cancer generally have a more severe depressed immune response, resulting in a prolonged postoperative recovery. Acute complications such as hemorrhage and infection can occur with any type of surgery. Postoperative infection remains a major problem, especially for patients with cancer who have received treatment before surgery (Ewer and Ali, 1990). Steroids delay wound healing because they decrease the immune system's inflammatory response. Cortisone in particular delays the development of normal tissue and slows the healing of the wound (Hotter, 1982; Robson, 1988).

Effects from Chemotherapy

Chemotherapy, especially in high doses, leads to myelosuppression because chemotherapeutic agents are most effective against both malignant and normal rapidly dividing cells (Guy, 1991; Raefsky and Wasserman, 1992; Rostad, 1991). The degree of suppression of the major cell lines is determined by the different effects from the drugs on the precursor cells and by the kinetics of the particular cell line in the peripheral circulation (Cawley, 1990; Gastineau and Hoagland, 1992). The degree of myelosuppression also depends on the drug, the dose, schedules, previous antineoplastic treatment, and concomitant therapy.

Acute myelosuppression is caused by the destruction of the proliferating progenitors of mature blood cells. This destruction leaves no cells to replace circulating mature cells as they die, so the blood cell count drops. The lowest point to which it drops is called the *nadir*.

Following chemotherapy administration, the nadir for white blood cells (WBCs) usually occurs in 8 to 12 days and the nadir for platelets usually occurs in 12 to 14 days (Table 22-2). Recovery takes 3 to 4 weeks (Maxwell and Maher, 1992). Thrombocytopenia occurs more slowly than leukopenia because of the significant difference in the half-lives of these two cell lines. With high-dose therapy or drug combinations, the nadir persists for several days to weeks because the stem cell population fails to repopulate quickly after the intense bone marrow damage.

Table 22-2 Hematologic Toxicity from Multimodal Treatment

Treatment	Hematologic Toxicity
Alkylating Agents (Cell Cycle Nonspecific)	
Altretamine	Neutropenia and thrombocytopenia are mild; anemia is rare; nadir in 3 to 4 weeks; recovery in 2 to 3 weeks
Busulfan	Leukopenia 100%*; nadir in 7 to 14 days; thrombocytopenia 70%; nadir in 11 to 30 days; recovery in 24 to 54 days; can be prolonged with high doses
Carboplatin	Leukopenia is mild; renal dysfunction increases severity; thrombocytopenia is severe and dose limiting; nadir in 21 days with recovery in 28 days; anemia is mild
Chlorambucil	Leukopenia 100%; nadir in 14 to 20 days; recovery in 28 to 42 days; thrombocytopenia 100%; nadir in 10 to 14 days; recovery in 21 days; anemia is rare
Cisplatin	Leukopenia 36%; nadir in 23 to 28 days; recovery in 40 days; increased severity with renal toxicity; thrombocytopenia 5%; nadir in 14 days; recovery in 21 days; anemia 25% to 30%; hemolytic anemia is rare
Cyclophosphamide	Leukopenia 100%; nadir in 8 to 15 days; recovery in 17 to 28 days; thrombocytopenia 20%; nadir in 10 to 14 days; recovery in 21 days; anemia is rare
Dacarbazine	Leukopenia 30% to 50%; nadir in 10 to 24 days; recovery in 2 to 3 weeks; thrombocytopenia 30% to 50%; anemia is rare
Ifosfamide	Leukopenia 12%; nadir in 10 days; recovery in 18 days; thrombocytopenia is 6%; anemia is rare; myelosuppression is dose-limiting in high doses
Mechlorethamine	Leukopenia 100%; nadir in 10 days; recovery in 21 to 28 days; thrombocytopenia 100%; nadir in 10 days; recovery in 21 to 28 days; anemia is rare
Melphalan	Leukopenia 65%; nadir in 21 to 25 days; recovery in 28 to 45 days; thrombocytopenia 75%; nadir in 21 to 25 days; recovery in 28 to 45 days; anemia 75%; nadir in 8 to 20 days; recovery in 42 to 50 days; myelosuppression can be dose limiting
Procarbazine	Leukopenia 100%; nadir in 25 to 26 days; recovery in 36 to 50 days; thrombocytopenia 100%; nadir in 21 days; recovery in 28 days; anemia 5%
Thiotepa	Leukopenia 40%; thrombocytopenia 80%; anemia 50%; nadir in 14 days; recovery in 28 days; myelosuppression can be cumulative

*The symbol % refers to the rate of toxicity occurrence.

Data from Guy, 1991; Fisher, Knobf, and Durivage, 1993; and Hoagland, 1992.

Continued

Table 22-2   Hematologic Toxicity from Multimodal Treatment—cont'd

Treatment	Hematologic Toxicity
Antimetabolites (S-Phase Specific)	
Cytarabine	Leukopenia 100%; nadir in 7 to 9 days; recovery in 12 days; second nadir in 15 to 24 days; recovery in 34 days; thrombocytopenia 100%; nadir in 15 days; recovery in 25 days; anemia is mild
Floxuridine	Leukopenia 57%; nadir in 21 days; recovery in 30 days; thrombocytopenia and anemia are rare
5-Fluorouracil	Leukopenia 100%; nadir in 9 to 14 days; recovery in 21 to 25 days; thrombocytopenia and anemia are mild; myelosuppression is less common with continuous IV infusion
Hydroxyurea	Leukopenia 70%; thrombocytopenia 20%; anemia 34%; nadir in 7 days; recovery in 14 to 21 days; megaloblastic erythropoiesis is frequent
Mercaptopurine	Leukopenia, thrombocytopenia, and anemia are mild; nadir in 14 days; recovery in 21 days
Methothrexate	Leukopenia 30%; first nadir in 4 to 7 days; recovery in 7 to 14 days; second nadir in 12 to 21 days; recovery in 15 to 29 days; thrombocytopenia 30%; nadir in 5 to 7 days; recovery in 15 to 27 days; anemia is rare; myelosuppression is more severe with nephrotoxicity
Thioguanine	Leukopenia 100%; nadir in 14 to 28 days; recovery in 6 weeks; thrombocytopenia 100%; nadir in 14 days; anemia is mild
Antitumor Antibiotics (Cell Cycle Nonspecific)	
Bleomycin	Myelosuppression is rare
Dactinomycin	Leukopenia 55%; thrombocytopenia 47%; anemia 50%; nadir in 14 to 21 days; recovery in 21 to 28 days
Daunorubicin	Leukopenia 90%; nadir in 8 to 10 days; thrombocytopenia 90%; nadir in 4 to 15 days; recovery in 15 to 21 days; anemia is rare
Doxorubicin	Leukopenia 100%; thrombocytopenia 40%; nadir in 10 to 14 days; recovery in 21 to 24 days; anemia is rare
Mitomycin-C	Leukopenia 50%; nadir in 25 days; recovery in 39 days; thrombocytopenia 40%; nadir in 28 days; recovery in 50 days; anemia 3%
Mitoxantrone	Leukopenia 50%; thrombocytopenia 12%; anemia 17%; nadir in 10 to 16 days; recovery in 21 days
Plicamycin	Leukopenia 6%; thrombocytopenia 6%; nadir in 5 to 10 days; recovery in 10 to 18 days; anemia is rare; bleeding episodes 12% with doses >30 μg/kg
Hormonal Agents	
Aminoglutethimide	Myelosuppression is rare
Buserelin	Myelosuppression is rare
Diethylstilbestrol	Myelosuppression is rare; thromboembolic disorders 18%; pulmonary emboli 5%
Estramustine	Myelosuppression is rare
Fluoxymestrone	Myelosuppression is rare; erythropoiesis is rare

Treatment	Hematologic Toxicity
Flutamide	Myelosuppression is rare; methemoglobinemia
Goserelin	Anemia 5%; myelosuppression is rare
Leuporlide	Myelosuppression is rare; thrombophlebitis, phlebitis, or pulmonary emboli 1%; anemia 3%
Medroxyprogesterone	Myelosuppression is rare; thromboembolic disorders
Megestrol acetate	Myelosuppression is rare
Mitotane	Myelosuppression is rare; leukopenia 7%
Tamoxifen	Transient leukopenia 10%; nadir in 10 days; transient thrombocytopenia 10%; nadir in 12 days; anemia 26%

Nitrosoureas (Cell Cycle Specific)

Carmustine	Leukopenia 100%; thrombocytopenia 100%; nadir in 5 to 6 weeks; can be cumulative; recovery in up to 60 days
Lomustine	Leukopenia 65%; nadir in 42 days; recovery in 49 to 56 days; thrombocytopenia 90%; nadir in 28 days; recovery in 35 to 42 days; anemia reaches nadir in 4 to 7 weeks; myelosuppression can be cumulative
Streptozocin	Leukopenia 5%; thrombocytopenia 5%; anemia 20%; nadir in 14 days; recovery in 21 days

Vinca Alkaloids (M-Phase Specific)

Etoposide	Leukopenia 60%; thrombocytopenia 28%; nadir in 7 to 16 days; recovery in 20 days; anemia is rare
Paclitaxel	Neutropenia can be dose-limiting; nadir in 8 to 10 days; recovery in 21 days; thrombocytopenia is moderate; anemia is rare
Vinblastine	Leukopenia 100%; thrombocytopenia 100%; nadir in 5 to 10 days; recovery in 12 to 24 days; anemia 50%
Vincristine	Leukopenia 5%; nadir in 4 to 5 days; recovery in 7 days; thrombocytopenia and anemia are rare

Biologicals

Interferon-α (Roferon-Alfa)	Leukopenia 69%; nadir in 22 days; thrombocytopenia 42%; nadir in 17 days; neutropenia 58%; anemia is rare
Interferon-α (Intron A)	Leukopenia 18%; thrombocytopenia 18%; granulocytopenia 20%; anemia 4%
Interferon-γ	Granulocytopenia is frequent; anemia is rare; thrombocytopenia is rare
Interleukin-2	Eosinophilia, thrombocytopenia, anemia, and leukopenia occur with prolonged treatment
Tumor necrosis factor	Leukopenia, eosinophilia, thrombocytopenia are rare
Levamisole	Leukopenia and thrombocytopenia are rare

Radiation Therapy

External-beam radiation	Myelosuppression occurs if large areas of bone marrow are in field; skull 10%, ribs/sternum 20%, pelvis 30%, vertebrae 25%, scapula 10%, proximal femur and humerus 5%

Effects from Radiation Therapy

The myelosuppressive effects from radiation therapy resemble the effects from chemotherapy. Irradiated fields of 20 Gy or more that involve the major bone marrow production sites of the ilia, the vertebrae, the ribs, the skull, the sternum, and the metaphyses of the long bones result in myelosuppression (see Table 22-2) (McDonald, 1992). Radiation administered to sites that include major blood vessels and lymphatic channels has a toxic effect on the mature lymphocytes (Haeuber and Spross, 1991).

Other than total nodal or total body irradiation, radiation does not usually cause the low blood counts that chemotherapy does. Radiation is a local therapy, and only affects the hematologic system when areas with large bone marrow are irradiated. Potential long-term effects result from damage to the pluripotential stem cell pool that is not actively proliferating (Raefsky and Wasserman, 1992). Chronic effects include aplasia (failure of the bone marrow to develop mature cells) of certain marrow segments and the development of various myelodysplastic syndromes such as leukemia (Fliedner, Northdurft, and Clavo, 1986; Frisch, Bartl, and Chiachuk, 1986).

Effects from Biotherapy

Because biological response modifiers modulate the immune system, the potential for hematologic toxicity exists (Wujcik, 1993b). Some investigators speculate that interferon (IFN) blocks release of blood components from the marrow and that the proliferation of hematopoietic progenitor cells is inhibited (Contino, Testa, and Dexter, 1986). Interleukin-2 (IL-2) administered for a prolonged period has produced anemia and thrombocytopenia (Caliendo, Joyce, and Altmiller, 1993). When IL-2 is discontinued, a temporary decrease in the WBC count occurs.

Effects from Multimodal Therapy

When chemotherapy or radiation therapy has been combined either sequentially or concomitantly, the bone marrow is compromised. Thoracic or pelvic radiation therapy with the sternum or iliac in the irradiated field with concomitant chemotherapy causes profound bone marrow suppression. Subclinical late effects of chemotherapy are now known to enhance seriously radiation-related toxicity.

The effects of chemotherapy and radiation therapy in combination are time-dependent. Hematologic toxicity is more profound when the two treatment modalities are administered simultaneously or when chemotherapy is administered after radiation (Thomas and Lindbald, 1988; von der Masse, 1994). Toxicity is more pronounced when chemotherapy is administered 1 to 3 days after radiation therapy (Raefsky and Wasserman, 1992). Often doses of chemotherapy must be reduced in patients who have previously received radiation treatment to large portions of the bone marrow, which compromises the patient's chance for cure (Khoury et al., 1991). Chronic hematologic toxicities can result when both chemotherapy and radiation have affected the bone marrow (Scofield, Liebman, and Popkin, 1991).

Studies have shown that interferon (IFN) has a synergistic effect with chemotherapy agents, increasing the degree of myelosuppression (Gastineau and Hoagland, 1992). Numerous preclinical studies have found the effect of myelosuppression enhanced by the combined action of IFN and chemotherapy agents such as doxorubicin, cyclophosphamide, the nitrosoureas, the vinca alkaloids, cisplatin, and 5-fluorouracil (Gilewski and Golomb, 1990).

In patients who have previously received radiation therapy, postoperative healing is delayed because of damage to the normal tissue. These tissues have an inability to elicit sustained cell-mediated response to bacteria; thus infection occurs (Conklin, Walker, and Hirsch, 1983).

❖ Nursing Management

A complete history and physical examination are paramount in determining the appropriate management of the patient with a hematologic toxicity. The nurse obtains a pretreatment, baseline, complete blood count with differential and usually monitors it at least weekly during treatment. Hematologic toxicities make the patient with cancer more susceptible to fatigue, infection, and bleeding.

Management of myelosuppression follows three basic principles: prevention, early detection, and aggressive management of complications. These three principles apply to all major forms of myelosuppression: anemia, thrombocytopenia, and neutropenia. The dose levels of each treatment modality may be decreased or limited when the blood counts indicate that the patient is unable to withstand additional toxicity from treatments (Fischer, Knobf, and Durivage, 1993; Rostad, 1990).

Anemia

Anemia is the reduction of the number of circulating RBCs and is reflected in a fall of the hemoglobin and hematocrit values (Rostad, 1990). Because the RBCs have a long life span of 120 days, anemia does not occur as often or become a dose-limiting factor of treatment (Gastineau and Hoagland, 1992). Signs and symptoms of anemia include fatigue, headaches, dizziness, irritability, tachycardia, tachypnea, hypotension, shortness of breath, dyspnea on exertion, and tissue hypoxia.

Nursing management for patients with anemia focuses on supportive care (see Patient Education Guidelines for Fatigue due to Anemia on page 376). Patients should be advised to adjust their activity levels to include provisions for rest periods to lessen fatigue. Encourage the patient to assign tasks to family and friends who often feel helpless and want to help with activities. Consistent periodic exercise should be encouraged to maintain muscle tone and to prevent secondary fatigue. The patient should report shortness of breath or the occurrence of palpitations to the physician or nurse immediately (Mayer, 1990). Oxygen should be provided to assist with shortness of breath.

In the past, the hemoglobin or hematocrit value was the key factor in determining the patient's need for RBC transfusion. Although this may be the most objective assessment tool, it is not necessarily the most accurate. Signs of tissue oxygenation (pulse, blood pressure, respiratory rate, color) and activity level should also be used

Patient Education Guidelines for

Fatigue due to Anemia

◆ Eat a well balanced nutritious diet.
  ◆ Eat foods high in iron such as potatoes, red meats, dark green leafy vegetables, and carrots.
  ◆ Eat high-protein and high-carbohydrate foods such as peanut butter, milk products (cottage cheese, cheese, milk, ice cream, yogurt, cream cheese), rice, pudding, custard, macaroni, pasta, potatoes.
  ◆ Try nutritional supplements such as Nutra Shake, Ensure, or Carnation Instant Breakfast.
  ◆ Add a tablespoon of powdered skim milk to fluids to provide more protein.

◆ Take naps or rest periods of 30 minutes to an hour, perhaps one in morning and one in the afternoon.
  ◆ Sleep later in the morning or go to bed earlier at night.
  ◆ Resting all day, however, will increase feelings of fatique.

◆ Plan consistent exercise periods, such as walking to a specific designation once a day.
  ◆ For extreme fatigue, prevent tissue breakdown by ambulating short distances three times a day, sitting on the side of the bed three times a day, or turning in bed.
  ◆ Provide skin care with water-based skin lotion.

◆ Don't be afraid to ask for help. Seek assistance with activities such as housework, child care, or meal preparation when experiencing fatigue.

◆ Tell your physician or nurse if you have pain, trouble sleeping, or difficulty catching your breath.

Permission granted to reproduce these guidelines for educational purposes only.

to determine transfusion requirements. After the hemoglobin value falls below 8 gm/100 ml, the hematocrit value falls below 25%, or the patient becomes symptomatic, packed RBCs should be transfused (Camp-Sorrell, 1993; Pavel, 1990). In the absence of active bleeding, 1 unit of packed RBCs should increase an adult's peripheral hematocrit level by 3% and hemoglobin by 1 g/100 ml (Pavel, 1990).

The administration of erythropoietin growth factor for erythroid progenitor cells may relieve chemotherapy-induced chronic anemia (Platanias et al., 1991). Erythropoietin is a glycoprotein hormone normally found in the body that promotes the proliferation of mature RBCs (Spivak, 1992). Administration of erythropoietin has proven effective in alleviating transfusion dependency in chemotherapy-induced anemia (Abels, 1992; Spivak, 1992). The dose is 100 to 150 units per kg subcutaneously three times a week. The efficacy of treatment is measured by the hemoglobin or hematocrit values. The minimum response time is 2 weeks; however, it can take as long as 4 to 6 weeks before an effect is seen. Potential adverse effects of erythropoietin include hypertension, headache, arthralgia, nausea, fatigue, low-grade fever, and clotted venous access device. Mild hypertension is the most common side effect, noted with a significant rise in hematocrit levels over a short period of time, which responds to antihypertensive drugs (Doweiko and Goldberg, 1991).

It is important to maintain adequate levels of iron, folic acid, and vitamin B_{12}, because these are essential for RBC development. If adequate levels of iron are not available for erythropoiesis, the patient will not respond to erythropoietin. Laboratory values for components such as vitamin B_{12}, folate, serum iron, total iron-binding capacity, serum ferritin, and transferrin saturation should be checked before and during therapy. The patient may need iron supplements and vitamins. Patients should be encouraged to eat a well-balanced diet rich in iron, vitamins, and minerals. Cultural and ethnic practices must be explored to ensure that recommendations do not interfere with patients' life-styles.

Neutropenia

To provide the best defense against bacterial invasion, the body needs adequate numbers of functioning neutrophils and macrophages (Fischer, Knobf, and Durivage 1993; Hoagland, 1992; Wujcik, 1993a). The major predictor of bacterial infection in patients with cancer is neutropenia, defined as the state when the absolute neutrophil count (ANC) is less than 1000 per mm³. The ANC is calculated by multiplying the total WBC by the percentage of neutrophils and the percentage bands (Box 22-1). The ANC indicates the number of cells capable of fighting infection by phagocytosis, the process of ingesting and digesting bacteria. When the ANC is less than 1000 the patient is neutropenic and at risk for infection. An ANC less than 500 increases the patient's risk for infection substantially, and phagocytic defenses are impaired. The incidence of gram-negative bacteremia and disseminated candidiasis is very high with an ANC less than 100 (Barry, 1989; Pizzo, 1993).

Box 22-1 Calculation of Absolute Neutrophil Count

The absolute neutrophil count (ANC) is calculated as follows:

$$ANC = \frac{(\% \text{ neutrophils} + \% \text{ bands})}{100} \times \text{white blood cell (WBC) count}$$

The example shows how to calculate the ANC of a patient with the following counts: neutrophils = 50%, bands = 8%, WBC = 4000.

$$ANC = \frac{(50\% + 8\%)}{100} \times 4000$$

$$ANC = (.50 + .08) \times 4000$$

$$ANC = 2320$$

Infection Risk

Not significant	ANC = 1500 to 2000
Minimal	ANC = 1000 to 1500
Moderate	ANC = 500 to 1000
Severe	ANC = <500

The most common sites for infection are the skin, the respiratory tract, the oral cavity, the sinuses, and the perianal area. Outward signs of infection are usually absent because the neutropenic patient cannot produce an adequate inflammatory response to create swelling, redness, or pus. Fever is usually the first and often the only sign of infection (Brandt, 1990; Finkbiner and Ernst, 1993). Fever is caused by the endogenous pyrogens produced by macrophages rather than the usual neutrophils (Schimpff, 1994). The diagnosis of infection is confirmed by physical assessments, chest radiographs, and cultures (such as blood, urine, stool, or sputum).

Infection and resultant complications are major causes of death in patients with cancer. General neutropenic guidelines (see Nursing Management of the Hospitalized Neutropenic Patient on page 379) are commonly recommended; however, there is no conclusive evidence that they reduce life-threatening infections or improve outcomes (Brandt, 1990; Camp-Sorrell, 1993; Fischer, Knobf, Durivage, 1993; Wujcik, 1993a). As the ANC decreases, more intensive, frequent assessment and monitoring are required to prevent sepsis. With care moving to the outpatient setting and into the home, the nurse is responsible for teaching the patient and family members about potential side effects and complications. Instructions must include how to monitor for complications, how to treat complications, and when to call the physician or nurse (see Patient Education Guidelines for High Risk for Infection on page 380).

The nurse identifies patients at risk for neutropenia and teaches them to take their temperature daily, preferably after 4 P.M. when the body temperature is usually higher, and to call the physician or nurse if it is greater than 100°F. The nurse assesses breaks in the skin from wounds or intravenous devices and takes measures to prevent further breakdown, because the skin is the first line of defense. The patient should bathe daily with meticulous personal hygiene and perineal care and perform oral care four times a day. To prevent perineal infections, patients and their significant others should be taught sexual hygiene. Hand washing should be followed strictly, as well as strict aseptic technique for all invasive procedures. Venipunctures for laboratory tests should be coordinated to limit the number of times they are done. Visitors should be limited to those without colds.

A patient must have adequate nutritional intake to supply the body the proteins and carbohydrates it needs for cell and tissue repair. However, fruits and raw vegetables should be avoided by patients experiencing a prolonged nadir of less than 500 ANC, as frequently happens to patients with bone marrow transplantations. *Pseudomonas aeruginosa, Enterobacter agglomerans, Enterobacter cloacae, Citrobacter, Serratia, Escherichia coli,* and *Klebsiella* have been cultured from uncooked foods. Several investigators hypothesize that ingestion of foods known to contain infectious organisms of various species will lead to colonization in the gut, subsequently causing an infection (Carter, 1993; Pinner et al., 1992).

Various techniques of protective isolation have been implemented to shield patients with neutropenia from nosocomial microbial flora (Donovan, 1982; Nauseef and Makie, 1981). These techniques range from complex total-protective environments to simple protective precautions. Total-protective environments include laminar-air-flow rooms or special-unit filtering with the use of sterile supplies and food. This type of isolation is reserved for patients who will experience

Nursing Management of

The Hospitalized Neutropenic Patient

Maintain a safe environment.
- Care for neutropenic patients first; avoid caring for other patients known to be infected and then caring for the neutropenic patient.
- Hand washing before and after patient contact must be followed strictly; use aseptic techniques when performing invasive procedures such as intravenous therapy, suctioning, or wound care.
- Avoid the insertion of indwelling catheters such as an intravenous or a urinary catheter.
- Limit visitors under the age of 12 to the patient's children and grandchildren; obtain a child's health history before the visit to ensure that contact with another child with a communicable illness such as chicken pox has not occurred.
- Avoid stagnant water that can harbor microorganisms.

Maintain accurate assessment data.
- Assess and document vital signs every 4 to 8 hours or more frequently as the ANC decreases.
  - If the patient's temperature increases above 101°F, a bacterial infection may be the cause.
  - If the patient's pulse is over 100 beats per minute and the blood pressure is dropping, the patient could be getting septic.
- Assess skin wounds and venous-access devices every 8 hours or more frequently as the ANC decreases. Redness, drainage, or edema are signs of infection.
- Monitor the CBC and differential. Calculate the ANC every day (see Box 22-1).
- Perform a physical exam, assessing for signs of infection, every 8 hours or more frequently as the ANC decreases.
  - Listen for abnormal breathing sounds, which could be a sign of infection.
  - Pain elicited during the physical exam could be a sign of infection.
  - Patches in the oral cavity could be a sign of infection.
  - Any orifice or open area that has redness, drainage, or edema may be infected.

Assist in the diagnosis and the management of infections:
- Culture the throat, urine, sputum, blood, and wounds when infection is suspected. Obtain a blood culture from a peripheral site and all venous-access devices to evaluate the source of infection.
- Administer antibiotics on a scheduled basis to ensure adequate blood levels for 10 to 14 days; rotate the site of antibiotic infusion into different ports of multilumen catheters in the event the source of infection is contained at the distal tip of the catheter.
- Administer acetaminophen every 4 hours to reduce fever; the maximum dose is 4000 mg in 24 hours.
- Promote cooling of the skin and mucous membranes by giving tepid sponge baths, reducing the amount of clothing worn by the patient, and reducing the temperature of the environment.
- Prevent the patient from catching a chill from a rapid reduction in body temperature by providing warm blankets or heating pads at the first sign of chilling, and change damp clothing immediately.

Implement specific measures to avoid infection in common sites.
- Encourage coughing and deep breathing every 4 hours or more frequently.

Continued

- Encourage patients to empty their bladders at least every 4 hours and avoid the use of douches and tampons.
- Use aseptic techniques with contact lens care.
- Perform oral care every 4 hours or more frequently.
- Encourage the patient to get out of bed every 8 hours and for meals during the day.
- Encourage the patient to keep fingernails clean and short to decrease the chance of scratching and compromising skin integrity.

Patient Education Guidelines for

High Risk for Infection

- Avoid using any type of container that has stagnant water such as humidifiers, flower vases, denture cups, and soap dishes. These are places microbes like to grow.
  - Add 1 teaspoon of chlorine bleach to each quart of water used in flower vases.
  - Add 1 teaspoon of vinegar to each quart of water or use saline for respiratory equipment; all equipment should be cleaned with 70% alcohol or chlorine bleach solution and vigorous scrubbing.
- Limit visitors to those without contagious illness such as colds, viruses, cold sores, influenzas, or chicken pox; do not allow visitors who have recently received vaccinations with living or attenuated microbes such as polio vaccine.
  - Avoid crowds as in shopping malls or grocery stores.
- Avoid cleaning bird cages or cat litter boxes because bacteria or fungi could lurk in the excreta.
- Eat a high-protein and high-carbohydrate diet.
- Use a mild soap such as Dove or Dial to wash each day; rinse the skin thoroughly and pat dry.
  - Cleanse the perianal area after each bowel movement and urination.
  - Perform skin care daily with a water-soluble lubricant to prevent dryness of the skin.
  - For personal hygiene, take a sponge bath, tub bath, or shower every day.
- Nails should be kept clean and short.
- Perform mouth care four times a day, as prescribed by your nurse or physician.
- Promote healing of all skin wounds by changing dressings every 8 hours or as instructed by your physician or nurse.
- Avoid enemas, suppositories, and rectal thermometers.
- If constipation is a problem, talk to your physician or nurse about putting you on a bowel regime.
- Drink at least eight 8-ounce glasses of fluid a day.
- If ordered to do so, take growth factors daily until told to stop by your physician or nurse.
  - Dispose of needles in a thick container such as a coffee can or egg carton.
  - Store in refrigerator at 36 to 45°F.
  - Keep appointments for blood work.
- Take your temperature daily in the late afternoon or early evening. Call your physician immediately if you have a temperature over 100°F.
- Call your physician immediately if you get severe chills, mouth sores, pain with swallowing, or fever.

transplantation. Simple, protective precautions are outlined in Nursing Management of the Hospitalized Neutropenic Patient on page 379.

Many principles of antibiotic therapy were developed for patients receiving high-dose chemotherapy for acute leukemia. However, with the increasing use of multimodal therapy for other cancers, prophylaxis is becoming more common. Generally patients who are neutropenic for less than a week and then become febrile require empirical oral antibiotic therapy and respond promptly (Pizzo, 1993).

Growth factors (colony-stimulating factors) are used to improve host defenses after chemotherapy or another multimodal treatment that induces neutropenia (Schimpff, 1994). Granulocyte CSF (G-CSF) helps accelerate myeloid recovery in patients receiving myelosuppressive chemotherapy, whereas granulocyte-macrophage CSF (GM-CSF) helps accelerate myeloid recovery after autologous bone marrow transplantation (Finkbiner and Ernst, 1993; Maxwell and Maher, 1992; Pizzo, 1993). CSFs are administered daily by subcutaneous injections. The recommended dose for G-CSF is 5 μg/kg/day and may be increased in increments of 5 μg/kg with each chemotherapy cycle according to the severity of the decrease in the ANC; the recommended dose for GM-CSF is 250 μg/m^2/day (Fischer, Knobf, and Durivage, 1993). CSFs are given for 10 to 14 days or until the ANC is greater than 10,000 per mm^3. Discontinuing daily doses of G-CSF or GM-CSF causes the count to drop quickly by 50%.

If the neutropenic patient experiences a fever, intravenous antibiotics are initiated with broad-spectrum coverage against gram-negative and gram-positive organisms. The goal of treatment is to use combination-antibiotic therapy with synergistic effects (Armstrong, 1991).

Infections can be caused by gram-negative bacteria (*Escherichia coli, Klebsiella pneumoniae, Enterobacter, Pseudomonas, Staphylococcus epidermidis, and Streptococcus*), fungi (*Candida albicans, Aspergillus, and Cryptococcus*), viruses, and parasitic infections. Often the infecting organism is difficult to detect, and consequently the patient can develop sepsis rapidly (Armstrong, 1991; Barry, 1989; Brandt, 1990; Pizzo, 1993; Sugar, 1990). If fever persists 3 to 5 days and no bacterial source has been identified, it is presumed the patient has a fungal infection and is treated with Amphotericin B (Sugar, 1990). *Herpes* viruses are a group of viruses that become latent in the body after a primary infection and reactivated after varying periods of time. For patients at a high risk for reactivation such as those with bone marrow transplantations, acyclovir is administered prophylactically (Zaia, 1990).

Thrombocytopenia

Signs and symptoms of thrombocytopenia include ecchymosis, petechiae, and bleeding from orifices. If the platelet count drops below 50,000, the risk of bleeding is high, and the patient is placed on bleeding precautions. A major risk for spontaneous bleeding not due to trauma arises when the platelet level is less than 20,000. A critical risk of fatal central nervous system bleeding, massive gastrointestinal hemorrhage, or respiratory tract hemorrhage exists with a platelet level lower than 10,000.

Bleeding precautions include testing all stools, urine, and vomitus for blood (see Nursing Management of Thrombocytopenia on page 382). The patient should avoid physical activity that could cause injury and should wear shoes during ambu-

Nursing Management of

Thrombocytopenia

◆ Monitor platelet counts before administering chemotherapy, biotherapy, or radiation therapy to areas where bone marrow is in the field.
  ◆ Monitor levels every 7 to 10 days after treatment.
  ◆ Monitor levels weekly or more often as indicated by the patient's platelet count.

◆ Assess for the presence of bleeding. Test the urine, stools, and vomit for blood.

◆ Avoid using a blood-pressure cuff or a tourniquet when a platelet level is less than 20,000.

◆ Monitor pad counts and amount of saturation during menses.

◆ Avoid intramuscular injections.

◆ Avoid invasive procedures such as enemas, suppositories, rectal thermometers, and indwelling catheters.
  ◆ If a device is necessary, use a small gauge, apply lubrication if possible, and insert it gently.
  ◆ After removing a needle, apply firm pressure to the venipuncture site for 5 minutes.
  ◆ Apply sandbags to the site if bleeding does not cease in 5 minutes.

◆ If the patient has an uncontrollable nose bleed, call the physician and obtain an order to insert cotton soaked with neosynephrine (1%) into the nose and continue to apply pressure. Neosynephrine will cause vasoconstriction of the blood vessels.

lation to maintain skin integrity. Drugs known to alter platelets or coagulation factors should be avoided. The patient should check with the pharmacist, the physician, or the nurse before using any over-the-counter drugs. Sharp objects such as a straight-edge razor should be avoided or handled carefully. If cuts occur, pressure applied to venipuncture sites for at least 3 to 5 minutes should stop the bleeding. Absorbable gelatin sponges or liquid thrombin can be applied to control bleeding if needed (Fischer, Knobf, and Durivage, 1993). The patient should also avoid constipation, and a bowel regimen may be initiated, especially if the patient has a tendency toward constipation or is taking narcotics. If the gums bleed during oral care, the patient should use toothettes or a soft toothbrush. Patient Education Guidelines for High Risk of Bleeding are presented on page 383.

If signs of bleeding are observed or if the platelet count falls below 20,000, platelets are usually transfused (Fuller, 1990). Patients who have multiple transfusions or have repeated febrile nonhemolytic transfusion reactions need leukocyte-poor platelet products, to decrease the chance of reactions (Fuller, 1990). As many as 70% of patients who receive repeated transfusions will become refractory or fail to increase the platelet count after a platelet transfusion. The use of human leukocyte antigens (HLA) may become necessary. Platelets with HLA typing have a

Patient Education Guidelines for

High Risk of Bleeding

◆ Avoid activities that have the potential for physical injury. Bleeding occurs more easily when the platelet count is low.
  ◆ Wear gloves while working in the garden.
  ◆ Wear shoes or slippers when out of bed.
  ◆ Avoid tight-fitting clothing.
◆ Use an electric razor or safety razor when shaving.
◆ Use an emery board or fine-mesh file for nail care.
◆ Eat soft, bland foods such as soup, yogurt, ice cream, and peanut butter. Avoid foods that are irritating such as hot, spicy, or rough dishes.
◆ Use a soft-bristle toothbrush or toothette for oral care, and avoid using dental floss when the platelet level is less than 50,000. Seek approval from the physician before having dental work.
◆ Avoid constipation. If you have difficulty, ask your nurse for a bowel regimen.
◆ Avoid blowing your nose forcefully. Only blow gently through both nostrils simultaneously, if necessary.
  ◆ If nose bleeding occurs, sit straight up and apply firm pressure to the nostrils below the bridge of the nose.
  ◆ If the bleeding does not stop, place an ice bag to the bridge of the nose and at the back of the neck.
  ◆ If bleeding continues, call your doctor.
◆ Do not take medications such as aspirin that have the potential to start or prolong bleeding. Ask your physician, nurse, or pharmacist if you are not sure of the contents of any of your medicines.
◆ Call your doctor or nurse for signs of bleeding such as nose bleeds, blood in your urine, black bowel movements, tiny purplish spots on your skin, or bruises that happen easily.

Permission granted to reproduce these guidelines for educational purposes only.

longer life span. Platelet infusions vary from 6 to 12 units, depending on where the platelets are obtained.

Specific written guidelines, such as the Patient Education Guidelines for High Risk of Bleeding above, need to be explained and given to the patient. Patients and families are taught how to recognize the presence of bleeding and are given phone numbers to contact the physician or the nurse immediately.

❖ Summary

Nursing care of patients receiving multimodal therapy is not intrinsically different from care of patients who receive single-modality treatment. However, the nurse should expect acute hematologic reactions earlier in the treatment course and also to a more severe degree. Nurses must anticipate side effects, perform ongoing patient assessments, and teach the patient and family how to monitor for problems at home. Early recognition and management of potential problems will enhance the patient's level of comfort during treatment and prevent major complications.

❖ *References*

Abels RI: Use of recombinant human erythropoietin in the treatment of anemia in patients who have cancer, Semin Oncol 19(3)(suppl 8):29–35, 1992.

Alkire K and Collingwood J: Physiology of blood and bone marrow, Semin Oncol Nurs 6(2):99–108, 1990.

Armstrong D: Empiric therapy for the immunocompromised host, Rev Infec Dis 13:S763–S769, 1991.

Barry SA: Septic shock: special needs of patients with cancer, Oncol Nurs Forum 17:31–35, 1989.

Brandt B: Nursing protocol for the patient with neutropenia, Oncol Nurs Forum 17(suppl):9–15, 1990.

Caliendo G, Joyce D, and Altmiller MC: Nursing guidelines and discharge planning for patients receiving recombinant interleukin-2, Semin Oncol Nurs 9(3)(suppl 1):25–31, 1993.

Camp-Sorrell D: Chemotherapy: toxicity management. In Groenwald SL, Frogge MH, Goodman M, and Yarbro CH, editors: Cancer nursing: principles and practice, ed 3, Boston, 1993, Jones & Bartlett Publishers, pp. 331–365.

Carter LW: Influences of nutrition and stress on people at risk for neutropenia: nursing implications, Oncol Nurs Forum 20:1241–1250, 1993.

Cawley MM: Recent advances in chemotherapy: administration and nursing implications, Nurs Clin No Am 25:377–392, 1990.

Conklin JJ, Walker RI, and Hirsch EF: Current concepts in the management of radiation injuries and associated trauma, Surg Gynecol Obstet 156:809–905, 1983.

Contino LH, Testa NG, and Dexter TM: The myelosuppressive effect of recombinant interferon (gamma) in short-term and long-term marrow cultures, Br J Haematol 63:517–524, 1986.

DiJulio J: Hematopoiesis: an overview, Oncol Nurs Forum 18(2)(suppl):3–6, 1991.

Donovan CT: Protective isolation, Oncol Nurs Forum 9(3):50–53, 1982.

Doweiko JP and Goldberg MA: Erythropoietin therapy in cancer patients, Oncology 5(8):31–37, 1991.

Erslev AJ and Weiss L: Structure and function of the marrow. In Williams WJ, Beutler E, Erslev AJ, and Lichtman MA, editors: Hematology, New York, 1983, McGraw-Hill, pp. 75–83.

Ewer MS and Ali MK: Surgical treatment of the cancer patient: preoperative assessment and perioperative medical management, J Surg Oncol 44:185–190, 1990.

Finkbiner KL and Ernst TF: Drug therapy management of the febrile neutropenic cancer patient, Canc Prac 1:295–304, 1993.

Fischer DS, Knobf MT, and Durivage HJ: The cancer chemotherapy handbook, ed 4, St. Louis, 1993, Mosby, pp. 217–246, 405–423.

Fliedner TM, Northdurft W, and Clavo W: The development of radiation late effects to the bone marrow after single and chronic exposure, Int J Radiat Biol 49:35–46, 1986.

Frisch B, Bartl R, and Chiachuk S: Therapy-induced myelodysplasia and secondary leukemia, Scandinavian J Haematol 36(suppl 45):38–47, 1986.

Fuller AK: Platelet transfusion therapy for thrombocytopenia, Semin Oncol Nurs 6:123–128, 1990.

Gastineau DA and Hoagland HC: Hematologic effects of chemotherapy, Semin Oncol 19:543–550, 1992.

Gilewski TA and Golomb HM: Design of combination biotherapy studies: future goals and challenges, Semin Oncol 17(1)(suppl 1):3–10, 1990.

Guy JL: Medical oncology: the agents. In Baird SB, McCorkle R, and Grant M, editors: Cancer nursing: a comprehensive textbook, Philadelphia, 1991, WB Saunders Co, pp. 266–290.

Haeuber D: Future strategies in the control of myelosuppression: the use of colony-stimulating factors, Oncol Nurs Forum 18(2 suppl):16–21, 1991.

Haeuber D and Spross JA: Alterations in protective mechanisms: hematopoiesis and bone marrow depression. In Baird SB, McCorkle R, and Grant M, editors: Cancer nursing: a comprehensive textbook, Philadelphia, 1991, WB Saunders Co, pp. 759–781.

Hoagland HC: Hematologic complications of cancer chemotherapy. In Perry MC, editor: The chemotherapy source book, Baltimore, 1992, Williams & Wilkins, pp. 498–507.

Hotter AN: Physiologic aspects and clinical implications of wound healing, Heart Lung 11:522–532, 1982.

Hrozencik SP and Connaughton MJ: Cancer-associated hemolytic uremic syndrome, Oncol Nurs Forum 15:755–759, 1988.

Khoury GG, Bulman AS, Joslin CA, and Rothwell RI: Concomitant pelvic irradiation, 5-fluorouracil and mitomycin-C in the treatment of advanced cervical carcinoma, Brit J Radiol 64:252–260, 1991.

Maxwell MB and Maher KE: Chemotherapy-induced myelosuppression, Semin Oncol Nurs 8:113–123, 1992.

Mayer DK: Biotherapy: recent advances and nursing implications, Nurs Clin No Am 25:291–308, 1990.

McDonald A: Altered protective mechanisms. In Dow KH and Hilderley LJ, editors: Nursing care in radiation oncology, Philadelphia, 1992, WB Saunders Co, pp. 96–125.

Nauseef WM and Makie DG: A study of the value of simple protective isolation in patients with granulocytopenia, N Eng J Med 304:448–453, 1981.

Pavel JN: Red blood cell transfusions for anemia, Semin Oncol Nurs 6:117–122, 1990.

Pinner R, Schuchat A, Swaminathan B, Hayes PS, Deaver KA, Weaver RE, Plikaytis BD, Reeves M, Broome CV, and Wenger JD: Role of foods in sporadic listeriosis: II. Microbiologic and epidemiologic investigation, JAMA 267:2046–2050, 1992.

Pizzo PA: Management of fever in patients with cancer and treatment-induced neutropenia, N Eng J Med 328:1323–1331, 1993.

Platanias LC, Miller CB, Mick R, Hart RD, Ozer H, McEvilly JM, Jones RJ, and Ratain M: Treatment of chemotherapy-induced anemia with recombinant human erythropoietin in cancer patients, J Clin Oncol 9:2021–2026, 1991.

Raefsky EL and Wasserman TH: Combined modality therapy. In Perry MC, editor: The chemotherapy source book, Baltimore, 1992, Williams & Wilkins, pp. 110–129.

Riboli EB, Terrizzi A, Arnulfo G, and Bertoglio S: Immunosuppressive effect of surgery evaluated by the multitest cell-mediated immunity system, Can J Surg 27(1):60–63, 1984.

Robson MC: Disturbances of wound healing, Ann Emer Med 17:1274–1780, 1988.

Rostad ME: Current strategies for managing myelosuppression in patients with cancer, Oncol Nurs Forum 18(2)(suppl):7–15, 1991.

Rostad M: Management of myelosuppression in the patient with cancer, Oncol Nurs Forum 17(1)(suppl 1):4–8, 1990.

Schimpff SC: Growth factors and empiric therapy with antibiotics: should they be used concurrently? Ann Int Med 121:538–540, 1994.

Scofield RP, Liebman MC, and Popkin JD: Multimodal therapy. In Baird SB, McCorkle R, and Grant M, editors: Cancer nursing: a comprehensive textbook, Philadelphia, 1991, WB Saunders Co, pp. 344–354.

Spivak JL: The application of recombinant erythropoietin in anemic patients with cancer, Semin Oncol 19(3)(suppl 8):25–28, 1992.

Sugar AM: Empiric treatment of fungal infections in the neutropenic host: review of literature and guidelines for use, Arch Int Med 150:2258–2264, 1990.

Thomas PRM and Lindbald AS: Adjuvant postoperative radiotherapy and chemotherapy in rectal carcinoma: a review of the Gastrointestinal Tumor Study Group experience, Radiother Oncol 13:245–252, 1988.

von der Masse H: Complications of combined radiotherapy and chemotherapy, Semin Rad Oncol 4(2):81–94, 1994.

Wujcik D: Infection control in oncology patients, Nurs Clin No Am 28:639–650, 1993a.

Wujcik D: An odyssey into biologic therapy, Oncol Nurs Forum 20:879–887, 1993b.

Zaia JA: Viral infections associated with bone marrow transplantation, Hematol Oncol Clin No Am 4:603–623, 1990.

Chapter 23

❖ *Organ Toxicities*

Dawn Camp-Sorrell

Although the literature lacks descriptions of specific side effects from multimodal therapy, it is known that multimodal therapy increases the onset, duration, and intensity of acute and chronic side effects. Toxicity of the organs (heart, lungs, kidneys, bladder, liver, and central nervous system) is a significant problem. It stands to reason that if an irradiated organ is radiosensitive, and if the same organ is chemotherapy-sensitive, the resultant side effect will be increased. For example, if bleomycin is administered and radiation is then administered to the mediastinum, pulmonary toxicity will occur earlier in the treatment plan and with a more intense presentation. Questions on how to minimize toxicity and maximize therapeutic effects are of major concern, because the most critical toxicity may be permanent, late organ damage rather than an acute reaction.

❖ Heart

The effects of cardiotoxicity can be acute, subacute, or chronic. Acute effects manifest as arrhythmias or electrocardiogram (ECG) changes, including nonspecific S-T segment abnormalities, loss of anterior electrical forces, various atrial and ventricular arrhythmias, and prolongation of the Q-T interval (Meister and Meadows, 1994). Rarely are these acute effects life-threatening or reason to discontinue therapy (Carlson, 1992). Subacute effects include myocarditis or pericarditis. These can lead to a rapid decrease in cardiac output that develops in days or weeks following therapy and that could be fatal. Chronic effects, which develop months or years after treatment, include congestive heart failure (CHF) or cardiomyopathy (Allen, 1992a; Steinherz and Steinherz, 1991).

Factors that increase the risk of cardiotoxicity include age (younger than 4 or older than 70), preexisting heart disease, hypertension, mediastinal irradiation, and poor nutritional status (Carlson, 1992). Other risk factors include a large chest-tumor mass or substantial mediastinal lymphadenopathy, concomitant use of cardiotoxic chemotherapy agents, and an elevated erythrocyte sedimentation rate (Lindower and Skorton, 1992). Up to 5% of patients will develop late cardiac failure and life-threatening abnormalities of cardiac conduction and rhythm. The incidence and severity of late cardiotoxicity appear to increase with time (Schober et al., 1993; Steinherz et al., 1991).

Effects from Surgery

Patients with preexisting congestive heart disease are at risk for cardiac decompensation as a result of stresses from surgery. Fluid overload can occur during or after surgery and can lead to heart failure and pulmonary edema.

Effects from Chemotherapy

The chemotherapeutic agents most often associated with cardiotoxicity are the anthracyclines, predominantly doxorubicin and daunorubicin. Doxorubicin and daunorubicin have an affinity for myocytes, the cells of the cardiac muscle. When myocytes are damaged, they are not easily replaced. This weakens the cardiac muscle and diminishes the heart's pumping capacity, resulting in congestive heart failure (CHF).

The risk for cardiotoxicity increases with the cumulative doses of anthracyclines. At a cumulative dose of 550 mg/m^2 of doxorubicin, there is a probability that 10% of patients will develop CHF. At a cumulative dose of 1000 mg/m^2, the probability of developing CHF increases to 50%. However, CHF has been seen in cumulative doses as small as 40 mg/m^2 and not seen in at least one patient who received more than 500 mg/m^2 (Allen, 1992a). Therefore the risk for cardiotoxicity exists throughout the course of treatment.

Other drugs that can cause cardiac toxicity include high-dose cyclophosphamide (greater than 1 g), 5-fluorouracil, paclitaxel, and ifosfamide. The cardiac effects from cyclophosphamide range from minor, transient ECG changes and asymptomatic increases of cardiac enzymes to fatal myopericarditis and myocardial necrosis. Cardiotoxicity from cyclophosphamide is not related to a cumulative dose but to the administration of high single doses. It usually occurs within 3 weeks of treatment (Allen, 1992b; Lindower and Skorton, 1992). Patients who do not develop heart failure appear to recover and return to their baseline.

5-Fluorouracil can cause cardiac symptoms ranging from angina pectoris to myocardial infarction with up to 12.5% mortality. Angina and infarction may be due to coronary spasms of the Prinzmetal's type responding to long-acting nitrates and calcium channel blockers (Allen, 1992b; Lindower and Skorton, 1992). Toxic effects generally occur within 24 hours after the last dose (Schober et al., 1993).

Paclitaxel can cause bradycardia, tachyrhythmia, bundle-branch blocks, and cardiac ischemia, which appear to be due to the Cremophor El (polyoxyethylated castor oil) with which paclitaxel is admixed (Rowinsky et al., 1991). These effects are self-limiting and abate immediately after the infusion is discontinued(Rogers, 1993). They can be minimized by premedication 6 and 12 hours before treatment with oral dexamethasone and diphenhydramine, with or without cimetadine. High-dose ifosfamide (10 to 18 g/m^2) has been reported to cause CHF, which responds to diuretics and vasodilator agents (Quezado et al., 1993).

Effects from Radiation Therapy

Radiation affects the fine capillary (vasculoconnective) stroma of the myocardium and can cause pericardial effusion and fibrosis with doses greater than 45 Gy (Rubin, 1984). The effects depend on the volume of heart irradiated and the total radiation dose (Kreuser et al., 1993). Most commonly the pericardium is affected, although the myocardium, the endocardium, the papillary muscles, valvular structures, and coronary arteries can also be adversely affected. Acute effects are noted in the first 48 hours after radiation therapy begins. The late phase develops approximately 70 days after radiation as a progressive thickening and fibrosis of the pericardium with or without accompanying effusion or tamponade (Gottdiener et al., 1983).

The incidence of symptomatic cardiac disease is as high as 68% of adults who receive mediastinal irradiation (Meister and Meadows, 1994). Acute pericarditis develops in about 3% of patients who have received radiation to the internal mammary chain for breast carcinoma or to the mediastinum for Hodgkin's disease. Pericarditis can occur weeks or even years after treatment is completed (Tabbarah, Lowitz, and Casciato, 1992). Delayed pericarditis occurs up to 15 years later in 10% to 15% of patients with Hodgkin's disease who received radiation to the mediastinum (Makinen et al., 1990). It has been estimated that when the heart is in the radiation field, 42% of patients have valvular thickening, 39% have pericardial thickening, 18% have reduced fractioned shortening, and 14% have reduced ejection fraction (Gottdiener et al., 1983).

Several studies have reported endocardial change resembling fibroelastosis with focal valvular thickening, with mitral valve insufficiency cited as the most common valvular defect. Mitral regurgitation may result from papillary dysfunction and aortic insufficiency secondary to valvular thickening (Lindower and Skorton, 1992). Damage to the capillary endothelium with ensuing microvascular obliteration results in ischemia and ultimately pericardial and myocardial fibrosis (Lindower and Skorton, 1992; Rubin, 1984).

Effects from Biotherapy

Capillary leak syndrome (CLS) is a major dose-related, dose-limiting toxicity of interleukin-2 (IL-2) that involves the cardiac and vascular systems (Siegel and Puri, 1991). This syndrome is characterized by an increase in capillary (vascular) permeability, which causes leakage of fluid into the tissue spaces, decreasing vascular resistance. As the intravascular volume decreases, the perfusion of blood to organs also decreases, leading to organ failure.

Arrhythmias and myocardial infarctions associated with interferon (IFN), IL-2, and tumor necrosis factor (TNF) have been attributed to significant alterations in fluid balance. A hyperdynamic state and an increased demand on the heart results (Allen, 1992a).

Hypotension can occur with INF, IL-2, and TNF. Hypotension is more common with IFN-γ than IFN-α or IFN-β and usually occurs 1 to 2 hours after administration. One type of IFN-related hypotension is usually due to peripheral vasodilation and responds well to fluid replacement. Another type is secondary to fever and insidious fluid imbalances that occur with chronic administration of IFN.

Hypotension associated with IL-2 can be profound and may be accompanied by tachycardia and arrhythmias as part of CLS. Hypotension can occur within several hours after administration of TNF and is a dose-limiting toxicity (i.e., TNF must be discontinued or the dose must be decreased if this occurs) (Brophy and Sharp, 1991; Moldawer and Figlin, 1988). Episodes of mild hypertension accompanied by tachycardia have occurred shortly after bolus administration of TNF, but these may be secondary to an acute febrile reaction (Feinberg et al., 1988).

Effects from Multimodal Therapy

Combinations of cardiotoxic chemotherapy with mediastinal irradiation have been reported to cause vascular damage (Schober et al., 1993). Although each modality targets different cells, the two modalities together can result in heart damage. Doxorubicin-induced CHF can be precipitated by volume load, surgical trauma, and general anesthesia (Ferrans, 1978). Doses ranging from 12.6 to 34 Gy to various radiation therapy ports (thoracic, upper spine, lung, and mediastinum) will enhance this effect (Meister and Meadows, 1994). In addition, 60 Gy to the heart apex can potentiate the effect (Allen, 1992a). Mediastinal irradiation and chemotherapy with subsequent thrombocytosis are possibly major pathogenic factors for the development of an acute myocardial infarction (MI) in young patients with Hodgkin's disease (Schober et al., 1993).

Accumulated doses of doxorubicin increase the risk of the chronic late effect of myocardial necrosis when mediastinal radiation is administered. Radiation recall can occur anytime after thoracic radiation when doxorubicin is administered. The effect is cardiac decompensation 4 to 10 years after thoracic radiation is given (Rubin, 1984).

Several preclinical studies have shown an enhanced effect from IFN combined with doxorubicin, cyclophosphamide, nitrosoureas, vinca alkaloids, cisplatin, or 5-fluorouracil. After patients received a combination of interferon-γ and vinblastine, hyponatremia, hypotension, and arrhythmias have occurred (Gilewski and Golomb, 1990).

Nursing Management of Cardiotoxicity

Nursing management begins with assessing for signs and symptoms of cardiac damage (see Nursing Management of the Patient at Risk for Cardiotoxicity on page 390). Signs and symptoms of acute CHF include a nonproductive cough, dyspnea, hepatomegaly, distended neck veins, tachycardia, peripheral edema, weight gain, and oliguria. A chest X ray will reveal an enlarged heart or cardiomegaly. ECG changes include a decrease in QRS voltage, nonspecific S-T segment abnormalities, T-wave changes, and prolongation of the Q-T interval.

Signs and symptoms of acute or chronic pericarditis include pleuritic chest pain, pericardial friction rub, ECG abnormalities, decreased ventricular systolic function, pericardial effusion, dyspnea on exertion, orthopnea, paroxysmal nocturnal dyspnea, and an enlarged heart on a chest X ray (Lindower and Skorton, 1992; Tabbarah, Lowitz, and Casciato, 1992). Endomyocardial fibrosis is manifested clinically as con-

Nursing Management of

The Patient at Risk for Cardiotoxicity

◆ Identify risk factors and assess the degree of cardiac impairment.
  ◆ Cumulative doses of doxorubicin greater than 550 mg/m² (greater than 450 mg/m² if combined with thoracic irradiation)
  ◆ Thoracic irradiation
  ◆ Preexisting cardiac disease or hypertension
  ◆ Elderly
  ◆ Malnutrition

◆ Assess for signs and symptoms such as tachycardia, shortness of breath, a nonproductive cough, neck vein distension, galloping heart rhythm, rales, high blood pressure, poor skin color, poor capillary refill, weak or absent peripheral pulse, and peripheral edema. Serum cardiac enzymes or an electrocardiogram may be ordered by the physician.

◆ Diuretics may be ordered to decrease pulmonary and systemic edema.

◆ Digoxin may be ordered to enhance cardiac output.

◆ Vasodilators may be ordered to reduce cardiac afterload.

◆ Oxygen may be ordered to help the patient breathe better.

◆ Daily aspirin or warfarin may be ordered to prevent thrombus formation.

◆ Antiarrhythmic drugs, an implantable cardioverter, or a pacemaker may be ordered to manage arrythmias.

◆ Cardiac transplantation could be an option for patients who have survived cancer and are considered cured.

◆ If the patient is hospitalized for treatment, assess the following conditions:
  ◆ Monitor weight daily
  ◆ Measure intake and output every 4 to 8 hours for signs of fluid overload
  ◆ Monitor vital signs every 4 to 8 hours to detect changes
  ◆ A cardiac monitor may be ordered
  ◆ Chemoprotectants such as ICRF-187 may be administered to prevent development of doxorubicin toxicity
  ◆ f the patient becomes hypotensive, colloid or crystalloid solutions may be ordered; monitor blood pressure in lying, sitting, and standing positions to detect or evaluate orthostatic hypotension

duction abnormalities, restrictive cardiomyopathy, or valvular incompetence. Symptoms that occur as a result of lost vascular tone after treatment with biologicals include hypotension, tachycardia, renal insufficiency, respiratory distress, peripheral edema, diarrhea, and weight gain (White, 1992).

Detection of cardiotoxicity is based on signs and symptoms and diagnostic tests. Radionuclide ventriculography or multiple-gated acquisition (MUGA) is a noninvasive test that measures cardiac output and determines the ejection fraction of the left ventricular function (Allen, 1992a). This is the most reliable noninvasive method to measure the cardiac contractile function. Chemotherapy should be discontinued when the ejection fraction at rest falls by more than 15% from the baseline measure (Carlson, 1992). Because clinical decompensation can occur 12 to 14 years after therapy, even in patients with no early symptoms, patients need to be followed closely for a prolonged period of time (Meister and Meadows, 1994; Steinherz and Steinherz, 1991), probably for the rest of their lives.

Nursing interventions are based on supportive care when heart damage occurs. Patients and their families need to be informed on how to provide this supportive care in the home (see Patient Education Guidelines for Heart Damage below). Treatment can include the use of digoxin, vasodilators, and diuretics. These agents alleviate symptoms and help to improve the patient's quality of life. Treatment of pericarditis includes corticosteroids, antipyretics, and pericardiocentesis. The disease is usually self-limiting but may become chronic. In the chronic phase, a pericardial window for symptomatic effusions or a pericardiectomy for constrictive pericarditis may become necessary.

Cardioprotective agents are a new strategy being developed to prevent cardiotoxicity. Drugs such as ICRF-187, verapamil, liposomal doxorubicin, alpha tocopherol, histamine blockers, alpha blockers, beta blockers, and cromolyn sodium are being used (Carlson, 1992; Speyer et al., 1992). Alternative chemotherapy drugs that offer similar efficacy but fewer cardiotoxic effects have been developed; these include epirubicin, mitoxantrone, and idarubicin (Allen, 1992a; Nielsen et al., 1990). Techniques have improved to block radiation from striking the heart. A cardiac silhouette excludes the heart as much as possible from the

---

 Patient Education Guidelines for

Heart Damage

◆ Avoid drinking alcohol, smoking, lifting heavy weights, or using illicit drugs such as cocaine.
◆ Maintain the diet recommended by your doctor or nurse.
◆ Your doctor or nurse may restrict your fluid intake to decrease the swelling.
◆ Call your doctor if you are unable to catch your breath, if your heart feels like it is running away, or if you become dizzy when you stand.
◆ Move slowly when going from a lying position to sitting or standing positions.
◆ Be sure to keep all your doctor appointments.
◆ Be sure to take frequent rest periods such as one nap in the morning and one in the afternoon to help you feel rested.
◆ Gauge your activities according to your energy level.
◆ Have emergency phone numbers available close to the phone (ambulance service, physicians, or treatment center).

Permission granted to reproduce these guidelines for educational purposes only.

primary beam, and radiation is delivered through anterior and posterior ports with judicious use of subcarinal blocks.

❖ *Lungs*

Pulmonary toxicity ranges from dyspnea and dry cough to fatal pulmonary fibrosis. Damage can be caused by direct effects on the lung parenchyma, by a hypersensitivity reaction, by idiosyncratic process, or by a combination of these factors. Whatever the mechanism, there is usually an initial inflammatory response followed by a fibrotic change in the interstitial tissue. The incidence of pulmonary toxicity increases with patients over the age of 70; patients who have had chest irradiation; patients who have had pulmonary toxic chemotherapeutic agents, preexisting lung disease such as chronic obstructive lung disease, or pulmonary infiltrates; patients who smoke; and patients who have previously received oxygen therapy (Todd et al., 1993).

Effects from Surgery

Resection for lung cancer decreases the amount of lung tissue in the body, affecting alveolar ventilation and gas exchange, which may already be compromised. With any type of surgery, pneumonia is possible and can be caused by the anesthesia, hypoventilation, or patient immobility. Whenever the chest is opened, air and fluid can settle into the space between the pleura. This causes the lung on that side to collapse.

Effects from Chemotherapy

Bleomycin causes pulmonary toxicity probably because of direct and indirect damage to cells. Bleomycin concentrates in the pulmonary capillary endothelium and alveolar type I cells, where the initial injury occurs. An inflammatory-type reaction follows the injury of the endothelial cells. Fibrotic changes in the lung result in diminished pulmonary capacity (Kreisman and Wolkove, 1992), with a decrease in carbon monoxide–diffusing ability. The incidence of symptomatic pulmonary disease is dose-related. In adults, with a cumulative dosage of more than 450 units of bleomycin, the incidence of toxicity is 5% to 10% (Meister and Meadows, 1994).

Carmustine causes pulmonary toxicity in up to 50% of patients who receive cumulative doses greater than 1500 mg/m^2. Patients can suffer a sudden onset of dyspnea and then progress rapidly to death; this occurs anywhere from 9 days to 12 years after the patient reaches the cumulative dose (Weiss, Poster, and Penta, 1981). Methotrexate can cause endothelial injury, capillary leak syndrome, pulmonary edema, and pulmonary fibrosis, and these can occur from days after treatment up to 5 years later. The toxicity can be acute, with pulmonary edema producing adult respiratory distress syndrome (ARDS) or it can be more gradual, with a systemic toxicity such as fever, chills, and malaise (Kreisman and Wolkove, 1992).

High doses of cytarabine (>3 gm/m^2) can cause capillary leak syndrome 2 to 21 days after the initial dose and can develop into ARDS. Procarbazine causes a hypersensitivity pneumonia that produces a fever, a skin rash, and blood and tissue eosinophilia (Kreisman and Wolkove, 1992).

Effects from Radiation Therapy

Toxicity of radiation is related to the volume of lung irradiated, the total radiation dose, and the fractionation schedule. Despite improvements in lung shielding and techniques for shrinking fields, damage occurs mainly in rapidly dividing cells such as bronchial epithelial cells, capillary endothelial cells, and type II alveolar pneumocytes. Radiation pneumonitis, which often progresses to pulmonary fibrosis, occurs 2 to 3 months after the initiation of radiation therapy (Meister and Meadows, 1994).

A latent symptom-free period can follow and ultimately progress to irreversible fibrosis 6 months to 1 year later, when more than 30 Gy are administered. In 5% to 15% of patients, signs and symptoms of pulmonary toxicity will develop. Some degree of damage occurs in the lung parenchyma when radiation is administered to the chest wall, the mediastinum, and the esophagus, as well as the lung itself (Lindower and Skorton, 1992). Radiation destroys the cells lining the alveoli, and the alveoli become inflamed and then accumulate exudative fluid. This process inhibits the diffusion of oxygen and carbon dioxide within the alveoli. If more than 25% of the lung tissue is exposed to radiation, the patient will exhibit a dry, hacking, persistent cough, fever, dyspnea after exertion, and weakness.

Effects from Biotherapy

Pulmonary toxicity often results from the large volume of colloid solutions used to manage capillary leak syndrome in patients receiving high-dose IL-2 therapy. Pulmonary distress is caused by a fluid shift from the extravascular spaces into the pulmonary vasculature. An intrinsic mechanism of IL-2 may account for the direct effects on pulmonary function. Chest X rays can show pleural effusions (Caliendo, Joyce, and Altmiller, 1993).

The incidence and severity of ARDS vary with the brand of IL-2, the dose administered, and the route of administration. In patients with ARDS, 9% to 77% exhibit weight gain, 12% to 100% develop pulmonary edema, and up to 31% have pleural effusion. Despite the increased cardiac output, the marked fall in peripheral resistance combined with pulmonary hypertension results in marked hypotension and must be supported by vasopressors rather than fluid. Mechanical ventilation may be necessary with supportive care using albumin, vasopressors, and oxygen. After discontinuation of IL-2, recovery is rapid. Tumor necrosis factor (TNF) stimulates production of superoxides and hydrogen peroxide by the neutrophils, and it may produce acute cytotoxic effects on alveolar capillary endothelium (Wujcik, 1993).

Effects from Multimodal Therapy

Pulmonary edema and/or fibrosis as a result of chemotherapy and radiation therapy increase surgical risk. Impaired pulmonary reserves result from pulmonary fibrosis, radiation effects, or loss of viable lung tissue from resection (Ewer and Ali, 1990). Bleomycin, carmustine, cyclophosphamide, and mitomycin-C combined with total body irradiation can cause pulmonary venoocclusive disease. Histologically there is a narrowing of the pulmonary veins and venules by loose fibrous material.

Dactinomycin, doxorubicin, bleomycin, and cyclophosphamide cause pronounced damage when administered with large-field thoracic radiation. Radiation pneumonitis is exaggerated in the patient who has previously received bleomycin or dactinomycin (von der Masse, 1994). The risk of symptomatic pneumonitis has been shown to increase with the combination of cyclophosphamide and 5-FU with or without methotrexate concurrently with radiation (Fu, Rayner, and Lam, 1984).

Nursing Management of Pulmonary Toxicities

Assessment begins with monitoring for signs and symptoms of pulmonary dysfunction (Box 23-1). Pulmonary toxicities are manifested as pulmonary fibrosis, chronic pneumonitis, ARDS, and pulmonary edema. Symptoms consist of an insidious onset of dyspnea, hypoxia, pulmonary hypertension, and a nonproductive cough, resembling restrictive lung disease. If left untreated, the damage can rapidly progress to severe restrictive lung disease with resultant poor oxygen exchange (Doll and Yarbro, 1992). Diagnosis of pulmonary toxicity can be difficult because many early symptoms can be confused with other processes commonly associated

---

Box 23-1 Nursing Assessment of Pulmonary Toxicity

Identify the patient's risk factors and assess the degree of pulmonary impairment.

♦ Risk factors include prior mediastinal irradiation, a history of pulmonary toxic chemotherapeutic agents (such as bleomycin), a history of smoking, previous heart disease, renal disease, or pulmonary disease such as chronic obstructive lung disease.

♦ Assess the patient's respiratory function for the quality of respirations and breath sounds.

♦ Assess for the use of accessory muscles, chest wall expansion, and pain on inspiration, which are signs of pulmonary dysfunction.

♦ Assess for the following symptoms of pulmonary toxicity before treatment and during follow-up visits:
  ♦ Radiation pneumonitis symptoms such as a dry, hacking, persistent cough, fever, dyspnea after exertion, and weakness; steroids may be ordered to decrease the symptoms
  ♦ Chemotherapy-induced pneumonitis produces a dry cough, dyspnea, tachypnea, rales, and asymmetric chest expansion

♦ Pulmonary function tests may be ordered to assess lung capacity, obstruction, and restriction.

♦ Pulse oximetry may be ordered to assess oxygen saturation to determine the need for supplemental oxygen.

♦ Postural drainage may be ordered to facilitate drainage of the lungs. Percussion is the rhythmic tapping of the chest wall for 1 to 2 minutes with cupped hands over the area of retained secretions.

with cancer. Diagnostic measures include pulmonary function tests, transbronchial biopsy, and pulmonary exercise testing (Ngan et al., 1993).

The treatment of pulmonary toxicity usually involves discontinuation of the offending treatment and the administration of relatively high doses of corticosteroids. Other measures are based on supportive care to help the patient to a comfortable state. The patient and family must learn how to provide this supportive care at home (see Patient Education Guidelines for Breathing Techniques below). Measures to facilitate expectoration of secretions and decrease shortness of breath are important lessons to teach. For instance, pursed-lip breathing helps to increase exhalation, which decreases shortness of breath.

❖ *Kidneys*

The principal excretory mechanisms of the kidneys include glomerular filtration and active and passive transport. Filtration of a drug is determined by molecular size, protein binding characteristics, glomerular integrity, and the number of nephrons. The amount of drug actually filtered depends on renal blood flow and is also affected by the rate of nonrenal metabolism.

Effects from Surgery

Nephrectomy can limit the use of aggressive hydration for chemotherapy and biotherapy protocols because the patient's ability to maintain fluid homeostasis is

---

Patient Education Guidelines for

Breathing Techniques

◆ Take a deep breath, cough, and change your position every 2 hours while awake if you are in bed. Try to sit in the chair or on the side of the bed three times a day.
◆ Try to drink eight 8-ounce glasses of fluid a day unless your doctor or nurse has restricted your fluids.
◆ Humidify the air with a cold-water vaporizer.
◆ Drink warm fluids or suck on a cough drop when coughing becomes persistent.
◆ Elevate the upper part of your body with pillows to help you breathe better.
◆ To help you when you cannot catch your breath, lean over a table with your shoulders slightly forward and your head and back bent forward. Relax and support your arms on the table. Place your feet firmly against a flat surface.
◆ Try pursed-lip breathing when you cannot catch your breath. Breathe in slowly through your nose and breathe out slowly through pursed lips.
◆ Your doctor may want you to receive a pneumococcal vaccine and yearly influenza vaccine to decrease the chance of infection.
◆ Prioritize your daily activities to decrease shortness of breath and fatigue.

Permission granted to reproduce these guidelines for educational purposes only.

compromised. Use of contrast dye for diagnostic tests may be limited or prohibited because the dye may have toxic effects on the remaining kidney. Renal shutdown of the opposite kidney could occur.

Effects from Chemotherapy

The renal tubules are vulnerable to chemotherapy toxicity because the majority of drugs is collected, concentrated, metabolized, and excreted through the kidneys. The tubules extract toxic drugs and their byproducts from the glomerular filtrate. Damage can occur as a result of higher levels of uric acid, glomerular necrosis, inadequate electrolyte reabsorption, loss of protein, acid-base disturbances, and elevated levels of blood urea nitrogen (BUN) (Gootenberg and Pizzo, 1991).

Serious fluid and electrolyte imbalances, which can progress to renal failure, are the result of direct and indirect effects of chemotherapeutic agents on the kidneys. The causes associated with metabolic disturbances include hyperuricemic nephropathy, rapid tumor-lysis syndrome, and direct toxic effects on the kidney. Hyperuricemic nephropathy occurs when excessive uric acid forms crystals that deposit in the renal tubules and collecting ducts. When the amount of uric acid exceeds that which can be filtered by the kidney, hyperuricemic nephropathy results. Rapid tumor-lysis syndrome starts with the rapid release of intracellular ions from dead malignant cells, and this results in hyperkalemia, hyperphosphatemia, and hypercalcemia (Lawton et al., 1991).

Cisplatin, a heavy metal, can damage the proximal tubule in an acute or a chronic form. The acute form occurs as a result of inadequate hydration and is exhibited as azotemia, increased serum creatinine, and oliguria. The chronic form is manifested as a decrease in the glomerular filtration rate that persists for years and is often identified only by sensitive measures of renal function (Vogelzang, 1991). Cisplatin commonly induces hypomagnesemia as a result of the kidney's inability to reabsorb magnesium following damage to the proximal tubule (Meister and Meadows, 1994). Sodium and calcium are also lost in the urine, although less frequently than magnesium (Patterson and Reams, 1992; Wujcik, 1992).

Carmustine has a nephrotoxicity that usually occurs late after treatment, eventually causing patients to develop renal failure and require dialysis. This toxicity is usually associated with a cumulative lifetime dose of 1 g/m^2, and the incidence increases significantly in those who are administered more than 1.5 g/m^2 (Vogelzang, 1991).

Streptozocin damages the renal tubules, causing atrophy and tubulointerstitial nephritis, and it is associated with renal dysfunction in more than 65% of patients. It appears that the dose of streptozocin at the time it is given is the cause rather than the cumulative dose. Total weekly doses of 1 to 1.5 g/m^2 have been documented to be safe and effective (Patterson and Reams, 1992; Vogelzang, 1991).

Vincristine and high-dose cyclophosphamide can result in the syndrome of inappropriate antidiuretic hormone (SIADH). SIADH causes hyponatremia because of the kidney's inability to dilute the urine. Fluids are retained and the extracellular fluid is expanded without edema. Vincristine acts through a central neuropathic effect and cyclophosphamide through a toxic effect on the distal tubules and collecting ducts.

Methotrexate (MTX) administered in high doses can crystallize in the renal tubules and collecting ducts as a result of an acid-base problem in the urine (Relling et al., 1994). To avoid this toxicity, the patient must be adequately hydrated and must maintain an alkaline urine pH of 7.0 or greater (Patterson and Reams, 1992; Relling et al., 1994; Vogelzang, 1991). In addition, leucovorin rescue is administered based on the MTX plasma concentrations to counteract MTX toxicity.

Ifosfamide, a renal tubule toxin, has been known to produce Fanconi's syndrome and glomerular damage in young children. Fanconi's syndrome is a generalized disorder of the proximal renal tubule characterized by excess renal excretion of glucose, amino acids, phosphate, bicarbonate, uric acid, sodium, potassium, magnesium, and low-molecular-weight proteins (DeLaat and Lampkin, 1992). Complications range from subclinical and clinical tubular nephrotoxicity to frank renal failure. Ifosfamide can also cause a reduction of the glomerular filtration rate, tubular defects, renal tubular acidosis, SIADH, and diabetes insipidus (Patterson and Reams, 1992).

Effects from Radiation Therapy

Doses of radiation to the kidney are limited to 12 to 15 Gy, but this may be excessive when the patient also receives dactinomycin or doxorubicin (Meister and Meadows, 1994). Radiation nephritis consists of a variety of syndromes produced by arteriolo-nephrosclerotic process. The clinical signs and symptoms develop 6 to 24 months after treatment as subacute renal failure, chronic nephritis manifested as proteinuria, and hypertension. Complete obliteration of the glomeruli can occur at a single dose above 5 Gy (Rubin, 1984).

Effects from Biotherapy

Oliguria and transient increased serum creatinine levels are common with IL-2, which can be a major dose-limiting factor (Siegel and Puri, 1991). At low doses, IL-2 causes progressive weight gain and peripheral edema followed by a decrease in urine output. High-dose IL-2 regimens cause oliguria and azotemia and increase serum creatinine levels up to five times normal. Renal dysfunction appears to be related to CLS; however, it could be a direct renal effect. The dysfunction is characterized by intravascular depletion and hypovolemia, which causes hypoperfusion to the kidneys. Intensive hemodynamic monitoring is necessary to check the fluid status closely. Discontinuing the therapy usually results in spontaneous diuresis with a normalization of serum creatinine levels after 2 to 3 days. Interferon can cause proteinuria and increase renal enzymes.

Effects from Multimodal Therapy

Both carmustine and cisplatin worsen renal damage when radiation to the kidneys is administered before, simultaneously with, or after chemotherapy (von der Masse, 1994). Furthermore, renal damage becomes more severe as the administration intervals for radiation and cisplatin therapy increase (Moulder and Fish, 1991; Stewart,

Oussoren, and Bartelink, 1989). Concomitant chemotherapy and biotherapy, such as the treatment used for melanoma, also increases the risk of nephrotoxicity.

Nursing Management of Nephrotoxicity

Monitoring for renal damage is imperative during multimodal treatment. Renal damage is often measured by serum creatinine level, creatinine clearance, or the glomerular filtration rate (GFR). An increase in serum creatinine or a decrease in urine creatinine clearance usually indicates renal toxicity. Sensitive determinants of proximal tubular dysfunction include aminoaciduria, phosphaturia, and increased excretion of urate. Distal tubular dysfunction can be characterized by polyuria and renal tubular acidosis. Signs and symptoms include azotemia, decreased creatinine clearance, enzymuria, and protein in the urine.

    The goal of nursing management is to prevent or minimize urinary dysfunction (see Nursing Management of the Patient at Risk for Nephrotoxicity below).

 Nursing Management of

The Patient at Risk for Nephrotoxicity

- Monitor urine creatinine clearance and serum electrolytes, creatinine, and BUN levels before each treatment and as ordered.
- When creatinine clearance falls below 50 mg/ml, hold treatment and inform the physician. Expect doses to be decreased for a low glomerular filtration rate (GFR):
    - If GFR is 30–50 ml/min, expect to give 75% dose of bleomycin, plicamycin, or mitomycin-C; 50% of cisplatin or methotrexate, and omit nitrosoureas
    - If GFR is 10–30 ml/min, expect to also omit cisplatin and methotrexate
    - If GFR is less than 10 ml/min, expect to give a 50% dose of bleomycin, cyclophosphamide, plicamycin, or mitomycin-C
- Assess for edema (periorbital, sacral, or peripheral edema; ascites).
- Administer sodium bicarbonate to ensure urinary alkalinization. Maintain the urine at a pH of 7.0 or higher before high-dose methotrexate treatments. Administer leucovorin rescue according to plasma concentration.
- Monitor serum bicarbonate levels as ordered. Less than 14 mmol/l indicates poor tissue perfusion and requires treatment with intravenous sodium bicarbonate.
- Administer additional hydration before and after chemotherapy when giving nephrotoxic agents.
- Administer diuretics as ordered to ensure adequate urine output.
- Allopurinol may be ordered to enhance uric acid excretion. Assess for symptoms of crystallization from uric acid (dysuria, frequency, urgency, bladder spasm, pain, or uric acid itch).
- If the patient is hospitalized, monitor the patient's intake and output every 4 to 8 hours, and maintain a minimum output of 100 ml of urine per hour.

Fluid intake should be increased to at least 3 liters a day, and if possible the patient should be instructed to drink at least a liter of fluid every 8 hours. Optimal renal function is maintained during nephrotoxic treatment by administering aggressive hydration (1 to 2 liters before chemotherapy) and diuretic administration. When giving MTX, especially high-dose MTX, sodium bicarbonate is administered intravenously to alkalinize the urine to maintain the pH greater than 7 to lower the level of uric acid. Allopurinol may be ordered to inhibit the synthesis of uric acid to prevent crystallization from occurring in the renal tubules.

When impaired renal function occurs, the patient's fluid intake will be restricted according to the previous day's intake and output. The daily intake of protein will also be restricted (usually 20 to 40 grams daily). Patients who receive other nephrotoxic drugs such as aminoglycosides must be monitored closely for nephrotoxicity.

❖ *Bladder*

Effects from Chemotherapy

Cyclophosphamide and ifosfamide are associated with hemorrhagic cystitis. The mechanism or damage involves the chemical acrolein, which is produced when cyclophosphamide or ifosfamide are metabolized in the liver to their active form. It is the acrolein that damages the epithelial lining of the bladder, causing hemorrhagic cystitis and scarring. The fibrotic changes can lead to a permanently contracted bladder and chronic urinary difficulties such as dysuria, frequency, or bleeding (Stillwell and Benson, 1988).

High-dose cyclophosphamide treatment can cause hemorrhagic cystitis in up to 70% of patients (Shepherd et al., 1991). The best method for preventing this toxicity is vigorous hydration before and during chemotherapy (Gootenberg and Pizzo, 1991). Mesna, a uroprotectant, is recommended with the administration of ifosfamide and high-dose (more than 2.5 g) cyclophosphamide. The inactive form, disulfide dimesna, circulates through the renal tubules where it is converted to the active mesna. Mesna binds to the chemical acrolein and blocks any damage to the bladder (Wujcik, 1992).

Effects from Multimodal Therapy

Cyclophosphamide has an enhanced effect when administered 9 months before or after radiation. Cisplatin has been shown to worsen bladder damage when administered at the same time as radiation therapy or after radiation (Stewart, 1986).

Radiation delivered to the pelvis and the bladder can induce hemorrhagic cystitis with a higher incidence when both cyclophosphamide and radiation are given concurrently (Stillwell and Benson, 1988).

Cystectomy can be complicated by uretero-cutaneous fistula, small bowel obstruction, and wound infection. A urinary diversion, with the ileum used as a conduit, can absorb and recirculate methotrexate, resulting in a higher serum concentration and clearance time, which yields an increase in toxicity (Bowyer and Davies, 1987). A transurethral bladder resection followed by intravesical chemotherapy or biotherapy increases the risk of chemical cystitis.

Nursing Management of Hemorrhagic Cystitis

Assessment begins with monitoring for signs and symptoms of cystitis such as urgency, frequency, and hesitancy of urination. The patient's urine should be checked for blood by using a reagent dipstick or by performing a urinalysis. A cystoscopic exam can confirm the findings that the mucosa is erythematous, inflamed, ulcerated, and necrosed.

Treatment for hemorrhagic cystitis begins with continuous saline irrigations of the bladder (see Nursing Management of the Patient at Risk for Cystitis below). Intravesical instillation of alum, silver nitrate, or formalin may be needed to stop the bleeding. If bleeding continues, a vasopressin drug such as Amicar can be given intravenously; if bleeding still cannot be controlled, a cystectomy with urinary diversion is performed (Stillwell and Benson, 1988). Bladder analgesics such as opioid suppositories can be administered to relieve pain. Patients must be taught to report any signs of cystitis or of blood in the urine. Patients must be encouraged to maintain hydration and to urinate frequently to prevent urine stasis.

Nursing Management of

The Patient at Risk for Cystitis

- ◆ Assess for urinary impairment:
  - ◆ The physical examination should include observation of urine quality and inspection of the perineal area for signs of vaginitis and skin breakdown.
  - ◆ The signs and symptoms of cystitis include frequent voiding with low urinary volume, pain on urination, low back pain, cloudy urine, hematuria, suprapubic pressure, fever, and foul-smelling urine.

- ◆ Interventions to prevent cystitis include the following:
  - ◆ A Foley catheter may be ordered for high-dose cyclophosphamide to prevent stasis within the bladder. If the patient does not have a catheter, the patient should be encouraged to empty his or her bladder every 2 hours when awake and every 4 hours when asleep.
  - ◆ Sodium bicarbonate may be given intravenously or orally to maintain urine pH at 7.0 or higher to prevent crystallization.
  - ◆ Encourage the patient to drink the equivalent of eight glasses of 8 ounces of fluid daily unless contraindicated.

- ◆ If cystitis is suspected, obtain an order for urinalysis to determine if blood is present.

- ◆ Cystoscopy may be performed to evaluate damage to the bladder.

- ◆ Hyperbaric oxygen therapy may be ordered for chronic radiation-induced cystitis refractory to conventional therapy. Instruct the patient that he or she will have to sit in a special chamber for approximately 2 hours while receiving 100% oxygen to promote vascularization and formation of granulation tissue in the bladder. The patient can expect to have up to 60 treatments.

- ◆ If bleeding occurs, continuous fluid irrigations of saline or formalin should decrease clots and bleeding. If bleeding still continues, cystoscopy with fulguration of bleeding points may be ordered. The last resort for uncontrolled bleeding is cystectomy.

❖ *Liver*

Effects from Surgery

Complications from liver resection include hemorrhage and infection. As a result of the resection, drug metabolism and excretion slow. Therefore, toxicity to other organs and tissue occurs (Beare and Myers, 1994).

Effects from Chemotherapy

Chemotherapy drugs metabolized in the liver increase the risk for liver damage. Damage can range from transient elevated enzyme levels to permanent cirrhosis. When the liver loses the ability to metabolize drugs, the level of bilirubin increases. In the presence of liver damage, levels of liver enzymes such as serum glutamic-oxaloacetic transaminase (SGOT), also called aspartate aminotransferase (AST), can be elevated.

In addition to elevated liver enzymes, specific hepatotoxicities include hepatitis, ascites, hepatomegaly, hepatocellular necrosis, venoocclusive disease (VOD), and secondary hepatic tumors (Wujcik, Ballard, and Camp-Sorrell, 1994). These toxicities can lead to loss of albumin, decrease in blood-clotting factors, edema, and an inability to detoxify other chemicals that pass through the liver.

Carmustine induces abnormalities in liver function in up to 26% of patients. Increases in levels of serum transaminase, alkaline phosphatase, and bilirubin are usually mild and revert to normal within brief periods. Methotrexate in high doses results in acute hypertransaminasemia, which is transient and reversible (Meister and Meadows, 1994).

Nitrosoureas can produce severe or fatal damage by causing diffuse hepatocellular necrosis and fatty replacement of hepatocytes. Hepatic dysfunction, manifested by elevated levels of alkaline phosphatase, serum total bilirubin, and SGOT, also occurs (Rubin, 1984).

Effects from Radiation Therapy

Radiation therapy of the whole abdomen or of the liver in patients with Wilm's tumor or neuroblastomas can cause acute radiation hepatitis (DeLaat and Lampkin, 1992). Doses higher than 20 Gy to the whole organ are known to produce hepatic dysfunction. Central vein thrombosis at the lobular level results in retrograde congestion, leading to hemorrhage and secondary alteration in surrounding hepatocytes. Severe acute changes often advance to progressive fibrosis or cirrhosis and liver failure (Rubin, 1984).

Effects from Biotherapy

Recombinant interferon-α produces increases in hepatocellular enzymes that are reversible but can be dose-limiting in higher dosages (Perry, 1992). Interferon-γ can cause a transient increase in transaminase and triglycerides. Tumor necrosis factor causes mild and transient hyperbilirubinemia and an increase in hepatic enzymes. Interleukin-2 can cause hyperbilirubinemia in 43% to 89% of patients. Growth factors can produce mild increases in hepatic enzymes.

Effects from Multimodal Therapy

Radiation to the liver, combined with any of the following—cisplatin, busulfan, cyclophosphamide, carmustine, cytarabine, dacarbazine, dactinomycin, or etoposide, has also been reported to cause VOD (Moertel et al., 1993). VOD is the non-thrombotic obliteration of the small intrahepatic branches of the hepatic veins by a reticular and collagenous intimal thickening (Doll and Yarbro, 1992). Vascular engorgement results in signs and symptoms of hepatomegaly, epigastric or upper-right-quadrant pain, ascites, weight gain, and production of abnormal liver enzymes (Dulley et al., 1987; Grandt, 1989; Rollins, 1986).

Nursing Management of Hepatotoxicity

Assessment of signs and symptoms of hepatotoxicity is the first step in identifying damage. Signs of damage include jaundice, right-upper-quadrant pain, fatigue, anorexia, and nausea. Third spacing (the shift of fluid from the vascular space to the interstitial space) can occur. Albumin can be administered to replace lost plasma protein and can help the kidney reabsorb fluids. It is recommended that liver function tests be performed before administering chemotherapy, and if there is evidence of hepatic dysfunction or damage, the dose of any hepatotoxic drug should be reduced or eliminated (Moertel et al., 1993). However, liver function tests do not always adequately reflect the degree of hepatic injury. The presence or absence of liver disease is best assessed by serial liver biopsies (Perry, 1992). Other supportive-care measures include giving diuretics, decreasing protein intake, administering lactulose, and providing emotional support.

❖ Nervous System

The central nervous system (CNS) is made up of collections of neurons and their connections that are organized into the brain and spinal cord. Neurotoxicities can affect the CNS, the peripheral nervous system, the cranial nerves, or a combination of all three. Some toxicities such as peripheral neuropathies can be reversible, whereas others such as hearing loss can be permanent. Common neurotoxicities include encephalopathies, peripheral neuropathies, cerebellar dysfunction, meningitis, hearing loss, leukoencephalopathy, arachnoiditis, and autonomic neuropathies.

Damage to the CNS strikes the cerebellum in particular, causing altered reflexes, unsteady gait, ataxia, and confusion. The peripheral nervous system is basically a set of communication channels located outside the CNS that consists of the cranial and spinal nerves. Damage to the peripheral nervous system produces paralysis or loss of sensation to those areas affected by that nerve. The autonomic nervous system includes those peripheral nerves that regulate functions occurring automatically in the body such as the cardiovascular, respiratory, or endocrine systems. Damage to the autonomic nervous system causes ileus, impotence, or urinary retention (Meehan and Johnson, 1992). The risk factors for developing neurotoxicity include the patient's age (elderly or young patients are at higher risk), impaired kidney function (inhibiting excretion of the drug), cranial irradiation, and neurologic complications related to the cancer.

Effects from Surgery

Surgery on any organ—for example, proctectomy—has the potential to affect nerve function. Lymph node dissection can decrease the feeling in an extremity or the surgical area for up to 6 months after surgery. In some cases, the numbness can be permanent, as occurs with radical neck dissection. The patient who has had a craniotomy must be observed for signs of increasing intracranial pressure and brain herniation.

Effects from Chemotherapy

The central and peripheral nervous systems are protected against potential neurotoxic effects from chemotherapy by the blood-brain barrier and the blood-nerve barrier. If intact, these barriers exclude most chemotherapeutic agents, which are water-soluble, relatively large molecules. The severity of the neurotoxicity is usually dose-related, with symptoms exhibited in a variable and unpredictable fashion. Neuropathies of the cranial nerve tend to be bilateral and are reversible on discontinuation or interruption of therapy (Meehan and Johnson, 1992). Patients receiving intrathecal chemotherapy risk developing neurotoxicities as a result of chemical irritation of the meninges or the ventricles. Significant neurotoxicity usually requires holding the treatment until the symptom resolves and reinstituting it at half the previous dose or discontinuing the drug entirely.

Cisplatin causes neurotoxicity by impairing DNA synthesis (Forman, 1990). Ototoxicity induced by cisplatin appears to be dose-dependent, with risk rising at total doses of 300 mg/m² to 400 mg/m². Other risk factors for ototoxicity are poor renal status, rapid administration of the drug, dehydration, and concurrent administration of diuretics or aminoglycosides. The mechanism of action is believed to be related to the loss of hair cells in the organ of Corland (Forman, 1990).

Vincristine affects the peripheral nervous system, causing myalgia, distal paresthesia, jaw pain, and muscle cramps shortly after administration. Patients who are elderly and patients who receive unit doses greater than 2 mg run a heightened risk for neurotoxicity. Vincristine is rapidly cleared from the blood but binds extensively to tissue, which accounts for the accumulation of the drug in the body and the typical delay of neurotoxicity until 3 to 10 days after administration. Severe pain at the angle of the jaw can appear as early as a few hours after the first dose and usually represents trigeminal nerve toxicity, which resolves spontaneously within a few days. Peripheral neuropathy progresses in a pattern from sensory changes to asymptomatic loss of Achilles tendon reflexes and paresthesia, evident in the fingers and toes. If therapy continues, the neuropathy can progress to more severe muscle weakness and then foot drop (Meehan and Johnson, 1992).

High-dose cytarabine treatments (3 gm/m²) can cause nystagmus and ataxia as initial signs of the cerebellar syndrome that can precede dysarthria (difficulty in speech) as well as personality changes and attention disturbances (Anderson and Holmes, 1993). Ocular toxicity results in conjunctivitis accompanied by photophobia, ocular burning pain, lacrimation, and decreased visual acuity. One possible explanation for the mechanism of damage could be that the cerebellar degeneration occurs as a result of cytarabine metabolites penetrating the blood-brain barrier into the cerebrospinal fluid (CSF). During infusion, the concentration of cytarabine in the CSF reaches 60% and accumulates in the CSF in 40 to 48 hours. Within 5 days after discontinuing the drug, the neurotoxicity resolves, although 30% of patients will not regain normal function.

Paclitaxel can cause numbness and paresthesia in a glove-and-stocking distribution. The onset is usually rapid and can occur within 1 day of administration, becoming progressively worse after multiple courses of higher doses (Rogers, 1993). Ifosfamide can produce confusion, lethargy, and weakness progressing to a comatose state. These symptoms occur with increased frequency with dosages of 3 to 5 g/m² and tend to resolve within 24 to 48 hours following discontinuation of the drug (Anderson and Deepak, 1991).

Methotrexate given intrathecally or intraventricularly can result in confusion, somnolence, behavioral changes, seizures, and hemiparesis. Acute meningitis or arachnoiditis can occur with symptoms of headache, fever, vomiting, or increased intracranial pressure. The onset occurs within 2 to 4 hours after injection, and the effects resolve in a few days. More serious encephalopathy is characterized by cranial-nerve palsies or cerebellar signs occurring 30 minutes, 2 days, or 2 weeks following administration. Symptoms can be subacute, chronic, reversible, or permanent.

Toxicity from 5-fluorouracil appears to be related to the drug concentration rather than the cumulative dose given. Cerebellar syndrome can occur 2 to 6 months after initiation of treatment, when the drug is given by weekly intravenous bolus administration. Cerebellar syndrome includes ataxia of the extremities, difficulty walking, nystagmus, and hypotonia. Symptoms resolve when treatment is discontinued (Anderson and Deepak, 1991).

Effects from Radiation Therapy

Cranial radiation therapy produces structural changes such as white matter abnormalities and calcification. The severity of effects from cranial irradiation varies greatly from individual to individual, depending on the dose, the dose schedule, the size and location of the radiation field, the amount of time elapsed after treatment, and the patient's age. As a rule, the larger the dose of radiation, the greater the effect.

Cranial irradiation can cause headache, nausea, lethargy, low-grade fever, and herniation of the brain. Subacute reactions can occur 4 to 15 weeks after treatment, and they generally follow a pattern of transient deterioration in function followed by a gradual improvement. Chronic effects begin 16 weeks after treatment with symptoms of memory loss, loss of motivation, poor judgment, and irritability (Anderson and Holmes, 1993). Radiation necrosis is a rare, devastating, late effect that occurs in 1% of patients who receive 50 to 60 Gy to the whole brain. The symptoms include headache, personality change, ataxia, or obtundation and appear 6 months to 3 years after treatment (Meister and Meadows, 1994).

Radiation myelopathy leaves the patient with a devastating neurological deficit. In the first few weeks after radiation, the patient complains of sensations like electric shock in the spine and the extremities when flexing the neck. The symptoms gradually abate within 3 to 4 months, leaving no permanent sequelae (Choucair, 1991).

Irradiation of the spinal cord produces a chronic effect called the Brown-Sequard syndrome, which progresses steadily over months to years to complete and permanent myelopathy. Paresthesias are the earliest symptoms, and patients usually do not have localized findings. Sensory loss and weakness almost always begin in the lower extremities and are often asymmetric, reflecting the patchy distribution of lesions in the spinal cord (Choucair, 1991).

Occasionally, myelography shows an intradural or extradural lesion due to swelling of the spinal cord from radiation necrosis or arachnoid or extradural scarring. The most specific myelographic sign of radiation damage is cord atrophy. The incidence of this atrophy is related to the total dose and the fractionation of the radiation, and the risk is very low in patients who receive less than 60 Gy per week. The thoracic spinal cord is more prone to damage because of its rich vascular supply. The maximum tolerable dose for the spinal cord is 50 Gy when 3 to 5 vertebrae are irradiated (Choucair, 1991).

Amyotrophy is a rare form of radiation-induced spinal cord injury that has a latency period of 3 to 26 months. The patient complains of weakness in the lower extremities, which may progress to atrophy and involuntary contraction or twitching of the muscles. Although amyotrophy continues to progress slowly, ultimately it is self-limited.

Effects from Biotherapy

Biological response modifiers can cause memory loss, disorientation, attentional and concentration deficits, and difficulty with abstract thinking and decision making. Cognitive function refers to those mental functions that are involved in the acquisition, processing, storage, and retrieval of information about one's body and environment. Components of cognitive function include orientation, attention, concentration, memory, and abstract thinking (Bender, 1994).

Interferon and IL-2 are strongly associated with cognitive dysfunction, which is dose-dependent and increases over time during treatment with those drugs. The mechanism of action is unclear, but researchers speculate that a direct effect on the frontal lobe or other structures of the CNS results in a diffuse toxic encephalopathy.

Neurotoxicity may occur with IFN-α, IL-2, and TNF. Central nervous system toxicities such as headache and alteration in speech, level of consciousness, and memory have been observed with IL-2 and TNF, and to a lesser degree with IFN-α. Neuropsychiatric side effects associated with IFN are primarily systemic: lethargy and hypersomnia, affective disorders (depression), and cognitive changes (confusion, hallucinations, and impaired memory). Although these neurobehavioral symptoms may persist, they usually resolve promptly following cessation of therapy (Bender, 1994; Irwin, 1987, Zimberg and Berenson, 1990).

CNS toxicity is common with treatment involving high-dose recombinant IL-2, particularly when concomitantly administered with LAK cells. Common neuropsychiatric side effects are related to changes in behavioral, psychomotor, and cognitive function, including confusion, disorientation, drowsiness, combativeness, hallucinations, and restlessness. Extending the infusion time and/or decreasing the total dose delivered can reduce symptoms in the CNS. While uncommon, hallucinations, delirium, and psychosis may occur (Zimberg and Berenson, 1990). Generally, side effects resolve when therapy is discontinued.

Nursing Management of

The Patient at Risk for Neurotoxicity

- ◆ Assess the patient's neurologic status to detect abnormalities:
  - ◆ Conduct a comprehensive assessment of neurologic symptoms, mental status, and physical status.
  - ◆ Repeat neurologic exams at frequent intervals during therapy to identify side effects promptly.
  - ◆ Use a standardized neurobehavioral assessment tool.
  - ◆ Assess gait, sensation in the extremities, gross motor skills, deep tendon reflexes, and speech alterations. Gait changes such as flapping of the feet or a broad-based stance are early signs of the motor effects of neuropathy.
  - ◆ Assess sensory manifestations by the patient's responses to pain, touch, temperature, vibration, and position.
  - ◆ Assess for headache, vertigo, slurred speech, hoarseness, blurred vision, papilledema, jaw pain, and facial palsies, which may indicate cranial nerve defects.
  - ◆ Observe the patient's ability to perform fine motor skills such as buttoning a shirt to assess his or her functioning.
  - ◆ A baseline audiometric assessment may be ordered before initiating chemotherapy with an ototoxic drug such as cisplatin.
  - ◆ Measure vibratory sensation with a low-pitched tuning fork (128 Hz) on the distal phalanx of the third middle finger and on the great toe.
- ◆ Consult physical therapy to develop an exercise program and to use assistive devices such as splints, orthotic braces, high-top sneakers, bedside commodes, raised toilet seats, and foot boards to prevent or control foot drop.
- ◆ Pyridoxine may be ordered to decrease the degree of neurotoxicity.
- ◆ Use supportive measures such as zipper ring pulls and triangular pencil grips when teaching the patient fine motor skills. Occupational therapy and vocational rehabilitation may be consulted if appropriate.
- ◆ CNS depressants such as sedatives, tranquilizers, and antiemetics must be used with caution because they can increase toxicity.

Effects from Multimodal Therapy

Combination effects from cytarabine and cranial irradiation cause headaches, acute arachnoiditis or meningitis, paraplegia, and necrotizing leukoencephalopathy. When cranial irradiation is administered, methotrexate or cytarabine given intrathecally seem to potentiate or enhance neurotoxic effects (Crossen et al., 1994). Necrotizing leukoencephalopathy produces symptoms of dementia, spasticity, ataxia, seizures, hemiplegia, and pseudobulbar paresis approximately 4 to 12 months after the completion of whole-brain irradiation. Combined use of cranial irradiation and intrathecally administered methotrexate increases the incidence (Meister and Meadows, 1994).

Nursing Management of Neurotoxicity

Neurotoxicity is detected by assessing each area of the CNS system. The first symptoms of peripheral neuropathy reported are usually numbness or tingling of the hands or feet. Ototoxicity is manifested as tinnitus and bilateral sensorineural hearing loss that increase with the patient's age, the dosage, and the administration schedule of cisplatin. The gastrointestinal tract is the major site of autonomic neuropathy with constipation, colicky abdominal pain, paralytic ileus, and sphincter incontinence. Symptoms of CNS dysfunction include dizziness, truncal dysmetria, dysarthria, and diadochokinesis (inability to perform rapid, alternating movements). In a physical examination, peripheral neuropathy is evaluated by testing vibratory sensation and deep tendon reflexes, which are decreased or absent. The examination should reveal a sharp sensory response to pain and temperature, which arises weeks or months later to the upper thoracic or cervical spine as a result of spinal cord irradiation.

If neurotoxicity occurs, management begins with the institution of safety measures to protect the patient from harm. For other measures, see Nursing Management of the Patient at Risk for Neurotoxicity on page 406. The family must be educated to follow these safety measures at home (see Patient Education Guidelines for Neurotoxicity on page 408). In an attempt to decrease this toxicity, a radioprotective compound, WR-2721, has been investigated and has proven that it can partially protect the peripheral nerves from cisplatin toxicity (Mollman et al., 1988).

❖ Summary

Much of the progress in the treatment of cancer has been achieved by the introduction of intensive multimodal regimens. Unfortunately these regimens are often accompanied by toxicities. It is imperative to anticipate toxicities to prevent or minimize them. Complications should be treated aggressively. Recent improvements in supportive care help decrease acute toxicity. However, chronic effects and permanent organ dysfunction can be dose-limiting.

The success of long-term monitoring of the patient treated with multimodal therapy will depend on providing patients with updated knowledge about their disease and treatment and on ensuring that they understand survivorship issues.

Patient Education Guidelines for

Neurotoxicity

◆ Institute safety measures in the home such as lowering the setting on water heaters to 110°F so that the patient will not get burned when bathing.
  ◆ Inspect affected sites for burns, cuts, or abrasions. Use rubber gloves or gardening gloves to protect affected hands from injury.
  ◆ Avoid the use of heating pads.
  ◆ Wear foot coverings all the time to protect the feet.
  ◆ Avoid extreme temperatures; use tepid bath water.

◆ Perform range-of-motion exercises in all the extremities to prevent immobility and atrophy.

Permission granted to reproduce these guidelines for educational purposes only.

Because long-term effects vary and may only become evident years after treatment ends, regular medical evaluation of survivors is an extremely important aspect of health care.

❖ *References*

Allen A: The cardiotoxicity of chemotherapeutic drugs, Semin Oncol 19:529–542, 1992a.

Allen A: The cardiotoxicity of chemotherapeutic drugs. In Perry MC, editor: The chemotherapy source book, Philadelphia, 1992b, Williams & Wilkins, pp. 582–597.

Anderson B and Holmes W: Altered mental status: an algorithm for assessment of delirium in the cancer patient, Curr Issues Cancer Nurs Prac Updates 2:1–10, 1993.

Anderson NR and Deepak ST: Ifosfamide extrapyramidal neurotoxicity, Cancer 68:72–75, 1991.

Beare PG and Myers JL: Adult health nursing, ed 2, St. Louis, 1994, Mosby, pp. 1763–1790, 1895–1932.

Bender CM: Cognitive dysfunction associated with biological response modifier therapy, Oncol Nurs Forum 21:515–523, 1994.

Bowyer GW and Davies TW: Methotrexate toxicity associated with ileal conduit, Brit J Urol 60:592, 1987.

Brophy L and Sharp E: Physical symptoms of combination biotherapy: a quality of life issue, Oncol Nurs Forum 18:23–40, 1991.

Caliendo G, Joyce D, and Altmiller MC: Nursing guidelines and discharge planning for patients receiving recombinant interleukin-2, Semin Oncol Nurs 9(suppl 1):25–31, 1993.

Carlson RW: Reducing the cardiotoxicity of the anthracyclines, Oncol 6:95–107, 1992.

Choucair AK: Myelopathies in the cancer patient: incidence, presentation, diagnosis, and management, Oncol 5:25–37, 1991.

Crossen JR, Garwood D, Glatstein E, and Neuwelt EA: Neurobehavioral sequelae of cranial irradiation in adults: review of radiation-induced encephalopathy, J Clin Oncol 12:627–642, 1994.

DeLaat CA and Lampkin BC: Long-term survivors of childhood cancer: evaluation and identification of sequelae of treatment, CA-Cancer J Clin 42:263–282, 1992.

Doll DC and Yarbro JW: Vascular toxicity associated with antineoplastic agents, Semin Oncol 19:580–596, 1992.

Dulley FL, Kanfer EF, Appelbaum FR, Amos D, Hill RS, Buckner CD, Shulman HM, McDonald GB, and Thomas ED: Venoocclusive disease of the liver after chemoradiotherapy and autologous bone marrow transplantation, Transplantation 43:870–873, 1987.

Ewer MS and Ali MK: Surgical treatment of the cancer patient: preoperative assessment and perioperative medical management, J Surg Oncol 44:185–190, 1990.

Feinberg B, Krurzrock R, Talpaz M, Blick M, Saks S, and Gutterman JU: A phase I trial of intravenously administered recombinant tumor necrosis factor-alpha in cancer patients, J Clin Oncol 6:1328–1334, 1988.

Ferrans VJ: Overview of cardiac pathology in relation to anthracycline cardiotoxicity. Cancer Treat Rep 62:955–961, 1978.

Forman A: Peripheral neuropathy in cancer patients: clinical types, etiology, and presentation, Oncol 4:85–89, 1990.

Fu KK, Rayner PA, and Lam KN: Modification of the effects of continuous low-dose-rate irradiation by concurrent chemotherapy infusion, Int J Radiat Oncol Biol Phys 10:1473–1478, 1984.

Gilewski TA and Golomb HM: Design of combination biotherapy studies: future goals and challenges, Semin Oncol 17(1)(suppl 1):3–10, 1990.

Gootenberg J and Pizzo PA: Optimal management of acute toxicities of therapy. Pedia Clin No Am 38:269–297, 1991.

Gottdiener JS, Katin MJ, Borer JS, Bacharach SL, and Green MV: Late cardiac effects of therapeutic mediastinal irradiation: assessment by echocardiography and radionuclide angiography, N Eng J Med 308:569–572, 1983.

Grandt NC: Hepatic venoocclusive disease following bone marrow transplantation, Oncol Nurs Forum 16:813–817, 1989.

Irwin MM: Patients receiving biological response modifiers: overview of nursing care, Oncol Nurs Forum 14(suppl):32–37, 1987.

Kreisman H and Wolkove N: Pulmonary toxicity of antineoplastic therapy, Semin Oncol 19:508–520, 1992.

Kreuser ED, Voller H, Behles C, Schroder K, Uhrig A, Besserer A, and Thiel E: Evaluation of late cardiotoxicity with pulse doppler echocardiography in patients treated for Hodgkin's disease, Br J Haematol 84:615–622, 1993.

Lawton CA, Cohen EP, Barber-Derus SW, Murray KJ, Ash RC, Casper JT, and Moulder JE: Late renal dysfunction in adult survivors of bone marrow transplantation, Cancer 67:2795–2800, 1991.

Lindower PD and Skorton DJ: The cardiovascular system and anticancer therapy. In Armitage JO and Antman KH, editors: A high-dose cancer therapy: pharmacology, hematopoietins, stem cells. Baltimore, 1992, Williams & Wilkins, pp. 505–517.

Makinen L, Makipernaa A, Rautonen J, Heino M, Pyrhonen S, Laitinen LA, and Siimes MA: Long-term cardiac sequelae after treatment of malignant tumors with radiotherapy or cytostatics in childhood, Cancer 65:1913–1917, 1990.

Meehen JL and Johnson BL: The neurotoxicity of antineoplastic agents, Curr Issues Cancer Nurs Prac Updates 1:1–11, 1992.

Meister LA and Meadows AT: Late effects of childhood cancer therapy, Curr Prob Pedia 23:102–131, 1994.

Mitchell MS: Principles of combining biomodulators with cytotoxic agents in vivo, Semin Oncol 19(suppl 4):51–56, 1992.

Moertel CG, Fleming TR, Macdonald JS, Haller DG, and Laurie JA: Hepatic toxicity associated with fluorouracil plus levamisole adjuvant therapy, J Clin Oncol 11:2286–2390, 1993.

Moldawer NP and Figlin RA: Tumor necrosis factor: current clinical status and implications for nursing management, Semin Oncol Nurs 4:120–125, 1988.

Mollman JE, Glover DJ, Hogan M, and Furman RE: Cisplatin neuropathy: risk factors, prognosis, and protection by WR-2721, Cancer 61:2192–2195, 1988.

Moulder JE and Fish BL: Influence of nephrotoxic drugs on the late renal toxicity associated with bone marrow transplant conditioning regimens, Int J Radiat Oncol Biol Phys 20:333–337, 1991.

Ngan HYS, Liang RHS, Lam WK, and Chan TK: Pulmonary toxicity in patients with non-Hodgkin's lymphoma treated with bleomycin-containing chemotherapy, Cancer Chem Pharm 32:407–409, 1993.

Nielsen D, Jensen JB, Dombernowsky P, Munck O, Fogh J, Brynjolf I, Havsteen H, and Hansen M: Epirubicin cardiotoxicity: a study of 135 patients with advanced breast cancer, J Clin Oncol 8:1806–1810, 1990.

Patterson WP and Reams GP: Renal toxicities of chemotherapy, Semin Oncol 19:521–528, 1992.

Perry MC: Chemotherapeutic agents and hepatotoxicity, Semin Oncol 19:551–565, 1992.

Quezado AMN, Wilson WH, Cunnion RE, Parker MM, Reda D, Bryant G, and Ognibene FP: High-dose ifosfamide is associated with severe, reversible cardiac dysfunction, Ann Int Med 118:31–36, 1993.

Relling MV, Fairclough D, Ayers D, Crom WR, Rodman JH, Pui CH, and Evans WE: Patient characteristics associated with high-risk methotrexate concentrations and toxicity, J Clin Oncol 12:1667–1672, 1994.

Rogers BB: Paclitaxel: a promising new drug of the 90s, Oncol Nurs Forum 20:1483–1489, 1993.

Rollins BJ: Hepatic venoocclusive disease, Am J Med 82:297–301, 1986.

Rowinsky EK, McGuire WP, Guarnieri T, Fisherman JS, Christian MC, and Donehower RC: Cardiac disturbances during the administration of paclitaxel, J Clin Oncol 9:1704–1712, 1991.

Rubin P: Late effects of chemotherapy and radiation therapy: a new hypothesis, Int J Radiat Oncol Biol Phys 10:5–34, 1984.

Schober C, Papageorgiou E, Harstrick A, Bokemeyer C, Mugge A, Stahl M, Wilke H, Poliwoda H, Hiddermann W, Kohne-Wompner CH, Weiss J, Preiss J, and Schmoll HJ: Cardiotoxicity of 5–fluorouracil in combination with folinic acid in patients with gastrointestinal cancer, Cancer 72:2242–2247, 1993.

Shepherd JD, Pringle LE, Barnett MJ, Klingemann HG, Reece DE, and Phillips GL: Mesna versus hyperhydration for the prevention of cyclophosphamide-induced hemorrhagic cystitis in bone marrow transplantation, J Clin Oncol 9:2016–2020, 1991.

Siegel JP and Puri RK: Interleukin-2 toxicity, J Clin Oncol 9:694–704, 1991.

Speyer JL, Green MD, Zeleniuch-Jacquotte A, Wernz JC, Rey M, Sanger EK, Ferrans V, Hochster H, Meyers M, Blum RH, Feit F, Attubao M, Burrows W, and Muggia FM: ECRF-187 permits longer treatment with doxorubicin in women with breast cancer, J Clin Oncol 10:117–127, 1992.

Steinherz LJ, Steinherz PG, Tan CTC, Heller G, and Murphy L: Cardiac toxicity 4 to 20 years after completing anthracycline therapy, JAMA 266:1672–1677, 1991.

Steinherz LJ and Steinherz PG: Delayed anthracycline cardiac toxicity, Princ Prac Oncol 5:1–15, 1991.

Stewart FA, Oussoren Y, and Bartelink H: The influence of cisplatin on the response of mouse kidney to multifraction irradiation, Radiother Oncol 15:93–102, 1989.

Stewart FA: Mechanism of bladder damage and repair after treatment with radiation and cytostatic drugs, Brit J Cancer 53(suppl 6):280–291, 1986.

Stillwell TJ and Benson RC: Cyclophosphamide-induced hemorrhagic cystitis: a review of 100 patients, Cancer 61:451–457, 1988.

Tabbarah HJ, Lowitz BB, and Casciato DA: Intrathoracic complications. In Casciato DA and Lowitz BB, editors: Manual of clinical oncology, ed 2, Boston, 1992, Little, Brown & Co, pp. 435–452.

Todd NW, Peters WP, Ost AH, Roggli VL, and Plantadosi CA: Pulmonary drug toxicity in patients with primary breast cancer treated with high-dose combination chemotherapy and autologous bone marrow transplantation, Am Rev Respir Dis 147:1264–1270, 1993.

Vogelzang NJ: Nephrotoxicity from chemotherapy: prevention and management, Oncol 5:97–112, 1991.

von der Masse H: Complications of combined radiotherapy and chemotherapy, Semin Rad Oncol 4(2):81–94, 1994.

Weiss RB, Poster DS, and Penta JS: The nitrosoureas and pulmonary toxicity, Cancer Treat Rev 8:111–125, 1981.

White CL: Symptom assessment and management of outpatients receiving biotherapy: the application of a symptom report form, Semin Oncol Nurs 8(suppl 1):23–28, 1992.

Wujcik D: Current research in side effects of high-dose chemotherapy, Semin Oncol Nurs 8:102–112, 1992.

Wujcik D: An odyssey into biologic therapy, Oncol Nurs Forum 20:879–887, 1993.

Wujcik D, Ballard B, and Camp-Sorrell D: Selected complications of allogeneic bone marrow transplantation, Semin Oncol Nurs 10(1):28–41, 1994.

Zimberg M and Berenson S: Delirium in patients with cancer: nursing assessment and intervention, Oncol Nurs Forum 17:529–538, 1990.

Chapter 24

❖ *Gonadal Toxicities*

Judith A. Shell
Mary L. Dougherty
Kathleen E. Bell

❖ *Components of Sexual Health*

The increasing success of multimodal treatment has extended the survival of many patients, even those with advanced malignancies. Because of many triumphs, quality of life is now an important issue. This includes the quality of sexual life, sense of self-esteem, role as male or female, and ability to procreate. A satisfying sexual relationship is an important aspect of life for many people and can augment communication, sharing, warmth, tenderness, and a secure self-concept. If the couple is homosexual, the issue of propagation may not be as significant, although an intimate relationship during and after cancer treatment is just as important. Presently patients are better educated concerning human sexuality, are more receptive to information, and demand an open discussion of potential sexual side effects from treatment. Nursing practice must ensure that the patient's sexuality is addressed.

Patients have many questions about how their disease and treatment will affect their roles as men and women, children, siblings, friends, and most important, as parents, partners, or lovers. Not only do they have psychosocial concerns, but many have physiologic fears. Men have concerns regarding impotence, sterility, retrograde ejaculation, loss of libido, and decreased masculinity. Women worry about vaginal stenosis, dryness, atrophy, menstrual irregularities, early menopause, sterility, decreased libido, and femininity (Balducci et al., 1988). Although all are important, this chapter primarily deals with many of the physiologic toxicities encountered during treatment.

Body Image

The way we view ourselves as sexual beings goes beyond the physical act of sexual intercourse. The World Health Organization (WHO) defines the essence of maleness and femaleness as one that integrates the somatic, emotional, intellectual, and social aspects of the sexual being to enrich and enhance personalities, communication, and love (WHO, 1976). Sexuality often changes its focus from procreation to recreation as we grow older, with an emphasis on companionship, physical nearness, intimate communication, and a pleasure-seeking relationship (Bates-Johnson, 1989). Human sexuality involves love, trust, and a sharing relationship with or without intercourse (Shell, 1990).

The image that we develop of ourselves begins early in life (during the first 3 years) and continues to evolve until we die. Body image creates a personal picture of oneself. Body image is a crucial component of sexuality, central to a realistic perception or sense of self, developed by comparing self to others and eliciting their feedback. It is influenced through social interaction, others' perceptions and responses to one's body, and it is always changing (disease, aging, pregnancy) (Fogel, 1990).

For many people, the process of becoming ill may distort how they view their bodies and cast doubt on their sexual identity and response. This may result from physical changes in body size and shape, loss of control over bodily functions, and/or feelings of being diseased and unclean. Because of the patient's own negative perceptions, the partner may hold him or her in less regard and favor. Consequently, at a time when closeness and intimacy are most important in a couple's life, they may be avoided because of embarrassment or a decreased sense of adequacy.

Ultimately it is the nurse's responsibility to dispel sexual myths and misconceptions about the nature of cancer and its long-term side effects. By dispelling beliefs such as sexual abstinence will prevent recurrence of the cancer and cancer is contagious, so partners cannot engage in sexual activity (even kissing, holding, or fondling), a loving and close relationship will be encouraged at a most needful time in the patient's life. Stern (1990) declares that, "cancer's most severe damage may be to communication between patients and loved ones" (p. 503).

Physiologic Sexuality

The physiologic effects on the patient's sense of sexuality depend on the location of the cancer and the treatment modality employed. Permanent alterations caused by the disease such as chronic pain, disfigurement, and system malfunction will necessitate changes in how the patient interacts sexually. Interference with sexual expression may be associated with ulcerating lesions of the breast, the vulva, the rectum, the penis, and even the face. Urinary or reproductive system cancers may be responsible for infertility, impotence, or orgasmic dysfunction. Treatments for other nongenital cancers, such as Hodgkin's disease, can leave the patient sterile due to gonadal failure. Weakness, fatigue, weight loss, and hair loss are side effects from treatment that can indirectly affect sexuality and decrease libido and self-esteem, causing the patient to withdraw from the partner (Hogan, 1985). There may also be other concurrent problems contributing to sexual dysfunction such as diabetes, alcohol and drug abuse, physical and sexual abuse, or a history of sexual promiscuity (Shell, 1994).

The physiologic aspect of reproduction is an important dimension of human sexuality. Most individuals in a heterosexual relationship are interested in becoming parents at some point during their lifetime; cancer, however, can suddenly modify or nullify those plans. Basically, a woman must have intact and functioning ovaries, fallopian tubes, a uterus, and a cervix; and a man must have testes, vas deferens, seminal vesicles, a prostate, and a penis in order to produce a child. Nonmalignant disorders of the reproductive system may preclude conception in both women and men. Women can experience vaginal changes (bleeding, discharge, overlubrication, or inadequate lubrication), vaginal infections (etiology: intercourse, contamination from rectum, hands, clothing, or foreign substance in vagina), or pelvic and vaginal pain (trauma from childbirth or episiotomy, criminal abortion, rape, penile thrusting, increased pelvic congestion, and endometriosis). Men can experience urethritis and prostatitis (dysuria, frequent urination, and painful ejaculation), benign prostatic hypertrophy (enlargement that can cause impotence), Peyronie's disease (penile deformity due to fibrous plaque in the corpora cavernosa), phimosis (tightness of the foreskin causing pain with erection), or priapism (sustained erection without sexual desire) (Hogan, 1985). Although the aforementioned anomalies can cause reproductive problems, most can be remedied or reversed. Sadly this is often not the case with cancer-induced infertility. Impaired fertility can

---

 Patient Education Guidelines for

Sexual Intimacy When You Have a Low White Blood Cell Count or Low Platelet Count

◆ When your total white cell count drops below 1000 or when your absolute neutrophil count drops below 1000, you are at risk for infection. Avoid genital, oral, or anal intercourse to lower the chance of getting an infection. Mouth kissing should also be avoided, but hand holding, caressing, and touching is encouraged after hand washing.

◆ When your platelets drop below 20,000 you are at risk for bleeding. Avoid genital or anal intercourse to lower the chance of bleeding.

◆ Lubricants can help lessen friction during intercourse and thereby lessen irritation of the penis and the vagina. Use only water-soluble lubricants.

◆ You may want to bathe with your partner. A little candlelight and some wine can make the atmosphere more intimate. Warm water may help to ease some general aches and stress.

◆ If you are nauseated or having pain and a time for intimacy is planned, take antinausea and pain medications ½ to 1 hour beforehand so that they have time to work.

◆ Avoid consuming a heavy meal or alcohol before intercourse.

◆ You might have more energy if you take a nap before intercourse.

◆ If you look pale, try putting on makeup or wearing bright colors to brighten your appearance.

◆ Remember to use reliable birth-control methods, because lack of menstruation or a low sperm count are not a guarantee against pregnancy.

Permission granted to reproduce these guidelines for educational purposes only.

be caused by surgery or radiation to the gonads, the pelvis, the retroperitoneum, or the spinal cord, or by the use of certain chemotherapeutic drugs, which interfere with spermatogenesis, erection, or ejaculation, and with ovum maturation.

Sexual Response Cycle

Males and females experience the sexual response cycle (SRC) in the same manner. Technically there are four identified phases that actually overlap each other: excitement, plateau, orgasm, and resolution. The male sexual response (desire, subjective arousal, erection, emission, ejaculation, and orgasm) has separate mechanisms of control, which can be affected independently (von Eschenbach and Schover, 1984). Although cancer therapy can destroy a man's ability to have an erection, the pleasure of sexual arousal and orgasm often remain intact. This is important because men often worry about being able to function as before (Shell, 1994). Although more has been learned recently about the female sexual response (desire, subjective arousal, vaginal expansion and lubrication, and orgasm), it remains less well understood (Schover, Schain, and Montague, 1989). Women with cancer may lose sexual desire during debilitating treatment, especially if the therapy affects the structure or innervation of the clitoris or the vagina. Along with painful intercourse, these factors tend to interfere with orgasm, and they may cause feelings of rejection by the partner (Shell, 1994).

Masters and Johnson (1966) explained that both the male and the female experience two physiologic responses during the SRC: myotonia (increased muscle tension) and vasocongestion in the genital organs. These responses are similar whether

---

Box 24-1 Sexual Response Cycle

Desire	Influenced by a wide variety of environmental stimuli, including psychosocial and cultural factors and physiology; that which causes one to initiate or be receptive to sexual activity.
Excitement	Develops from any bodily or psychic stimuli; with adequate stimulation, intensity increases rapidly; can be interrupted, prolonged, or ended by distracting stimuli.
Plateau	A consolidation period, with maintenance of stimulation; sexual tension becomes intensified to orgasm; can be affected by distracting stimuli.
Orgasm	Involuntary climax of increased sexual tension; usually lasts only a few seconds; vasocongestion and myotonia decrease; there is greater variation of intensity and duration of orgasm among females; the total body is involved, with a focus in the pelvic area.
Resolution	Involutional changes return body to preexcitement state; females, when adequately stimulated, may begin another sexual response cycle before sexual excitement totally resolves; males cannot be restimulated during the refractory period.

stimulated by intercourse, manual or mechanical manipulation, or by fantasy. Lauver and Welch (1990) added a fifth phase at the beginning of the SRC, because it seemed unlikely that an individual would automatically go from a resting phase to one of sexual arousal without acknowledging the psychological component. The fifth phase, desire, recognizes the important dimension of emotion, which can be monumentally affected in the individual with cancer. Box 24-1 summarizes the sexual response cycle.

❖ *Gonadal Toxicities*

Cancer therapy can adversely affect normal human sexual response; however, some side effects can be prevented or modified. Because of more sophisticated treatment measures (e.g., nerve-sparing surgery for prostate cancer and better gonad-shielding techniques in radiation therapy), people being treated for cancer can look forward to a better quality of life, which may include enhanced sexual self-worth and a better sexual relationship.

Effects from Surgery

Various types of cancer surgeries may cause sexual dysfunction, which can lead to infertility. This occurs directly by altering genital organs or indirectly by damaging the vascular or nerve supply in the pelvis or by reducing the levels of necessary hormones (Table 24-1). Sexual dysfunction with an organic basis is precipitated by surgeries such as radical prostatectomy, orchiectomy, radical cystectomy, or pelvic exenteration (see Figure 24-1). These procedures often lead to infertility problems and are the most difficult to manage because they remove sexual organs and/or their nerve supply (Yarbro and Perry, 1985). Other surgeries such as mastectomy or those for head and neck cancer will obviously cause a cosmetic change, altering self-image and sexual identity. Clearly, the most severe consequences to sexual response capabilities are due to radical pelvic surgeries. Detailed effects on female and male sexual physiology are described in Tables 24-2 and 24-3.

Effects from Pelvic Radiation on Female Function

External-beam radiation and intracavitary radiation (brachytherapy) are administered by the stage, cell type, and grade of the cancer. The use of external-beam radiation and the implantation of radioisotopes can result in temporary or permanent sexual alterations or dysfunction and the loss of ovarian function (Dembo and Thomas, 1994). Recent studies describe women who have experienced sexual dysfunction following radiation therapy for gynecologic tumors (Brunner et al., 1993; Thranov and Klee, 1994). Thranov and Klee (1994) found that sexual activity was not related to diagnosis or stage of disease. Of all patients with a partner (107 in this study), 22% expressed dissatisfaction with their sexual life after treatment. Despite a considerable decrease in sexual desire and frequent dyspareunia (difficult or painful coitus), many patients with gynecologic cancer continue to be sexually active.

Table 24-1   Cancer Surgeries That Cause Sexual Dysfunction

Type of Surgery	Sexual Dysfunction	Fertility Capability
Radical hysterectomy	♦ Radical surgery includes removal of all reproductive organs, including up to one half of the vagina and the broad ligaments, which causes possible discomfort with intercourse ♦ Feelings of lost femininity	Ovaries, fallopian tubes, and uterus are removed; patient is infertile and incapable of becoming pregnant
Radical vulvectomy	♦ Radical surgery may include removal of the clitoris, fatty and connective labial tissue, the urethra, the distal third of the vagina, the vulva, the anus, and lymph node dissection; this leads to narrowing of vaginal introitus, vaginal stenosis, perineal numbness, pain in scar area during intercourse ♦ Feelings of lost femininity and reduced acceptance of own body image	Usually occurs in postmenopausal women; pregnancy possible but discouraged due to extensive mutilation of perineum and lymph node dissection
Pelvic extenteration	♦ In total pelvic extenteration, organs removed include the distal sigmoid colon, the rectum, the bladder and distal portion of the ureters, all pelvic reproductive organs, the pelvic lymph nodes, the pelvic peritoneum, the levator muscles, and the perineum (McKenzie, 1988) ♦ Dysfunction manifested by creation of neovagina (Figure 24-1) and difficulty with dyspareunia, ability to have orgasm, and dry vagina (Beemer, Hopkins, Morley, 1988) ♦ Decreased femininity due to mutilation of genitals ♦ Decreased sexual desire due to multiple stomas	Because all reproductive organs are removed, sterility is complete
Radical prostatectomy	♦ Radical surgery includes removal of prostatic capsule, seminal vesicles, and a portion of the bladder neck; the vas deferens is tied off ♦ Erectile dysfunction occurs because of damage to the autonomic nerve plexus ♦ No ejaculate due to removal of seminal vesicles and transection of vas deferens ♦ If surgery is nerve-sparing, erectile capability usually remains (Waxman, 1993) ♦ Feelings of lost masculinity	After radical surgery, patient is infertile and unable to father a child because ejaculation is not possible

Penectomy	◆ Total penectomy involves amputation of the penis and dissection of surrounding lymph nodes ◆ Erection of remaining penile shaft, orgasm, and ejaculation still possible ◆ After a total penectomy, touch and friction in the perineal area promotes orgasm and ejaculation through perineal urethrostomy (Smith and Babian, 1992) ◆ Feelings of embarrassment and lost masculinity	Fertility not affected if partial penectomy is done; orgasm and ejaculation still occur; if penile shaft inadequate for vaginal penetration, artificial insemination can be substituted (Smith and Babian, 1992)
Orchiectomy	◆ *Unilateral* orchiectomy can cause decrease in orgasmic intensity, premature ejaculation, erectile dysfunction, and reduced sexual drive (Blackmore 1988) ◆ *Bilateral* orchiectomy causes loss of testosterone, decreased sexual desire, erectile dysfunction, atrophy of penis, and decreased body hair (Blackmore, 1988) ◆ Feelings of embarrassment, especially in young boys, and of lost masculinity	Fertility not affected in unilateral orchiectomy if endocrine function is adequate and normal sperm count and motility remain (Smith and Babian, 1992) Patient is infertile in bilateral orchiectomy due to loss of sperm production
Retroperitoneal lymph node dissection (RPLND)	◆ RPLND responsible for damage to sympathetic nerves, which affect ejaculation ◆ Patient may be unable to achieve erection ◆ Feelings of lost masculinity	If nerve-sparing surgery is done successfully, fertility is maintained. If not, patient is unable to achieve erection and/or ejaculation
Abdominal perineal resection (Female)	◆ After ostomy surgery, sexual dysfunction is rare due to nerve impairment; clitoral innervation is usually not disturbed; sensitivity remains ◆ Dyspareunia may result from removal of lower rectum and adhesion formation on posterior vaginal wall ◆ Decreased sexual desire and difficulty reaching an orgasm may occur	Fertility unaffected; pregnancy possible, although stoma may swell and become tender (Hogan, 1985)

Continued

Table 24-1 Cancer Surgeries That Cause Sexual Dysfunction—cont'd

Type of Surgery	Sexual Dysfunction	Fertility Capability
Abdominal perineal resection (Male)	◆ Possible nerve damage may result in erectile dysfunction, ejaculatory failure, or retrograde ejaculation ◆ Sexual desire may be decreased due to presence of ostomy (Cosimelli et al., 1994)	Fertility affected if unable to ejaculate; alternative is to salvage sperm by urinating immediately into a sterile container after retrograde ejaculation; viable sperm cells are centrifuged out and placed in a nutrient solution preparatory to use in artificial insemination (vonEschenbach and Schover, 1984)
Radical cystectomy (Female)	◆ Organs removed are the bladder, the urethra, the ureters, the ovaries, the fallopian tubes, and the interior vaginal wall (Schover, 1987) ◆ Dyspareunia due to reduced vaginal depth ◆ Decreased feelings of attractiveness and sexual desire due to loss of reproductive ability, urinary stoma, and surgical scars ◆ Atrophy and loss of vaginal secretions due to obliterated ovarian hormones ◆ Difficult reaching orgasm (Schover and vonEschenbach, 1985)	All reproductive organs are removed; sterility is complete
Radical cystectomy (Male)	◆ Organs removed include the bladder, the prostate, and the seminal vesicles ◆ Dysfunction is manifested by decreased masculinity due to dry orgasm ◆ Erectile dysfunction may occur due to injury to the pelvic autonomic plexus during dissection around the prostate and the urethra ◆ Orgasm possible with adequate stimulation and normal levels of sexual desire (Schover, Gonzales, and vonEschenbach, 1986)	Men experience dry orgasm because the prostate and seminal vesicles are removed; sterility is complete; sperm banking is recommended if children are desired

Table 24-2 Effects from Surgery for Pelvic or Genital Cancer on Female Sexual Physiology

Surgical Procedure	Hormonal Basis of Sexual Desire	Capacity for Pleasure with Genital Touch	Capacity for Vaginal Lubrication	Ease of Reaching Orgasm	Sensation of Orgasm	Dyspareunia
Radical hysterectomy	Unchanged*	Unchanged	Unchanged	Unchanged	Unchanged	Rare; must adjust to shallower vagina
Radical cystectomy	Unchanged*	Unchanged	Reduced	Unchanged, despite loss of anterior vaginal wall	Unchanged	Frequent, but can be reduced
Abdominoperineal resection	Unchanged*	Unchanged	Unchanged	Probably unchanged; no research available	Unchanged	Frequent, but can be reduced
Total pelvic exenteration and vaginal reconstruction using myocutaneous gracilis flaps	Unchanged*	Some loss of erotic zones, vagina, and occasionally part of vulva; erotic sensations still occur in remaining genital area; neovagina can develop erotic sensitivity	Lost; must use artificial lubricants in neovagina and daily douches to reduce odor	Often must relearn how to reach orgasm	Unchanged, or mild loss of intensity	Occasional, but can be reduced
Radical vulvectomy	Unchanged	Some loss of erotic zones; erotic sensations still occur in remaining genital area	Unchanged	Often must relearn how to reach orgasm	No research data available	Frequent, because of urethral irritation or stenosis of vaginal entrance; can be reduced

*Even if bilateral oophorectomy is included, adrenal androgens should maintain an adequate degree of desire. Some clinicians recommend a combination of androgen and estrogen replacement therapy. "Hot flashes" from estrogen deficiency may interfere with sexual pleasure. If bilateral oophorectomy is included, vaginal lubrication is reduced unless estrogen replacement therapy is prescribed. Dyspareunia is more common when surgery is combined with pelvic irradiation, which reduces vaginal lubrication even further and can promote vaginal atrophy and stenosis. Reprinted with permission from Schover LR and Fife M: Sexual counseling with radical pelvic or genital cancer surgery, J Psychosoc Oncol 3:21–41, 1985.

Table 24-3　Effects from Surgery for Pelvic or Genital Cancer on Male Sexual Physiology

Surgical Procedure	Hormonal Basis of Sexual Desire	Capacity for Pleasure with Genital Touch	Capacity for Erection	Sensation of Orgasm	Ejaculation	Dyspareunia
Radical prostatectomy	Unchanged	Unchanged	Usually impaired;* men younger than 60 are more likely to recover; full recovery takes 6 months	Unchanged, or mild loss of intensity	No semen produced; dry orgasm	Rare
Radical cystectomy	Unchanged	Unchanged	Usually impaired;* men younger than 60 are more likely to recover; full recovery takes 6 months	Unchanged, or mild loss of intensity	No semen produced; dry orgasm	Rare, but more likely after complete urethrectomy
Abdomino-perineal resection	Unchanged	Unchanged	Often impaired, but recovery rates are higher than for radical prostatectomy or cystectomy	Unchanged, or mild loss of intensity	Dry orgasm is common because of damage to presacral sympathetic nerves	Rare, but some perineal pain or phantom rectal sensations
Total pelvic exenteration	Unchanged	Unchanged	Almost always permanently impaired	Unchanged, or mild loss of intensity	No semen produced; dry orgasm	Occasional
Partial penectomy	Unchanged	Erotic sensations still occur in remaining genital area	Unchanged; penile shaft lengthens to permit coitus and (often) female orgasm	Unchanged	Unchanged	Rare; genital edema after groin dissection
Total penectomy	Unchanged	Erotic sensations still occur in remaining genital area	None	Unchanged, but need to relearn erotic zones	Unchanged, but semen is expelled through perineal urethrostomy	Occasional; genital edema after groin dissection

*With the development of new nerve-sparing surgical techniques, rates of erectile recovery are higher. However, a 6-month recovery period is still necessary. Reprinted with permission from Schover LR and Fife M: Sexual counseling with radical pelvic or genital cancer surgery, J Psychosoc Oncol 3:21–41, 1985.

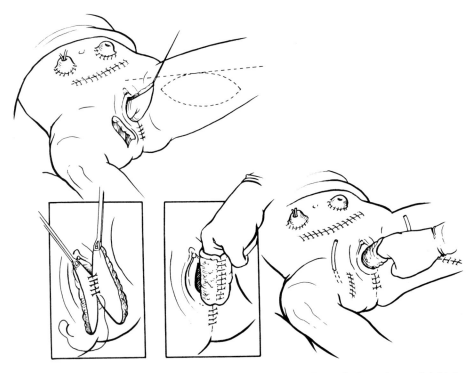

Fig. 24-1. Creation of a neovagina using full-thickness gracillis grafts from the medial thigh. From Rock J: TeLinde's operative gynecology, ed 7, Philadelphia, 1991, JB Lippincott Co.

Brunner et al. (1993) suggest that the increase in dyspareunia and decreased vaginal length may explain the decrease in sexual satisfaction, particularly in those treated for cervical carcinoma (see Patient Education Guidelines for Internal Radiation for Cervical Cancer on page 422). Although Brunner's study evaluated the length within the vaginal vault before and after treatment, no relationship was established.

During a 1-year follow-up, Schover and colleagues found that women who received radiation therapy experienced arousal-phase sexual dysfunction (Schover, Fife, and Gershenson, 1989). In addition, these women worked less outside the home, performed fewer household chores, took less care of their families, and socialized less, suggesting that the overall quality of life became worse within 1 year after radiation therapy. Table 24-4 describes the sexual dysfunction and fertility capability of women with a gynecologic malignancy after treatment with radiation therapy.

When whole-abdomen radiation is used, sterility is the most predominant long-term side effect. The effect of radiation on oocytes depends on the patient's age, the radiation dose, and the dose fraction. Oophoropexy can be performed as a means to preserve ovarian function. This procedure relocates the ovaries outside the area of radiation, thereby preventing exposure by (1) surgically suspending the ovaries within the pelvis outside treatment field, or (2) placing them midline behind the uterus. Shielding devices are sometimes used to protect ovarian function (Yarbro and Perry, 1985). Radiation therapy of the abdomen, the pelvis, and the

Patient Education Guidelines for

Internal Radiation for Cervical Cancer

♦ Intracavitary implants (radioactive sources placed directly into the vagina) require you to be admitted to the hospital into a private room.

♦ Be sure to bring reading material or an interesting hobby such as needlepoint to occupy your time.

♦ Visitors will have limited time to see you during your hospitalization. Instructions will be provided regarding the amount of time and the distance away from you visitors must stay to protect them from radiation. Visitors under 18 years of age and women who are or may be pregnant are not permitted to visit.

♦ The nursing staff will have limited time to spend caring for you. However, assistance is always readily available.

♦ Before the implantation, an enema will be given to reduce bowel activity while the radioactive source is in place. Medication will be given to prevent bowel activity during your hospitalization. A vaginal douche will be given to cleanse the vagina and a Foley catheter will be inserted into the bladder. Your diet will be restricted to liquids or low-residue foods.

♦ The applicators will be placed inside of you in the operating suite when you are under anesthesia. The procedure is not actually a surgical procedure but a placement of applicators within the pelvic cavity.

♦ After the applicator is determined to be in the correct position, you will return to your room and the implant will be placed in the applicator.

♦ During the time you have the implants, you must stay flat on your back, with the head of the bed elevated 20°. You can roll from side to side. The linen will not be changed unless it becomes soiled. You will receive a daily bath, but only from the waist up. This is to prevent dislodging the applicators.

♦ After the prescribed treatment, the implant will be removed. Afterwards the Foley catheter will be removed and a vaginal douche will be given. An enema is usually given to initiate bowel activity, and then you will be discharged from the hospital.

♦ After the implants are removed, you will not be radioactive. You will not have to take special precautions because your urine, feces, or vomitus will not be radioactive.

Permission granted to reproduce these guidelines for educational purposes only.

lymph nodes can cause short-term side effects such as fatigue, bone marrow depression, nausea, vomiting, diarrhea, enteritis, weight loss, dysuria, urinary frequency, and decreased vaginal lubrication and sensation. These can affect sexuality.

Pelvic radiation therapy also causes ovulation to cease and production of estradiol and progesterone to end (Dembo and Thomas, 1994). The oocyte in the premature follicle is more sensitive to radiation damage than the ovum of the mature follicle, and in the graafian follicle the oocyte may be more radiosensitive than the ovum.

Table 24-4 The Sexual/Fertility Effect of Irradiation on the Female Client

Region of Treatment	Sexual Dysfunction	Fertility Capability
External Beam Whole pelvis Abdomen Paraaortic lymph nodes Pelvic lymph nodes	Symptoms of bowel and bladder dysfunction may impede enjoyment of intercourse The management of side effects often diverts attention away from sexual activity and produces feelings of decreased sexual desirability and reduced frequency Hormonal imbalance, vaginal dryness, hot flashes, and dyspareunia The decline of sexual activity may be a temporary side effect	Loss of ovarian function, leading to sterility Age: Dependent <20 yr 70% chance of retaining regular cyclic menses 30 yr 20% chance of normal ovarian function >40 yr women are virtually sterile and 100% experience amenorrhea; ovaries can be repositioned with oophoropexy
Intracavitary Implant within vaginal vault and/or into the uterine cavity	As above Predominantly, vaginal lubrication and sensation are decreased Change in coital position may be necessary May take longer to reach orgasm Vaginal soreness after coitus may be present Postcoital bleeding Vaginal stenosis and atrophy or necrosis	"Scatter" radiation may affect ovarian function

Data from Bruner et al., 1993; Hellman, 1993; Lamb, 1985; Peck, McGrier, and Kretchmer, 1940; Schover, Schain, and Montague, 1989; Thranov and Klee, 1994.

Radiation for cervical cancer causes an acute mucosal reaction of moist desquamation about 4 to 6 weeks after initiation of therapy. The area becomes sore and sensitive to touch.

Late effects of pelvic radiation, which develop over 2 to 5 years, tend to obliterate the cervix, shorten the vagina, and cause fibrosis and stenosis of the vaginal wall. Chronic mucosal ulceration with bleeding, sepsis, or fistula formation can occur. Edema and vascular changes can occur in the submucosa and myometrium of the uterine corpus. The secondary changes occur because of ovarian obliteration with hormonal depletion.

Effects from Pelvic Radiation on Male Function

The testicle is very sensitive to radiation due to the prolonged cell cycle of the germinal epithelium. Mutations occur in the process of spermatogenesis and the semen volume decreases. Doses of 0.3 to 1 Gy cause temporary oligspermia with 25% recovery in a year; 2 to 3 Gy cause azoospermia with 75% recovery within 40 months; and 4 Gy or more can cause permanent sterility (Rowley, Leach, and Warner, 1986). External-beam radiation to the pelvis can cause fibrosis of the pelvic vascular system and interfere with penile blood flow needed for erectile function, resulting in the inability to achieve or maintain an erection.

Recovery of sexual function as well as spermatogenesis is thought to occur in 1 to 5 years after treatment, although some studies have shown residual oligospermia and a decrease in seminal volume even after fertility returns. Using questionnaires, Schover, Gonzales, and vonEschenbach (1986) interviewed 84 men who had received radiation therapy for seminoma testicular cancer about sexual function, marital status, and fertility. In response, 12% reported low sexual desire, 15% reported erectile dysfunction, and 49% reported a reduced semen volume at an average of 9.7 years after diagnosis.

Approximately 40% to 60% of those who receive external-beam radiation for prostate cancer report a gradual loss of ability to achieve or maintain an erection over a period of 6 to 12 months after treatment (Banker, 1988; Beiler, Wright, and Reddy, 1981; Hanks, Myers, and Scardino, 1993). These figures appear highly dependent on the individual's level of sexual activity before diagnosis and treatment. Banker (1988) surveyed 100 men regarding impotence after they received external-beam radiation therapy for prostate cancer, and he asked them to rank their degree of sexual activity. Those who had intercourse more than three times per month before diagnosis regained potency 73% of the time, while those who had sex less frequently reported a 40% to 46% rate of potency. Patients who receive radiation to the pelvis for bladder or colorectal cancer experience problems with impotence similar to those experienced by patients treated for prostate cancer.

Prostate cancer may also be treated with interstitially placed, sealed radioactive isotopes. This form of treatment leaves only 15% of patients impotent, as compared to 40% to 50% when treated with external-beam radiation, due to decreased exposure to radiation of the entire pelvis (Hanks, Myers, and Scardino, 1993). Other side effects from this treatment resemble side effects from external-beam radiation.

Hodgkin's lymphoma accounts for 1% to 7% of all testicular tumors (American Cancer Society, 1991). Treatment for this disease often involves irradiation of the pelvic lymph nodes, which subsequently produces toxicities such as fibrosis of the pelvic vasculature, glandular tissue atrophy, and blood vessel changes. Many bone marrow transplant treatment regimens, especially those for lymphoma and leukemia, include the use of total body irradiation. Azoospermia was almost universal in male bone marrow transplant patients treated with 10 Gy of total body irradiation in a single fraction, with only 2 of 41 patients recovering normal sperm counts 6 years after transplantation (Deeg, Storb, and Thomas, 1984; Sanders, 1982).

Effects from Chemotherapy and Hormone Therapy

Chemotherapy and hormone therapy cause problems in the reproductive system and affect the endocrine capability of the gonads, causing hormone deficiencies that increase the risk of heart disease, bone fractures, and emotional distress. Gonadal toxicity after treatment with chemotherapy depends on the type of drug (Table 24-5) (alkylating agents are the most destructive), the dosage, and the age and sex of the patient (Kreuser et al., 1990). Rivkees and Crawford (1988) explained that because chemotherapeutic agents usually affect cells with a high mitotic rate, it is understandable that damage occurs more often in sexually mature males than in prepubescent males and females. Specifically, gametogenesis has not yet begun in children, and men experience greater mitotic activity in the testis than women do in the ovary.

A useful marker to assess reproductive function (i.e., production of sperm and ova) during and after chemotherapy administration is the level of serum follicle-stimulating hormone (FSH). After the depletion of testicular germinal stem cells and ovarian follicles, a rise in the FSH level occurs. The level of luteinizing hormone (LH) can also be a helpful indicator of toxicity; however, these levels tend to rise in women before they do in men. LH in men indicates Leydig cell activity, and these cells tend to remain essentially intact during chemotherapy (Sherins and Mulvihill, 1989).

Clinically, ovarian dysfunction is progressive, and women will experience menopausal symptoms such as amenorrhea or irregular menses, hot flashes, decreased libido, and possibly nervousness, anxiety, and depression (Ingle, 1990). Unlike the gradual increase of effects on the ovary, testicular damage happens abruptly, with resulting oligospermia or azoospermia. Testosterone levels, however, usually remain unaffected because Leydig cell function remains unimpaired (Ingle, 1990).

Although many agents cause specific effects on fertility in men and women, they can also cause severe general systemic effects that interfere with sexual expression. These include gastrointestinal and pulmonary toxicity, neurotoxicity, cardiotoxicity, alopecia, fatigue, and bone marrow suppression. It is important to remember how devastating these toxicities and effects can be to a sexual relationship and especially to the patient's self-esteem. Remedies to relieve these side effects are discussed in other chapters.

Effects from Biotherapy

Biological response modifiers (BRMs) are being used with increasing frequency. Unfortunately, little is known about their toxic effects on gonadal function. In one

Table 24-5 The Effect of Chemotherapy Drugs on Fertility

Disease	Chemotherapy	Sexual Dysfunction	Fertility Capability
Hodgkin's disease	MOPP (Mustargen, Oncovin, procarbazine, prednisone) ABVD (Adriamycin, bleomycin, vinblastine, dacarbazine)	Female: Ovarian failure that leads to dry vagina and dyspareunia; systemic effects (e.g., alopecia and fatigue) lead to poor body image and possible decreased sexual desire. Male: Decreased testicular function leads to decreased sense of masculinity and possible difficulty with erection; systemic side effects lead to decreased sexual desire	Female: Ovarian failure reported with MOPP therapy in 28% of patients under age 24 and 86% over age 24 (Kreuser et al., 1990); patient infertile; fewer problems with ABVD regimen. Male: Decreased testicular function affects spermatogenesis (ranging from oligospermia to azospermia); infertility reported in 70–100% of patients treated with MOPP; toxicity markedly less with ABVD (Kreuser et al., 1990; Carde et al., 1993)
Leukemia	Cytarabine, daunomycin, methotrexate, asparaginase, vincristine, prednisone, 6-mercaptopurine	Female: Ovarian function not appreciably disturbed; systemic effects will cause decreased sense of self-image and consequent loss of sexual desire. Male: Acute gonadal toxicity and systemic effects may affect masculinity with possible erection problems and decreased sexual desire	No chronic ovarian toxicity; fertility maintained. No chronic testicular failure; sperm production is normalized and fertility maintained
Testicular cancer	Cisplatin, vinblastine, bleomycin	Vascular or neurotoxicities may affect erectile capability; knowledge that azospermia occurs after chemotherapy and fear of systemic effects may decrease self-concept and sense of masculinity	Spermatogenesis returns in approximately 48 months after therapy is complete; fertility is retained (Kreuser et al., 1990)
Prostate cancer	(Hormone) LHRH antagonist (Lupron); antiandrogen (Flutamide); estrogen therapy (rarely used today)	Low levels of testosterone will result, leading to a lowered level of sexual desire, erectile dysfunction, less pleasurable orgasm, decreased semen production, diminished spermatogenesis; estrogen therapy leads to gynecomastia (breast enlargement), feminization, erectile dysfunction, penile and testicular atrophy, decreased spermatogenesis; decreased sense of masculinity	Because these men usually must stay on these hormones to reduce the risk of reoccurrence, they will usually be infertile
Breast cancer	Methotrexate or doxorubicin, cyclophosphamide, 5-fluorouracil	Decreased sense of femininity and self-worth due to systemic side effects; ovarian failure may cause vaginal lubrication problems; decreased sexual desire	Ovarian function returns; fertility remains

study, sexual dysfunction occurred in 81 males with hairy-cell leukemia who received alpha interferon (IFN-α) (Schilsky et al., 1987). Many of these patients experienced low testosterone levels, along with elevated FSH levels. However, Schilsky et al. (1987) reported that after further follow-up "prospective analysis of testicular function in a larger number of patients receiving IFN failed to confirm our initial impression that IFN may produce significant gonadal toxicity" (p. 180). Reiger (1994) mentions decreased libido associated with IFN administration but not with administration of other BRMs. Information available in the package inserts of many of the BRMs instruct patients to use contraceptive methods to avoid pregnancy while taking the drug. Recent nursing literature available on these drugs, however, makes no mention of gonadal toxicities (Brophy and Sharp, 1991; Dudjak, 1993; Sharp, 1993; Shelton, 1993). Even though these agents may not cause concern about sterility, sexuality issues will most likely surface related to their systemic side effects, especially fatigue.

Effects from Multimodal Therapy

Myers and Schilsky (1992) found that women who received MVPP (mechlorethamine, vinblastine, procarbazine, and prednisone) for Hodgkin's disease reported a higher incidence of menopausal symptoms and menstrual irregularities when treated with total nodal irradiation. Autopsies of girls who received at least one alkylating agent for extragonadal tumors found that more than 50% had a decrease in the number of ovarian follicles and an increase in stromal fibrosis. When radiation therapy had been given in addition to chemotherapy, the results were more severe (Myers and Schilsky, 1992).

In another review of literature on combined chemotherapy and radiation therapy, von der Masse (1994) focused on several studies of the effects on the testis. When given before radiation, bleomycin, carmustine, cyclophosphamide, procarbazine, and vincristine each enhanced the effects of radiation. When given concomitantly with radiation, bleomycin, carmustine, cyclophosphamide, hydroxyurea, procarbazine, and vincristine each greatly enhanced the effects of radiation. Carmustine, cyclophosphamide, hydroxyurea, procarbazine, and vincristine also enhanced radiation effects to the testis when given after radiation.

Radical prostatectomy or cervical surgery followed by adjuvant pelvic radiation therapy caused sexual dysfunction and rectal stenosis. Radiation therapy followed by adjuvant chemotherapy also causes increased sexual dysfunction.

Effects from Other Factors

Anxiety, stress, and depression can have an indirect effect on gonadal function. Whether or not the relationship becomes dysfunctional often depends on how stable the relationship was before the cancer diagnosis (Shell, 1994). Anxiety and stress can accentuate a treatment-induced problem such as impotence or painful intercourse and can be a devastating occurrence that adversely affects the patient's sense of femininity or masculinity. The nurse must acknowledge each patient's unique sexual identity and promote various methods of sexually relating other than penile-vaginal intercourse. This will help to overcome the patient's feelings of unattractiveness and decreased desirability, which in turn will help to decrease the stress and anxiety of illness. Although sexual expression may be altered by disease, sexuality itself is not destroyed by cancer or its treatment (Smith and Babian, 1992).

❖ Nursing Management

Key elements of a comprehensive and timely assessment are provided in Table 24-6. These elements enhance the nurse's and the patient's comfort during this most sensitive discussion. It is important to be able to provide open, honest information and to establish trust and rapport with the patient and partner. Many nurses inquire about how to "get started" talking about sexuality with their patients. The literature provides various approaches, including the PLISSIT method and Schain's (1988) PLEASURE model. Some approaches are simple, while others include very comprehensive and in-depth questions. One of the easiest methods to use includes a few simple questions, such as those in Box 24-2, which can be directed to the patient during a bath, a chat about chemotherapy and its side effects, or any other conversation about psychosocial matters. These questions are non-gender-based and are appropriate to use with either heterosexual or homosexual patients and couples.

Table 24-6   Nursing Assessment Guidelines

Necessary Elements	How to Accomplish
Provide privacy	If the patient is not in a private room, move to another area such as an office or a conference room. If this is not possible, pull the curtain and speak in low tones.
Ensure patient confidentiality	Assure the patient and his or her partner that your conversation is private. Meet privately with the patient first, then include the partner, if possible. If the patient reveals a homosexual preference, strict confidentiality is essential, unless the patient has made this public knowledge.
Determine patient goals and priorities	Remember that all patients do not experience sexual satisfaction in the same way. They may not have a partner or want one. Ascertain their preferences and have various suggestions ready to explain.
Address sexual concerns early	Establish a relationship with the patient (you may have only one meeting) that will permit open discussion of any sexual concerns. Initiate discussion early in the relationship. This implies that sexuality is an important component of good health.
Avoid overreaction	Listen to the patient with genuine interest, which conveys acceptance. Do not reveal shock or surprise with your facial expressions. Keep personal feelings to yourself.
Refer patients for complex problems	Know your referral options and use them if a problem is too complex or beyond the scope within which you can be helpful.

Adapted from Shell J: Impact of cancer on sexuality. In Otto S, editor: Oncology nursing, ed 2, St. Louis, 1994, Mosby.

Box 24-2 Questions to Ask Patients Related to Sexuality

◆ Does your cancer (or its treatment) change the way you see yourself as a man (woman)?
◆ Do you have a special or significant person, partner, or lover?
◆ Who lives at home with you?
◆ Patients who are beginning treatment for cancer often worry about how these treatments can affect the physical part of the relationship with their partner. Do you have any concerns about that?
◆ Do you expect your sexual function to change in any way after your cancer treatments?

After these questions become incorporated into the nurse's assessment, the nurse's comfort level about discussing sexuality will increase. When nurses begin to incorporate these questions into their assessment vocabulary, the author often advocates soliciting assistance from the nurse's significant other, a friend, or a patient the nurse knows well. This can help ease feelings of uncertainty and promote increased articulation and the satisfaction of acquiring a new skill.

Psychosocially there are many elements of the cancer experience that may affect sexuality. However, first it is important to ascertain the patient's sexual life-style status. Is the patient involved in any type of sexual relationship, and, if so, is it homosexual, heterosexual, a monogamous relationship in a familial environment, or perhaps one of multiple casual relationships? If patients do not have a sexual partner, it cannot be assumed that they will be unaffected by the sexual complications of the disease; treatment can still cripple their self-image.

A homosexual relationship will encounter much of the same stress and strain as a heterosexual relationship during the cancer experience. After the relationship is disclosed to the nurse, a discussion about emerging sexual dysfunction should take place with the patient and partner. As with heterosexual couples, gays and lesbians are nurtured by a strong spiritual closeness and find sexual satisfaction in ways that do not necessarily involve direct genital activity.

Whether heterosexual or homosexual, individuals who engage in multiple sexual encounters should be counseled that this life-style is likely to change. At this crucial and frightening time, it is imperative to have a strong bond with someone capable of providing emotional support such as a trusted friend or a close sexual partner. Research has shown that if partners are supportive before diagnosis, they tend to be supportive after diagnosis (Anderson and Jochimsen, 1985; Renshaw, 1986). Timely discussion of possible or probable sexual dysfunction and ways to manage it can help all couples tolerate treatment with less stress. Also, the confidence that sexual problems have been recognized, or being dealt with, and may be satisfactorily overcome could inspire greater compliance with therapy.

Many factors influence sexuality during treatment for cancer, and patients must be made aware that effective interventions are available to preserve their masculinity and femininity. Patients must learn about the possible sexual changes that occur during or after therapy and receive counseling about options for preventing or correcting problems of sexual dysfunction and about any myths they may have related to their sexuality and the cancer experience (Smith and Babian, 1992). If the patient is currently in a relationship, the love, support, intimacy, and understanding of the partner can help restore the patient's self-confidence and determination to survive the disease and the treatment. Specific interventions on how to adapt to sexual changes can be communicated to the patient and partner if they express a desire to know. These are presented in Nursing Management of Specific Sexual Changes on page 431. Some patients may hesitate to ask questions about sexual function, or perhaps they are no longer interested or involved in a sexual relationship. A couple's values and beliefs are significant to the success of any suggested intervention, and what may be acceptable expression for some may not be for others (Shell, 1994). Often, however, once permission is given to the couple by the nurse to consider alternatives to their sexual expression or their sexuality, they may eagerly accept these suggestions with anticipation. Not only will rehabilitation of some of their sexual concerns begin but their self-image and self-esteem will be restored as well.

Contraception

Many women patients assume that they cannot become pregnant if they stop menstruating during chemotherapy administration. Males assume they cannot impregnate their partners if the physician has told them that their sperm count will drop or that sperm production will cease during treatment. This should be emphatically refuted and contraceptive measures should be explained to the patient and the partner. Although teratogenic effects are not noted in chemotherapy patients after the first trimester, effective contraception is recommended to avoid the possibility of this type of complication. Hormone manipulation (birth control pills) can be useful if this is not deleterious to the disease process. Otherwise, barrier methods (condoms, sponge, cervical cap, and diaphragm) with a spermicide are recommended.

Sperm Banking

Sperm banking and artificial insemination are now feasible alternatives for most men undergoing treatment for cancer. This is due to the advent of several assisted reproductive technologies (ART) such as in vitro fertilization (IVF), gamete intrafallopian transfer (GIFT), and zygote intrafallopian transfer (ZIFT), which allow men with lower than normal sperm concentrations to take advantage of semen cryopreservation.

The IVF program has four steps:

- Development of ovarian follicles (sacs containing the eggs) and ripening of the eggs
- Collection of the oocytes (eggs)
- Fertilization of an egg and growth of the embryo (it takes about 18 hours for fertilization to be completed and approximately 12 more hours for the fertilized cell to divide into two cells)
- Replacement of the embryo into the uterus (Michigan Reproductive and IVF Center, 1993).

Nursing Management of

Specific Sexual Changes

Female-Specific Sexual Changes

If the patient had a radical hysterectomy, suggest the following interventions to increase sexual intimacy:

◆ A change in the angle of penile thrust can be accomplished by elevating the hips on one or two pillows.

◆ A deeper vaginal barrel can be mimicked by enclosing the penis in one or both palms (Donahue and Knapp, 1977).

◆ Vaginal penetration from behind, between closely adducted thighs, may increase pleasure for both partners.

◆ If coitus is not possible, the basic mechanics of cunnilingus (application of tongue or mouth to the vulva) and/or fellatio (sexual gratification by intromission of the penis into another individual's mouth) should be explained.

◆ Vaginal lubricants (e.g., Lubrin, Replens, Gyne-Moistrin, and Astroglide) can be purchased over the counter and be used to decrease irritation and dyspareunia. These vaginal moisturizers are odorless, greaseless, and tasteless and last longer than substances such as KY jelly. Patients should be cautioned against the use of Vaseline, because it is greasy and can block the urethra. Flavored lubricants are also available if the couple is interested in oral-vaginal loveplay.

◆ If an indwelling catheter remains after hospitalization, it can be placed up over the lower abdomen and taped in place.

◆ Expressing love in alternative oral, anal, and digital styles can be fulfilling and pleasurable for some couples.

◆ Any time ovaries are removed, hot flashes, sweats, and restlessness will probably follow. To relieve these symptoms, Bellergal-S tablets may be prescribed.

If the patient had a pelvic exenteration, suggest the following interventions to increase sexual intimacy:

◆ Regarding adaptation to a bowel or bladder conduit and worries about appearance, appliance fit, possible leakage and odor, please see recommendations under ostomies.

◆ Sexual stimulation of other erotic areas such as the anus, the urethra, the ostia of the ileal conduit or colostomy, and the scar tissue in the area of the vulva is encouraged.

◆ Mutual masturbation may also be arousing.

If the patient had a colorectal resection, suggest the following interventions to increase sexual intimacy:

◆ Prepare the pouch (empty and deodorize it) and verify that the seal is intact before engaging in sexual activity. If the ostomy is dry (controllable with irrigation), a cover or patch can be used instead of a bag.

◆ Patients should avoid foods that cause gas or loose stool at least 6 to 12 hours before intercourse. Because there is no control over flatus from the stoma, it may be helpful to rehearse a response to avoid an uncomfortable moment.

◆ Attractive camouflage such as an opaque pouch cover, a cummerbund, lingerie, underwear with an opening up the center, or modified satin boxer shorts can be worn. Lingerie and underwear are also available with inside pockets to hold the pouch. (Ask local ostomy associations where these are available in your area.)

Continued

◆ A rubber sheet can be placed under the bedsheet and a towel on top of it to protect the mattress in case of leakage. It is important that the patient and partner have a sense of humor regarding the pouch and to expect that it will probably leak sometime during sexual activity.
◆ Various sexual positions may need to be tried because a stoma may get rubbed or irritated during sex in the traditional missionary position.
◆ Patients and partners should be warned not to put anything in the stoma (including a penis) because this will cause a dangerous tear. The stoma can be stimulated carefully during sexual activity or masturbation, but objects should not be placed inside it.

If the patient had a vulvectomy, suggest the following interventions to increase sexual intimacy:
◆ Comfort during intercourse will be enhanced if the female sits astride the male because she can then control penile penetration to her tolerance.
◆ With a vaginal lubricant, finger manipulation can help stretch the vaginal orifice during foreplay, which decreases the discomfort of immediate penetration with a penis or a dildo.
◆ Patients can do exercises to prevent vaginismus. Kegel exercises, usually taught to obstetrical patients to help gain control over the pubococcygeal muscles, can increase muscle tone. These exercises involve tightening and relaxing the muscles of the perineum several times a day, and they can even be done while driving a car or sitting at a desk.

If the patient had a radical cystectomy, many of the aforementioned interventions can help increase sexual intimacy.

If the patient had radiation therapy for any of the above disease sites, suggest the following interventions to increase sexual intimacy:
◆ Sexual intercourse to tolerance during treatment is encouraged to decrease possible adhesion development. If the area becomes tender because of a radiation reaction, intercourse must cease, but it can resume after healing occurs.
◆ A water soluble lubricant will most likely need to be used at all times after radiation is finished to decrease vaginal irritation and discomfort. This can be applied as a part of foreplay or privately.
◆ The female superior position can be used to allow more control but may not be as comfortable. Rear entry can also be used.
◆ Vaginal dilators must be used for at least the first three years after completion of radiation if the patient is not sexually active. Patients with partners may also use dilators if intercourse is too exhausting or uncomfortable during and immediately after treatment. Sensitivity to patient and partner is necessary when explaining the importance of dilator use (Dow, 1992).

Male-Specific Sexual Changes
If the patient had a prostatectomy, suggest the following interventions to increase sexual intimacy:
◆ Although the frequency of sexual arousal can decrease, the patient may still be aroused by the correct stimulus. Arousal can be stimulated by erotic books, pictures, or movies. Long periods of foreplay (e.g., romantic dinners, bathing together, a different environment) can also be stimulating.

◆ If the patient is unable to have an erection with enough stiffness for penetration, mutual masturbation can allow the patient to reach orgasm and ejaculation. The partner should massage the penis by pushing down with pressure at the base of the penis. The penis should not be pulled up toward the abdomen or it can lose blood. A female partner can assist erection by inserting a partially erect penis into the vagina and flexing her perineal muscles.

◆ If urinary incontinence is a problem, the patient should always urinate before intercourse, and perhaps wear a condom if the partner is bothered by this occurrence. Remind the couple that urine is sterile and can be washed off immediately.

◆ Penile implants are available in several varieties (rigid, semirigid, and inflatable), and the risks and benefits should be explained to the patient and his partner. (For an in-depth explanation, see Shell, 1994.) Currently patients are given the option of having an implant done at the time of surgery or of waiting until approximately 6 months after surgery to ascertain erectile damage.

◆ Penile self-injection to stimulate erection is another option (Figure 24-2). The dose is titrated to produce an erection with satisfactory tumescence (circumference) and rigidity for vaginal penetration (Pierce et al., 1991). Two frequently used drugs are Papaverine, a smooth muscle relaxant that produces vasodilation, and Phentolamine, an adrenergic blocker that also produces vasodilation (Al-Juburi and O'Donnell, 1987). An injection of Alprostadil diluted with normal saline can also be used.

◆ Vacuum devices to provide for erection are another alternative. There are two products currently available on the market that produce an erection by using negative pressure to draw blood into the penis and create tumescence. A constricting device placed around the base of the penis keeps the blood in the penis (Figure 24-3).

If the patient had an orchiectomy or a retroperitoneal lymph node dissection, suggest the following interventions to increase sexual intimacy:

◆ If a retroperitoneal lymph node dissection has destroyed erectile capabilities, the preceding suggestions may serve this patient population also.

◆ Although sexual desire may decrease at this time because of surgery and/or chemotherapy, serum testosterone levels may have decreased too, and replacement therapy may be required.

◆ If absence of ejaculation is a problem, alpha-adrenergic drugs Entex LA or Ornade can be tried. These drugs can also intensify orgasm for some patients (Schover, 1987; Shell, 1994).

◆ If the loss of a testicle causes embarrassment, a silicone prosthesis can be placed, often at the time of surgery (Gritz et al., 1989). These can also be used for patients with prostate cancer who have had both testicles removed to promote hormonal manipulation of their disease.

◆ Sexual relations may resume approximately 6 weeks after surgery if physiologically possible. If patients have permanent erectile dysfunction, sperm banking is available (see page 430).

If the patient had a penectomy, suggest the following interventions to increase sexual intimacy:

◆ After the penectomy, if the remaining stump is not sufficient for penetration, the couple may wish to use a phallic vibrator as a penis substitute.

Continued

◆ If a total penectomy has occurred, stimulation of the mons pubis, the perineum, and the scrotum can produce orgasms with pleasurable contractions in the remaining cavernous musculature.

If the patient had a radical cystectomy, suggest the following interventions to increase sexual intimacy:
◆ Suggestions for ostomy patients and the aforementioned male-specific recommendations apply to this patient population.

If the patient had a colorectal cancer, refer to the female-specific interventions described above to increase sexual intimacy.

Neutropenia and Thrombocytopenia
For male or female patients experiencing neutropenia or thrombocytopenia, see the Patient Education Guidelines on sexual intimacy on page 413.

The GIFT procedure is somewhat different in that the sperm and eggs are mixed and injected into one or both fallopian tubes. After the gametes have been transferred, fertilization can take place in the fallopian tube as it does in natural reproduction. ZIFT is another procedure in which the egg is fertilized in vitro and the zygote is transferred to the fallopian tube at the pronuclear stage before cell division takes place. The eggs are harvested and fertilized in one day, and the embryo is transferred the following day (Michigan Reproductive and IVF Center, 1993). In 1988 reported pregnancy rates that resulted in live births were about 12% for IVF and approximately 17% to 22% for GIFT (American Fertility Society, 1989; Levran

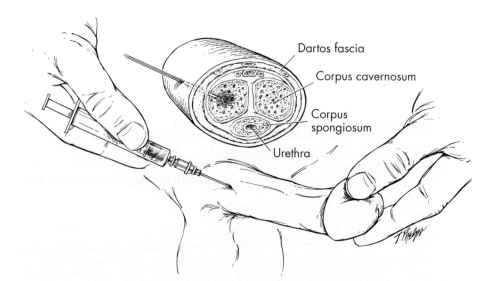

Fig. 24-2. Method of penile self-injection to stimulate erection. Reprinted with permission of American Family Physician, March 1988, vol. 37, no. 3, and Tim Phelps, illustrator, Georgetown University Medical Center.

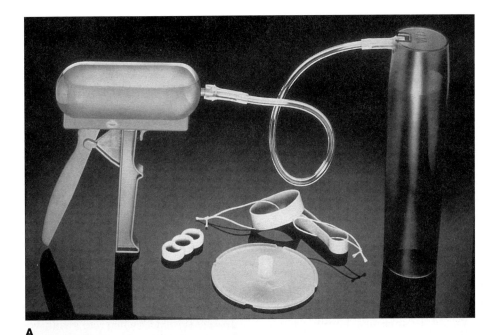

A

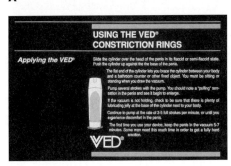

**USING THE VED®
CONSTRICTION RINGS**

Applying the VED®

B

Fig. 24-3. **A,** The vacuum erection device (VED) is used to help a man with impotence problems attain an erection. **B,** Directions for application of the vacuum erection device (VED). Reprinted with permission of Mission Pharmaco Co.

et al., 1990). The patient will undoubtedly have questions about this and other matters when he and his partner are considering sperm banking and any of the ART procedures. The patient should be helped to evaluate all the options available to him.

Before ART was available, men interested in sperm banking had to have 20 million sperm per ml of semen with 60% motility (Smith and Babian, 1992). This was often difficult, especially for those men who had a diagnosis of testicular cancer or Hodgkin's disease, because they often had low sperm counts at the time of diagnosis. Recently Sanger, Olson, and Sherman (1992) reported 115 live births after artificial insemination with semen from men having various cancers, some of whom had as few as 500,000 motile spermatozoa. Of these 115 births, there were no reports of birth defects.

Cryogenic Laboratories, Inc. (CLI) reports that semen from patients with cancer can be stored in liquid nitrogen on a long-term basis (up to 16 to 18 years) and still result in normal live births. However, cryobanking may not be feasible for all men because sperm motility may be adversely affected by the freezing process and may decline after thawing. CLI requires that a complete post-thaw analysis be performed routinely on all semen specimens to determine cryosurvival parameters (Cryogenic Laboratories, Inc., 1993). Fees for sperm banking usually include laboratory semen analysis ($170 per specimen) and an annual storage fee ($120 per account). If a man wants to bank two specimens, it costs $340 for analysis and $120 for storage.

Oocyte Banking

The options for women are somewhat different than for men. Oocytes cannot be cryopreserved because of their fragility, but embryos can, with the intent of thawing and transferring them to the uterus at a later date. Therefore embryos are created using the spouse's or partner's sperm. Theoretically the cryopreserved embryos can remain in this state indefinitely, although most are used within a 2-year period. After the decision is made to thaw the embryos, each one is examined to determine whether it is medically appropriate (normal-looking) to transfer to the uterus. Usually about 50% of embryos will survive the freezing-and-thawing process. "Usual success rate with frozen embryos transferred in the human has not been well-established, however, it is approximately 5% to 15% when 3 to 4 embryos are transferred back," (Michigan Reproductive and IVF Center, 1993).

Oral Contraceptives and Luteinizing-Hormone-Releasing Hormone (LHRH) Agonists

Because chemotherapy can be particularly devastating to the female and male gonads, researchers have been looking at the possibility of using oral contraceptives and LHRH agonists to halt spermatogenesis in men and ovulation in women, thereby protecting gonadal function from chemotherapy-induced adverse events. However, the administration of testosterone to men, oral contraceptives (estrogen-progesterone) to women and gonadotropin-releasing hormone (GNRH) to men and women does not seem particularly useful or effective (Sherins and Mulvihill, 1989). Unfortunately, current evidence suggests that gonadal function in men and women (spermatogenesis and ovulation) does not completely return to pretreatment normal standards and seems unaffected by the use of contraceptives or LHRH agonists as possible protective agents (Kreuser et al., 1990; Rivkees and Crawford, 1988).

Oophoropexy

Oophoropexy, an additional method to protect fertility, is discussed on page 421.

❖ Pregnancy During and Following Cancer Treatment

In pregnant women, the most common cancers that occur include breast, cervical, ovarian, lymphoma, and colorectal cancers (Harris, 1990). Several factors must be considered when deciding whether or not to treat the patient during pregnancy, especially during the first trimester, because the potential for fetal loss or malformation is greatest during this period (Harris, 1990). These factors include gestational age of the fetus; maternal and fetal health at the time of diagnosis; the mother's prognosis and likelihood of having future pregnancies after treatment; and the known teratogenic effects of chemotherapeutic agents. Mulvihill et al. (1987) reported fetal loss or fetal abnormality in 28% of women who received therapy at conception or during early pregnancy for lymphoma, Hodgkin's disease, or leukemia. During the second and third trimester, chemotherapy is generally not associated with fetal malformation.

Radiation therapy can cause teratogenic effects throughout pregnancy. If the fetus is exposed, especially during the first 2 to 9 weeks, fetal loss or major malformation may result. Abnormal development of the central nervous system, retarded growth, hypogonadism, and sterility can occur if the fetus is exposed later in pregnancy.

Women should be counseled to use contraception during treatment, because in addition to the trauma of the cancer diagnosis it is devastating to have to decide whether or not to terminate a pregnancy. However, patients may wish to terminate an abnormal pregnancy because of treatment-related effects detected on a fetal ultrasound monitor or through cytogenetic testing of amniotic fluid.

Pregnancy after treatment for cancer is usually not discouraged, but there is no consensus on how long a woman should wait before becoming pregnant. The "old rule" specified a waiting period of 2 years, but this has not been substantiated in the literature (Kreuser, et al., 1990). If fertility returns and the couple wants to try for a child before the end of the 2-year waiting period, they should be informed that there appears to be no increased risk of fetal complications (Kreuser et al., 1990). Pregnancy after treatment for Hodgkin's disease was studied by Andrieu and Ochoa-Molina (1983). They found that the incidence of fetal abnormalities did not increase if the patient had previous chemotherapy or radiation therapy.

❖ Summary

Because matters of sexuality are important and patients with cancer deserve the necessary assistance to relieve anxieties related to therapy, nurses must be able to see beyond the disease and continue to improve patients' knowledge related to all aspects of cancer care. Worthiness and a sense of belonging are often equated with receiving and giving sexual pleasure and experiencing closeness with a partner. During the most difficult times of diagnosis and treatment, people with cancer should be afforded as many elements as possible to maintain their sexual health. Clearly, their quality of life related to sexuality will be enhanced through the assessment, education, interventions, support, and understanding only a nurse can give.

❖ References

Al-Juburi A and O'Donnell P: Penile self-injection for impotence in patients after radical cystectomy-ileal loop, Urology 30(1):29–30, 1987.

American Cancer Society: Facts and figures, New York, 1991, American Cancer Society.

American Fertility Society: IVF and GIFT: A patient's guide to assisted reproductive technology, 1989, The American Fertility Society, under the direction of the Patient Education Committee and the Publications Committee.

Anderson B and Jochimsen P: Sexual functioning among breast cancer, gynecologic cancer, and healthy women, J Consult Clin Psych 53:25–32, 1985.

Andrieu JM and Ochoa-Molina ME: Menstrual cycle, pregnancies and offspring before and after MOPP therapy for Hodgkin's disease, Cancer 52:435–438, 1983.

Balducci L, Phillips M, Gearhart J, Little D, Bowie D, and McGehee R: Sexual complications of cancer treatment, AFP 37:159–171, 1988.

Banker F: The preservation of potency after external beam irradiation for prostate cancer, Int J Radiat Oncol Biol Phys 15:219–220, 1988.

Bates-Johnson B: Sexuality and the elderly, Enterostomal Therapy 16:158–163, 1989.

Beemer W, Hopkins M, and Morley G: Vaginal reconstruction in gynecologic oncology, Obstetrics and Gynecol 72:911–914, 1988.

Beiler D, Wright D, and Reddy G: Radical external radiotherapy for prostate carcinoma, Int J Radiat Biol Phys 7:885–893, 1981.

Blackmore C: The impact of orchidectomy upon the sexuality of the man with testicular cancer, Cancer Nurs 11:33–40, 1988.

Brophy L and Sharp E: Physical symptoms of combination biotherapy: a quality of life issue, Oncol Nurs Forum 18(1) (suppl 1991):25–30, 1991.

Brunner DW, Lancicano R, Keegan M, Corn B, Martin E, and Hanks G: Vaginal stenosis and sexual function following intracavitary radiation for the treatment of cervical and endometrial carcinoma, Int J Radiat Oncol Biol Phys 27:825–830, 1993.

Carde P, Hagenbeek A, Hayat M, Monconduit M, Thomas J, Burgers M, Noordijk E, Tanguy A, Meerwaldt J, Le Fur R, Somers R, Kluin-Nelemans H, Busson A, Breed W, Bron D, Holdrinet A, Rutten E, Michiels J, Regnier R, Debusscher L, Musella R, Fargeot P, Thyss A, Cattan A, Rigal-Huguet F, Roth S, Caillou B, Dupouy N, and Henry-Amar M: Clinical staging versus laparotomy and combined modality with MOPP versus ABVD in early-stage Hodgkin's disease: the H6 twin randomized trials from the European Organization of Research and Treatment of Lymphoma Cooperative Group, J Clin Oncol 11:2258–2272, 1993.

Cosimelli M, Mannella E, Giannarelli D, Casaldi V, Wappner G, Cavaliere F, Consolo S, and Appetecchia M: Nerve-sparing surgery in 302 resectable rectosigmoid cancer patients: genitourinary morbidity and 10 year survival, Diseases: rectum 37(2)(suppl):42–26, 1994.

Cryogenic Laboratories, Inc: Cryopreservation of human semen, Roseville, Minnesota, 1993, Cryogenic Laboratories, Inc.

Deeg J, Storb R, and Thomas E: Bone marrow transplantation: a review of delayed complications, Br J Haematol 57:185–208, 1984.

Dembo A and Thomas G: The ovary. In Cox J, editor: Moss's radiation oncology: rationale, technique, and results, ed 7, St. Louis, 1994, Mosby, pp. 712–733.

Donahue V and Knapp R: Sexual rehabilitation of gynecologic cancer patients, Obstectrical Gynecology 49:118–121, 1977.

Dudjak L: Rationale and therapeutic basis for patients receiving recombinant interleukin-2, Semin Oncol Nurs 9(3)(suppl 1):3–7, 1993.

Fogel K: Human sexuality and health care. In Fogel K and Lauver DD, editors: Sexual health promotion, Philadelphia, 1990, WB Saunders Co, pp. 1–18.

Gritz E, Wellisch D, He-Jing W, Siau S, Landsverk J, and Cosgrove M: Long-term effects of testicular cancer on sexual functioning in married couples, Cancer 64:1560–1567, 1989.

Hanks GE, Myers CE, and Scardino PT: Cancer of the prostate. In DeVita VT, Hellman S, and Rosenberg SA, editors: Cancer: principles and practice of oncology, ed 3, Philadelphia, 1993, JB Lippincott Co, pp. 1073–1125.

Harris B: Issues in nursing care of pregnant patients with cancer. In Lowdermilk D, editor: NAACOGs clinical issues in perinatal and women's health nursing 1(4), Philadelphia, 1990, JB Lippincott Co, pp. 423–436.

Hellman S: Principles of radiation therapy. In DeVita V, Hellman S, and Rosenberg SA, editors: Cancer: principles and practice of oncology, ed 3, Philadelphia, 1993, JB Lippincott Co, pp. 247–275.

Hogan R: Cancer and cancer therapy. In Human sexuality: a nursing perspective, Norwalk, Connecticut, 1985, Appleton-Century-Crofts, pp. 373–384.

Ingle R: Cancer and sexuality. In Fogel K and Lauver DD, editors: Sexual health promotion, Philadelphia, 1990, WB Saunders Co, pp. 313–324.

Kreuser ED, Hetzel WD, Billia DO, and Thiel E: Gonadal toxicity following cancer therapy in adults: significance, diagnosis, prevention, and treatment, Canc Treat Rev 17:169–175, 1990.

Lamb M: Sexual dysfunction in the gynecologic oncology patient, Semin Oncol Nurs 1:9–17, 1985.

Lauver D and Welch M: Sexual response cycle. In Fogel K and Lauver DD, editors: Sexual health promotion, Philadelphia, 1990, WB Saunders Co, pp. 39–52.

Levran D, Dor J, Rudak E, Nebel L, Ben-Schlomo I, Ben-Rafael Z, and Mashiach S: Pregnancy potential of human oocytes—the effect of cryopreservation, N Eng J Med 323:1153–1156, 1990.

Masters W and Johnson V: Human sexual response, Boston, 1966, Little, Brown & Co.

McKenzie F: Sexuality after total pelvic exenteration, Nurs Times 84(20):27–30, 1988.

Michigan Reproductive and IVF Center: Patient education handouts, 1993, Michigan Reproductive and IVF Center.

Mulvihill J, McKeen E, Rosner F, and Zarrabi M: Pregnancy outcome in cancer patients: experience in a large cooperative group, Cancer 60:1143–1150, 1987.

Myers SE and Schilsky RL: Prospects for fertility after cancer chemotherapy, Semin Oncol 19:597–604, 1992.

Peck WS, McGrier JT, and Kretchmar NR: Castration of the female by irradiation, Radiol 34:176–186, 1940.

Pierce A, Whittington R, Hanno P, English W, Wein A, and Goodman R: Pharmacologic erection with intracavernosal injection for men with sexual dysfunction following irradiation: a preliminary report, Int J Radiat Oncol Biol Phys 21:1311–1314, 1991.

Reiger P: Biotherapy. In Otto S, editor: Oncology nursing, ed 2, St. Louis, 1994, Mosby, pp. 526–560.

Renshaw D: Sexual and emotional needs of cancer patients, Clin Ther 8:242–246, 1986.

Rivkees S and Crawford J: The relationship of gonadal activity in chemotherapy-induced gonadal damage, J Am Med Assoc 259:2123–2125, 1988.

Rowley J, Leach E, and Warner G: Effect of graded doses of ionizing radiation on the human testis, Radiat Res 59:665–678, 1986.

Sanders J: Effects of cyclophosphamide and TBI on ovarian and testicular function, Exp Hematol 10(suppl 11):49, 1982.

Sanger W, Olson J, and Sherman J: Semen cryobanking for men with cancer—criteria change, Fertility Sterility 58:1024–1027, 1992.

Schain W: A sexual interview is a sexual intervention, Innov Oncol Nurs 4:2, 1988.

Schilsky R, Davidson H, Magid D, Daiter S, and Golomb H: Gonadal and sexual function in males with hairy cell leukemia: lack of adverse effects of recombinant 2-interferon treatment, Cancer Treat Rep 71(2):179–181, 1987.

Schover L: Sexuality and fertility in urologic cancer patients, Cancer 60:553–558, 1987.

Schover L and Fife M: Sexual counseling with radical pelvic or genital cancer surgery, J Psychosoc Oncol (3):21-41, 1985.

Schover L, Fife M, and Gershenson D: Sexual dysfunction and treatment for early stage cervical cancer, Cancer 63:204–212, 1989.

Schover L, Gonzales M, and vonEschenbach A: Sexual and marital relationships after radiotherapy for seminoma, Urology 27(2):117–122, 1986.

Schover L, Schain W, and Montague D: Sexual problems of patients with cancer. In DeVita V, Hellman S, and Rosenberg SA, editors: Cancer: principles and practice of oncology, ed 3, Philadelphia, 1989, JB Lippincott Co, pp. 2206–2224.

Schover L and von Eschenbach A: Sexual function and female radical cystectomy: a case series, J Urology 134:465–468, 1985.

Schover L and von Eschenbach A: Sexual and marital counseling with men treated for testicular cancer, J Sex Marital Ther 10(1):29–40, 1984.

Sharp E: Case management of the hospitalized patient receiving interleukin-2, Semin Oncol Nurs 9(3)(suppl 1):14–19, 1993.

Shell J: Sexuality for patients with gynecologic cancer. In Lowdermilk D, editor: NAACOGs clinical issues in perinatal and women's health nursing 1(4), Philadelphia, 1990, JB Lippincott Co, pp. 479–494.

Shell J: Impact of cancer on sexuality. In Otto S, editor: Oncology nursing, ed 2, St. Louis, 1994, Mosby, pp. 737–760.

Shelton B: Clinical pharmacological research with interleukin-2: implications for nursing, Semin Oncol Nurs 9(3)(suppl 1):8–13, 1993.

Sherins R and Mulvihill J: Gonadal dysfunction. In DeVita V, Hellman S, Rosenberg SA, eds. Cancer: principles and practice of oncology, ed 3, Philadelphia, 1989, JB Lippincott Co, pp. 2170–2180.

Smith D and Babian R: The effects of treatment for cancer on male fertility and sexuality, Canc Nurs 15:271–275, 1992.

Stern C: Body image concerns, surgical conditions, and sexuality. In Fogel K and Lauver DD, editors: Sexual health promotion, Philadelphia, 1990, WB Saunders Co, pp. 498–516.

Thranov I and Klee M: Sexuality among gynecologic cancer patients—a cross-sectional study, Gynecol Oncol 52:14–19, 1994.

von der Masse H: Complications of combined radiotherapy and chemotherapy, Semin Radiat Oncol 4:81–94, 1994.

vonEschenbach A and Schover L: The role of sexual rehabilitation in the treatment of patients with cancer, Cancer 54:2662, 1984.

Waxman E: Sexual dysfunction following treatment for prostate cancer: nursing assessment and interventions, Oncol Nurs Forum 20:1567–1571, 1993.

World Health Organization: Education and trends in human sexuality: the training of health care professionals. Technical report series no. 572. Geneva, Switzerland, 1976. World Health Organization.

Yarbro C and Perry M: The effect of cancer therapy on gonadal function, Semin Oncol Nurs 1:3–8, 1985.

Chapter 25

❖ *Other Side Effects*

Kimberly A. Rumsey

In addition to the side effects discussed in previous chapters, multimodal therapy can also cause fatigue, flulike syndrome, hypersensitivity, lymphedema, and secondary malignancies. This chapter discusses nursing assessment, management, and issues regarding these side effects.

❖ Fatigue

Fatigue is difficult to define because of its complex nature and subjectivity. For many people, fatigue means feeling tired and weak, which generally resolves with rest and sleep (Pickard-Holley, 1991). For the cancer patient, fatigue is characterized by feelings of tiredness and discomfort that result in a decreased ability to perform daily activities (Pickard-Holley, 1991; Piper et al., 1989).

Acute fatigue is expected, and normal tiredness that protects the individual from exhaustion can usually be attributed to an identifiable cause such as a specific activity or exertion. Acute fatigue has rapid onset, short duration, and can usually be relieved with rest. In contrast, chronic fatigue does not serve a specific purpose and is generally related to several contributing factors. Chronic fatigue has a gradual onset, is cumulative, and persists for several weeks or months (Piper, 1991). In Piper's Integrated Fatigue Model (Piper, Lindsey, and Dodd, 1987)(Figure 25-1), Piper outlines potential causes of fatigue and emphasizes the importance of considering all aspects that can contribute to the manifestation of fatigue.

Effects from Multimodal Therapy

Fatigue has been estimated to occur in 82% to 96% of patients receiving chemotherapy (Cassileth et al., 1985; Meyerowitz, Watkins, and Sparks, 1983). Fatigue is also common in patients receiving biotherapeutic agents such as interleukin-2 (IL-2), interferon (IFN), tumor necrosis factor (TNF), and colony-stimulating factors (CSF) (Piper et al., 1989). Radiation therapy commonly results in fatigue, which increases in intensity over the course of treatment but gradually improves once therapy has ended (Irvine et al., 1991). As these treatment modalities are combined, the incidence of fatigue increases (Brophy and Sharp, 1991).

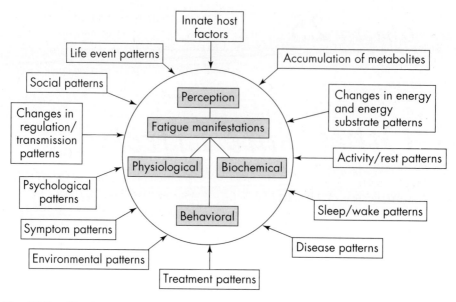

Fig. 25-1. Piper's Integrated Fatigue Model. From Piper BF, Lindsey AM, and Dodd MJ: Fatigue mechanisms in cancer patients: developing nursing theory, Oncol Nurs Forum 14(6):17–23, 1987.

Nursing Management

Successful management of fatigue begins with an accurate and complete assessment. Various components of this assessment include the pattern of fatigue and the patient's usual activities, as well as additional data.

Many patients with cancer believe that fatigue is an unavoidable consequence of their illness and its treatment and therefore do not report the full impact that fatigue has on their daily lives. The intensity of fatigue can be measured with a visual analog scale. The nurse can ask "On a scale of 0 to 10, with 0 representing no fatigue and 10 representing the most fatigue imaginable, how much fatigue are you experiencing now?" (Winningham et al., 1994). The onset and duration of fatigue, the association between fatigue and the treatment regimen, and exacerbating and alleviating factors should also be assessed (Aistars, 1987; Nail and Winningham, 1993; Piper, 1991; Winningham et al., 1994).

The nurse should ask patients to describe a typical day in which they do not experience fatigue and to compare that to a day in which they do experience fatigue. This includes the times they awaken and go to bed, the number of hours they sleep each night, the number of times they wake during the night, the activities (physical and mental) they perform during the day, and the times and duration of rest periods during the day (Nail and Winningham, 1993). Patients should also discuss the impact of fatigue on their ability to complete usual activities (Aistars, 1987; Nail and Winningham, 1993).

Chronic illnesses such as diabetes and congestive heart failure can contribute to fatigue. Laboratory data should be examined for evidence of anemia or electrolyte imbalances that could exacerbate fatigue, and a nutritional assessment should be conducted to eliminate dietary factors. Stress, depression, and pain should also be eliminated as possible causes of fatigue (Piper, 1991; Rumsey, Rieger, and Harle, 1992).

The primary goals of nursing management of fatigue are to promote independence in the activities of daily living and to utilize measures to prevent further disability (Rumsey, Rieger, and Harle, 1992). Only minimal research on nursing interventions exists. Current nursing care is focused on effective utilization of energy, nutritional management, stress management, and management of other contributing factors (Aistars, 1987; Piper, 1991; Piper et al., 1989). Nursing Management of Fatigue is outlined below.

The nurse can help patients achieve effective utilization of energy by advising them how to balance energy expenditure and energy conservation. Based on each patient's usual activities and pattern of fatigue, the nurse can help him or her pace activities and incorporate scheduled rest periods. Patients can prioritize their activities and identify those they want to continue doing themselves and those they can delegate to others (Piper, 1991; Rumsey, Rieger, and Harle, 1992).

Adequate caloric and vitamin intake can also help alleviate fatigue. Patients should be encouraged to write down everything they eat and drink for an accurate appraisal of dietary and fluid intake. A consultation with a dietician may also be appropriate (Piper, 1991).

Stress management involves assisting patients and family members to identify and to use resources appropriately. Relaxation and distraction techniques can help patients cope with stressful situations and may help them to rest better at night.

 ### Nursing Management of

Fatigue

Assess the parameters of fatigue.
- Patterns
- Usual activities
- Causative factors

Provide treatment for those factors that can be controlled or eliminated.
- Control pain, nausea, and constipation
- Administer oxygen, blood, and/or epoetic alfa if appropriate

Provide suggestions for effective utilization of energy.
- Assist patients to prioritize their activities and to pace themselves
- Encourage scheduled rest periods and normal sleep patterns
- Encourage patients to seek assistance with their activities as necessary

Encourage stress management.
- Assist patients to identify and to utilize available resources
- Encourage the use of relaxation and distraction techniques
- Encourage patients to follow a low-intensity exercise program
- Initiate appropriate referrals to mental health workers, social workers, chaplains, or dieticians

Exercise is an important part of stress management, even for patients with fatigue. Low-intensity walking programs can be effective for these patients; however, patients should be advised to consult a physician before beginning such a program (Winningham, 1991).

Patient education is imperative for patients with cancer who experience chronic fatigue. The goal is to teach patients to identify fatigue and to empower them to manage fatigue adequately (Skalla and Lacasse, 1992). The Patient Education Guidelines below describe appropriate material to teach patients about fatigue as a side effect of multimodal treatment. Nurses should be explicit when explaining fatigue and should emphasize that it is a common, chronic problem experienced by most patients with cancer. Through adequate education, patients gain a clear understanding of the problems associated with fatigue and their personal role in managing the problem.

❖ Flulike Syndrome

Flulike syndrome (FLS), also known as *constitutional symptoms,* is a group of symptoms that includes fever, chills, rigors, myalgias, and headaches. The pathophysiology of fever forms the basis for explaining the pathophysiology of FLS. Fever is defined as an increase in body temperature in response to an alteration in the set point that governs temperature (Haueber, 1989). There are two types of *pyrogens* (substances that can stimulate the resetting of the temperature set point). *Exogenous pyrogens* originate outside the body and include substances such as bacterial

---

Patient Education Guidelines for

Fatigue

◆ Fatigue is a common side effect of cancer and its treatment. A number of things can add to your feelings of fatigue, including pain, stress, low blood cell counts, and interrupted sleep at night.

◆ You may need to plan rest periods during the day, decide which activities you need to do yourself, which ones others can do, and which ones can be left undone. Your nurse can assist you to contact a home care nurse in your area if you need help caring for yourself.

◆ A diet high in protein and carbohydrates helps combat fatigue. Drink eight 8-ounce glasses of fluid every day unless your nurse or physician tells you otherwise. Ask your nurse or physician about vitamin supplements and helpful hints to improve your nutritional status.

◆ Notify your nurse or physician if you have pain (especially if it disrupts your sleep) or are short of breath.

◆ Stress and depression can also contribute to fatigue. Sharing your thoughts with a trusted family member, a friend, clergy, your nurse, or a cancer support group may be helpful.

◆ Gentle exercise such as walking can also help relieve fatigue. Contact your nurse or physician before starting an exercise regimen.

Permission granted to reproduce these guidelines for educational purposes only.

endotoxins, fungi, and viruses. *Endogenous pyrogens* are proteins produced by the patient's cells and are termed cytokines. The endogenous pyrogens play a central role in the etiology of FLS (Dinarello, Cannon, and Wolf, 1988).

Effects from Biotherapy

FLS is commonly experienced by patients receiving certain biotherapeutic agents such as interferon-α or interleukin-2 (IL-2). Colony-stimulating factors (CSFs) sometimes cause mild FLS symptoms. Interleukin-1 (IL-1) is the prototype cytokine used to illustrate their effect on fever because it can directly affect the temperature set point. IL-1 stimulates fibroblasts and monocytes to release prostaglandins, which diffuse across the blood-brain barrier into the preoptic anterior hypothalamus, which controls temperature in the body (Stitt, 1986). The prostaglandins directly cause an increase in the temperature set point. Chills and rigors produce heat as the body attempts to attain this new temperature. Prostaglandins also stimulate pain receptors, causing the myalgia and headaches generally associated with FLS (Dinarello, Cannon, and Wolf, 1988; Haeuber, 1989).

Some of the biological agents such as interferon-α are cytokines or endogenous pyrogens. Others such as IL-2 are known to induce the release of IL-1, resulting in FLS (Haeuber, 1989).

Effects from Chemotherapy

Several chemotherapeutic agents cause FLS. Paclitaxel produces flulike myalgias that may last up to a week after therapy. FLS caused by dacarbazine usually begins a week after treatment and can last as long as 3 weeks (Wilkes, Ingwersen, and Burke, 1994). Procarbazine is also associated with FLS, but the effect is limited to the first dose of therapy (Dorr and Von Hoff, 1994). Bleomycin can cause fever with or without chills during the first 24 hours after administration. Other chemotherapeutic agents associated with FLS include 5-azacytidine, carboplatin, and cytarabine (Dorr and Von Hoff, 1994).

Effects from Multimodal Therapy

Biotherapy is a relatively new treatment modality and is only beginning to be used with other modalities. Patients with metastatic melanoma may sometimes receive an investigational regimen that combines chemotherapy (dacarbazine with or without cisplatin) with biotherapy (IL-2). Side effects for each treatment cycle of a regimen using all three agents were measured, and in almost all instances "fever/chills" were present (Flaherty et al., 1993).

Nursing Management

Nursing assessment of FLS focuses on the signs and symptoms of fever. The nurse should not assume that all fevers are side effects related to the treatment agents. Other variables to be assessed include the length of time the patient has been receiving the agent, the fever pattern compared with the usual fever patterns, and signs and symptoms of infection (Rieger, 1994). Fevers higher than 100°F that persist despite administration of antipyretics or other control measures should be reported immediately.

The ideal method of managing FLS has yet to be established. Current recommendations focus on alleviation of the discomfort associated with FLS and patient education. Treatment can sometimes be manipulated by altering the timing of administration. For example, if interferon-α is administered a couple of hours before bedtime, the fever will generally occur in the middle of the night when the patient is asleep, resulting in minimal discomfort. Patients also frequently receive premedication with prostaglandin inhibitors (ibuprofen, acetaminophen, or indomethacin) and an antihistamine. Meperidine or other narcotics can also be administered to control rigors (Caliendo, Joyce, and Altmiller, 1993; Rieger, 1994; Viele and Moran, 1993). Antihistamines, nonsteroidal antiinflammatory drugs, or acetaminophen can be given for headaches. For persistent temperatures greater than 102°F, a tepid sponge bath or shower, ice packs, or hypothermia blanket may be needed.

Patient education is a vital component of the nurse's role in caring for patients who receive FLS-producing agents. This education often alleviates anxiety and results in increased feelings of control for the patient and family because therapy is sometimes administered at home (Rumsey, 1995). Instruction includes information about specific side effects, self-management, and reportable signs and symptoms. Patients are also taught how to take their temperature correctly, to read a thermometer, and to document the results. Nurses, in collaboration with physicians, should establish guidelines for interventions for reportable fevers (Rieger and Rumsey, 1992; Rumsey, 1995). Patients can also be taught relaxation techniques that could prevent or diminish other symptoms associated with FLS (Haeuber, 1989).

❖ Hypersensitivity Reactions

Hypersensitivity reactions result from overstimulation of the immune system. The agent administered is recognized by the immune system as an antigen, antibodies are formed, and T-cells and macrophages are sensitized. Table 25-1 lists four types of hypersensitivity reactions.

The most common and life-threatening hypersensitivity reactions seen in oncology patients are type I or anaphylactic reactions. In type I reactions, IgE antibodies develop as a result of exposure to the antigen or drug. Antigen-antibody complexes bind to mast cells, causing the release of vasoactive amines, such as histamines, leukotrienes, and prostaglandins. The resultant increase in vasodilation, capillary permeability, and smooth muscle contraction causes the signs and symptoms associated with hypersensitivity reactions (Weiss, 1992). The symptoms may be localized or generalized.

All drugs have the potential to initiate hypersensitivity reactions, but asparaginase and paclitaxel are the agents most commonly associated with severe reactions (Weiss, 1992; Wilkes, Ingwersen, and Burke, 1994). Table 25-2 provides the names of other drugs associated with hypersensitivity reactions.

Patients receiving biotherapy occasionally have hypersensitivity reactions. These reactions occur most commonly in patients receiving monoclonal antibodies and usually include urticaria, pruritis, bronchospasm, and anaphylaxis (Rieger, 1992).

Table 25-1   Types of Hypersensitivity Reactions

Type	Major Signs and Symptoms	Mechanism
I	Urticaria, angioedema, rash, bronchospasm, abdominal cramping, extremity pain, agitation and anxiety, hypotension	Antigen interaction with IgE bound to mast cell membrane causes degranulation Drug binding to mast cell surface causes degranulation Activation of classic or alternative complement pathways produces anaphylatoxins Neurogenic release of vasoactive substances
II	Hemolytic anemia	Antibody reacts with cell-bound antigen and activates complement
III	Deposition of immune complexes in tissues results in various forms of tissue injury	Antigen-antibody complexes form intravascularly and deposit in or on tissues
IV	Contact dermatitis, granuloma formation, homograft rejection	Sensitized T-lymphocytes react with antigen and release lymphokines

From Weiss RB: Hypersensitivity reactions. In Perry MC, editor: The chemotherapy source book, Baltimore, 1992, Williams & Wilkins.

Table 25-2   Drugs Associated with Hypersensitivity Reactions

Highest Reported Incidence*	Case Reports
Asparaginase	Diaziquone
Paclitaxel	Etoposide
Cisplatin	Methotrexate
Teniposide	Trimetrexate
Elliptinium	Cytarabine
Procarbazine	Cyclophosphamide
Melphalan (IV)	Ifosfamide
Mechlorethamine (topical)	Chlorambucil
Anthracycline antibiotics	5-Fluorouracil
(e.g., doxorubicin, daunorubicin)	Mitoxantrone
	Mitomycin-C
	Bleomycin
	Dacarbazine
	Vinca alkaloids
	Didemnin B

*Reports of >5% incidence in the literature.
From Oncology Nursing Society: Cancer chemotherapy guidelines: recommendations for the management of vesicant extravasation, hypersensitivities, and anaphylaxis, Pittsburgh, 1992, Oncology Nursing Press.

Nursing Management

Before administering a drug known to cause hypersensitivity reactions, the nurse should review the patient's history for allergic reactions and record baseline vital signs (Oncology Nursing Society [ONS], 1992). During the administration of the agent, the patient should be monitored for signs and symptoms associated with localized or generalized hypersensitivity reactions. Localized reactions usually manifest as urticaria, wheals, or localized erythema. Subjective signs for generalized hypersensitivity or anaphylactic reactions include generalized itching, chest tightness, agitation, light-headedness or dizziness, abdominal cramping, anxiety, burning or tingling sensations, and chills (ONS, 1992). Objective signs and symptoms include urticaria that may be localized or generalized; angioedema of the face, neck, eyelids, hands, and feet; respiratory distress with or without wheezing; hypotension; and cyanosis (ONS, 1992).

Localized hypersensitivity reactions are generally treated with diphenhydramine and/or hydrocortisone, and vital signs are monitored frequently for several hours following treatment. The drug may be discontinued, or if critical to the treatment plan, it may be continued but with premedication of antihistamines and corticosteroids.

Generalized hypersensitivity reactions are considered a medical emergency and require immediate action. When they occur, drug administration is stopped immediately. The nurse documents the reaction in the patient's medical record. Many times, subsequent treatments do not include the drug; however, other options such as physician-guided desensitization, premedication, increased dilution of the drug, and increased infusion time can also decrease the incidence of another anaphylactic reaction (ONS, 1992).

Education for patients receiving any type of drug therapy includes discussion of the incidence and the signs and symptoms of hypersensitivity reactions. Before administration of the drug, the patient is encouraged to report pain or tightness in the chest, shortness of breath, or generalized itching. If a reaction to a drug should occur, the patient is taught the exact name of the drug and the type of reaction that occurred. If the reaction is severe and life-threatening, the nurse should encourage the patient to wear a medi-alert bracelet or necklace.

❖ Lymphedema

Lymphedema is the accumulation of fluid in the tissues of an extremity. The lymph system returns fluid and plasma from the interstitial spaces into the circulatory system. Lymph, which is composed of fluid and proteins, enters the lymphatic system via the lymphatic capillaries. Lymph flows through the capillaries into progressively larger lymphatic vessels and eventually into the thoracic duct, which empties into the subclavian veins.

Lymphedema occurs when the proteins cannot move out of the interstitial spaces and increased amounts of fluid are drawn into these spaces (Whitman and McDaniel, 1993). Lymphedema is usually caused by a vascular insufficiency of the lymphatic system. In dynamic insufficiency, the lymphatic load exceeds the transport capacity. The function and anatomy of the lymph system are normal but unable to handle the large volume of lymph. Mechanical insufficiency occurs when the anatomy of the lymph system has been disturbed, as in lymph node dissection, resulting in a reduction of the lymphatic transport capacity.

Cancer treatment can cause lymphedema. Several factors associated with lymphedema risk include infection, metastatic involvement of the lymph node area, trauma to the affected extremity, obesity, and local or general application of heat to the extremity (Granda, 1994; Kennelly and Yurkovic, 1991; Whitman and McDaniel, 1993).

Effects from Surgery

Lymphedema occurs in 6% to 12% of all patients with breast cancer (Whitman and McDaniel, 1993), but it also may occur following surgery for gynecologic malignancies, prostate cancer, lymphoma, or melanoma. The type of surgery performed influences the risk of developing lymphedema. Patients who have extensive lymph node dissection (levels I, II, and III) have a higher risk of developing lymphedema than those who have more conservative lymph node surgeries (Crane, 1994; ReJohnson, 1994). An increased incidence has been reported in patients with breast cancer who had an oblique versus a transverse incision for axillary lymph node dissection (Granda, 1994).

Effects from Multimodal Therapy

Treatment with radiation therapy after lymph node dissection increases the risk of lymphedema (McGrath, 1992; Whitman and McDaniel, 1993). Several studies indicate a slight increase in lymphedema in the affected arm of patients with breast cancer who receive cyclophosphamide, methotrexate, and 5-fluorouracil (CMF) in addition to axillary lymph node dissection and breast irradiation (McGrath, 1992); however, further study is needed before a definitive statement can be made.

Nursing Management

Assessment for lymphedema continues for the duration of the patient's life, because lymphedema can occur weeks or years after treatment. Preoperative assessment involves complete physical and functional assessment of the extremity (Granda, 1994), including skin integrity, sensation and circulation, girth, and range of motion. The data collected serve as a baseline used for comparison postoperatively.

The nurse should also assess for subjective signs and symptoms of lymphedema. Frequently the first sign of increasing edema is a change in sensation. The patient may report that the extremity feels tight or heavy (Whitman and McDaniel, 1993). In addition, the nurse should ask if the patient has noticed a change in the size of the extremity or in the fit of clothing.

Increased girth of the affected extremity usually indicates lymphedema. An increase of 1 inch or 3 cm from the preoperative girth indicates lymphedema (Granda, 1994; Whitman and McDaniel, 1993). Lymphedema during the first 6 weeks after surgery does not cause concern because edema related to the surgery will take approximately that long to dissipate.

The patient can also experience circulatory changes related to lymphedema. The circulation of the affected extremity should be assessed, including peripheral pulse, temperature, color of the skin, and capillary refill. These results are compared with the preoperative assessment and with the assessment of the opposite extremity (Granda, 1994; Whitman and McDaniel, 1993).

Nursing care of the patient with lymphedema focuses on assessment and prevention. Patient education begins preoperatively and includes discussion of the incidence, etiology, and symptoms associated with lymphedema. The nurse should emphasize the role of exercise in the prevention and treatment of lymphedema. Exercises should start during the immediate postoperative period, beginning with isometric exercises and progressing to active, full-range-of-motion exercises (Granda, 1994; Kennelly and Yurkovic, 1991; ReJohnson, 1994; Whitman and McDaniel, 1993). Initially the patient may need assistance and encouragement to perform these exercises, but with time they become easier and can be adapted to the patient's life-style.

If lymphedema occurs, the extremity should be elevated for at least 30 minutes three times a day (Crane, 1994; Granda, 1994; Kennelly and Yurkovic, 1991). The patient can use a decompression device to decrease the edema by mechanically massaging the extremity and facilitating lymph drainage (Kennelly and Yurkovic, 1991). Once the edema has decreased, the extremity can be fitted with an external elastic support that the patient can wear continuously under clothing. The patient should continue exercises of the extremity, although a consultation with a physical therapist may be necessary. In severe cases of lymphedema, the patient may need albumin and diuretics to reduce the edema (Kennelly and Yurkovic, 1991).

❖ Secondary Malignancies

Secondary malignancies are a serious, long-term complication associated with cancer therapy. A second malignancy means that a new primary tumor has occurred, rather than a recurrence of the original cancer. Pathologists can distinguish between a recurrence and a second cancer when they view different histologic types of cells under the microscope (Heyne et al., 1992).

The development of a second malignancy can be attributed to treatment-related risk factors such as the type of treatment and the dose. Chemotherapy and radiation therapy cause cellular damage to the DNA molecules, resulting in the death of tumor cells. At the same time, mutagenic alterations may occur in the DNA, increasing the risk of second malignancy (Little, 1993; Shulman, 1993).

Researchers have also investigated age at the time of treatment as a potential risk factor. Results have indicated an increased incidence of secondary malignancy after age 40, which corresponds to the increased incidence of first or primary malignancy in the same age group (Henry-Amar and Dietrich, 1993). Another factor thought to contribute to the risk of second malignancy includes common underlying predisposing factors such as smoking, which is associated with both bladder and lung cancers.

Effects from Chemotherapy

The alkylating agents such as cisplatin, cyclophosphamide, dacarbazine, mechlorethamine, and thiotepa are the most common agents associated with the development of second malignancies (Shulman, 1993). Hematologic malignancies are the most common second malignancy, and acute myelogenous leukemia (AML) is the most prevalent (Henry-Amar and Dietrich, 1993; Tucker et al., 1988). Incidence of a secondary AML peaks 5 years following treatment of the initial malignancy. Patients treated with MOPP (mechlorethamine, vincristine [Oncovin], procarbazine, and prednisone) for Hodgkin's disease have the highest risk of developing a secondary AML (Shulman, 1993; Tucker et al., 1988). Treatment-related AML has also occurred in patients previously treated for multiple myeloma, non-Hodgkin's lymphoma, breast cancer, gastrointestinal cancer, lung cancer, germ cell tumors in men, ovarian cancer, and survivors of childhood cancers (Moore and Ruccione, 1993).

The most frequent secondary cancers other than AML include non-Hodgkin's lymphoma, lung cancer, stomach cancer, melanoma, and sarcoma (Tucker, 1993). The risk of developing non-Hodgkin's lymphoma or a solid tumor varies according to the time since treatment.

Effects from Radiation Therapy

Malignant transformation from radiation is known to occur at doses ranging from 40 to 60 Gy (Little, 1993; Tucker et al., 1988). Cancers resulting from radiation therapy appear near or within the treated area and usually do not occur until 10 years after treatment, with increasing risk associated with longer follow-up time (Fraser and Tucker, 1989). Breast cancer after mantle radiation for Hodgkin's disease occurs four times more often than in the general age-matched population (Hancock, Tucker, and Hoppe, 1993). Tumors occur at a younger-than-expected age, are frequently bilateral, and are often medial (on the inner half of the breast) (Yahalom et al., 1992). Lung cancer on the irradiated side occurs three times as often in women treated for breast cancer than in those with no history of breast cancer. For women whose breast was irradiated and who continued to smoke, the risk for lung cancer is 32.7 times that of age-matched nonsmokers who have no previous history of breast cancer (Neugart et al., 1994). Sarcomas of various sites have also been noted after radiation therapy (Mark et al., 1994). Solid tumors noted after pelvic irradiation include bladder, rectal, and bone cancers (Fraser and Tucker, 1989).

Effects from Multimodal Therapy

Overall, patients who received multimodal therapy involving chemotherapy and radiation therapy have an increased cumulative risk of secondary malignancies (Henry-Amar and Dietrich, 1993; Tucker et al., 1988). One study reports increased incidence of second solid tumors but not acute leukemia when chemotherapy and radiation therapy are combined (Biti et al., 1994).

Nursing Management

At the time of a routine medical follow-up exam, assessment should include life-style factors that may increase the risk of developing a second malignancy. The assessment should include smoking history, dietary habits, and knowledge of breast, testicular, and skin self-examination techniques (Robinson and Mertens, 1993; Tucker, 1993).

Patient Education Guidelines for

Secondary Malignancies

♦ Several factors may increase your risk for developing another type of cancer, including the type of treatment and dose used to treat this cancer, your age at the time of treatment, and your life-style. Your physician or nurse will discuss your risk with you.

♦ You may need to make some changes in life-style that will help decrease your risk of developing a second cancer, such as smoking cessation, following a low-fat, high-fiber diet, and beginning self-examination of your breasts, testicles, or skin. Your physician or nurse can refer you to support groups and nutritionists to help with these changes.

♦ You will have follow-up appointments for the rest of your life. It is important that you keep all of these appointments to detect any cancer early.

Permission granted to reproduce these guidelines for educational purposes only.

The major role of the nurse in managing second malignancies involves education and encouragement of the patient. Teaching includes the incidence and etiology of second malignancies; life-style changes necessary to decrease risk such as diet modification or smoking cessation; and the need to continue follow-up appointments for life. If, for example, the patient practiced breast self-examination, the nurse should assess the patient's technique and provide information as necessary. However, if the patient did not previously practice breast self-examination, more complete teaching is necessary, including a demonstration and return demonstration of proper technique. Patients are also taught the warning signs of cancer and encouraged to report any concerns or suspicions immediately. Patient Education Guidelines for Secondary Malignancies are presented above.

❖ Summary

Multimodal therapy has improved the outcome of many different types of malignancies; however, major side effects are often associated with these therapies. It is important that the nurse understand these side effects in order to assess them and accurately manage them. As more multimodal treatments become standard, nurses will be challenged to assess the side effects, to design appropriate interventions, and to teach the patient adequately.

❖ References

Aistars J: Fatigue in the cancer patient: a conceptual approach to a clinical problem, Oncol Nurs Forum 14(6):25–30, 1987.

Biti G, Cellai E, Magrini SM, Papi MG, Ponticelli P, and Boddi V: Second solid tumors and leukemia after treatment for Hodgkin's disease: an analysis of 1121 patients from a single institution, Int J Radiat Oncol Biol Phys 29:25–31, 1994.

Brophy LR and Sharp EJ: Physical symptoms of combination biotherapy: a quality-of-life issue, Oncol Nurs Forum 18(suppl 1):25–30, 1991.

Caliendo G, Joyce D, and Altmiller MC: Nursing guidelines and discharge planning for patients receiving recombinant interleukin-2, Semin Oncol Nurs 9(suppl 1):25–31, 1993.

Cassileth BP, Lusk EJ, Bodenheimer BJ, Farber JM, Jochimsen PJ, and Morrin-Taylor B: Chemotherapeutic toxicity. The relationship between patient's pretreatment expectations and post-treatment results, Am J Clin Oncol 8:419–425, 1985.

Crane R: Breast Cancer. In Otto S, editor: Oncology nursing, ed 2, St. Louis, 1994, Mosby, pp. 90–129.

Dinarello CA, Cannon JG, and Wolf SM: New concepts on the pathogenesis of fever, Rev Inf Dis 10(1):168–189, 1988.

Dorr RT and Von Hoff DD: Cancer chemotherapy handbook, ed 2, Norwalk, Connecticut, 1994, Appleton & Lange.

Flaherty LE, Robinson W, Redman BG, Gonzalez R, Martino S, Kraut M, Valdivieso M, and Rudolph AR: A phase II study of dacarbazine and cisplatin in combination with outpatient-administered interleukin-2 in metastatic malignant melanoma, Cancer 71:3520–3525, 1993.

Fraser MC and Tucker MA: Second malignancies following cancer therapy, Semin Oncol Nurs 5:43–55, 1989.

Granda C: Nursing management of patients with lymphedema associated with breast cancer therapy, Cancer Nurs 17:229–235, 1994.

Haeuber D: Recent advances in the management of biotherapy-related side effects: flulike syndrome, Oncol Nurs Forum 16(suppl):35–41, 1989.

Hancock SL, Tucker MA, and Hoppe RT: Breast cancer after treatment of Hodgkin's disease, J Nat Cancer Inst 85:25–31, 1993.

Henry-Amar M and Dietrich PY: Acute leukemia after the treatment of Hodgkin's disease, Hemat Oncol Clin North Am 7:369–387, 1993.

Heyne KH, Lippman SM, Lee JJ, Lee JS, and Hong WK: The incidence of second primary tumors in long-term survivors of small-cell cancer, J Clin Oncol 10:1519–1524, 1992.

Irvine DM, Vincent L, Bubela N, Thompson L, and Graydon J: A critical appraisal of the research literature investigating fatigue in the individual with cancer, Cancer Nurs 14:188–199, 1991.

Kennelly LF and Yurkovic CA: Altered tissue perfusion, peripheral, related to lymphedema. In McNally JC, Somerville ET, Miaskowski C, and Rostad M, editors: Guidelines of oncology nursing practice, Philadelphia, 1991, WB Saunders Co, pp. 387–391.

Little JB: Cellular, molecular, and carcinogenic effects of radiation, Hemat Oncol Clin No Am 7:337–351, 1993.

Mark RJ, Poen J, Tran LM, Fu YS, Selch MT, and Parker RG: Postirradiation sarcomas, Cancer 73:2653–2662, 1994.

McGrath EB: Lymphedema. In Dow KH and Hilderley LJ, editors: Nursing care in radiation oncology, Philadelphia, 1992, WB Saunders Co, pp. 323–333.

Meyerowitz BE, Watkins IK, and Sparks FC: Quality of life for breast cancer patients receiving adjuvant therapy, Am J Nurs 83:232–235, 1983.

Moore IM and Ruccione KS: Late effects of cancer treatment. In Groenwald SL, Goodman M, Frogge MH, and Yarbro CH, editors: Cancer nursing: principles and practice, ed 3, Boston, 1993, Jones & Bartlett, pp. 840–858.

Nail LM and Winningham ML: Fatigue. In Groenwald SL, Goodman M, Frogge MH, and Yarbro CH, editors: Cancer nursing: principles and practice, ed 3, Boston, 1993, Jones & Bartlett, pp. 608–619.

Neugart AI, Murray T, Santos J, Amols H, Hayes MK, Flannery JT, and Robinson E: Increased risk of lung cancer after breast cancer radiation therapy in cigarette smokers, Cancer 73:1615–1620, 1994.

Oncology Nursing Society: Cancer chemotherapy guidelines: recommendations for the management of vesicant extravasations, hypersensitivities, and anaphylaxis, Pittsburgh, 1992, Oncology Nursing Press.

Pickard-Holley S: Fatigue in cancer patients: a descriptive study, Cancer Nurs 14:13–19, 1991.

Piper BF: Alterations in energy: the sensation of fatigue. In Baird SB, McCorkle R, and Grant M, editors: Cancer nursing: a comprehensive textbook, Philadelphia, 1991, WB Saunders Co, pp. 894–908.

Piper BF, Lindsey AM, and Dodd MJ: Fatigue mechanisms in cancer patients: developing nursing theory, Oncol Nurs Forum 14(6):17–23, 1987.

Piper BF, Rieger PT, Brophy L, Haeuber D, Hood LE, Lyver A, and Sharp E: Recent advances in the management of biotherapy-related side effects: fatigue, Oncol Nurs Forum 16(suppl):27–34, 1989.

ReJohnson J: Caring for the woman who has had a mastectomy, Am J Nurs 94(5):24–31, 1994.

Rieger PT: Biotherapy. In Otto S, editor: Oncology nursing, ed 2, St. Louis, 1994, Mosby, pp. 526–556.

Rieger PT: The pathophysiology of selected symptoms associated with BRM therapy. In Sergi JS, Jassak P, and Mayer DK, editors: Biological response modifiers: perspectives for oncology nurses (issue 2), San Francisco, 1992, Cetus Corporation.

Rieger PT and Rumsey K: Responding to the educational needs of patients receiving biotherapy. In Carrol-Johnson RM, editor: The biotherapy of cancer V, Pittsburgh, 1992, Oncology Nursing Press, Inc (monograph), pp. 8–10.

Robinson LL and Mertens A: Second tumors after treatment of childhood malignancies, Hemat Oncol Clin No Am 7:401–415, 1993.

Rumsey KA: Patient education. In Rieger PT, editor: Biotherapy: a comprehensive review, Boston, 1995, Jones & Bartlett, pp. 271–289.

Rumsey KA, Rieger PT, and Harle M: Nursing management of the patient receiving biological response modifiers. In Rumsey KA and Reiger PT, editors: Biological response modifiers: a self-instruction manual for health professionals, Chicago, 1992, Precept Press, Inc, pp. 55–75.

Shulman LN: The biology of alkylating-agent cellular injury, Hematol Oncol Clin No Am 7:325–335, 1993.

Skalla KA and Lacasse C: Patient education for fatigue, Oncol Nurs Forum 19:1537–1541, 1992.

Stitt JT: Prostaglandin e as the neural mediator of the febrile response, Yale J Biol Med 59(2):137–149, 1986.

Tucker MA: Solid second cancers following Hodgkin's disease, Hematol Oncol Clin No Am 7:389–400, 1993.

Tucker MH, Coleman CN, Cox RS, Varghese A, and Rosengerg SA: Risk of second cancers after treatment for Hodgkin's disease, New Eng J Med 318(2):76–81, 1988.

Viele CS and Moran T: Nursing management of the nonhospitalized patient receiving recombinant interleukin-2, Semin Oncol Nurs 9(suppl 1):20–24, 1993.

Weiss RB: Hypersensitivity reactions. In Perry MC, editor: The chemotherapy source book, Baltimore, 1992, Williams & Wilkins, pp. 553–569.

Whitman M and McDaniel RW: Preventing lymphedema. An unwelcome sequel to breast cancer, Nursing 23(12):36–39, 1993.

Wilkes GM, Ingwersen K, and Burke MB: Oncology nursing drug references, Boston, 1994, Jones & Bartlett.

Winningham ML: Walking program for people with cancer. Getting started, Cancer Nurs 14:270–276, 1991.

Winningham ML, Nail LM, Burke MB, Brophy L, Cimprich B, Jones LS, Pickard-Holley S, Rhodes V, St. Pierre B, Beck S, Glass EC, Mock VL, Mooney KH, and Piper B: Fatigue and the cancer experience: the state of the knowledge, Oncol Nurs Forum 21:23–36, 1994.

Yahalom J, Petrek JA, Biddinger PW, Kessler S, Dershaw DD, McCormick B, Osbourne MP, Kinne DA, and Rosen PP: Breast cancer in patients irradiated for Hodgkin's disease: a clinical and pathologic analysis of 45 events in 37 patients, J Clin Oncol 10:1674–1681, 1992.

SPECIAL CONSIDERATIONS AND FUTURE TRENDS

Chapter 26

❖ *Patient Education*

Debra J. Luce

Education is one of the most important aspects of care that nurses provide. Education of patients with cancer focuses on increasing knowledge, skills, and self-care abilities to change behavior and to obtain control over a situation that may seem hopeless (Villejo and Meyers, 1991). The benefits of patient education include prevention or minimization of treatment side effects; decreased anxiety with fewer phone calls or visits to the nurse or treatment center; fewer or shorter hospitalizations; increased feelings of control and improved quality of life with increased productivity at work, school, and home (Fernsler and Cannon, 1991; Villejo and Myers, 1991).

Multiple factors affect the ability of patients and families to receive consistent, meaningful learning opportunities. Variation in health care settings, educational resources, and the amount of time available for teaching influences patient education throughout the continuum of cancer care.

❖ *Issues Related to Patient Teaching*

Age

More than 70% of all cancers occur in people over the age of 60 (Steele et al., 1995). The methods and materials used to teach patients must overcome factors that may hinder elderly patients' ability to understand and to incorporate new information and skills into daily life. Most of today's elderly do not have the same level of formal education as younger people. For instance, in 1960 only 20% of older people graduated from high school (Kick, 1989). Many people had to leave school to learn a trade and to provide income for their families. In contrast, statisticians have predicted that 64% of older people will be high school graduates by the year 2000 (Kick, 1989).

Physical changes associated with aging must be considered. Changes in vision, taste, touch, smell, and hearing can lead to difficulties in understanding instructions.

Only pieces of words or sentences may be heard or seen, making the performance of skills such as maintaining a vascular access device difficult. Neurologic changes may lead to (or cause) longer reaction times, increase the time needed to process new information, and decrease the ability to react to multiple or complex stimuli (Kick, 1989).

Teaching is more effective when the elderly can relate what is being taught to previous experiences and/or perceive the new information or skill as personally relevant (Kick, 1989). For example, when teaching a lady whose hobby is gardening it may be helpful to compare colony-stimulating factors to fertilizer. The decreased length of hospital stays and the increased expectation that patients will perform technical skills and self-monitoring throughout complex therapies also affect the elderly's "need to know" (Stevenson and Crosson, 1991).

When teaching children, their age and developmental stage must be considered. A child's ability to comprehend must be taken into account when questions are asked. Brief, simple explanations related to the disease, the treatment, potential side effects, and self-care must be presented without long technical discussion. Use of play therapy and multimedia such as the American Cancer Society's video, "Why Charlie Brown, Why?," aid in teaching the child, and his or her siblings, friends, schoolmates, teachers, school nurse, and family. All of these individuals need to have information on what to expect, how to monitor the child, and how to adapt the school setting, if necessary.

Culture

In working with patients and families from diverse cultural backgrounds, areas to assess include specific beliefs and values and the degree to which the patient practices those beliefs. It is important to assess cultural factors that may interfere with or contradict recommended treatment without stereotyping (such as assuming that all Jewish patients eat only kosher food). If diet modifications are needed, the patient's usual dietary practices and willingness to modify them must be explored (Tripp-Reimer and Afifi, 1989). Establishment of rapport is crucial to positive interaction. Addressing the patient as "Mr." or "Mrs." and involving an interpreter or significant other enhances the patient's comfort level. Box 26-1 depicts an example of a learning needs assessment tool that includes cultural influences on learning. When teaching patients who don't speak English, present information in the same order as for English-speaking patients and utilize pictures, but do not assume that lack of English means lack of intelligence (Tripp-Reimer and Afifi, 1989).

Education and Reading Level

Assessment of educational level requires caution because incorrect assumptions can be made. Many adults who did not complete high school have been self-taught through the media and job-related training. Conversely, there are high school graduates who cannot read or comprehend at a high school reading level or lower. Some educators estimate that 17 million people in the U.S. are marginally functionally literate (Wong, 1992). *Functional literacy* is defined as the ability to read well enough

---

Box 26-1 Format for Learning Needs Assessment

1. Primary language spoken
   _____ English
   _____ Other (specify) _____ . Has an interpreter been requested?
   _____ yes _____ (name)

2. Desire or motivation to learn
   _____ Total disinterest or defers to family member
   _____ (name of family member)
   _____ Minimal information desired
   _____ Moderate information desired
   _____ Desires all there is to know
   _____ Willing to answer questions

3. How does patient like to learn? (check all that apply)
   _____ Discussion and verbal explanation
   _____ Reading
   _____ Movie or demonstration
   _____ Other (explain) _____

4. Formal education level _____ (grade)

5. Barriers to learning (check all that apply)
   _____ Cannot read English   _____ Cannot write English
   _____ Pain or discomfort   _____ Sedation
   _____ Sleep deprivation   _____ Anxiety
   _____ History of noncompliance   _____ Multiple misconceptions
   _____ Family   _____ Other (specify) _____

6. Religious, cultural, or life-style barriers
   _____ None
   _____ Barriers (specify) _____

7. Sensory deficits (check all that apply)
   _____ Hard of hearing   _____ Poor vision
   _____ Poor sensation in hands   _____ Other (specify) _____

8. Previous education
   _____ Understands reason for hospitalization or appointment
   _____ Understands planned treatment program

Adapted from and used with permission of the Patient Education Task Force, Candler Hospital, Savannah, Ga., 1994.

---

to understand and interpret what is read and the ability to use the information (Hussey and Gilliland, 1989). Asking questions such as "How much do you read?," "What kinds of things do you enjoy reading?," and saying "People learn in different ways—reading, watching television or videos, and through talking: which way works best for you?" assists the nurse in selecting the best teaching method(s) for an individual patient. Caution must be exercised in teaching patients who have college education. Health care professionals often incorrectly assume that a highly educated person wants volumes of technical information and will absorb it readily. It must be recognized that these people are patients first. They must be assessed for what they know, want to know, and need to know and for barriers to learning like other patients.

Stage of Disease

During the time before and at actual diagnosis, patients often feel acutely anxious (Welch-McCaffrey, 1985). The term *cancer* is overwhelming and terrifying to most people: their ability to understand what is being said during the initial conversation is minimal.

Appointments with a variety of specialists to discuss treatment options can increase anxiety and confusion because of the massive amount of new terminology and the potential for conflicting treatment recommendations. During the workup and before initiation of treatment, patients often express anxiety and concern that nothing is being done to treat the cancer and that they feel in limbo. Anxiety levels tend to decrease when active treatment begins because patients feel that something positive is being done to combat the disease (Adams, 1991; Welch-McCaffrey, 1985). Throughout treatment it is important to reassess what the patient understands and provide appropriate teaching to decrease the amount of physical distress. This results in an increased sense of control (Welch-McCaffery, 1985).

If the disease reoccurs, patients' anxiety and emotional needs may actually be greater than at the time of initial diagnosis. This can affect learning because the patient will also have to cope with feelings of defeat: "I did everything right but it came back." Patients need to be reassured that they did not cause the recurrence.

Learning needs for patients with prolonged disease-free survival can also be affected by frustration, confusion, or anger if they encounter obstacles such as employability, insurability, and the long-term effects of treatment (Mullin, 1985).

Informed Consent

The content and terminology of informed-consent documents are often technical and require combined teaching efforts by physicians and nurses. Topics to be addressed include treatment-plan options, risks and potential benefits, alternative treatments, and how response from cancer treatment will be evaluated (Schulmeister, 1991). The informed-consent document should have short sentences, content outlined in a logical manner, simple terminology, and reiteration of previous discussions with the patient. With this approach, the informed-consent document becomes another teaching tool rather than an intimidating legal paper. (See Chapter 7, Clinical Trials, for additional information on informed consent.)

Assessment of Readiness to Learn

All of the factors presented above can affect the patient's readiness to learn. Anxiety can have a positive effect on learning through motivation. Information seeking is one of the most basic forms of coping for some people (Cohen and Lazarus, 1979). Pain, nausea, fatigue, and other physical symptoms decrease the patient's participation in learning activities. When symptoms are under control, patients can better focus on the information presented. Psychologic factors such as motivation, attitude, beliefs about cancer or illness in general, and patients' emotional response to their diagnosis can also affect the patient's readiness to learn. Negative aspects of these factors can be difficult for the nurse to minimize (Ruzicki, 1989).

Availability of Significant Others

Family or significant others have a crucial role in patient education. When patients have skills to learn, it is often the significant other who oversees or actually performs the task. This can occur if the patient lacks the ability or desire to perform self-care or because the loved one wants to participate in the patient's care. Family members can coordinate meals and monitor for signs and symptoms of treatment complications. Increased understanding about the patient's care can reduce stress and feelings of helplessness. Cancer diagnosis and treatment affect the life-styles and emotions of the patient and the significant other, and therefore both should be considered as a unit. Teaching patients and significant others together provides both with consistent information. Together they can help each other generate questions, concerns, and areas for further instruction.

When a significant other is not available, alternative support and increased attention to the patient's educational needs and to the evaluation of knowledge and skills learned is necessary. Alternative support includes friends, volunteer agencies, home health care services, or other community services.

❖ Aspects of Patient Education

Teaching Along the Cancer Continuum

The cancer continuum includes diagnosis, treatment, follow-up, and survival, or else recurrence and death. Education continues during all phases. A multitude of health professionals provide information across a variety of settings that are usually not coordinated and that may be at different levels and locations, especially if patients are receiving multimodal therapy. Unfortunately, many health care professionals teach differently, and this can confuse the patient. The amount of new and unfamiliar experiences encountered by patients with cancer is phenomenal. Patients can expect to see multiple physicians, nurses, and other health care providers across a wide array of settings, sometimes simultaneously or over a span of time. When patients receive multimodal therapy, communication among the different health professionals and the patient is crucial to avoid fragmentation, contradiction, and misunderstanding. Nurses must ensure that patients have the information needed for management of side effects and for knowing what symptoms to report and to whom.

Diagnosis

At the time of diagnosis, patients need to know about evaluative tests and treatment options (Mullin, 1985; Welch-McCaffrey, 1985). Explanations about the purpose of each test, how it is performed, what the patient can expect to see and hear, and the anticipated information from the tests will help minimize anxiety and enhance understanding. For example, explaining the purpose of a bone scan to a woman with newly diagnosed breast cancer will help her understand that the bone scan establishes a baseline for staging and for future reference, whereas without explanation she may assume that her disease is advanced because she is having a test done in areas far from her breasts. Box 26-2 presents an example of how to explain the purpose of a staging test. Explanations can be supplemented with pamphlets, diagrams, or fact sheets. Other areas of discussion include preparing for tests (e.g., eating nothing after midnight), the approximate time needed to conduct the test, the follow-up after the test (e.g., taking a laxative after a barium enema), and the date when patients can expect to receive the results.

Patients experience heightened anxiety during "limbo" time (between initial symptoms and test results). Prompt and clear explanations of test results and their meaning enhances understanding and coping. Confusion occurs when a patient does not understand differences among tests. Repeated explanations and the use of a variety of methods that stimulate different senses increases retention and understanding (Chaisson, 1980; Kick, 1989). Box 26-3 outlines guidelines for teaching.

Treatment
Educating patients who receive multimodal treatment is a greater challenge than educating those who receive single-modality treatment. The facets of multimodal treatments that require discussion include the purpose of recommended treatments, the timing of the various modalities (including the anticipated total time), and the expected outcome from the treatments. Other subjects to teach include potential side effects and topics related to self-care (Adams, 1991). Coordination of teaching by nurses from each modality when the patient is receiving concurrent treatment is crucial.

Empowering the Patient
In generations past, patients simply relied on their physicians without questioning or becoming actively involved in treatment options or self-care. Americans today are more empowered as a result of the information explosion, and many want to be

---

Box 26-2 Example of an Explanation for Staging Tests

"Mrs. Jones, Dr. X has ordered a bone scan. This is a test that will show what your bones look like right now. There are two reasons to do this test. One is to make sure that no signs of cancer are in your bones. If the scan shows that the cancer had spread to your bones, the treatment Dr. X would recommend for your cancer is different than if there is no indication of disease spread. The second reason for the test is to look for any unusual areas in your bones that could be from arthritis or an old, healed broken bone. That way we know what is normal for you. If the test is repeated at a later date, it can be compared with today's test. This test is performed on all women at our hospital who have breast cancer."

Box 26-3 Guidelines for Patient Education

◆ Assess learning needs. Assume that you don't have the patient's chart and ask the patient to describe what has been happening—to assess for misconceptions.

◆ Assess barriers to learning (see Box 26-1).

◆ Ask the patient what he or she wants to know.

◆ Present "critical elements" first (the most important facts the patient needs to have).

◆ Categorize—provide information in blocks in a short, logical progression.

◆ Teach when symptoms are controlled, after rest. Make sure the patient is comfortably seated, bedpans and urinals are empty, and the patient doesn't need to use the bathroom.

◆ Use lay terms to explain concepts and medical terms.

◆ Remind the patient that the information about the cancer and its treatment is new, overwhelming, and impossible to retain at one time. Assure the patient that the information will be repeated and that each time he or she will remember more.

◆ Encourage the patient to ask questions. Besides helping to clarify items for the patient, this is a good way to assess his or her understanding.

◆ Present yourself as a patient advocate. Let your words and actions give the patient the sense that you care and want to help.

◆ Relate the new information to the patient's past experiences or show the direct usefulness of the information to the patient's current situation.

◆ Individualize teaching content and methods to the patient's abilities, needs, and desires.

◆ Use a multimedia approach, including the following:
  ◆ Discussion
  ◆ Written materials
  ◆ Visual aids: flip charts, diagrams, bold print, color
  ◆ Combined visual and auditory aids: videotapes, slides and audio cassettes, films
  ◆ Combined visual and tactile aids: anatomical models, demonstrations with return demonstrations

◆ Dispel myths; provide perspective. Bring up some of the myths yourself. "Many people think of cancer as a punishment for things done or not done in the past. Do you think of cancer that way?"

◆ Ensure privacy when teaching. Turn off TVs, radios, or anything else that may distract the patient or interfere with hearing you.

◆ Try to find a block of time for teaching. Let co-workers know what you are doing so they can try to cover your other assignments.

◆ Document the patient's needs, desires, and barriers to learning; the information provided and the methods used; and the level of comprehension, the patient's response, and any comment on further teaching or reinforcement needed.

◆ Give or send a copy of the documentation to the patient, and send a copy to other health care providers who will be following the patient.

Adapted from Wong M: Self-care instructions: do patients understand educational materials?, Focus on Critical Care 19(1):47–49, 1992; and Morra ME: Teaching strategies: public education. In Groenwald SL, Frogge MH, Goodman M, and Yarbro CH, editors: Cancer nursing: principles and practice, ed. 3, Boston, 1993, Jones & Bartlett.

an integral part of their health decisions. Education provides patients with information to enhance their ability to make informed decisions about treatment and self-care. A patient who truly understands the benefits, risks, and rationale for treatment becomes a more active, less anxious member of the health care team. A patient may express negative feelings about treatment and its effect, but active participation offers a patient a sense of increased control.

The resources available in each health care setting dictate how much information patients receive and its degree of accuracy. Resources include people, media, privacy, space, and time. A guideline to assess what the patient already knows and what areas require further teaching is found in Box 26-4. Sample questions are included under each section to help the nurse identify the patient's understanding, misconceptions, and information related to the specific health care setting. If necessary, the nurse can refer the patient to appropriate resources.

Follow-up
The follow-up teaching phase of the cancer continuum usually does not require the same intensity of patient education as the diagnostic and treatment phases. Patient education in this phase relates to the importance of follow-up tests and appoint-

---

Box 26-4 Patient Knowledge and Teaching Assessment

Brief History. Assess what the patient currently understands is happening: "What brings you here (to this office or hospital)?" or "What occurred to make you seek medical attention?"

Understanding by the Patient or Significant Other of the Disease, Treatment Plans, and Prognosis. "What have the doctors told you?" or "What is your understanding of what you have?" or "What do you think is happening?"

Feelings the Patient or Significant Other Has About the Diagnosis. "How did you feel when you found out your diagnosis?" "Have you known anyone with cancer? How are they doing?" (This can stimulate much conversation if the person died or is not doing well.)

Concerns Felt by the Patient or Significant Other. "Most people have concerns, fears, and questions about the effects of cancer and its treatment. What kinds of things are you concerned or worried about?" (Work? Finances? Side effects?)

Knowledge that the Patient or Significant Other Needs. This may vary with the particular setting. For example, the significant other may need to understand why the patient is receiving both chemotherapy and radiation therapy at the same time and to know the schedule of treatments and the expected side effects.

Support Needs of the Patient or Significant Other. This may vary. As an example, the patient may want to talk to someone who has been through the same multimodal treatment for his or her type of cancer.

Adapted from COPES (Candler Oncology Patient Education and Support), Candler Hospital, Savannah, Georgia, 1992.

ments, signs and symptoms of recurrence, and long-term adverse effects of treatment. Patients may also require education related to issues such as adapting lifestyles or changing jobs.

If the patient is cured and treatment becomes part of an ever more distant past, education is still needed. Although follow-up appointments become less frequent, education about rehabilitation, new technology, the politics of health care, follow-up visits, employability, and insurability should continue.

In the event that the cancer is not controlled or recurs, the focus of patient education is on issues related to new treatments or to supportive care. For example, nurses may have to teach families how to bathe and turn patients, to provide oral and skin care, and to change an occupied bed. Symptoms of impending death may also need to be discussed. Families often need information regarding community resources.

Evaluating the Effectiveness of Teaching

There are several ways to evaluate the effectiveness of teaching. If a skill has already been taught, repeat verbalization and actual demonstration of the skill validates the learning. To verify that patients and significant others understand what treatment side effects to report, ask questions such as "What would you call the doctor about when you are at home?" or "Tell me what you remember about how chemotherapy affects your blood." Follow-up phone calls after therapy using a prepared survey can also validate learning (Pruitt, 1993).

Evaluating Educational Materials

Evaluating the quality of educational materials is an important aspect of patient education. It is easy to order pamphlets and videotapes that are available for free and to indiscriminately order inexpensive items with titles that "sound good." Good judgment is needed to evaluate their accuracy, currentness, and appropriateness for the population being served. The language must be understandable and the reading level appropriate. Box 26-5 presents the SMOG formula, a simple tool to assess the reading level of written materials.

Videos that express basic concepts in short time frames will be better understood than long, technical ones. The kind of script and actors (or real people) in a video can affect how patients assimilate the information. For example, a video that talks in general terms about multimodal cancer treatments but features only breast cancer survivors who are elderly, white women may make it difficult for a young black male with lung cancer to relate to the information presented, whereas a video with actors representing a variety of cancers, ages, and ethnic backgrounds would keep the interest of a more diverse group of viewers.

Resources

Many areas offer formal teaching programs such as the American Cancer Society's program, "I Can Cope." "I Can Cope" consists of 1½- to 2-hour educational sessions, usually conducted once a week over 6 to 8 weeks (Johnson, 1982). Topics

Box 26-5 The SMOG Readability Formula

To calculate the SMOG reading grade level, begin with the entire written work that is being assessed, and follow these four steps:

1. Count off 10 consecutive sentences near the beginning, in the middle, and near the end of the text.
2. From this sample of 30 sentences, circle all of the words containing 3 or more syllables (polysyllabic), including repetitions of the same word, and total the number of words circled.
3. Estimate the square root of the total number of polysyllabic words counted. This is done by finding the nearest perfect square, and taking its square root.
4. Finally, add a constant of 3 to the square root. This number gives the SMOG grade, or the reading grade level that a person must have reached if he or she is to understand fully the text being assessed.

A few additional guidelines will help to clarify these directions:

- A sentence is defined as a string of words punctuated with a period (.), an exclamation point (!), or a question mark (?).
- Hyphenated words are considered one word.
- Numbers that are written out should also be considered, and if in numeric form in the text, they should be pronounced to determine if they are polysyllabic.
- Proper nouns, if polysyllabic, should be counted, too.
- Abbreviations should be read as unabbreviated to determine if they are polysyllabic.

Not all pamphlets, fact sheets, or other printed materials contain 30 sentences. To test a text that has fewer than 30 sentences:

1. Count all of the polysyllabic words in the text.
2. Count the number of sentences.
3. Find the average number of polysyllabic words per sentence as follows:

$$\text{Average} = \frac{\text{Total number of polysyllabic words}}{\text{Total number of sentences}}$$

4. Multiply that average by the number of sentences *short of 30*.
5. Add that figure to the total number of polysyllabic words.
6. Find the square root and add the constant of 3.

Perhaps the quickest way to administer the SMOG grading test is by using the SMOG conversion table. Simply count the number of polysyllabic words in your chain of 30 sentences and look up the approximate grade level on the chart.

SMOG Conversion Table*

Total Polysyllabic Word Counts	Approximate Grade Level (+ 1.5 Grades)
0–2	4
3–6	5
7–12	6
13–20	7
21–30	8
31–42	9
43–56	10
57–72	11
73–90	12
91–110	13
111–132	14
133–156	15
157–182	16
183–210	17
211–240	18

*Developed by Harold C. McGraw, Office of Educational Research, Baltimore County Schools, Towson, Maryland.

From: United States Department of Health and Human Services: Pretesting in Health Communications (NIH pub. no. 89-1493), Washington D.C., 1989, U.S. Government Printing Office.

covered include cancer detection and treatment, nutrition, coping with symptoms related to cancer and its treatment, activity, and psychosocial issues. Many "I Can Cope" programs include a panel discussion on topics related to insurance, financial, and legal issues. The sessions require in-depth planning, because they include handouts, speakers from the community, and multimedia presentations. Patients and families receive the most benefit if they attend all of the sessions.

Some hospitals, cancer centers, and other organizations offer periodic programs for patients and the community on cancer-related topics. One hospital offers a weekly 1-hour class that covers one of four broad areas related to cancer on a rotating basis: "What is cancer and how is it diagnosed?"; "What you need to know about treatments for cancer"; "Nutrition and symptom management"; and "Psychosocial issues related to cancer." Participants can start any week and continue until they attend all four sessions, repeating as many as needed.

Local units of the American Cancer Society, hospitals, and other facilities often sponsor support groups. Some are general support groups, open to anyone with cancer. Multiple specialized support groups may also be available. Support groups sometimes offer educational programs with various speakers on preselected topics in addition to emotional support.

Educational Tools

Written and multimedia materials for patient education are becoming increasingly available. Companies that provide products for cancer patients often develop free or low-cost educational materials. Nurses need to review all material to ensure that the information and reading level are appropriate and accurate. Beware of brochures, videos, and other materials that promote a specific product.

❖ Summary

Patient education is crucial for a successful journey through the cancer experience. Assessing what the patient already knows, wants to know, and needs to know at each encounter directs the nurse in what the patient understands and what the patient still needs to learn. Evaluation of barriers to learning helps the nurse choose appropriate educational materials to enhance comprehension and retention. Assessment and access to quick-and-easy educational resources provides an arsenal of teaching options. Comprehensive education for the patient receiving multimodal therapy is challenging but attainable. The improved patient outcomes, especially quality of life, are well worth the effort.

❖ References

Adams M: Information and education across the phases of cancer care, Semin Oncol Nurs 7:105–111, 1991.

Chaisson GM: Patient education: whose responsibility is it and who should be doing it, Nurse Admin Quart 4(2)1–11, 1980.

Cohen F and Lazarus RS: Coping with the stresses of illness. In Cohen F and Adler NE, editors: Health psychology: a handbook, San Francisco, 1979, Jossey-Bass, pp. 217–254.

Fernsler J and Cannon C: The whys of patient education, Semin Oncol Nurs 7:97–104, 1991.

Hussey L and Gilliland K: Compliance, low literacy, and locus of control, Nurs Clin No Am 24:605–611, 1989.

Johnson J: The effects of a patient education course on persons with chronic illness, Cancer Nurs 5:117–123, 1982.

Kick E: Patient teaching for elders, Nurs Clin No Am 24:681–686, 1989.

Morra ME: Teaching strategies: public education. In Groenwald SL, Frogge MH, Goodman M, and Yarbro CH, editors: Cancer nursing: principles and practice, ed 3, Boston, 1993, Jones & Bartlett, pp. 1553–1575.

Mullin F: Seasons of survival. Reflections of a physician with cancer, N Eng J Med 313:270–273, 1985.

Pruitt S: Quality assurance plan promotes effective patient teaching, Oncol Nurs Forum 20:825, 1993.

Ruzicki D: Realistically meeting the educational needs of hospitalized acute and short-stay patients, Nurs Clin No Am 24:629–637, 1989.

Schulmeister L: Establishing a cancer patient education system for ambulatory patients, Semin Oncol Nurs 7:118–124, 1991.

Steele GD, Jessup LM, Winchester DP, Murphy GP, and Mencec HR: Clinical highlights from the National Cancer Data Base: 1995, CA Cancer J Clin 45:102–111, 1995.

Stevenson E and Crosson K: Patient education: history, development and current directions of the American Cancer Society and National Cancer Institute, Semin Oncol Nurs 7:135–142, 1991.

Tripp-Reimer T and Afifi L: Cross-cultural perspectives on patient teaching, Nurs Clin No Am 24:613–619, 1989.

U.S. Department of Health and Human Services: Pretesting in health communications (NIH pub. no. 89-1493), Washington, D.C., 1989, U.S. Government Printing Office.

Villejo L and Meyers C: Brain function, learning styles, and cancer patient education, Semin Oncol Nurs 7:97–104, 1991.

Welch-McCaffrey D: Evolving patient education needs in cancer, Oncol Nurs Forum 12(5):62–65, 1985.

Wong M: Self-care instructions: do patients understand educational materials? Focus Crit Care, 19(1):47–49, 1992.

Chapter 27

❖ *Psychosocial Issues*

Robyn Rebl Mundy

In the past, the hospital staff nurse had time to develop care plans to assist patients with cancer and their families in regard to psychosocial issues. In the managed-care environment of today, however, many patients with cancer are discharged before the nurse can adequately identify psychosocial needs (Leigh, 1992). In addition, hospitals that regularly use agency or "float pool" nurses rarely provide the opportunity for the patient to interact with the same nurse. The result is often a psychosocial assessment resembling a snapshot, which captures a moment in time but lacks the clarity provided by the same nurse assessing the patient over an extended period. Multimodal cancer treatment compounds the situation when the patient receives services from several doctors and possibly from several agencies, thus having little consistency across the continuum of care.

As seen in the preceding chapters, multimodal cancer treatment significantly improves survival. However, the goal of most patients with cancer is to go beyond mere survival and to maximize the quality of their lives. Although difficult to define, Cella and Tulsky (1990) described quality of life as the patient's appraisal of and satisfaction with current level of functioning as compared to what is perceived to be possible or ideal.

❖ *Psychologic Sequelae of Cancer and Treatment*

A diagnosis of cancer often sets the stage for intense psychologic distress. Major psychosocial issues include accepting the loss of the healthy self, changes in body image, role conflict, feelings of isolation, and changes in social, occupational, and spiritual structure (Welch-McCaffrey, 1989). Recognizing pathologic behavioral responses among patients with cancer can be difficult, especially for a nurse who is unfamiliar with the individual's history. The stress associated with assimilating a cancer diagnosis can present a significant challenge for even the most emotionally stable individual.

A major part of dealing with this type of stress involves understanding feelings of grief and loss. It is important for the nurse to listen carefully to what the patient

469

says. If the conversation seems to dwell heavily on issues of loss, it may signal psychologic distress. Not all psychologic distress is bad, however; some psychologic distress is an expected or normal reaction to a cancer diagnosis.

As with other situations involving extreme variability of response, the nurse facilitates adaptive coping by listening in a nonjudgmental fashion. Actively listening for the basic theme of a conversation will cue the nurse in identifying the patient's psychosocial state. The nurse can often glean valuable information by using appropriate open-ended statements that facilitate communication (Box 27-1).

Depression

Although statistics on the prevalence of depression among cancer patients range from 6% to 58% (Bukberg, Penman, and Holland, 1986; Massie and Holland, 1990), it is generally agreed that patients with cancer are at significant risk for depression. A critical function of the nurse is to distinguish between symptoms of normal or expected depression and pathologic or serious depression. Common symptoms of depression include changes in eating and sleeping habits (more or less than normal), chronic sadness, difficulty with memory and concentration, distraction, irritability and crying episodes, and the inability to make decisions (Massie and Holland, 1990). Some level of depression at the time of diagnosis is appropriate. Recommended nursing interventions include encouraging verbalization to help the individual regain a sense of self-worth, to correct misconceptions about the past and present to regain a sense of perspective, and to integrate the illness into a continuum of life experiences.

The patient may need assistance making treatment decisions, especially if multimodal therapy is recommended. To hear that more than one therapy is needed may add to the patient's feeling of being overwhelmed. If modalities are given sequentially, the patient has to reconsider the decision to accept recommended cancer treatment each time a new modality begins. Having experienced difficult

---

Box 27-1 Tips for Communicating with Open-ended Statements

◆ Listen carefully to the patient's dialogue.

◆ Cue your responses with statements like, "Tell me more about that," or "How did that make you feel?" Responding to these types of statements requires more than a "yes" or "no" reply, thus facilitating a richer response.

◆ Avoid any responses that could close communication such as "Would you like to . . ." or "Are you feeling sad about . . . ." These responses lead to the "yes" or "no" reply.

◆ Practice these techniques by role playing on a frequent basis. Although they often feel stilted and artificial in the beginning, you can easily reach a high level of proficiency at facilitating open-ended statements.

side effects from chemotherapy, he or she can be reluctant to start radiation therapy, anticipating more side effects. This may be especially difficult if the patient pushed himself through the first therapy by counting the number of remaining treatments (which is common). Starting a new treatment modality can make therapy seem endless.

Nurses can sometimes help patients and family members minimize feelings of isolation and despair simply by encouraging participation at meetings of cancer support groups. Sometimes this is all a patient needs. Some patients or family members, however, may need more structured psychologic intervention. For instance, any time a patient or family member brings up the issue of suicide, even in a joking manner, the nurse should immediately request a psychiatric consultation. Generally the nurse should consider referral for specialized services when severe depressive symptoms last longer than a week, when they worsen rather than improve, or when they interfere with the patient's ability to function or cooperate with treatment (Massie and Holland, 1990). Referral should also be considered if mild symptoms do not improve within a month. Box 27-2 presents risk factors for psychopathology among patients with cancer.

Depression among the elderly is common, and this becomes a significant issue because more than 50% of all cancers occur in this age group (American Cancer Society, 1996). Goldberg and Cullen (1986) discussed the issue of depression among geriatric cancer patients (those over the age of 65). They asserted that the prevalence of depression in this group was associated with premorbid history and personality.

Psychiatric medications such as antidepressants may be effective in treating depression for some patients with cancer (Massie, Holland, and Straker, 1989). Antidepressant therapy should be carefully monitored in persons receiving multimodal therapy because of the risk of interactions with other drugs (Massie and Holland, 1990). For instance, patients receiving procarbazine for the treatment of Hodgkin's disease should not take an MAO-inhibitor antidepressant.

Box 27-2 Risk Factors for Psychopathology Among Cancer Patients

- Preexisting psychiatric history
- Dysfunctional psychosocial support systems
- Recent (within 1 year) or ongoing psychosocial crises:
  - Death of a spouse or loved one
  - Divorce
  - Illness of spouse or loved one
  - Financial crisis created by the cancer
  - Employment problems
- Randomization to clinical trials for experimental treatment:
  - Anxiety about the randomization process
  - Pressure from family members to participate
- Long-term survivors with fear of recurrence

Fear of Recurrence

Another serious psychosocial challenge is controlling the fear of recurrence. The recommendation of multimodal therapy reinforces this ("My disease must be bad if I need more than one kind of treatment"). Welch-McCaffrey (1989) identified fear of recurrence, uncertainty about the future, and fear of reentry into work situations as major psychosocial issues in survivorship. Dow (1991) described the recurrence of cancer as a potentially devastating experience if patients associate recurrence with failure or the feeling that they were the source of the failure. Patients need to be reassured that many times multimodal therapy is recommended to decrease the chance of recurrence. If multimodal therapy is recommended to maintain quality of life (e.g., chemotherapy and radiation therapy instead of laryngectomy), patients need to understand that disease recurrence after multimodal therapy is not more common than if radical surgery were performed.

Patients also have a high risk for psychologic distress at the end of therapy. This is because many patients feel that when the treatment has stopped, so has any active method of fighting the cancer. It is important to encourage patients completing therapy to continue attending support-group meetings or to seek individual counseling to help control excessive fear of recurrence.

❖ Multiple Providers and Treatment Settings

The patient with cancer receiving multimodal therapy challenges the nurse to provide smoothly coordinated services. Multimodal therapy frequently results in multiple-specialty physicians managing a case simultaneously. For example, a woman with breast cancer may have a surgeon, a medical oncologist, and a radiation oncologist providing treatment at the same time. Her primary physician may also be involved in her care. Other caregivers might include the clinical nurse specialist, the staff nurse, the dietician, the social worker, the rehabilitation counselor, the physical therapist, and the pastoral care representative. When care is delivered in multiple-treatment settings, the team members multiply.

Who does the patient with cancer contact for symptom management? This should be clearly communicated to the patient and clarified whenever new providers become involved with the patient. The nurse promotes appropriate resource management by providing a comprehensive list of all the patient's providers (including telephone numbers) and any other information pertinent to his or her treatment. This information should include a simple explanation of the responsibility or role of each physician or provider. For example, the patient should know who to contact for treating a throat infection: the primary physician, the medical oncologist, or the radiation oncologist?

Ideally there should be an atmosphere of cooperation and communication among team members. However, philosophical differences may exist that sometimes make cooperation and communication difficult. The result may be confusion and increasing levels of anxiety for the patient, who may not understand the nature of this conflict and who may develop a negative attitude about treatment and perhaps even question the competence of providers.

Coordinating communication among providers in multimodal cancer treatment is an essential function of the oncology nurse. The skillful nurse supports the patient with cancer receiving multimodal therapy in several ways. First, the nurse can facilitate communication among medical providers. This can sometimes require arranging for multidisciplinary meetings so that members of the health care team can confer directly. If that cannot be physically arranged, telephone conference calls often prove useful. It is important to include the patient with cancer as a participant in this process.

Second, the nurse can serve as a constant across multiple treatment settings. The nurse supports the patient with cancer across all modalities of treatment by developing effective communication to identify concerns. Skillful patient interviews rest on a foundation of culturally and individually appropriate attending behavior, which includes assessing patterns of eye contact, body language, vocal qualities, and tracking verbal cues (Ivey, 1988). Developing these skills helps facilitate trust, decrease anxiety, and assist patients and their loved ones in communicating needs.

Third, the nurse's role as case coordinator becomes critical in rural settings where patients may live long distances from treatment centers and oncology specialists. Curtiss (1993) discussed cancer care issues in rural areas. She proposed various models for rural oncology care that included visiting/consulting oncology clinics, satellite clinics, oncology services via management contracts, and regionalized oncology programs. Although improvement in technology and telecommunication will enhance services available in rural areas, they will not replace the important function of the professional nurse as a community case coordinator.

Community Support Services

It is important that patients with cancer and their families learn how to access community services. As consumers of health care, they can take responsibility for their choices. This philosophy of personal responsibility and self-determination evolved from a trend toward empowerment of the patient. Empowerment refers to any process that enables people to "own their own lives" (Church, 1990).

Bernie Siegel (1986) promoted acceptance of autonomy and patient empowerment. He argued that controlling negative attitudes about cancer would significantly improve the quality and quantity of life for cancer survivors. He emphasized the need for positive cognitive reframing of the cancer treatment experience through mutual support, counseling, guided imagery, and alternative treatment methods.

Spiegel (1990) presented an important study about the potential benefit of attending cancer support groups. In an investigation of quality-of-life parameters for survivors of metastatic breast cancer, he serendipitously found that regular attendance at cancer-support-group meetings lengthened median survival time from 18 to 36 months. The reason for such a significant increase in survival has yet to be empirically determined. However, it may be speculated that stress and stress management could hold the key to fostering healthy behaviors that lead to improved survival.

Family Dynamics

Multimodal therapy, like treatment for other chronic illnesses, often requires significant physical, psychosocial, and spiritual contributions by family members. The ability of families to function well is often tested when a member is diagnosed with cancer. For the purpose of this discussion, *functionality* is the degree to which families can pull together, pool resources, and plan for the care of the patient with cancer. Family functional status is so important that it alone can significantly contribute to the success or failure of any cancer treatment plan (Quinn and Herndon, 1986).

The quality of family life as a distinct concept was explored by Jassak and Knafl (1990). They contended that although family life and relationships are acknowledged as important dimensions of the quality of life, research has focused predominantly on the concept of the individual's quality of life. Furthermore, they asserted that the oncology nurse has the unique opportunity and ability to assess the quality of family life and to develop strategies that promote family adaptation to illness.

The development of appropriate nursing interventions for families begins by assessing the structure of the family, identifying strengths and limitations within the family, and determining attitudes and beliefs about cancer within the family. This is often best accomplished by interviewing the family members separately. Gross inconsistencies in response among individuals may signify the potential development of significant conflict among the family members. It also helps to interview family members together to determine the power structure within the family unit. Attitudes of powerful family members may unduly influence patients in making decisions about treatment options. Box 27-3 presents tips on facilitating communication with family members.

Besides assessing family structure, boundaries, and functions, Welch-McCaffrey (1989) emphasized that the nurse should evaluate the primary caregiver to determine his or her perception of the situation. A full range of support services, including individual, group, and peer counseling, should be offered to all members of the family during this stressful time.

Families cope with stressful situations in a variety of ways. With relationship to illness, Quinn and Herndon (1986) focused on two major styles of adaptation, *separateness* and *connectedness*. Separateness refers to the degree to which members

---

Box 27-3 Tips on Facilitating Communication with Family Members

- ◆ Determine the power structure of the family unit.
  - ◆ Who makes the decisions for the family?
  - ◆ How are personal decisions for individual members made?
- ◆ Analyze how members communicate with one another.
  - ◆ Do members share information with each other?
  - ◆ Do they share information accurately?
- ◆ Listen for opportunities to find a compromise during conflict.
- ◆ Avoid intruding in a dialogue between family members.
- ◆ Stress the positive characteristics of each family member.

establish distinct boundaries from one another. For example, families with overly rigid boundaries often fail to provide intimacy during a crisis with cancer. Families at the extreme of this type often cannot talk about the disease and may demonstrate a maladaptive form of denial until the disease is advanced. Denial is not always a pathologic response, but it becomes maladaptive when the patient with cancer suppresses feelings in order to promote family harmony. An appropriate nursing intervention in this situation might involve arranging a professionally facilitated meeting between health care providers and family members to promote positive coping skills.

Connectedness refers to the degree to which members' boundaries may merge or overlap one another. Enmeshment may result, and this may lead members of this type of family to over-identify with the experience of having cancer. When members experience the same stressors under these circumstances, it becomes difficult to support each other.

Whatever the family type, it is important for the nurse to remember that each family has a unique functional style. The expected outcome is to assist members in achieving the highest functional level possible in order to facilitate a healthy relationship with the patient receiving multimodal cancer therapy.

❖ *Employment and Insurance Discrimination*

Although there is some discrepancy of opinion about the prevalence of discrimination issues (Hoffman, 1991), many authors argue that employment and insurance discrimination issues abound in the cancer population (Brown and Tai-Seale, 1992; Mellette and Franco, 1987; Rebl-Mundy, Moore, and Mundy, 1992). The National Institutes of Health (1990) estimated that about 25% of persons with cancer experience employment discrimination.

If modalities are given sequentially, multimodal therapy may involve a longer time commitment to therapy and may result in a longer absence from work or a longer period of part-time attendance at a full-time job. Concurrent therapy, with increased side effects, may make it more difficult for the patient to remain working and may necessitate unexpected or unwanted work absence.

Assessing employment- and insurance-related issues can often be accomplished by asking if the patient is having any difficulties on the job as a result of the diagnosis and treatment. For example, fatigue as a result of cancer treatment might exclude persons from certain job tasks. Some employers find modifying jobs difficult and resist making necessary accommodations to retain employees receiving multimodal therapy despite the fact that they are mandated by law to do so.

No other piece of legislation has had the impact of the Americans with Disabilities Act of 1990 on the employment and discrimination issues facing patients with cancer (Glajchen, 1994). It basically states that an entity is prohibited from discrimination toward an individual based on the existence of a disability. Because cancer was recognized as a severe disability in the Vocational Rehabilitation Act of 1973, the law provides legal protection from discriminatory behavior by employers toward employees with a diagnosis of cancer. However, a person who is trying to cope with cancer treatment and side effects may not have the energy to fight employer discrimination.

Many patients with cancer return to work after treatment is completed (Brown and Tai-Seale, 1992). However, some authors question the view that it is always better for persons with cancer to return to work as soon as possible. Glajchen (1994) recommended caution in assuming that continued employment is always the right answer for a person with cancer. She asserted that each individual's case possesses unique characteristics that make it inappropriate to set forth generalized occupational recommendations.

Many individuals with cancer need to work for a variety of reasons. For instance, a patient with cancer might lose health insurance benefits by giving up a job. The inability to quit or change jobs because of fear of losing benefits is often referred to as *job lock* (Glajchen, 1994). In this case, the patient with cancer is forced to maintain employment, sometimes to the detriment of physical health. Glajchen asserted that persons with cancer who are forced to remain in a job can become psychologically devastated and angry. In addition, job lock can frustrate career advancement and undermine the ability to ask for raises or improved working conditions.

Some employers perpetuate a belief that patients with cancer are too sick to work. Although the reason for their quasipaternalism may vary, the result for the patient can be the development of *disability syndrome*. Disability syndrome occurs when individuals become psychologically too "disabled" to work when they are medically able to do so (Rebl-Mundy et al., 1994). Disability syndrome occurs most often among cancer patients who have been externally pressured to perceive themselves "disabled" by employers, family, and others for a variety of reasons.

Nursing interventions for patients with cancer who have complex employment and insurance issues should include referral for rehabilitation counseling. Every state is mandated by the federal government to operate a department or division of vocational rehabilitation. The department is often staffed with certified rehabilitation counselors who are trained therapists with expertise in assisting individuals with disabilities in finding or maintaining suitable gainful employment. Referrals should be made as early as possible to minimize anxiety and stress during treatment (Brown and Tai-Seale, 1992).

Another piece of legislation that has direct implications for persons and families with cancers is the Family Medical Leave Act of 1993 (Chira, 1993). The law guarantees 12 weeks of unpaid leave for medical emergencies, childbirth, or adoption. This law can be enormously helpful for patients with cancer and family members who must travel long distances for multimodal therapy if one of the treatment modalities is not available at an institution near home. However, the loss of income during this time remains a significant problem.

❖ Selected Ethical Issues

Several ethical dilemmas can affect patients with cancer who are receiving multimodal therapy. A dilemma is a situation that requires a choice between two or more difficult or even conflicting courses of action; it is a problem seemingly incapable of a satisfactory solution (Whitman, 1980). Many of the multimodal therapy protocols are investigational. This means signing on to a clinical trial and consenting to be randomized to a treatment. Randomization is quite scary; letting a computer decide one's treatment is not something a lot of people feel comfortable about. Having the oncologist not recommend a specific treatment (other than to partici- pate in the clinical trial) increases the feeling of loss of control. Clinical trials may not be psychologically appropriate for all eligible patients.

A frequently encountered ethical dilemma for patients with cancer considering multimodal therapy occurs when the person must decide whether or not to pro- ceed with exceedingly expensive treatment options. The dilemma in this situation is that the treatment may increase the patient's period of survival but leave the patient or family financially compromised in the process. Outside large urban areas, the accessibility of radiation therapy and biotherapy may be a problem. The patient who needs to travel to obtain recommended treatment has to weigh the benefit of treatment against the expense of travel, which in many cases includes nonreim- bursable costs such as hotels and food. If a family member is to accompany the patient, that family member may experience loss of income or may have to find someone else to assume that person's normal functional role (e.g., mother, home- maker). The role of the nurse is to assist the patient and family to identify available financial and human resources, prioritize needs, and make decisions.

The decision of when to stop or withhold treatment presents another fre- quently encountered ethical dilemma. Many side effects are intensified in multi- modal therapy, and each time the patient faces severe side effects, he or she has to evaluate the worth of continuing treatment. The President's Commission for the Study of Ethical Problems in Medicine and Biomedical and Behavioral Research (1983) stated that when there is a conflict between the patient and the health care providers, the patient's *autonomy* (right to privacy and self-determination) takes precedence over the health provider's *beneficence* (desire to act in the best interest of the patient).

Thomasma (1989) asserted that a balance should be struck between patient wishes and traditional health care paternalism, where patients have had little or no say about when to start or stop treatment. He recommended that the best way for nurses to handle these types of professional practice issues is through the establish- ment of advance directives and intensive dialogue with the patient or surrogates about the patient's values throughout the course of treatment. *Advance directives* are legal documents that outline specifically what medical treatment the patient will accept in the event that the patient cannot at some future time speak for himself or herself. Every patient should be offered the opportunity to develop advance direc- tives for their care.

There are also important ethical issues for the nurse to consider when obtain- ing informed consent for multimodal therapy. The basic role of the nurse in this sit- uation is to support the patient by providing information that should include immediate and long-term risks and benefits (Varricchio and Jassak, 1989). Items to be disclosed when obtaining informed consent include the diagnosis, the nature and purpose of proposed treatment, the risks and consequences of the proposed treatment, the probability that the proposed treatment will be successful, feasible treatment alternatives, and the prognosis if the treatment is not given. Although it is the physician's role to provide this information, the nurse is also responsible for ensuring that the patient understands it.

The law requires that the patient or surrogate be judged able to comprehend information being presented (Silva and Zeccolo, 1986). The nurse should assess and identify the existence of psychosocial barriers such as difficulties with language, cognitive deficits, anxiety, educational limitations, or cultural differences that may diminish the patient or surrogate's ability legally to give informed consent. It is the nurse's responsibility to advocate for all patients in this matter.

This position of advocacy is based on the principle that individual self-determination is the highest value in the patient-nurse relationship (Gadow, 1989). Gadow asserted that the nurse's partnership role is ideally suited to assist patients in discerning and clarifying their beliefs, values, and goals as they examine available options. Appropriate decisions about pain control, treatment choice, research participation, family involvement, withdrawal of treatment, and the degree to which the patient with cancer wants to be informed can be enhanced by the presence of the nurse as a partner and advocate.

❖ Summary

Patients with cancer receiving multimodal therapy and their families face a number of significant psychosocial issues that impact the quality of their lives. These include, but are not limited to, issues related to the psychological sequelae of cancer and treatment, multiple providers and treatment settings, family dynamics, employment and insurance discrimination, accessing community support services and resource management, and selected ethical issues. It is hoped that discussion of these issues will assist the nurse in providing better psychosocial outcomes when working with patients receiving multimodal cancer therapy.

❖ References

American Cancer Society: Cancer facts and figures, Atlanta, 1996, American Cancer Society.

Brown HG and Tai-Seale M: Vocational rehabilitation of cancer patients, Semin Oncol Nurs 8:202–211, 1992.

Bukberg J, Penman D, and Holland JC: Depression in hospitalized cancer patients, Psychosom Med 46:199–212, 1986.

Cella DF and Tulsky DS: Measuring quality of life today: methodological aspects, Oncology 4:29–38, 1990.

Chira S: Family leave is law: will things change? New York Times, August 15, 1993.

Church K: Systems advocacy and empowerment: definitions and relationships, Toronto, Ontario, 1990, Psychiatric Patient Advocate Office.

Curtiss CP: Trends and issues for cancer care in rural communities, Nurs Clin of No Am 28:241–251, 1993.

Dow KH: The growing phenomenon of cancer survivorship, J Prof Nurs 7(1):54–61, 1991.

Gadow S: An ethical case for patient self-determination, Semin Oncol Nurs, 5:99–101, 1989.

Glajchen M: Psychosocial consequences of inadequate health insurance for patients with cancer, Cancer Prac 2:115–120, 1994.

Goldberg RJ and Cullen LO: Depression in geriatric cancer patients: guide to assessment and treatment, Hospice J 2(2):79–98, 1986.

Hoffman B: Employment discrimination: another hurdle for cancer survivors, Cancer Investigation 9:589–595, 1991.

Ivey AE: Intentional interviewing and counseling, Pacific Grove, California, 1988, Brooks/Cole.

Jassak PF and Knafl KA: Quality of family life: exploration of a concept, Semin Oncol Nurs 6:298–302, 1990.

Leigh SA: Cancer rehabilitation, Semin Oncol Nurs 8:164–166, 1992.

Massie MJ and Holland JC: Depression and the cancer patient. J Clin Psychiatry 51(7):12–17, 1990.

Massie MJ, Holland JC, and Straker N: Psychotherapeutic interventions. In Holland JC and Rowland JH, editors: Handbook of psychooncology: psychological care of the patient with cancer, New York, 1989, Oxford University Press, pp. 455–469.

Mellette SJ and Franco MS: Psychosocial barriers to employment of the cancer survivor. J Psychosoc Oncol 5(4):97–115, 1987.

National Institutes of Health: Facing forward—a guide for cancer survivors (NIH pub. no. 90–2424), Washington D.C., 1990, U.S. Department of Health and Human Services.

President's Commission for the Study of Ethical Problems in Medicine and Biomedical and Behavioral Research: Making health care decisions, Washington D.C., 1983, U.S. Government Printing Office.

Quinn WH and Herndon A: The family ecology of cancer. J Psychosoc Oncol 4(1/2):45–59, 1986.

Rebl-Mundy R, Moore SC, Corey JB, and Mundy GD: Disability syndrome: the effect of early vs. delayed intervention. Am Assoc Occ Health Nurs J 42:379–383, 1994.

Rebl-Mundy R, Moore SC, and Mundy GD: A missing link: rehabilitation counseling for persons with cancer, J Rehab 58(2):47–49, 1992.

Siegel BS: Love, medicine and miracles, New York, 1986, Harper & Row.

Silva MC and Zeccolo PL: Informed consent: the right thing to know and the right to choose. Nurs Manage 17(4):18–19, 1986.

Spiegel D: Can psychotherapy prolong cancer survival? Psychosomatics 31:361–365, 1990.

Thomasma DC: Ethics and professional practice in oncology, Semin Oncol Nurs 5:89–94, 1989.

Varricchio CG and Jassak PF: Informed consent: an overview, Semin Oncol Nurs 5:95–98, 1989.

Welch-McCaffrey D: Family issues in cancer care: current dilemmas and future directions, J Psychosoc Oncol 6(1/2):199–211, 1989.

Whitman H: Ethical issues in cancer nursing. II. Impediments to ethical nursing practice, Oncol Nurs Forum 7(2):40–42, 1980.

Chapter 28

❖ *Continuity of Care*

Norma J. Fenerty

Continuity of care is an important element of health care. With chronic illnesses such as cancer, continuity of care becomes a complex concern because patients generally receive multimodal therapy in several settings (Fenerty, 1993a). Collaborative efforts by the health care team across settings help assure the patient's transition through the health care environment (Preston and Hannigan-Maloney, 1990).

Discharge planning is defined as a sequence of events initiated after a person is admitted to a health care setting to facilitate continuity of care (Kelly and McClelland, 1985). Discharge-planning activities utilize the nursing process (McCarthy, 1988) and are most effective when an interdisciplinary approach is used (Corkery, 1989). *Continuity of care* is defined as a coordinated series of activities that involve the client and the health care team working together to facilitate the transition of health care from one institution, agency, or individual to another (McKeenan and Coulton, 1985).

Discharge planning is the process; continuity of care is the goal (Buckwalter, 1985; O'Hare, Yost, and McCorkle, 1993). Continuity of care can only be achieved when the patient works with the health care professionals to accomplish mutually agreed upon goals (McCarthy, 1988). The concept of continuity of care ideally encompasses a lifetime of health care (Farren, 1991).

Recent innovations that affect the continuity-of-care process are collaborative care models—often referred to as *critical* or *clinical pathways*–which extend from preadmission to postdischarge. The emphasis is on open communication and coordination among all members of the health care team, including the patient (Jones and Mulliken, 1994).

❖ *Ambulatory Care*

The majority of individuals with a suspected or confirmed cancer diagnosis enter the health care continuum by way of ambulatory care. The ambulatory care nurse begins evaluation of the patient's present health care status using a standardized patient assessment form. To save time and to assess what the patient understands, the patient may be asked to complete most of the form. Afterwards the nurse reviews the form with the patient to determine the patient's unmet health needs. At that time, patient needs are addressed and referrals are made to appropriate support services. This information becomes part of the permanent medical record and accompanies the patient to other settings in the same institution. Prescribed medications and continuing-care instructions are documented, and a written copy of all instructions, including appointments, is given to the patient.

For legal reasons, all follow-up telephone contact should be part of the permanent record. A standardized form like the one in Figure 28-1 can be used for documentation of telephone communication. Copies of this form are sent to appropriate team members for their information. Alternative methods of documentation exist. In one institution a notebook is kept by the phone in the respective outpatient areas of ambulatory care, the chemotherapy clinic, and the radiation clinic. This notebook contains a progress-note page for each patient. "Telephone contact" is written on the top of the page on which all calls are documented. When the page is full, it is sent to medical records for placement in the chart (Liebman, in press a). This prevents the need to retrieve the chart from the medical records department for every phone call and also ensures that the information is recorded.

TELEPHONE DOCUMENTATION

Call received by: _____ Date: _____ Time: _____

Call initiated by: ❑ Patient ❑ Family ❑ Pharmacy ❑ Home Health RN ❑ Family MD ❑ Other

Patient name: _____ Medical Record #: _____ Phone Number: _____

Attending MD/Fellow: _____ Primary RN: _____

Allergies: _____ Treatment: ❑ Chemo ❑ XRT ❑ Surgery ❑ F/U

PURPOSE OF CALL: Patient Problem/Question: _____

_____

_____

Prescription: _____

_____

Tests/ Appointments: _____

ACTION TAKEN: ❑ Handled by RN ❑ Secretary ❑ Physician/Fellow ❑ Other _____

_____

_____

Prescription called ❑ Lab Results Given ❑ Attending MD Notified ❑ Yes Time _____ ❑ No

See Progress Notes _____ Dr. _____

Signature _____

Fig. 28-1. Telephone Documentation. Courtesy of Fox Chase Cancer Center, Philadelphia, Pennsylvania.

❖ Preadmission

A nurse in the preadmission setting promotes continuity of care by providing information and coordinating arrangements for care. Nurse-to-nurse referrals are often generated for preoperative education or for preadmission discussion of available home health supports for postdischarge care when requested by the patient. Because of managed care and other insurance-provider restrictions, increasing numbers of patients have preadmission testing done by outside labs or facilities. It is vital that the nurse in the preadmission setting obtain and review this information in a timely manner.

❖ Admission

Although discharge planning requires a team approach, the primary nurse usually initiates the discharge process at the time of admission (Corkery, 1989). Discharge planning is best accomplished through the use of a comprehensive standardized assessment followed by an individualized plan that outlines action needed to implement the continuity of care process (Kelly and McClelland, 1985).

The nurse completes an admission assessment of the patient or updates the ambulatory care assessment, which identifies the patient's problems. A plan of care is developed utilizing standards of nursing care and standards of nursing practice. The standards are based on nursing literature derived from research. A discharge-planning assessment tool can provide a quick reference to the primary nurse; ideally it should be located on the front of every nursing care plan. "Thinking about H.O.M.E." (Box 28-1) outlines discharge-planning activities from admission to discharge.

When a nurse identifies a patient who requires assistance with complex discharge-planning needs, a referral is made to the discharge-planning nurse. The discharge-planning nurse provides information about available resources and makes necessary referrals (Chielens and Herrick, 1990). The primary nurse communicates discharge-planning activities to other nurses through the use of a nurse discharge-planning record.

One benefit of discharge planning initiated early in the admission phase is that the patient and caregivers become aware that the health care team is working toward the patient going home. This may have a positive effect on a patient's confidence in recovery (Farren, 1991). Another benefit is that the patient and family know that the patient is not expected to remain in the hospital until completely well; discussing after-discharge care means that some of the recovery of health will occur at home.

❖ Discharge

Appropriate health care professionals identified by the primary nurse provide discharge instructions. Identifying and meeting the continuing-care needs of persons with cancer requires the knowledge and expertise of the interdisciplinary team members. The nurse may request a pharmacist to provide patient education materials for a new medication or chemotherapy. The nutritionist may write dietary

---

Box 28-1 Thinking About H.O.M.E.

How was the patient managing prior to admission?
◆ Discuss with patient and caregiver(s)
◆ Evaluate resources per nursing admission history sheet
  ◆ Prehospitalization place of residence
  ◆ Family (caregiver)
  ◆ Community resources being utilized at time of admission such as home health, adult day-care centers, friends, or neighbors

Offer the services of discharge-planning coordinators (DPCs)
◆ Informational
  ◆ Insurance coverage for continuing-care needs
  ◆ Access to choice of services: individual-counseling format versus family-meeting format
◆ Concrete
  ◆ Home care nurses
  ◆ High-tech therapies
  ◆ Private-duty help

Management problems at time of discharge
◆ Communicate continuing-care needs to DPC (discharge-planning coordinator)

Educational needs and equipment needs
◆ Educational needs for home care nurse follow-up
  ◆ Reinforce discharge instructions
  ◆ Monitor chemotherapy and radiation therapy side effects
  ◆ Pain management
  ◆ Wound care
  ◆ Tube or drain care
  ◆ Nutrition
  ◆ Ostomy and skin care
  ◆ Oxygen
◆ Equipment needs
  ◆ Assess level of functioning and need for rehabilitation
  ◆ Equipment needs communicated to DPC

From Fenerty, NB: Discharge planning guide for primary nurses, Oncol Nurs Forum 20:117, 1993. Reprinted from the Oncology Nursing Forum with permission from the Oncology Nursing Press, Inc.

---

instructions or a home enteral feeding regimen for the patient, or the respiratory therapist may perform noninvasive testing to evaluate if home oxygen is indicated. The social worker may arrange ambulance transportation home, provide counseling about financial concerns, recommend outpatient support groups, or arrange transfer to a skilled nursing facility or rehabilitation center. The rehabilitation therapists (e.g., physical therapist, occupational therapist) provide instructions on individualized home exercise programs and subsequent medical equipment needed.

The physician communicates information about needed posthospital care, including outpatient therapies and laboratory monitoring (Fenerty, 1993a).

The discharge instruction sheet is completed at the time of patient discharge. Standardized discharge instruction sheets following chemotherapy (Figure 28-2) or surgery provide the nurse with tools to assist the patient in a safe transition from hospital or clinic to home.

❖ *Referral*

Referrals communicate information about patients' continuing-care needs between health care organizations. This information assists in transferring responsibility for providing care and linkage across settings (Anderson and Helms, 1993, 1994). When the referral form has inadequate information, a barrier in communication arises between health care providers and results in gaps in patient care (Anderson and Helms, 1994; Fritsch-deBruyn and Cunningham, 1990).

Using a standardized patient referral form, which includes detailed information about diagnoses, medical interventions during the current hospitalization, allergies, caregiver support, functional abilities, discharge medications, equipment arrangements, and continuing-care needs, assists the home health nurse in providing continuity of care. The home health nurse depends on this information to initiate a plan of care and to justify interventions to third-party payers (Corkery, 1989; Fenerty, 1993a; Preston and Hannigan-Maloney, 1990). The person completing the referral should sign the form and include a phone extension. This identifies a source who can clarify orders or receive feedback (Anderson and Helms, 1994). Patient education forms used by the referring agency can be attached to the referral form to ensure continuity of care from one agency to another (Preston and Hannigan-Maloney, 1990).

❖ *Establishing Linkages*

Home and Ambulatory Care

One way to maximize the limited contact that a patient may have with the health care team in an ambulatory setting is to provide each patient with a follow-up assessment form (Figure 28-3) at their return appointment after completion of therapy. The information obtained helps the nurse to identify potential problem areas requiring nursing interventions and to prioritize care.

The ambulatory care nurse can utilize a triage documentation form (Figure 28-4) when a patient comes in with an urgent problem. Documentation of the various cancer treatments the patient received or is receiving can clarify a complex treatment history. If hospitalization results, this baseline data helps the nurse in the inpatient setting develop the patient's care plan. If the patient is not hospitalized but is followed by a home-care agency, a copy of this form sent to the patient's home health nurse will help provide continuity of care. If the patient is not followed by a home health nurse and more than one unscheduled visit a week occurs in either ambulatory care or the emergency room, the cancer team should consider a home health referral.

CHEMOTHERAPY PATIENT DISCHARGE INSTRUCTIONS
(Check appropriate space or write in information)

Patient Addressograph

Mode of Discharge: _____ Ambulatory _____ Wheelchair _____ Stretcher

Discharged to: _____ Own Home _____ Other Facility Accompanied by _____

If inpatient, Pre-Admission Medications Returned to Patient/Family _____

Belongings Returned to Patient/Family _____

Follow-Up Appointments: _____

Telephone Contact:

_____ Medical Clinic 728-2600 _____ Surgical Clinic 728-2601 _____ Radiation Clinic 728-2581

_____ Emergency Evening, Night, Weekend, Holidays 728-6900

_____ Home Care _____

_____ Durable Medical Equipment _____

_____ Discharge Planning Coordinator _____

_____ Social Worker _____

_____ Other _____

Home Medications	Dose	Route	Times Daily	Purpose of Medication
1.				
2.				
3.				
4.				
5.				
6.				

(If more than six medications, use second sheet)

Patient allergies: _____

Chemotherapy medications received in clinic/hospital _____

DISCHARGE INSTRUCTIONS
(Check appropriate spaces)

ACTIVITY:

__ As tolerated. Take rest periods as needed, pace yourself, do not over tire.

__ Avoid crowds, people with colds or infections.

__ Avoid strong sunlight, use sunblock and sunglasses for protection.

DIET:

__ High protein and high caloric foods as tolerated.

__ If nausea/vomiting, try small frequent meals.

__ Drink 6–8 glasses of fluid/day. Replace fluids if vomiting or diarrhea.

__ If mouth sores, avoid spicy and acidic foods and fluids; avoid foods/fluids at extremes of temperature; use S & S mouthwash at least four times/day (using S & S mouthwash before meals may make food more palatable).

CALL MD IF:

__ Temperature is 100.5° or greater.

__ Increased shortness of breath and/or mucus/sputum production.

__ Pain or burning with urination.

__ Any other signs of infection.

__ Unable to take fluids due to vomiting or sore throat for more than 24 hours.

__ Numbness/tingling in extremities; severe constipation; hearing loss and/or ringing in ears.

__ Unusual bleeding or bruising; blood in urine or BM; bleeding gums or nose bleeds.

__ Diarrhea for longer than 48 hours.

__ New and/or increase in existing pain level.

I understand these instructions and have received a copy

Patient or responsible person signature _____ Date _____

RN signature _____ Date _____

Figure 28-2. Chemotherapy Patient Discharge Instructions. Courtesy of Fox Chase Cancer Center, Philadelphia, Pennsylvania.

FOLLOW-UP SELF-ASSESSMENT FORM

To help us to know what problems, concerns, or questions you have we ask that you fill out this form. When you are finished, please bring this to your radiation oncology nurse.

Have you had any problems since your last visit?   YES _____ NO _____

   If YES, please explain _____

Have you been admitted to any hospital since your last visit?   YES _____ NO _____

   If YES, please explain _____

Please list all the medicines you are taking now.

_____   _____   _____

_____   _____   _____

_____   _____   _____

Do you understand the reason you are taking each of these
   medicines?   YES _____ NO _____

Do you have pain?   YES _____ NO _____

   If YES, please explain _____

Are you having any problems with your mouth or swallowing?   YES _____ NO _____

Has your weight changed?   YES _____ NO _____

If YES— Did you lose weight?   YES _____ NO _____

         Did you gain weight?   YES _____ NO _____

Do you have any problems with your skin?   YES _____ NO _____

Do you have any wound problems?   YES _____ NO _____

Are you having any problems with your bowels?   YES _____ NO _____

If YES— Is it constipation?   YES _____ NO _____

         Is it diarrhea?   YES _____ NO _____

Are you having any problems urinating?   YES _____ NO _____

If YES— Do you have burning?   YES _____ NO _____

         Do you have frequency?   YES _____ NO _____

Do you have any concerns or questions about your sexual activity?   YES _____ NO _____

Females—Do you examine your breasts each month?   YES _____ NO _____

Who lives with you?   I live alone   _____

                Spouse   _____

                Children   _____

                Parents   _____

                Other   _____

Who helps you at home?   I don't need help   _____

                I need help but no one helps me   _____

                Spouse   _____

                Children   _____

                Parents   _____

                Visiting Nurse   _____

                Other   _____

Do you have trouble with any of the following:

   Getting meals   Always   _____

                Sometimes   _____

                Never   _____

Washing and getting dressed	Always	_____
	Sometimes	_____
	Never	_____
Housekeeping	Always	_____
	Sometimes	_____
	Never	_____

Do you think your family wants or needs help caring for you? YES _____ NO _____
Do you need help caring for your children, spouse, or parents? YES _____ NO _____
Do you have concerns or questions about health insurance or other
    financial matters? YES _____ NO _____
Do you need help with rides to get to the doctor? YES _____ NO _____
Is there anything else you would like to say or ask?

_____

_____

_____

Fig. 28-3. Follow-up Self-Assessment Form. From Bruner DW and Slivjak A, editors: Documentation manual for radiation oncology nursing, Philadelphia, 1994, Fox Chase Cancer Center. Reprinted with permission from the Department of Radiation Oncology.

Interinstitution Communication

Follow-up care can be as simple as a telephone call placed to a patient at home to evaluate the effectiveness of patient education (Nichols and Bennett, 1993). Conversely, it can present a major challenge when a cancer patient receives multimodal treatment in more than one setting.

An institution with a large bone marrow transplantation program offers a unique solution to communication between nurses in different settings. Each patient is asked to identify a primary nurse from the referring office or hospital who can assist in obtaining records, making appointments, and discussing patient and family issues. When the patient is discharged from the tertiary hospital, this nurse is notified by telephone and receives a nursing posttransplant flow sheet by mail. This form outlines the pretransplant regimen; date of transplant; complications; latest blood counts; the need for transfusions and premedications; supportive care issues, such as effective antiemetics; central line care; current medications; and any miscellaneous information needed to ensure a smooth transition from the tertiary care center to the patient's community setting (Nelson, 1993). This close communication also gives the nurse at the community hospital a resource to call if questions arise.

A patient health care diary helps provide continuity of care as the patient moves through different care settings. The use of a diary increases the patient's participation in care (Preston and Hannigan-Maloney, 1990). Information in a patient health care diary includes the names and telephone numbers of all health care personnel involved in care; a medical history, including the cancer problem and multimodal treatment; medication list; caregiver information; laboratory monitoring; chemotherapy scheduling calendar; venous-access-device care; nutrition, including a food diary; potential side effects of multimodal cancer treatment, including a symptom distress scale and pain diary (Martin and Preston, 1989).

One institution identified a need for improved patient care coordination between its inpatient units and outpatient clinics. Twice a month they now hold

---

AMBULATORY CARE NURSING TRIAGE DOCUMENTATION FORM

Patient Addressograph

Scheduled visit: _____   Drop in: _____
Date: _____   Allergies: _____
Diagnosis: _____

CURRENT TREATMENT

Radiation Therapy Site: _____   Surgery: _____

Current Medication List: _____   Chemotherapy Cycle   1   2   3   4   5   6

_____   _____

_____   _____

_____   _____

_____   _____

Time last medication taken: _____

PRESENTING PROBLEM *(circle all that apply)*

Information • Comfort • Protective Mechanisms • Elimination • Ventilation • Coping
Mobility Mechanisms • Sexuality • Circulation

1. _____   2. _____   3. _____

NURSING NOTES

_____

_____

_____

_____

LABS/RADIOLOGY DONE: Medications given:

_____   _____

_____   _____

See progress notes for more information:
❑ YES   ❑ NO   Patient Discharged: _____

Referral initiated: ❑ YES   ❑ NO   Inpatient Unit: _____
Social Service • Physical Therapy • Palliative Care   OPD Appt: _____
Home Care • Pain Management • Other

DISPOSITION OF PATIENT: NAME OF PHYSICAN NOTIFIED

Patient Admitted   ❑ YES   ❑ NO   NURSE'S SIGNATURE

Fig. 28-4. Ambulatory Care Nursing Triage Documentation Form. Courtesy of Fox Chase Cancer Center, Philadelphia, Pennsylvania, 1994.

formal nursing rounds to discuss patients who are seen in one area of the hospital and are expected to be seen in other areas (e.g., radiation therapy clinic, chemotherapy clinic, or inpatient unit). Nursing representatives from all oncology areas, a discharge-planning nurse, and a social worker attend the rounds. The group discusses areas of concern and develops nursing care plans. This provides consistency wherever the patient goes, as well as an introduction before the nurses actually meet the patient, improving continuity of care (Liebman, in press b).

Computerized Linkages

A perceived lack of nursing communication tools for patient information flow between the inpatient oncology unit, the medical oncology clinic, and the radiation oncology clinic led to the development of a computerized inpatient-outpatient flow sheet in one regional cancer center. Nurses from these areas developed a clinical data base that the nursing staff in its three distinct oncology areas could access. A nurse in any oncology department can initiate the form. Priority entry is assigned to patients to be admitted. Nurses enter updates into the computer on patients with venous access devices and on ill patients with a potential for admission after clinic hours (Case and Jones, 1989). A computerized nurse-to-nurse consultation system has been devised to enhance professional communication at the tertiary care level (Orchard and Swenson, 1993).

Computer technology allows health care professionals to capture, manipulate, and retrieve information in a timely, accessible manner. Computerization offers the potential for providing linkage between different health care settings (Reider and Houser, 1985). However, computerized linkage between settings raises unresolved issues such as securing and maintaining patient confidentiality. The future of computerization of all health care information is unknown.

❖ Summary

Continuity of care is every health care consumer's right. When a patient with cancer receives multimodal therapy in different settings, maintaining continuity of care presents a challenge to the nurse. An organized, multidisciplinary approach to continuing care fosters achievement of outcome criteria established by professional standards. Discharge-planning activities—once associated only with the inpatient setting—have evolved into formalized programs that span all settings. The development of computerized flow sheets may promote linkage between settings within an organization. Interagency communication by computer is a concept that warrants further exploration.

❖ References

Anderson MA and Helms L: An assessment of discharge planning models: communication in referrals for home care, Ortho Nurs 12:41–49, 1993.

Anderson MA and Helms L: Quality improvement in discharge planning: an evaluation of factors in communication between health care providers, J Nurs Care Qual 8(2):62–72, 1994.

Bruner DW and Slivjak A, editors: Department of radiation oncology follow-up self-assessment form. In Documentation manual for radiation oncology nursing, Philadelphia, 1994, Fox Chase Cancer Center.

Buckwalter KC: Exploring the process of discharge planning: application to the construct of health. In McClelland E, Kelly K, and Buckwalter KC, editors: Continuity of care: advancing the concept of discharge planning, Orlando, Florida, 1985, Grune & Stratton, Inc, pp. 5–10.

Case CL and Jones LH: Continuity of care. Development and implementation of a shared patient data base, Cancer Nurs 12:332–338, 1989.

Chielens D and Herrick E: Recipients of bone marrow transplants: making a smooth transition to an ambulatory care setting, Oncol Nurs Forum 17:857–862, 1990.

Corkery E: Discharge planning and home health care: what every staff nurse should know, Ortho Nurs 8(6):18–27, 1989.

Farren EA: Effects of early discharge planning on length of hospital stay, Nurs Economics, 9(1):25–30, 1991.

Fenerty NJ: Interdisciplinary discharge planning: a continuing care management model, Cancer Prac 1:147–152, 1993a.

Fenerty NB: Discharge planning guide for primary nurses, Oncol Nurs Forum 20:117, 1993b.

Fritsch-deBruyn R and Cunningham H: A check on nurses' knowledge and sense of responsibility for discharge planning, J Nurs Staff Develop 6:173–176, 1990.

Jones RA and Mullikin CW: Collaborative care: pathways to quality outcomes, J Healthcare Qual 16(4):10–13, 1994.

Kelly K and McClelland E: Discharge planning. In Bulechek G and McCloskey J, editors: Nursing interventions. Treatments for nursing diagnoses, Philadelphia, 1985, WB Saunders Co, pp. 385–400.

Liebman MC: Documenting telephone calls, Oncol Nurs Forum 22: in press, a.

Liebman MC: Nursing rounds enhance continuity of care, Oncol Nurs Forum 22: in press, b.

Martin V and Preston F: Patient health care diary, 1989, unpublished.

McCarthy SA: The process of discharge planning. In O'Hare PA and Terry MA, editors: Discharge planning: strategies for assuring continuity of care, Rockville, Maryland, 1988, Aspen Publishers.

McKeenan KM and Coulton CJ: A systems approach to program development for continuity of care in hospitals. In McClelland E, Kelly K, and Buckwalter K, editors: Continuity of care: advancing the concept of discharge planning, Orlando, Florida, 1985, Grune & Stratton, Inc.

Nelson JM: Interinstitution coordination smooths transitions, Oncol Nurs Forum 20:117, 1993.

Nichols M and Bennett MV: Follow-up phone call facilitates evaluation of learning, Oncol Nurs Forum 20:827, 1993.

O'Hare PA, Yost LS, and McCorkle R: Strategies to improve continuity of care and decrease rehospitalization of cancer patients: a review, Cancer Investigation 11:140–158, 1993.

Orchard MLH and Swenson GN: Enhancing professional communication: a formal computerized nurse-to-nurse consultation system, Nurs Admin Q 18(1):66–79, 1993.

Preston FA and Hannigan-Maloney C: Home care for the oncology patient. In Hubbard S, Greene P, and Knobf M, editors: Current issues in cancer nursing practice, Philadelphia, 1990, JB Lippincott Co, pp. 13–25.

Reider KA and Houser ML: Enhancing discharge planning: continuous care using an automated decision support system. In McClelland E, Kelly K, and Buckwalter KC, editors: Continuity of care: advancing the concept of discharge planning, Orlando, Florida, 1985, Grunne & Stratton, Inc, pp. 161–171.

Chapter 29

❖ *Future Trends in Oncology Nursing and Multimodal Therapy*

Anne E. Belcher

The future of oncology, with its emphasis on multimodal therapy, is interwoven with the future of health care. It is imperative that nurses understand the issues and trends underlying health care reform and respond in innovative and cost-effective ways while maintaining the quality of care that is the hallmark of the specialty. Boyle, Engelking, and Harvey (1994a) listed ten major predictions about cancer in the twenty-first century, emphasizing aggressive multimodal therapy, with care given by multiple agencies. McLaughlin-Hagan and Baird (1993) predict numerous future trends based on the costs of cancer, changes in hospital care, treatment options, and advances in education and research. These trends include but are not limited to an increasing use of case management and managed care for the delivery of services; greater emphasis on collaborative practice, entrepreneurship, and intrapreneurship (defined as entrepreneurship within a large organization); the expanding role of the nurse as advocate; greater nurse involvement in policy development; the changing focus of advanced practice; and preparation for oncology nursing as a specialty.

Engelking (1994) notes that

the ability to medically support patients undergoing intensive therapies and the evidence that more aggressive therapeutic approaches (e.g., chemotherapy dose intensification with stem cell or growth factor rescue) result in improved outcomes [which] will make the concept of combining multiple highly aggressive anticancer therapies to achieve cure a standard for treatment of many more tumor types (p. 67).

Harvey (1994) indicates that the multidisciplinary, multimodal nature of cancer treatment makes the economics of cancer care difficult to quantify because of the uncertainty of outcomes, the social-support needs of patients and families, the cost and appropriateness of clinical trials, and the long-term care needs of persons with cancer.

It is anticipated that the health care industry will view cancer care as one of the top money-makers in the future; however, increasing profits will adversely affect patients, employers, and insurance companies as health care organizations seek to increase profits further and to cut costs by such measures as hiring less-qualified care providers—that is, nonlicensed personnel—and adding other responsibilities to those initially employed in a more traditional role—that is, registered nurses providing respiratory therapy. At the regulatory level, states may deny a certificate of need to a hospital that wants to provide multimodal therapy (e.g., adding radiation therapy equipment and personnel to their services), basing the denial on cost containment. The impact on the patient is obvious: when different treatments are provided at different sites, patients and families have to coordinate travel, job responsibilities, child care, and other aspects of their lives in order to meet multiple schedules in multiple settings. The trend toward hospital mergers nationwide may further limit patient options as to where they receive treatment and the number of settings in which treatment is received.

Cancer centers will compete more aggressively for patients and treatment options by designing innovative marketing programs and networking arrangements, by using political strategies to gain support for certificates of need, and by merging with community hospitals, home-care agencies, and hospices to provide comprehensive services to their clients. In addition, long-distance clinical monitoring systems will enable patients to receive highly complex cancer treatments at home. For example, medications will be titrated at a base facility and administered by the patient or a family member; the patient's response to the drugs will be tracked in real time (as it occurs). Patients will be linked to a tertiary care facility that manages their care and to medical information systems; they will receive immediate advice and treatment when indicated. The role of acute-care facilities will obviously change from providing direct care to monitoring and regulating care from a distance (Harvey, 1994).

As the cost of cancer care rises and the number of cancer survivors increases, third-party payers also will ration payment and will require health care providers to document the cost effectiveness of cancer treatments. The benefit of this rationing will be more efficient care; the adverse effect will be caregivers' failure to deliver adequate care, particularly in acute-care settings because of third-party payers' denial of payment beyond specific parameters.

As medical schools increase the number of physicians prepared to provide primary care—that is, general practitioners and family practitioners—fewer specialists will be trained to meet the needs of persons with such diseases as cancer. It is anticipated that specialists such as oncologists will prescribe treatment that will be administered and monitored by the generalists in offices and clinics. Nurses must be prepared to bridge the gap in care that could occur as a result of this division of responsibility. One essential response to this change in the delivery of cancer care is the preparation of more advanced-practice nurses (APNs) who have the expertise to assess, diagnose, plan, intervene, and evaluate along the cancer continuum. For example, the APN will monitor patients' responses to therapy, identifying and managing symptoms that result from the disease and its treatment. Oncology nurses will be called upon as individuals and groups to describe their unique contributions to the care of persons with cancer, to provide evidence of their positive effect on cost control, and to assure the quality of care.

Persons with cancer who require hospitalization will need more skilled nursing care and comprehensive education in preparation for continuing care in the home. Although cancer centers will continue to focus on staging the disease and providing the major treatment modalities for complex cancers, the management of adverse effects of cancer and its treatment will move into ambulatory, community, and home settings. Alternative-care settings such as residential facilities and day centers will be used for care during the workday. Nurses will function as case managers, using established standards of care for the identification and prediction of patient care needs, appropriate care providers, and appropriate care settings. Home-care nurses will provide increasingly more acute care, and laypersons will require home nursing courses and support in order to participate effectively as caregivers at home and in hospices.

❖ *Case Management*

The term *case management* refers to a generic process that is made operational through a variety of models, implemented by an assortment of health care providers, and results in diverse outcome goals (Knollmueller, 1989). The American Nurses Association (1988) identifies the significant goals of case management as optimizing and increasing the client's self-care abilities; enhancing the patient's quality of life and adjustment to altered health states; preventing inappropriate hospitalizations and decreasing recidivism; providing quality health care with decreased fragmentation of care across settings; and promoting health care cost containment. Multimodal therapy, with its complex treatments, intense side effects, and high potential for fragmentation of care, brings out the need for case management.

Managed care is a system of resource utilization that can be applied to all patients in a health care institution; it is used to predict and to formulate a cost-effective plan of care and to track patient progress during hospitalization (Papenhausen, 1990). Managed care focuses on coordinating the activities of health care providers to address patients' physical, psychosocial, and family needs in a cost-effective manner.

The goal of case-managed care is to improve the quality of care by decreasing fragmentation of care and improving patients' quality of life. Studies suggest that managed care also achieves cost savings through patient education, self-management programs, and reductions in hospital admissions. Nurses play an important role in the activities that generate these savings, including primary care, utilization review, case management, quality improvement, and administration (Nelson, 1993). A major difference between managed care and case management systems is the degree and intensity of individual interaction between patients and health care providers. The role of the oncology nurse as case manager is emerging. As Zander (1994) has indicated:

Nurses are in a unique position to provide case management in collaboration with physicians and the institution because they have intimate access of patients and families over extended time periods. . . . They [nurses] are at the juncture of cost and quality, and they know the human implication of trade-offs such as early discharge, patient education in groups, or the use of new technology (p. 201).

Persons with cancer are in particular need of case management because they are high-risk/high-cost patients who need coordination between multimodal treatment settings and along the cancer care continuum. Oncology nurses are well suited to function as case managers and to develop plans of care that reflect the complex needs of persons with cancer.

❖ *Collaborative Practice*

Collaborative practice is defined by England (1986) as the integration of multidisciplinary professional practices into a comprehensive approach to meet the needs of the patient. The essential elements for effective collaborative practice are a common purpose, diverse professional skills and contributions, and effective communication. According to Dumont and Niziole (1991), collaboration

expresses the value that patient needs are multidimensional and should remain the focus of concern for all caregivers. Mutual respect among colleagues and open communication are the cornerstones of collaborative practice . . ." (p. 331).

Role negotiation is necessary at the time the team is formed and throughout the patient's movement toward predetermined outcomes. Team members must agree on interdependent and cooperative decision making, sharing of knowledge, consensus of goals, confidence in one another's ability, and mutual trust (Burchell, Thomas, and Smith, 1983), especially with multimodal treatment. Collaboration occurs when professionals work as a team, blending knowledge and skills to improve the quality of patient care. Nowhere is this more evident than in oncology care as nurses, physicians, social workers, nutritionists, physical therapists, and other members of the health care team use one another's skills and knowledge to meet individual patient needs. There is a long history of oncology nurses developing collaborative practices with physicians for symptom management (e.g., pain management). In the years to come, collaborative relationships inside and outside health care organizations will be needed to address the complex needs of persons with cancer and their families, particularly those receiving multimodal therapy.

❖ *Entrepreneurship and Intrapreneurship*

Aydelotte, Hardy, and Hope (1988) describe nurses in entrepreneurial roles as independent practitioners and as owners or proprietors of health care enterprises. *Intrapreneurship* refers to characteristics of entrepreneurial functioning within large organizations (Herron and Herron, 1991). Boyle, Engelking, and Harvey (1994b) describe intrapreneurs as dreamers who assume hands-on responsibility for fostering innovation inside their orga-nization. Characterized by energy, enthusiasm, self-confidence, motivation and acknowledgement of their personal strengths, intrapreneurs also are mentors and acknowledge personal and organizational limits, and they consciously cultivate key rela-tionships (p. 77).

A number of important conclusions are reached from an extensive review of the literature:

The essence of entrepreneurship appears to be innovation through reallocation or reconfiguration of resources for the purpose of creating benefit. . . . This reconfigura-tion implies an awareness of or alertness to the opportunity to do so for the purpose of creating benefit (Herron and Herron, 1991, p. 311).

Although numerous studies have attempted to describe the personality charac-teristics of the entrepreneurial nurse, Herron (1990) has shown that skills tend to be more important; they include product or service design, functional business and industry knowledge, leadership, networking, administrative planning, and oppor-tunity recognition and implementation.

With health care reform, hospitals and other organizations face increasing pres-sure to deliver care more efficiently. They will have to use the creative potential of their employees, especially nurses, by encouraging and supporting intrapreneur-ship. For example, the continuing trend toward work redesign to meet patient needs better and to save money will prompt hospitals to use nurses' knowledge and experience to meet these goals. Herron and Herron (1991) recommend that entre-preneurship theory be used by nurses "to build professional practice models which foster the joint realization of both nursing and organizational goals" (p. 315).

Oncology nurse entrepreneurs exemplify autonomous nursing in assuming the management and risk of a business; researching markets and analyzing potential clients; creating effective marketing strategies and product promotions; identifying and lowering costs; setting fees and setting up efficient accounting systems; paying strict attention to legalities; and continuously assessing consumer satisfaction. The nurse entrepreneur represents the ideal of the nurse in independent practice to meet the nursing needs of the person with cancer, an example of which is the owner of a cancer home-care agency. The nurse intrapreneur represents the ideal of the nurse in collaborative practice to meet the organization's needs for providing quality care during multimodal therapy in a cost-effective manner.

❖ Oncology Nurses as Advocates

The nurse as advocate "has moved from a posture of interceding, supporting, or pleading a case for the client to acting as guardian of the client's rights to auton-omy and free choice" (Nelson, 1988, p. 136). This shift in role has occurred in spite of nurses' perceived obligation to be loyal to personal values and beliefs, which can differ from the values and beliefs of a patient, a physician or group of physicians, or an employer. This shift presents a unique challenge to the oncology nurse, whose job description may include recruitment of patients into research protocols that place financial, logistical, and time demands on the subject and that create discomforting side effects. As persons with cancer become increasingly knowledgeable about cancer and its management, they are demanding more information and more detailed explanations. They look to nurses for such data and for support of their informed decisions.

Oncology nurses' advocacy for persons with cancer should focus on the following patient rights (Annas, 1974):

♦ Knowledge of research and experimental protocols and complete and accurate information regarding medical care and procedures
♦ Clear, concise explanations of all proposed procedures, including risks, mortality, and probability of success
♦ Clear, complete, and accurate evaluation of one's condition and of the prognosis without treatment
♦ Opportunity to refuse any drug, test, procedure, or treatment

An area of increasing complexity and concern in oncology is the potential impact of cost containment on the development of new therapeutic agents and techniques for multimodal treatment. For example, pharmaceutical companies are under pressure to bring new drugs to market more quickly and with fewer development costs, which they have traditionally passed on to patients. Although the benefit of increased governmental regulation of costs should be passed on to the patient in the form of less expensive drugs and earlier access to new and refined techniques and equipment, there is reason for concern that access will be rationed. Rationing may occur in terms of an upper limit on reimbursement for drugs, procedures, and so on or in terms of other criteria such as age, stage of disease, or geographical location. The oncology nurse as advocate must stay knowledgeable about trends in this and other such areas, speak knowledgeably with persons in policy-making positions, and serve as a resource to consumer groups, particularly those focused on cancer care. Another example of the oncology nurse's role as advocate is involvement in the breast cancer advocacy movement. Langer and Dow (1994) published a comprehensive description of advocacy development of the breast cancer advocacy movement, nurses as patient advocates, nursing's involvement with political advocacy, breast cancer advocacy into the future, and the forging of partnerships between breast cancer advocates and nursing.

Other examples of the nurse's role as advocate focus on helping patients to understand the importance of asking for consultation with other members of the health care team before making therapeutic decisions at the beginning of treatment or at various points along the care continuum. How often does a surgeon perform a laryngectomy on a patient with early laryngeal cancer when the patient's voice could have been preserved with an equal chance of a positive outcome? Patients need to know that surgery may not be the best or only treatment available for their diagnosis. Awareness of multimodal therapy and the options from which they can choose are critical knowledge for persons with cancer to obtain. Likewise, a surgeon may tell a patient "I have done all that I can," implying that he or she has done all that can be done and that there is nowhere else to go. Again, the nurse as advocate should inform the patient of adjuvant therapies that may be available and applicable to the diagnosis.

The essential aspects of oncology nurses' advocacy for persons with cancer are (1) informing patients adequately so that they can make knowledgeable decisions and (2) supporting them in whatever decisions they make. Patients also have the right not to know, if they do not want to know (Kohnke, 1982).

Issues identified by Miller, Mansen, and Lee (1983) as critical to the development of the oncology nurse as advocate include the following:

- Redefinition of the role of the physician as sole authority and decision maker
- Redefinition of the role of the nurse as caregiver or implementer of the physician's plan of care
- Dealing with colleagues' concern regarding nurse advocates as encouraging patient resistance and noncompliance
- Overcoming lack of nurse authority or power

To serve as patient advocates, oncology nurses must address each of these issues in an informed and proactive manner. This includes clarifying professional nursing's commitment to advocacy, becoming more socially and politically active, and developing negotiating skills. It is imperative that nurses assume this role, particularly in light of multimodal therapies and their implications for patients' quality of life.

❖ *Oncology Nurses' Role in Policy Development*

Policy evaluation must be based on the identification and assessment of policy consequences and outcomes. Oncology nurses are in an ideal position to provide such feedback, along with recommendations for policy renewal or revision, because they can provide information based on nursing research and expert opinion.

Policy formulation uses the input of individual oncology nurses, lay groups, and organizations, who can provide the policy makers with specific patient examples, expert opinions, and research reports. Given (1994) believes that understanding policy issues may be the most important aspect of the nurses' participation in public policy. This includes knowing the history and source of the problem, the proposed solutions, and the lobbying efforts and stakes of the interested parties.

❖ *Advanced Practice in Oncology Nursing*

Madden and Ponte (1994) describe advanced-practice nurses (APNs) as "expert practitioners" who

deliver care, manage patients and families, teach, consult, research, and do a range of other activities based on the needs of patients and the environment in which they practice (p. 56).

Traditionally the clinical nurse specialist (CNS) has practiced in secondary- and tertiary-care settings, whereas the nurse practitioner (NP) has practiced in community or primary-care settings. However, patient care needs have been changing the range of knowledge and skills required of the advanced-practice nurse and guiding the domain of service for advanced-practice-nurse specialization. For example, as acute-care hospitals extend service beyond their walls, APNs prepared as CNSs

need to acquire advanced assessment skills and prescriptive privileges for reimbursement purposes. Madden and Ponte (1994) believe that

> it no longer makes sense for academic institutions to prepare one or the other [CNS or
> NP]. For advanced nurse practitioners to succeed in meeting [health care] network
> needs, they must acquire both sets of skills (p. 57).

Madden and Ponte (1994) describe the need for APNs to play key roles in critical-
pathway teams and as consultants in clinical practice within the framework of health
care reform. Gioiella (1993) similarly believes that advanced-practice roles in nursing are converging as the commonalities between the CNS and NP roles are identified and described.

The APN has always played an important consultative role. Consultation may
focus on process, resources, and expert care. The process consultant diagnoses a situation and generates recommendations, while the client takes action. Areas of
process consultation include development of case-management models or clinical
paths, professional-practice models, or documentation processes. The resource
consultant presents alternatives for resolving a patient-family problem or meeting
complex patient care needs. The expert practitioner/consultant often carries a case-
load of patients across a continuum of care. The advanced-practice nurse who is not
"unit based" in a hospital, home, or ambulatory-care setting can work with the
patient and caregivers in different multimodal settings, ensuring that the patient
does not "fall through the cracks" if receiving treatment in various places.

Madden and Ponte (1994) suggest that APNs develop a portfolio that
describes the resources or assets of a group of APNs. The health care network or
health alliance manages the portfolio to meet the needs of the network or alliance.
Health care networks or alliances, as proposed by the American Nurses Association
(ANA), the American Hospital Association (AHA), and other interest groups are
viewed as a method for providing a continuum of care from screening to acute care
to chronic care in the home or in an institution (ANA, 1992). APNs use the portfolio analogy as a guide in marketing their clinical, consultation, management,
research, and teaching skills.

This is a time of great change in the education and practice of APNs in oncology and in other specialties. Oncology nurses need to be able to articulate the role
of the APN to policy makers, employers, colleagues, and consumers to assure the
continuing viability of the role. The Oncology Nursing Certification Corporation's
establishment of the Advanced Oncology Nursing Certification examination is a
useful credential for APNs as they pursue their practice in a wide variety of health
care settings.

❖ *Preparation for Oncology Nursing as a Specialty*

Nurse educators are being encouraged to devote more time and attention to cancer
as a chronic disease in generic nursing curricula. The American Cancer Society Pro-
fessors of Oncology Nursing recently completed a Cancer Nursing Curriculum
Guide for Baccalaureate Nursing Education (in press). The purpose of these curriculum guidelines is to provide a framework for educators to use in ensuring that
undergraduate nursing curricula include essential content in cancer nursing.

It is anticipated that programs in oncology nursing at the master's degree level will offer subspecialty tracks that reflect the needs of specific populations—that is, pediatric oncology, geriatric oncology, and persons with specific types of cancer. Doctorally prepared oncology nurses will be needed in larger numbers to direct the study of persons along the cancer care continuum. Nursing education at all levels should incorporate courses on economics, policy analysis, and comprehensive models of care delivery.

❖ Summary

The future of oncology nursing resembles its past: dynamic, challenging, and exciting. Issues that reflect health care reform are shaping nursing as a profession and oncology nursing as a specialty. The oncology nurse must be politically astute, well-educated, and clinically skilled in order to survive in the years to come.

Multimodal therapy will play a larger role in cancer treatment as surgical and radiation techniques are improved, as new chemotherapeutic agents and chemoprotectants are developed, and as biotherapeutic techniques are refined. This evolution of complex and multifaceted therapy will require more experienced and more educated nurses with specialization in oncology nursing.

❖ References

American Cancer Society: Cancer nursing curriculum guide for baccalaureate nursing education, Atlanta, in press, American Cancer Society.

American Nurses Association: Nursing case management, Kansas City, 1988, The Association.

American Nurses Association: Nursing's agenda for health care reform, Washington, D.C., 1992, American Nurses Publishing.

Annas GJ: The patient rights advocate: can nurses effectively fill the role? Supervisor Nurse 5:21–25, 1974.

Aydelotte MK, Hardy MA, and Hope KL: Nurses in private practice: characteristics, organizational arrangements, and reimbursement policy, Kansas City, 1988, American Nurses Foundation.

Boyle DM, Engelking C, and Harvey C: Making a difference in the 21st century: are oncology nurses ready? Oncol Nurs Forum 21:53–55, 1994a.

Boyle DM, Engelking C, and Harvey C: Taking command of the future: getting ready NOW for the 21st century, Oncol Nurs Forum 21:77–79, 1994b.

Burchell RC, Thomas DA, and Smith HL: Some considerations for implementing collaborative practice, Am J Med 74:9–13, 1983.

Dumont J and Niziole KC: The cornerstone of collaboration, Prof Nurs 7:331, 1991.

England D: Collaboration in nursing, Rockville, Maryland, 1986, Aspen Publishers.

Engelking C: New approaches: innovations in cancer prevention, diagnosis, treatment, and support, Oncol Nurs Forum 21:62–71, 1994.

Gioiella EC: Meeting the demand for advanced practice nurses, Prof Nurs 9(5):54–55, 1993.

Given B: How nurse researchers can influence policy, ONS News 9(5):4, 1994.

Harvey C: New systems: the restructuring of cancer care delivery and economics, Oncol Nurs Forum 21:72–77, 1994.

Herron DG and Herron L: Entrepreneurial nursing as a conceptual basis for in-hospital nursing practice models, Nurs Economics, 9:310–316, 1991.

Herron L: The effects of characteristics of the entrepreneur on new venture performance, doctoral dissertation, Columbia, S. Carolina, 1990, University of South Carolina.

Knollmueller R: Case management: What's in a name? Nurs Manage 20(10):38–42, 1989.

Kohnke MF: Advocacy: risk and reality, St. Louis, 1982, Mosby.

Langer AS and Dow KH: The breast cancer advocacy movement and nursing, Oncology nursing. Patient treatment and support 1(3), 1994.

Madden MJ and Ponte PR: Advanced practice roles in the managed care environment, Nurs Admin 24(1):56–62, 1994.

McLaughlin-Hagan M and Baird SB: Predicting future trends in oncology nursing, Nurs 93 23(5):55–56, 1993.

Miller BK, Mansen T, and Lee H: Patient advocacy: do nurses have the power and authority to act as patient advocate? Nurs Leadership 6:56–60, 1983.

Nelson ML: Advocacy in nursing, Nurs Outlook 36:136, 1988.

Nelson P: ANA to help develop managed care curriculum, Amer Nurse 25(5):25, 1993.

Papenhausen JL: Case management: a model of advanced practice, Clin Nurse Specialist 4:169–170, 1990.

Zander K: Case management a golden opportunity for whom? In McCloskey JC and Grace HK, editors: Current issues in nursing, ed 3, St. Louis, 1990, Mosby, pp. 199–204.

Glossary

Ablative Destructive, as in laser therapy or cryotherapy.

Accelerated fractionation Normal fractionated doses of radiation therapy given more frequently than 5 days a week. Also known as accelerated hyperfractionation.

Adenocarcinoma A cancer arising from the glandular or ductal tissue.

Additive effect The sum of the results of two or more treatment modalities.

Adjuvant therapy Therapy administered after initial treatment without demonstrable residual diseases.

Allogenic Having cell types that are antigenically distinct. Transplanting bone marrow from one person to another person who is of the same tissue type.

Alopecia Loss of hair resulting from destruction of or damage to the hair follicle.

Alternating therapy Treatment of one modality given within the treatment cycle of another modality (e.g., chemotherapy given once every 28 days, with radiation therapy starting 7 days after the chemotherapy dose and ending 7 days before the next chemotherapy dose). Also called interdigitating therapy.

Anemia Reduced quantity of erythrocytes and/or reduced hemoglobin in the circulating erythrocytes.

Anorexia Loss of appetite.

Antagonist That which counteracts the action of something else.

Antibody An immunoglobulin protein produced by plasma cells and B-cells in response to invasion by a foreign antigen, which has the ability to combine with the antigen that stimulated its production.

Antiemetic Preventing or relieving nausea and vomiting.

Antigen Any substance not normally found in the body that, when present, is specifically recognized by an antibody and by cells of the adaptive immune system.

Antineoplastic Anticancer, as in antineoplastic drugs.

Aplastic anemia Deficient red cell production caused by disorders of the bone marrow.

Autologous Derived from the same individual organism, especially products or components such as a patient's own bone marrow transplanted after ablative treatment.

Basophil A medium-size leukocyte, assists in inflammation.

B-cell (B-lymphocyte) A cell derived from a bone marrow stem cell in humans, capable of responding to an antigen by the production of an antibody.

Benign Nonmalignant, noncancerous.

Biological response modifier (BRM) An agent that can modify host reactions against disease.

Biopsy The removal and pathological examination of tissue from the body to determine if a tumor is malignant or benign.

Blast An immature leukocyte.

Blocks Devices used in radiation to prevent radiation beams from penetrating areas of the body that do not require treatment.

Blood-brain barrier The barrier that prevents or delays certain substances in the blood from entering brain tissue.

Body surface area A calculation of the quantity of surface area of an individual's body, expressed in square meters.

Bone marrow The spongelike tissue within the bone where red blood cells, white blood cells, and platelets develop.

Brachytherapy A type of radiation where the source is placed within the body or a body cavity.

Cachexia A condition of severe malnutrition.

Cancer A group of neoplastic diseases in which there is a transformation of a normal body cell into an uncontrolled proliferation of abnormal cells.

Capillary leak syndrome A shift of fluid from the intravascular space, resulting in accumulation of fluid in the extravascular space.

Carcinogen A physical, chemical, or biological stressor that causes neoplastic changes in normal cells.

Carcinogenesis The production of cancer.

Carcinoma A term used to describe cancer derived from epithelial tissues.

Cell cycle The reproductive cycle of all cells.

Cell-mediated immunity Immunity involving T-cells and cells of the natural immune system such as natural killer cells and monocytes, referring specifically to the body's defense against virally infected cells and malignant cells.

Centigray (cGy) 1/100 Gy. The centigray replaced the rad in 1985 as the unit of radiation dose (1 rad = 1 cGy).

Chemotherapy The use of drugs to combat disease; most commonly, drugs used against cancer.

Colony-stimulating factor (CSF) A group of hormonelike glycoproteins that stimulate growth of and maturation of hematopoietic cells.

Colostomy A surgical procedure in which an artificial opening is made on the surface of the abdomen for the purpose of evacuating the bowels. A surgical substitute for the rectum and the anus.

Commitment The process by which components of the hemopoietic hierarchy increasingly lose the potential to differentiate into alternative cell lines.

Comorbity The existence of more than one disease or illness at the same time.

Complete response All disease is eradicated for at least a month after the completion of treatment. The difference between complete response and cure is that when a patient is cured, the complete response is permanent.

Computerized axial tomography (CAT or CT) scan A diagnostic radiologic imaging technique that produces images of 1-cm-thick slices through a patient's body.

Concomitant therapy Two or more treatment modalities given at the same time.

Concurrent therapy See Concomitant therapy.

Conditioning or preparative regimen Doses of chemotherapy and/or radiation lethal to the bone marrow given to eradicate cancer cells from the body (ablative therapy).

Cure Eradication of all disease.

Cytokine One of a number of complicated proteins that regulate cells and govern the immune system function.

Cytotoxic agent An agent capable of specific destructive action on certain cells, usually referring to chemotherapy.

Debulking A surgical technique used to reduce the tumor burden to improve response to other treatment modalities.

Differentiated cells Cells with recognizable, specialized structures and functions.

Differentiation The process of having recognizable, specialized structures and functions.

Disease control Treatment given to keep cancer from continuing to grow when a cure is not possible.

Dysgeusia Impairment of taste, in which normal tastes are interpreted as unpleasant or completely different.

Dyspareunia Painful intercourse experienced by women.

Dysphagia Difficulty in swallowing.

Emetic An agent that produces vomiting.

Eosinophil A medium-size leukocyte normally constituting 1% to 2% of the leukocytes that is active in allergic reactions.

Erythrocyte A red blood cell.

Etiology The science of the cause of disease.

Fractionation Division of the total dose of radiation into small doses given at frequent (usually daily) intervals.

Grade A method of classifying cancer on a scale of I to IV based on the degree of cellular anaplasia observed under the microscope.

Granulocytopenia A decrease in granulocytes (neutrophils, eosinophils, and kasophils).

Gray (Gy) A unit of radiation dose. 1 Gray = 100 centigray (cGy).

Hematopoiesis The process by which blood cells are produced in the bone marrow.

Hematopoietic growth factor An alternate term for colony-stimulating factor.

Hemopoiesis The process by which the various components of the blood are formed and mature.

Histocompatibility The ability of cells to survive without immunological interference.

Histology The examination under the microscope of the function, structure, and composition of tissue.

Homeostasis A state of adaptive balance in the internal environment.

Human leukocyte antigen (HLA) An antigen present on the surface of white blood cells and platelets.

Humoral immunity Specific immunity activated by antibody found in blood and lymph, specifically in viral and bacterial organisms that have not invaded cells of the body.

Hyperfractionation Multiple daily treatments of radiation therapy given at doses less than the standard daily dose of 1.8 to 2 Gy, Associated with increased acute side effects.

Hyperthermia The use of heat to enhance the effects of radiation therapy.

Ileostomy A surgical procedure to create an opening into the ileum for evacuation of stool.

Immunity A protective mechanism that serves to maintain the integrity for the body against foreign substances or disease.

Immunoglobulin A glycoprotein composed of heavy and light chains that functions as antibody.

Immunosuppression Diminished functioning of the immune system.

Immunosurveillance A theory that the immune system plays an important role in the prevention of developing cancer.

Immunotherapy A treatment modality in which biologicals are administered in an attempt to stimulate the immune system to recognize malignant cells and destroy them.

Induction therapy Giving adjuvant therapy before giving the primary therapy. Also known as neoadjuvant therapy.

In situ A lesion with the histological characteristics of a malignancy except invasion. Confined to the site of origin.

Interferon (IFN) A class of cytokines that has immunoregulatory function, including enhancing the activities of macrophages and natural killer cells.

Interleukin A class of cytokines produced by lymphocytes and/or macrophages in response to antigenic or mitogenic stimulation that mediate communication between cells of the immune system.

Karnofsky scale An assessment tool used to evaluate the overall condition and performance ability of a patient.

Leukemia A diffuse cancer characterized by the abnormal proliferation and release of leukocyte precursors.

Leukocyte A white blood cell that defends the body against pathogenic microorganisms causing disease. Five types: lymphocytes, monocytes, neutrophils, eosinophils, and basophils.

Lymph node Lymphoid tissue organized as lymphatic organs along the course of the lymphatic vessels that filter and destroy invasive bacteria.

Lymphocyte A type of white blood cell that generally numbers from 20% to 50% of the total, further divided into B-cells and T-cells.

Lymphokine An activated killer cell capable of killing tumor cells, activated by cytokines derived from lymphocytes, particularly interleukin-2.

Lymphoma A nodular malignancy arising from lymphoid tissue.

Macrophages Any of the large, mononuclear, highly phagocytic cells derived from monocytes, stimulated by inflammation.

Magnetic resonance imaging (MRI) A noninvasive nuclear procedure for imaging tissues of high-fat-and-water content that cannot be seen with other radiologic techniques.

Malignant Cancerous; having the characteristics of disorderly, uncontrolled, chaotic proliferation.

Melanoma Malignant disease of the skin.

Meta analysis A statistical method of analyzing groups of research studies to provide more information about the topic being studied.

Metastasis The distant spread of the original cancer from the primary site.

Micrometastasis The distant spread of cancer from the primary site but of a size too small to be detected.

Monoclonal antibody (MoAb) An antibody produced from a single clone of cells.

Monocyte A type of white blood cell constituting 5% to 10% of the total.

Monokine A cytokine such as tumor necrosis factor released by mononuclear phagocytes.

Mucositis Inflammation of a mucous membrane.

Multimodal therapy The use of any combination of surgery, radiation therapy, chemotherapy, and biotherapy to treat cancer. Also known as combined-modality therapy.

Myelosuppression A reduction in bone marrow function, resulting in a reduced release of red blood cells, white blood cells, and platelets into the peripheral circulation.

Nadir A period of time when the blood cells reach their lowest number.

Natural killer cells A group of large, granular lymphocytes that have the intrinsic ability to recognize and destroy some virally infected cells and some tumor cells.

Neoadjuvant therapy Giving adjuvant therapy before giving the primary therapy. Also known as induction therapy.

Neoplasm New growth; may be benign or malignant.

Neutropenia An abnormally low quantity of neutrophils in the circulating blood.

Neutrophil The largest amount of white blood cells, constituting 60% to 70%.

Nitrogen balance The state of the body in regard to the ingestion and excretion of protein. *Positive:* The amount of nitrogen excreted is less than the quantity ingested, indicating adequate protein intake. *Negative:* The amount of nitrogen excreted is greater than the quantity ingested, indicating protein depletion and malnutrition.

Oncology The study of malignant diseases.

Palliation Treatment given for symptom control only when control or cure is not possible.

Partial response Reduction of 50% or more of tumor size, lasting at least 1 month after completion of treatment.

Platelet A blood cell primarily involved with coagulation of blood and clot formation. Also called a thrombocyte.

Pluripotent stem cell A primitive blood cell in the hematopoietic hierarchy, the forerunner of all cell lineages.

Precursor cell A nucleated cell that is morphologically recognizable as belonging to a specific lineage and that gives rise immediately to the mature components of the circulating blood.

Progenitor cell An early ancestor of the mature components of the blood.

Rad See Centigray.

Radiation enhancer An agent that has an antitumor effect when given alone. Given to make cancer cells more sensitive to radiation therapy.

Radiation recall The recurrence of side effects of previous radiation therapy. Can be induced by several chemotherapeutic agents.

Radiation sensitizer An agent that by itself has no antitumor effect but when given with radiation therapy makes cancer cells more radiosensitive.

Radiation therapy The treatment of cancer with ionizing radiation. *External beam:* Radiation therapy delivered by a machine external to the patient's body; teletherapy. *Internal beam:* The use of radioactive needles, seeds, or other implants to deliver radiation to a specific area; brachytherapy.

Radioresistant A cancer resistant to the effects of radiation and therefore not destroyed by radiation therapy.

Radiosensitive A cancer sensitive to radiation and therefore destroyed by radiation therapy.

Radiosensitivity The response of a tumor to ionizing radiation.

Refractory Resistant to treatment.

Relapse The return of a cancer after remission has been achieved.

Remission The abatement of signs and symptoms of a malignancy; without indication of the presence of cancer.

Sandwich therapy Giving a half course of one treatment modality, a full course of a second modality, and then completing treatment from the first modality.

Sarcoma A malignant solid tumor composed of tissues of mesodermal origin.

Sequential therapy Treatment from one modality after completion of treatment from another modality.

Side effect An unwanted but expected effect from antineoplastic therapy that occurs in normal cells.

Split-course radiation A "rest" period is provided during the treatment course to allow time for normal cells to recover from radiation damage. Also provides time for tumor cells to grow.

Stage, staging A method of classifying malignancies on the basis of the presence and extent of the tumor within the body, usually based on the TNM (tumor, nodes, metastases) system.

Stem cell A cell that gives rise to a specific type of cell.

Stereotactic surgery A surgical technique used to localize the tumor and to destroy it.

Stomatitis Mucositis of the mouth.

Survivorship The state of living with cancer in remission or having obtained a prognosis of cure.

Synergistic effect The effect of two or more treatment modalities when one also enhances the effect of the other. The synergistic effect is more than the expected additive effect.

Syngeneic Having identical matched cell types.

T-cell (T-lymphocyte) A thymus-dependent cell involved in a variety of cell-mediated immune responses.

Thrombocytopenia An abnormally low quantity of platelets in the circulating blood.

TNM classification A system of staging cancer where *T* stands for tumor size, *N* for lymph node involvement, and *M* for metastasis.

Toxicity An enhanced side effect reaction.

Tumor A neoplasm, a new growth of tissue in which cell growth is uncontrolled and progressive.

Tumor marker A product produced by a cancer cell or in response to the presence of cancer that may be released into the circulation or may remain associated with the cancer cell. Markers are used to follow the progression or regression of the cancer during and after treatment.

Undifferentiated cell A cell that has lost the capacity for specialized functions.

Xerostomia Dryness of the mouth.

Index

Page numbers followed by an *f* indicate figures. Tables are designated by a *t* and boxes by a *b*.